# Lecture Notes
# in Business Information Processing           **341**

More information about this series at http://www.springer.com/series/7911

Marinos Themistocleous · Paulo Rupino da Cunha (Eds.)

# Information Systems

15th European, Mediterranean,
and Middle Eastern Conference, EMCIS 2018
Limassol, Cyprus, October 4–5, 2018
Proceedings

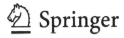 Springer

*Editors*
Marinos Themistocleous 🔘
University of Nicosia
Nicosia, Cyprus

Paulo Rupino da Cunha 🔘
University of Coimbra
Coimbra, Portugal

and

University of Piraeus
Piraeus, Greece

ISSN 1865-1348        ISSN 1865-1356   (electronic)
Lecture Notes in Business Information Processing
ISBN 978-3-030-11394-0        ISBN 978-3-030-11395-7   (eBook)
https://doi.org/10.1007/978-3-030-11395-7

Library of Congress Control Number: 2018966823

This Springer imprint is published by the registered company Springer Nature Switzerland AG
The registered company address is: Gewerbestrasse 11, 6330 Cham, Switzerland

# Preface

The European, Mediterranean, and Middle Eastern Conference on Information Systems (EMCIS) is an annual research event addressing the discipline of information systems (IS) from regional as well as global perspective. EMCIS has successfully helped bring together researchers from around the world in a friendly atmosphere conducive to the free exchange of innovative ideas. EMCIS is one of the premier conferences in Europe and the Middle Eastern region for IS academics and professionals, covering technical, organizational, business, and social issues in the application of information technology. EMCIS is dedicated to the definition and establishment of IS as a discipline of high impact for the methodology community and IS professionals – focusing on approaches that facilitate the identification of innovative research of significant relevance to the IS discipline following sound research methodologies that lead to results of measurable impact.

We received 108 papers EMCIS 2018 from 31 countries around the world. The papers were submitted through the EasyChair online system and were sent for double-blind review. The papers were reviewed either by members of the conference committee or by external reviewers. Papers submitted by the track chairs were reviewed by one conference co-chair and one member of the Executive Committee. The papers of the conference chairs and conference program chairs were reviewed by one senior external reviewer and one senior member of the Executive Committee. Overall, 42 papers were accepted for EMCIS 2018; 34 of them as full papers and another eight as short papers submitted to the following tracks:

- Big Data and Analytics
- Blockchain Technology and Applications
- Cloud Computing
- Digital Services and Social Media
- e-Government
- Health-Care Information Systems
- Management and Organizational Issues in Information Systems
- IT Governance

The papers were accepted for their theoretical and practical excellence and for the promising results they present. We hope that the readers will find the papers interesting and we are open for a constructive discussion that will improve the body of knowledge on the field of IS.

October 2018
Marinos Themistocleous
Paulo Rupino da Cunha

# Organization

## Conference Co-chairs

George Angelos
  Papadopoulos
Angelika Kokkinaki

University of Cyprus, Cyprus

University of Nicosia, Cyprus

## Conference Executive Committee

Marinos Themistocleous
  (Program Chair)
Paulo Rupino Cunha
  (Program Chair)
Gianluigi Viscusi
  (Publications Chair)
Muhammad Kamal
  (Public Relations Chair)

University of Nicosia, Cyprus and University
  of Piraeus, Greece
University of Coimbra, Portugal

École Polytechnique fédérale de Lausanne (EPFL),
  Switzerland
Brunel University, UK

## International Committee

Janice Sipior
Heinz Roland Weistroffer
Vincenzo Morabito
Piotr Soja
Peter Love
Gail Corbitt
Miguel Mira da Silva
Vishanth Weerakkody
Lasse Berntzen
Marijn Janssen
Stanisław Wrycza
Kamel Ghorab
Celina M. Olszak
Flora Malamateniou
Andriana Prentza
Inas Ezz

Ibrahim Osman
Przemysław Lech
Euripidis N. Loukis
Mariusz Grabowski
Małgorzata Pańkowska

Villanova University, USA
Virginia Commonwealth University, USA
Bocconi University, Italy
Cracow University of Economics, Poland
Curtin University, Australia
California State University, USA
University of Lisbon, Portugal
University of Bradford, UK
Buskerud and Vestfold University College, Norway
Delft University of Technology, The Netherlands
University of Gdansk, Poland
Alhosn University, UAE
University of Economics in Katowice, Poland
University of Piraeus, Greece
University of Piraeus, Greece
Sadat Academy for Management Sciences – SAMS,
  Egypt
American University of Beirut, Lebanon
University of Gdansk, Poland
University of the Aegean, Greece
Cracow University of Economics, Poland
University of Economics in Katowice, Poland

# Keynote Speakers

# An Enterprise View of Food Security: A Puzzle, Problem or Mess for a Circular Economy

Zahir Irani

University of Bradford, UK

**Abstract.** Interventions to provide food security are many, ranging from strategically leasing arable land from overseas Governments through to innovative approaches that seek increased levels of produce yield. The challenges and responses are not uniform and indeed are in many respects polarised, with those in resource-poor countries and some developing nations facing a lack of access to food and/or severe food shortages, right the way through to those in the West suffering increasingly higher levels of obesity (due to excessive over-consumption). The latter clearly represents an oversupply of food manifesting in overindulgence whereas the former is a product of food scarcity resulting ever too often in malnutrition or even starvation. The challenges around the safe and secure access to food as well as its production, supply and recovery are intimately connected with information, resources and policy and national/paranational political strategies; the effect of the macro- and meso-economic landscapes in terms of stability and access to funding; social attitudes to food, nutrition, well-being and food waste; technological innovations in agriculture; legal jurisdiction constraints (including tariffs); and food supply and sustainability within the broader climate change and environmental context.

The presentation explores the use, applicability and relevance of strategic planning as a process and tool when applied to exploring food security challenges, in the context of existing research on food security and food waste in the food supply chain. The issues associated with robust and resilient food supply chains within a circular economy are increasingly being seen as supportive of creating enhanced levels of food security but it is argued that this is only sustainable when strategically planned as part of a cross-enterprise, information-rich and complex supply chain. The presentation will navigate through the multiple strategic, tactical and operational challenges from an enterprise perspective around food security and postulate food security as a puzzle, problem or mess.

**Short bio:** Professor Zahir Irani is the Faculty Dean of Management, Law and Social Sciences at the University of Bradford, UK. Professor Irani has held several senior management positions at Brunel University London, the most recent of which being the Founding Dean of College (Business, Arts and Social Sciences – CBASS) which he set up following an organizational restructuring from eight schools into three colleges. Prior to this role, he was seconded full-time to Whitehall, where he was a Senior Policy

Advisor at the Cabinet Office during part of the coalition Government. He is however most proud of being Head of the Brunel Business School, which in 2013 was awarded the Times Higher Education Business School of the Year under his leadership.

He completed a BEng (Hons) at Salford University before then accepting a research position in industry where he finished his Master's degree by research. He has a PhD in the area of investment evaluation and undertook his leadership development at the Harvard Business School. He has an extensive list of 3 and 4 star publications in the area of information systems, Project Management and eGovernment, and has published in Journal of Management Information Systems, European Journal of Information Systems, Government Information Quarterly, Information Systems Journal, European Journal of Operational Research and IEEE Transactions on Engineering Management to mention a few. He has had significant grant income from national and international funding councils including H2020, Qatar Foundation, EPSRC, ESRC and FP7. His H-index is 71.

# Big Data Analytics and Artificial Intelligence Meet Human Brain: Towards a New Co-working Space in Research and Practice

Claudia Loebbecke

University of Cologne, Cologne, Germany

**Abstract.** The processing capacity of today's smartphone outperforms the computers that landed a man on the moon in 1969. Digitization, Big Data Analytics, and Artificial Intelligence (AI) are about to drive fundamentally transformed business models and management approaches, thereby challenge established economics. As impressive examples are gaining ground, the disruptive effects will not spare those who underestimate their increasing momentum. This presentation will outline how digitization, big data analytics, and AI can empower organizations and lead to emerging approaches of value creation in business, society, and research.

**Short bio:** Claudia Loebbecke holds the Chair of Media and Technology Management at the University of Cologne. She is a member of the European Academy of Sciences and Arts and serves on the editorial boards of various academic journals. Prior to her appointment at the University of Cologne, Claudia worked at INSEAD, McKinsey & Co., Hong Kong University of Science and Technology, Erasmus University and Copenhagen Business School. As a senior research-active academic, she has undertaken short-stay research visits to universities in the US, Australia, the UK, Italy, and France. Her research focuses on business models, business models, business transformation, and organizational management in light of digital and creative innovations. She has published over 250 internationally peer-reviewed journal articles and conference papers and contributed to the development of more than twenty in-depth case studies in eight different countries. Claudia holds master's and PhD degrees from the University of Cologne and an MBA from Indiana University in the US.

# Toward Programmable Money and Machine-to-Machine Commerce: Implications and Research Challenges

George Giaglis

University of Nicosia, Cyprus

**Abstract.** The invention of crypto-currencies, like Bitcoin, has paved the way for a revolution in how we perceive the notion and functions of money. For the first time in human history, we can program money and have it become active (i.e. decide for its own how to behave, where to and when to move, etc.). As money is being transformed, commerce is poised to change, too: coupled with blockchains, advances in artificial intelligence and the internet of things promise to create a world in which intelligent software will soon enter the economic landscape as quasi-independent agents in commercial transactions. This will pave the way for previously unheard-of types of commerce (like human-to-machine and machine-to-machine commerce) and methods of industrial organization (like decentralized autonomous organizations that employ no humans and exist only on the cloud in the form of smart contracts). In this talk, we will discuss the implications of such developments and offer thoughts for research challenges that need to be tackled, both technological and societal.

**Short bio:** Professor George M. Giaglis is Director of the Institute for the Future at the University of Nicosia, as well as a leading expert on blockchain technology and applications and advisor to many blockchain projects and technology start-ups. Prior to joining UNIC, he was Professor at the Athens University of Economics and Business (2002–2017), where he also served as Vice Rector (2011–2015). George has been working on digital currencies and blockchain since 2012, with his main focus being on new forms of industrial organization (programmable smart contracts, decentralized applications and distributed autonomous organizations) and new forms of corporate financing (token economy, crypto-economics and ICOs). He has been one of the first academics to research and teach on blockchain, having: designed the curriculum of the world's first full academic degree on blockchain (MSc in Digital Currency at the University of Nicosia); led the development of blockchain credentialing technology that has resulted in the first ever publishing of academic certificates on the blockchain; taught on the disruptive innovation potential of blockchain, both at academic programs and in executive seminars worldwide; organized a number of prominent blockchain conferences and events, including Decentralized. Throughout his career, he has published more than 10 books and 150 articles on leading scientific journals and conferences, while he is frequently interviewed by media and invited as keynote speaker or trainer in events across the globe. He is the Chief Editor for Blockchain Technology at the Frontiers in Blockchain Journal and member of the Editorial Board at Ledger.

# Contents

**Blockchain Technology and Applications**

The Relationship Between Bitcoin Trading Volume, Volatility,
and Returns: A Study of Four Seasons . . . . . . . . . . . . . . . . . . . . . . . . . . . 3
  *Angelika Kokkinaki, Svetlana Sapuric, and Ifigenia Georgiou*

Verify-Your-Vote: A Verifiable Blockchain-Based Online Voting Protocol . . . 16
  *Marwa Chaieb, Souheib Yousfi, Pascal Lafourcade, and Riadh Robbana*

To Chain or Not to Chain? A Case from Energy Sector . . . . . . . . . . . . . . . 31
  *Marinos Themistocleous, Kypros Stefanou, Christos Megapanos,
  and Elias Iosif*

Continuance Intention in Blockchain-Enabled Supply Chain Applications:
Modelling the Moderating Effect of Supply Chain Stakeholders Trust . . . . . . 38
  *Samuel Fosso Wamba*

**Big Data and Analytics**

Big Data Analysis in UAV Surveillance for Wildfire
Prevention and Management . . . . . . . . . . . . . . . . . . . . . . . . . . . . . . . . . . 47
  *Nikos Athanasis, Marinos Themistocleous, Kostas Kalabokidis,
  and Christos Chatzitheodorou*

Harnessing Cloud Scalability to Hadoop Clusters . . . . . . . . . . . . . . . . . . . 59
  *Arne Koschel, Felix Heine, and Irina Astrova*

For What It's Worth: A Multi-industry Survey on Current and Expected
Use of Big Data Technologies . . . . . . . . . . . . . . . . . . . . . . . . . . . . . . . . . 72
  *Elisa Rossi, Cinzia Rubattino, and Gianluigi Viscusi*

A Step Foreword Historical Data Governance in Information Systems . . . . . . 80
  *José Pedro Simão and Orlando Belo*

Parliamentary Open Big Data: A Case Study of the Norwegian Parliament's
Open Data Platform . . . . . . . . . . . . . . . . . . . . . . . . . . . . . . . . . . . . . . . . 91
  *Lasse Berntzen, Rania El-Gazzar, and Marius Rohde Johannessen*

Data Requirements Elicitation in Big Data Warehousing . . . . . . . . . . . . . . 106
  *António A. C. Vieira, Luís Pedro, Maribel Yasmina Santos,
  João Miguel Fernandes, and Luís S. Dias*

Towards Integrations of Big Data Technology Components . . . . . . . . . . . .   114
  *Kalinka Kaloyanova*

Experimental Evaluation of Big Data Analytical Tools. . . . . . . . . . . . . . . .   121
  *Mário Rodrigues, Maribel Yasmina Santos, and Jorge Bernardino*

**Cloud Computing**

Model for Improved Load Balancing in Volunteer Computing Platforms . . . .   131
  *Levente Filep*

Towards a Formal Approach for Verifying Dynamic Workflows
in the Cloud. . . . . . . . . . . . . . . . . . . . . . . . . . . . . . . . . . . . . . . . . . . . . . . .   144
  *Fairouz Fakhfakh, Hatem Hadj Kacem, and Ahmed Hadj Kacem*

Investigating the Factors Affecting the Adoption of Cloud Computing
in SMEs: A Case Study of Saudi Arabia . . . . . . . . . . . . . . . . . . . . . . . . . .   158
  *Fahad Alghamdi, Dharmendra Sharma, and Milind Sathye*

CSCCRA: A Novel Quantitative Risk Assessment Model
for Cloud Service Providers . . . . . . . . . . . . . . . . . . . . . . . . . . . . . . . . . . .   177
  *Olusola Akinrolabu, Steve New, and Andrew Martin*

Mobile Number Portability Using a Reliable Cloud Database Appliance
to Match Predictable Performance . . . . . . . . . . . . . . . . . . . . . . . . . . . . . .   185
  *Katelaris Leonidas, Themistocleous Marinos, and Giovanni Roberto*

**Digital Services and Social Media**

Exploratory Research to Identify the Characteristics of Cyber Victims
on Social Media in New Zealand . . . . . . . . . . . . . . . . . . . . . . . . . . . . . . .   193
  *Varun Dhond, Shahper Richter, and Brad McKenna*

The Novel Online Comparison Tool for Bank Charges
with User-Friendly Approach . . . . . . . . . . . . . . . . . . . . . . . . . . . . . . . . . .   211
  *Ivan Soukal*

An In-Store Mobile App for Customer Engagement: Discovering Hedonic
and Utilitarian Motivations in UK Grocery Retail . . . . . . . . . . . . . . . . . . .   225
  *Joanne Pei-Chung Wang and Anabel Gutierrez*

Information Quality of Web Services: Payment Account Online
Comparison Tools Survey in the Czech Republic and Slovakia. . . . . . . . . . .   244
  *Ivan Soukal*

An Organizational Scheme for Privacy Impact Assessments . . . . . . . . . . . .   258
  *Konstantina Vemou and Maria Karyda*

How Social Media Can Afford Engagement Processes . . . . . . . . . . . . . . . . .   272
    *Xiaoxiao Zeng, Brad McKenna, Shahper Richter, and Wenjie Cai*

**e-Government**

GE-government: A Geographic Information Based E-government
Citizens' Adoption Framework . . . . . . . . . . . . . . . . . . . . . . . . . . . . . . .   283
    *Hassan K. Dennaoui and Angelika I. Kokkinaki*

Factors Affecting Intention to Use E-government Services: The Case
of Non-adopters . . . . . . . . . . . . . . . . . . . . . . . . . . . . . . . . . . . . . . . .   302
    *Stellios Rallis, Dimitrios Chatzoudes, Symeon Symeonidis,*
    *Vasillis Aggelidis, and Prodromos Chatzoglou*

Agile Development in Bureaucratic Environments: A Literature Review . . . .   316
    *Gerald Onwujekwe and Heinz Weistroffer*

Transparency Driven Public Sector Innovation: Smart Waterways
and Maritime Traffic in Finland . . . . . . . . . . . . . . . . . . . . . . . . . . . . . . .   331
    *Vaida Meskauskiene, Anssi Öörni, and Anna Sell*

**Healthcare Information Systems**

Analysis of the Readiness for Healthcare Personnel Adopting
Telerehabilitation: An Interpretive Structural Modelling (ISM) Approach . . . .   353
    *Mahadi Bahari, Tiara Izrinda Jafni, Waidah Ismail, Haslina Hashim,*
    *and Hafez Hussain*

An Ontological Model for Analyzing Liver Cancer Medical Reports . . . . . . .   369
    *Rim Messaoudi, Taher Labidi, Antoine Vacavant, Faiez Gargouri,*
    *Manuel Grand-Brochier, Ali Amouri, Hela Fourati, Achraf Mtibaa,*
    *and Faouzi Jaziri*

The Road to the Future of Healthcare: Transmitting Interoperable
Healthcare Data Through a 5G Based Communication Platform . . . . . . . . . .   383
    *Argyro Mavrogiorgou, Athanasios Kiourtis, Marios Touloupou,*
    *Evgenia Kapassa, Dimosthenis Kyriazis, and Marinos Themistocleous*

**IT Governance**

Agile Requirement Engineering Maturity Framework for Industry 4.0 . . . . . .   405
    *Samaa Elnagar, Heinz Weistroffer, and Manoj Thomas*

Exploring Determinants of Enterprise System Adoption Success in Light
of an Ageing Workforce . . . . . . . . . . . . . . . . . . . . . . . . . . . . . . . . . . . .   419
    *Ewa Soja and Piotr Soja*

Limiting the Impact of Statistics as a Proverbial Source of Falsehood ...... 433
*Yiannis Kiouvrekis, Petros Stefaneas, Angelika Kokkinaki,*
*and Nikos Asimakis*

Comparison of the Non-personalized Active Learning Strategies Used
in Recommender Systems .................................... 443
*Georges Chaaya, Jacques Bou Abdo, Elisabeth Métais, Raja Chiky,*
*Jacques Demerjian, and Kablan Barbar*

Board Interlocking and IT Governance: Proposed Conceptual Model ....... 457
*Allam Hamdan, Abdalmuttaleb Musleh Al-Sartawi, Reem Khamis,*
*Mohammed Anaswah, and Ahlam Hassan*

Business Model Representations and Ecosystem Analysis: An Overview .... 464
*Alejandro Arreola González, Matthias Pfaff, and Helmut Krcmar*

## Management and Organizational Issues in Information Systems

Strategy in the Making: Assessing the Execution of a Strategic
Information Systems Plan .................................... 475
*José-Ramón Rodríguez, Robert Clarisó, and Josep Maria Marco-Simó*

Information Flows at Inter-team Boundaries in Agile Information
Systems Development ...................................... 489
*Scarlet Rahy and Julian Bass*

Critical Factors of Strategic Information Systems Planning
Phases in SMEs .......................................... 503
*Maria Kamariotou and Fotis Kitsios*

Bargaining Between the Client and the Bank and Game Theory .......... 518
*Martina Hedvicakova and Pavel Prazak*

The Determinants of XBRL Adoption: An Empirical Study
in an Emerging Economy .................................... 532
*Tanja Lakovic, Biljana Rondovic, Tamara Backovic-Vulic,*
*and Ivana Ivanovic*

Mobile Technology Acceptance Model: An Empirical Study on Users'
Acceptance and Usage of Mobile Technology for Knowledge Providing .... 547
*Janusz Stal and Grażyna Paliwoda-Pękosz*

**Author Index** ............................................ 561

# Blockchain Technology and Applications

# The Relationship Between Bitcoin Trading Volume, Volatility, and Returns: A Study of Four Seasons

Angelika Kokkinaki[✉], Svetlana Sapuric, and Ifigenia Georgiou

University of Nicosia, Nicosia, Cyprus
{kokkinaki.a,sapuric.s,georgiou.i}@unic.ac.cy

**Abstract.** We study the relationship between Bitcoin trading volume, volatility, and returns using financial data for the period July 2010–November 2017. When we compare the raw annualized volatility of the Bitcoin exchange rate against common currencies, we observe that Bitcoin's is higher. However, when the volume of Bitcoin transactions is considered, the volatility of the Bitcoin stabilizes significantly. Then we divide our sample into four distinct time periods, defined by three important events, namely, the loss of public confidence in the banking system in 2013, the MtGox Bitcoin Exchange hack in early 2014, and the introduction of the Bitcoin legislation in Japan in April 2017. Using asymmetric EGARCH models with the lag of the natural logarithm of the volume of the Bitcoin both as a regressor in the mean equation as well as in the specification of the conditional variance as multiplicative heteroskedasticity we show that volume and volatility are related after 2013, and volume and returns are related before the MtGox hack, positively and significantly. Further, during the euphoric period between the beginning of 2013 and up to the MtGox hack an unexpected rise in Bitcoin returns increases Bitcoin volatility more than an unexpected, equally sized decrease (asymmetry).

**Keywords:** Bitcoin · Volume · Volatility · Asymmetric GARCH

## 1 Introduction

A simple look at the history of Bitcoin makes the bitcoin price seem like a roller coaster. From its inception in 2009 and the first transaction in 2010 when its price – its exchange rate to the US dollar - was just $0.008 up to the beginning of its rapid rise in 2013 - allegedly due to the loss of confidence in the existing banking system, followed by the substantial dive of the Bitcoin price during the first quarter of 2014 after the MtGox Exchange hack and closing, and its subsequent recovery in the second quarter of the year, it has been a thrilling ride[1]. The Bitcoin exchange rate had since continued to steadily rise and the year 2017 has been one of the most successful for Bitcoin

---

[1] During the first quarter of 2014 the exchange rate of Bitcoin had decreased to $298.73 from $1,128.47 since November 2013. Adverse events such as the closing of the Mount Gox Exchange and the negative outlook from the Chinese government have all played a role in damaging the performance of Bitcoin.

© Springer Nature Switzerland AG 2019
M. Themistocleous and P. Rupino da Cunha (Eds.): EMCIS 2018, LNBIP 341, pp. 3–15, 2019.
https://doi.org/10.1007/978-3-030-11395-7_1

investors so far. In the beginning of January 2017 Bitcoin had started with a price of just over $1,000 and has reached values of almost $7,500 by the beginning of November 2017, an increase of 650%, and a year-to-year increase of 947%. The price of Bitcoin on the 11th of November - our last data point - amounted to $6731.32; by the 17th of December 2017 it went up to a record $20,000, only to lose one third of its value in twenty-four hours, dropping below $14,000 on December 22th of the same year.

Bitcoin is widely perceived in the social media and fora as a substantially volatile and, thus a risky currency. In fact, a lot of discussion takes place on whether Bitcoin is money, or whether it can be considered a currency, and the main premise of these doubts is its enormous volatility. It has been noted that what is keeping Bitcoin from satisfying the criteria of being a currency - namely, being a medium of exchange, a unit of account, and a store of value - is its price volatility (Baur and Dimpfl 2018; Cermak 2017). Yermack (2015) asserts that Bitcoin behaves more like a speculative investment rather than a currency; its volatility imposed large short-term risk upon users being enormously higher compared to the volatilities of widely used currencies (Yermack 2015). Bitcoin volatility is even substantially higher than volatilities of currencies of least developed countries and also higher than the volatility of any other cryptocurrency (Kasper 2017).

An omission of previous studies – and of the media - is that the volume of transactions is not taken into account when talking about the volatility of Bitcoin. The relationship between volatility of returns and trading volume has been greatly explored in the literature (Karpoff 1987; Carroll and Kearney 2012). However, studies on Bitcoin volatility largely ignore the volume of transactions and its relation on volatility on the performance of the Bitcoin exchange rate. Balcilar et al. (2017) attempt to fill this gap by undertaking a study on the use of volume information to predict Bitcoin volatility, with the analysis being tailored towards the specification of the model and its non-linearity. They find that volume cannot be used to predict the volatility of Bitcoin returns at any point (Balcilar et al. 2017).

In our study we attempt to extend our understanding of these relationships by increasing the span of the time period of study to include the year 2017 in which both Bitcoin price and trading volume had reached unprecedented heights.

In this study we show that the value of the Bitcoin exchange rate is not as volatile as widely acclaimed once the low volume of trades are taken into account studying the period from July 2010 to November 2017.

Further, we divide our sample of the Bitcoin to US dollar observations into four distinct time periods, defined by three important events that pertain to the Bitcoin market. We study each period separately by employing asymmetric EGARCH models to show that volume and volatility are positively and significantly related after the beginning of the year 2013, and volume and returns are positively and significantly related before the MtGox hack. Further, we find that an unexpected rise in Bitcoin returns is expected to increase Bitcoin volatility more than an unexpected decrease of the same magnitude during the euphoric period between the beginning of 2013 and up to the Mt Gox hack in early 2014.

The paper is organized as follows: Sect. 2 provides a literature review through which we form a set of hypotheses. Methodological approaches employed in this paper as well as data examined in this study are described in Sect. 3. Section 4 presents findings with regards to the hypotheses. In Sect. 5 the empirical results and conclusions are discussed.

## 2  Background and Motivation of Hypotheses

It is widely acclaimed that Bitcoin is a very risky currency with high values of volatility. Yermack (2015) compares the annualized volatility of Bitcoin to different currencies from July 10, 2010 to November 29, 2013 to find that Bitcoin is highly volatile and that its zero correlations with the other traditional currency exchange rates deem Bitcoin unfitting for hedging purposes. Kasper (2017) studied the period from March 2014 to March 2017 to find that Bitcoin volatility was still substantially higher than volatilities of currencies of least developed countries. In fact, only five currencies were found to have higher volatility for more than 10% of the time period under study.

Baur and Dimpfl (2018) show that the volatility of Bitcoin prices is up to 30 times larger compared to major currencies for the time period 1 January 2014 to 25 January 2017 concluding that Bitcoin cannot function as a currency. These results agree with Cermak (2017) who uses a GARCH(1,1) model to study Bitcoin's volatility from August 18, 2010 to March 17, 2017 taking into consideration the macroeconomic variables of countries where Bitcoin is being traded the most. Cermak (2017) finds that Bitcoin currently does not satisfy the criteria of being a currency, its biggest obstacle being its price volatility. Bitcoin volatility prevents Bitcoin from functioning as a medium of exchange, a unit of account, and a store of value. However, they observe that Bitcoin volatility has been steadily declining throughout its lifetime, and they argue that if it follows this trend, Bitcoin volatility will reach the levels of fiat currencies in 2019–2020 and Bitcoin will eventually become a functioning alternative to fiat currencies (Cermak 2017).

We would like to verify that Bitcoin is more volatile than other currencies for the time period we examine in this study. So, our first hypothesis becomes:

*H1: Bitcoin is more volatile than other currencies.*
In a market such as the Bitcoin market where investors rely on technical analysis since there is no reliable fundamental technique to quantity its intrinsic value, the relationship between volume, returns, and volatility seems to be of particular importance (Balcilar et al. 2017). These relationships have been investigated for other markets and recently, Balcilar et al. (2017) investigated these relationships for the Bitcoin market. They use a nonparametric causality-in-quantiles approach for the period December 2011 to April 2016 to find that the volume of transactions can be used to predict the Bitcoin returns except for the bull and bear periods; their results further indicate that the volume does not have any predictive power on the volatility of Bitcoin, pointing out that the relationship between the two variables may not be linear (Balcilar et al. 2017).

The direction of the relationship between volume and volatility is not so straightforward. From one point of view, a higher trading volume can imply higher liquidity, a situation that makes it easier for investors to abandon the investment, introducing instability and boosting volatility in the market (O'Hara 1995). Furthermore, a higher volume can draw attention to an asset and this can in turn trigger additional trading (Miller 1977); Herd behavior has a role to play into all this, too (Schwert 1990). Urquhart (2018) shows that trading volume and volatility both drive market's attention to the Bitcoin. Furthermore, Baur and Dimpfl (2018) find a positive volume - volatility relationship and they argue that this suggests that the majority of Bitcoin trading is noise trading. Thus, a *positive* relationship between volume and volatility can be expected.

On the other hand, based on the Market Microstructure Theory, the higher liquidity – that according to O'Hara (1995) is implied by high volume - is considered to be negatively correlated to price volatility (Li and Wu 2011). This suggests that a higher trading volume is related to lower volatility in securities prices. Thus, according to this theory, a *negative* relationship is expected between trading volume and price volatility.

We expect that in the case of Bitcoin, volume will be positively associated with volatility during the period starting 2013 onwards, and that the effect will be particularly pronounced during the period ending with the MtGox hack in early 2014. Therefore, our next hypothesis becomes:

*H2: Bitcoin Volatility and Bitcoin Volume are positively related during the period before the MtGox hack.*

Regarding the relationship between volume and returns, Gervais et al. (2001) find that increased trade volume creates a return premium; they find that stocks experiencing unusually high (low) trading volume over a period of one day to a week tend to appreciate (depreciate) over the course of the following month. Trading volume can be viewed as a measure of liquidity, which is significantly related to future stock returns (see for example Amihud and Mendelson 1986; Amihud 2002; Liu 2006). Moreover, as mentioned earlier, higher volume means increased attention to the asset (Miller 1977). Balcilar et al. (2017) find that Bitcoin trading volume can predict its returns – except in Bitcoin bear and bull market conditions. Thus, our next hypothesis becomes:

*H3: Bitcoin Returns and Bitcoin Volume are positively related.*

Another point of interest is whether the reaction of return volatility to unexpected changes in returns ("news") is symmetric for rises and decreases of returns ("good" and "bad" news, respectively). It has been demonstrated by several studies that "bad news", i.e. an unexpected fall in returns may increase volatility more - the so-called "leverage effect", while 'good news' i.e. an unexpected rise in returns may lead to decreased volatility, called the "volatility feedback effect" (see Koutmos 1995; Nam 2001; Bollerslev et al. 2009). In other words, the reaction to bad vs. good news is usually asymmetric, and an unexpected fall in returns is expected to increase volatility more than an unexpected increase of the same magnitude. Furthermore, the asymmetry is more pronounced in bear markets: bad news during a bear market has a bigger negative impact than bad news during a bull market (Parker and Li 2006).

For Bitcoin, at least for the "euphoric" period between the beginning of 2013 and the closing of MtGox we would expect the opposite effect, namely, we expect that an unexpected rise in returns would increase volatility more than an unexpected decrease of the same magnitude. This so-called "anti-leverage effect" has been observed in other studies (see Harrison and Zhang 1999; Ghysels et al. 2005; Ludvigson and Ng 2007; Wu 2017) and its possibility has been theoretically argued by Nelson (1991) and Glosten et al. (1993). Wu (2017) describes how this is the case in Chinese markets, associating this partly with the prevalence of "retail investors" behaving like short-term speculators. So, for the Bitcoin market, we would expect that "euphoric buying" when there is a rise in returns would be more prevalent than "panic selling" when returns decrease. The reason we expect this is that the main motivation for Bitcoin enthusiasts is ideological (Khairuddin et al. 2016; Bouri et al. 2017). Thus, our fourth hypothesis becomes:

*H4: At least during the "euphoric" Bitcoin time period, an unexpected rise in Bitcoin returns is expected to increase Bitcoin volatility more than an unexpected decrease of the same magnitude.*

## 3 Data and Methodology

To examine the first hypothesis that the Bitcoin is more volatile than other currencies we use descriptive statistics and graphs of Raw Vs. Returns divided by Volume (in USD) and compare the Bitcoin exchange rate against the US dollar to the midnight exchange rates of the Euro, the British Sterling Pound, the Chinese Yuan, the Japanese Yen, the Russian Ruble, the Swiss Franc, and the London price of gold, for the period from the 19th of July 2010 up to the 11th of November 2017, gathering a total of 2,673 observations[2].

In order to develop the daily change in the exchange rates for each currency of analysis, the following computation was employed:

$$\Delta \text{ in Exchange Rate} = \left( \frac{\text{ER}_t - \text{ER}_{t-1}}{\text{ER}_{t-1}} \right) \tag{1}$$

This calculation gave us a sample size of 2,054 observations. Following Yermack (2015) we compute the annualised volatility for each of the currency changes in exchange rates and gold as shown in Eq. 2[3]:

$$\text{Annualised Volatility} = \text{Standard Deviation} * \text{SQRT}(252) \tag{2}$$

---

[2] The data for the Bitcoin exchange rate as well as the exchange rate of all other currencies was used from the Federal Reserve, www.quandl.com and www.oanda.com. Volume data is available from the 14th of September 2011.

[3] Assuming that there are 252 trading days in the year.

We construct a standardised value of the daily change in the exchange rate of Bitcoin by dividing it by the natural logarithm of the daily volume of trades as shown in Eq. 3:

$$\text{Adjusted Return} = \frac{\Delta \text{ Exchange Rate}}{\ln(\text{Volume of Trades})} \tag{3}$$

To examine our second, third, and fourth hypotheses, we model the volatility of Bitcoin returns for the time period of interest in order to assess the relationship between volume and returns, and volume and the volatility of returns. Because we hypothesize that the reaction to bad vs. good news is asymmetric (Hypothesis 4), we use the Exponential GARCH, the EGARCH (Nelson 1991) to model Bitcoin volatility, a model that places no restrictions on the parameters.

Our mean equation (to examine Hypothesis 3) is:

$$Return = \text{ c } + \text{ b}_{1\ (\textit{ln Volume BTCUSD}_{t-1})} * ln\ Volume\ BTCUSD_{t-1} + \varepsilon_t$$

Where $ln\ Volume\ BTCUSD_t$ is the natural logarithm of the volume of the Bitcoin at time t, expressed in US Dollars, and $\varepsilon_t$ denotes error terms (return residuals), subject to a mean process.

The form of the variance depends on the GARCH model assumed, but in order to examine Hypothesis 2 we also include in the specification of the conditional variance the natural logarithm of the volume of the Bitcoin at time t−1 as multiplicative heteroskedasticity (see Judge et al. 1985).

The Exponential GARCH (EGARCH) model assumes a specific parametric form for the conditional heteroskedasticity that may be present (Hypothesis 4), described by the equation below:

$$\ln\left(\sigma_t^2\right) = \omega + \alpha(|z_{t-1}| - \mathrm{E}[|z_{t-1}|]) + \gamma z_{t-1} + \beta\ln\left(\sigma_{t-1}^2\right)$$

We ran this model for four distinct time periods (data subsets), defined by important events that pertain to the bitcoin market.

## 4 Empirical Results

### 4.1 Performance of Bitcoin

In July 2010 Bitcoin began to trade on a Japanese-based online exchange, MtGox, and started to attract interest and gain popularity. In the beginning of 2013 due to the loss of public faith in the traditional banking system, the performance of the Bitcoin exchange rate picked up. This can be seen in Fig. 1.

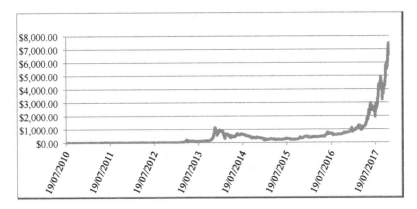

**Fig. 1.** Bitcoin-Dollar exchange rate

Nonetheless, as Fig. 1 shows the first quarter of 2014 has somewhat been unsteady in terms of the Bitcoin-Dollar exchange rate. The lowest value traded was on the date MtGox closed down after its hack. During the next couple of years, the value of Bitcoin exhibited a steady rise. This has been mainly attributed to the increased adoption of Bitcoin in the Asian markets. The above observations were also used to inform the division of our sample into the four sub-time-periods described in the previous section.

Figure 2 shows the daily change in the Bitcoin exchange rate to the US dollar; the change in the value of Bitcoin exhibited high variations throughout the period of analysis. From 2015 and up until the end of our analysis period the return performance of Bitcoin had shown a steadier trend. In comparison to the other currencies of analysis, the performance of the change in the Bitcoin exchange rate is the most radical, which can be seen in Table 1.

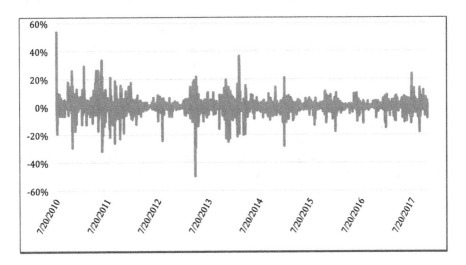

**Fig. 2.** Percentage change in Bitcoin exchange rate in US dollars

**Table 1.** Average percentage change in exchange rates of all currencies and gold

| Currency/Gold | Average change | Maximum | Minimum |
|---|---|---|---|
| Euro | −0.0097% | 7.4953% | −7.5651% |
| GBP (Sterling Pound) | −0.0101% | 2.7821% | −8.1694% |
| Yaun | −0.0013% | 1.8161% | −0.6871% |
| Yen | 0.0101% | 3.3428% | −3.4977% |
| Ruble | −0.0102% | 3.2790% | −3.1933% |
| Franc | −0.0015% | 4.5441% | −13.0222% |
| Bitcoin | **0.4424%** | **53.5962%** | **−49.7501%** |
| Gold | 0.0072% | 4.2775% | −4.3418% |

## 4.2   Volume of Bitcoin Trades

The volume of Bitcoin trades has to some extent experienced a similar trend as to the value and daily percentage change of the Bitcoin-Dollar exchange rate. This can be clearly seen in Fig. 3, which shows the daily volume of Bitcoin trading in US dollars. Up to 2013, over two years since Bitcoin trading had begun, the volume of trades was significantly low, even though the value of the Bitcoin-Dollar exchange rate was at its lowest points. This coincides with the general lack of confidence and fear of the 'unknown' that investors had with the Bitcoin. It is in the first quarter of 2013 that the volume of trades of Bitcoin had started to depict higher amounts, with amount of trades reaching more than $72 million by the end of 2013. Taking into consideration the uncertain and crisis-prone European markets, the investors' confidence in a centralised banking system had reversed, which demonstrates the increase in volume during 2013. Nonetheless, the volume of trades does decrease in the first quarter of 2014, which coincides with the closedown of MtGox in February. Many investors and traders that were holding Bitcoin had continued to do so, because no one wants to sell at the lowest value. The anticipation of a value increase had led to a decision to hold. Inevitably, holding Bitcoins over longer periods will decrease the volume of trades and ultimately drive the price down. This has been the case for the following two years 2015–2016, where the volume of trades had been at a relatively lower, stable level. During 2017, the volume had increased substantially. A number of Asian exchanges, predominantly from China, have introduced trading of Bitcoin and cryptocurrencies which has seen the rally of volume of trades. At that point there had been 16.7 million Bitcoins mined[4], which shows that Bitcoin was still well into circulation, except that investors had been holding them. Therefore, the decrease in value of Bitcoin-Dollar exchange rate during the various periods of our analysis is not due to its uncertainty or riskiness, but due to the low volume of trading as the majority are had chosen to hold their Bitcoins.

---

[4] www.cryptocoinsnews.com.

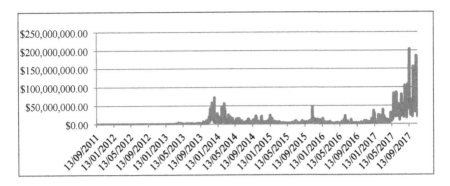

**Fig. 3.** Bitcoin trading volume in US dollars

### 4.3 Is Bitcoin as Risky as Perceived?

In concurrence with Yermack (2015), we also find that the value of Bitcoin exhibits the highest annualised volatility even when adding more currency exchange rates in comparison and extending the sample period. Figure 4 demonstrates the annualised volatility of the percentage change in daily exchange rates for six major currencies, gold and Bitcoin, all measured against the US dollar, during our period of analysis. Without a doubt, studying the 'raw' annualised volatility deduces that the Bitcoin's exchange rate has been the most volatile during our sample period in comparison to gold and other major currencies.

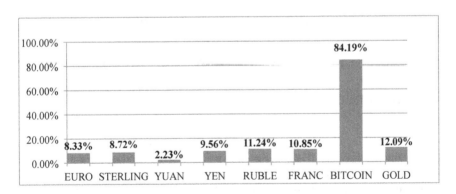

**Fig. 4.** Annualised volatility of Bitcoin and major currencies

Figure 5 presents the results with the standardised value of the daily percentage change in the Bitcoin-Dollar exchange rate by dividing it by the natural logarithm of the daily volume of trades. Compared to Fig. 2, the trend and general performance of the Bitcoin is to a greater extent more stabilised.

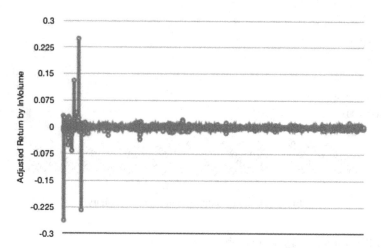

**Fig. 5.** Daily percentage changes in the Bitcoin-Dollar exchange rate divided by the natural logarithm of the daily volume of trades for the time period 19/09/2011–11/11/2017.

Furthermore, as shown in Table 2, the average percentage change of Bitcoin is very close to zero (0.00016%) and the range between the maximum and minimum percentage changes in the Bitcoin exchange rate is now considerably smaller as opposed to the initial difference in the maximum and minimum percentage changes in Bitcoin (103.3%) in Table 1.

**Table 2.** Average percentage change of Bitcoin divided by change in volume.

| Currency | Average % change | Maximum | Minimum |
|----------|------------------|-----------|------------|
| Bitcoin  | 0.00016%         | 0.249218% | −0.262607% |

### 4.4    EGARCH Results

As shown in Table 3, the coefficient of the variable lnVolumeBTCUSDt−1 that represents the natural logarithm of the volume of the Bitcoin at time $t-1$ in the specification of the conditional variance (Hypothesis 2) is positive and statistically significant in all periods but the period before 2013. Thus, Hypothesis 2 that BTC Volatility and Bitcoin Volume are related cannot be rejected for the last three time periods under study.

The coefficient of the variable lnVolumeBTCUSDt−1 that represents the natural logarithm of the volume of the Bitcoin at time $t-1$ in the specification of the mean equation (Hypothesis 3) is positive and statistically significant in the first two time periods under study that are ending before the hack of the MtGox exchange. The coefficient is positive but insignificant after the MtGox hack.

Further, the asymmetry term, i.e. the so-called "leverage effect", $\gamma$ (Hypothesis 4), although relatively small and in no case dominating the arch effect, $\alpha$, is positive and statistically significant during the time period of the beginning of 2013 up to the time of the MtGox hack, revealing that volatility increases more when there are unexpected

**Table 3.** EGARCH models. *, **, **: Statistically significant at the 0.10, 0.05, and 0.01 level of significance, respectively. Distribution: Student t, Sandwich estimators.

| Time periods: | | Before 2013 | Beginning of 2013 to MtGox hack | MtGox - hack, before Japanese legislation | After Japanese legislation |
|---|---|---|---|---|---|
| Sample dates: | | 9/14/2011–12/31/2012 | 1/1/2013–2/21/2014 | 2/22/2014–3/31/2017 | 4/1/2017–11/11/2017 |
| *Mean equation* | | *Coef. (P > \|z\|)* | *Coef. (P > \|z\|)* | *Coef. (P > \|z\|)* | *Coef. (P > \|z\|* |
| Coefficient of the lag of lnVolumeBTCUSD in the Mean equation | **H3** | 0.0009** (0.0460) | 0.0011* (0.0840) | 0.0011 (0.1410) | 0.0004 (0.8120) |
| Mean Equation Constant | | −0.0049 (0.1980) | −0.0063 (0.4220) | −0.0155 (0.1700) | 0.0024 (0.9350) |
| *Variance equation (EGARCH model)* | | | | | |
| Coefficient of lnVolumeBTCUSDt-1 (Multiplicative Heteroskedasticity) | **H2** | −0.0600 (0.4630) | 0.2026** (0.0300) | 0.0764* (0.0800) | 0.1041* (0.0840) |
| $\omega$ | Constant | −0.3175 (0.6330) | −4.6030** (0.0250) | −1.6040* (0.0520) | −2.7397* (0.0500) |
| $\gamma$ | Asymmetry term/Leverage effect (**H4**) | 0.0043 (0.9700) | 0.2102** (0.0140) | 0.0192 (0.6710) | −0.0317 (0.6280) |
| $\alpha$ | ARCH term | 0.8246** (0.0440) | 0.9229*** (0.0000) | 0.5149*** (0.0000) | 0.2495*** (0.0090) |
| $\beta$ | GARCH term | 0.8548*** (0.0000) | 0.6830*** (0.0000) | 0.9068*** (0.0000) | 0.8478*** (0.0000) |
| Number of obs | | 475 | 417 | 1131 | 225 |
| Wald chi2(1) | | 4 | 2.99 | 2.16 | 0.06 |
| Prob > chi2 | | 0.0456 ** | 0.0837 * | 0.1413 | 0.8119 |
| AIC | | −2087.158 | −1383.795 | −5058.234 | −783.1486 |
| BIC | | −2053.852 | −1351.531 | −5017.987 | −755.8198 |

increases in returns than it does to decreases in returns during that period of time. Thus, for this specific period, Hypothesis H3 is not rejected. For the period before 2013 as well as for the period after the MtGox hack and before the Japanese legislation, $\gamma$ is positive but not statistically significant. For the period after the Japanese legislation, $\gamma$ becomes negative but it is still not statistically significant.

# 5   Discussion

In this study, we examined the hypothesis regarding the volatility of Bitcoin exchange rate against common currencies by collecting and analysing financial data from July 2010 until November 2017.

Initially, the raw annualized volatility of Bitcoin has been compared to conventional and major exchange rates. The first set of results indicated a high value of annualized volatility for the Bitcoin exchange rate in accordance with previous literature (Yermack 2015; Kasper 2017; Cermak 2017; Baur and Dimpfl 2018). However, when the volume of Bitcoin transactions was taken into consideration, the volatility of the Bitcoin exchange rate stabilized significantly.

Furthermore, we divided the sample observations into four distinct time periods, defined by three important events that pertained to the cryptocurrency market. We used the asymmetric EGARCH models that include the lag of the natural logarithm of the volume of the Bitcoin at time t−1 both as a regressor in the mean equation as well as in the specification of the conditional variance as multiplicative heteroskedasticity to find some interesting results.

First, we find that lagged volume and volatility are positively and significantly related after the beginning of 2013, but before that, the two variables are unrelated. This could be because attention had been drawn to the Bitcoin in 2013, and this has triggered additional trading (Miller 1977; Schwert 1990).

Second, we find that volume and returns are positively and significantly related before the MtGox hack and closing down in February 2014. This could be due to a return premium, according to Mingelgrin (2001). It could also be because of the increased attention to the asset (Miller 1977).

Further, we find that the price volatility of Bitcoin increases as a result of good news in comparison to bad news during the euphoric period between the beginning of 2013 and up to the MtGox hack. This is consistent with Bouri et al. (2017) who studied this from August 18, 2011 to April 29, 2016 and they give a "safe haven" explanation for this, arguing that in this respect, Bitcoin behaves like gold. This is also consistent with Bitcoin being considered as a speculative asset, as this so-called "anti-leverage effect" can be present in speculative markets characterised by short-termism (Wu 2017). On the other hand, it could be that adopters of Bitcoin that motivated by Bitcoin's possible role in a monetary revolution, users' increased empowerment, and their perception that Bitcoin has a "real" value (Khairuddin 2016) would view good news as "confirming" their expectations and the enthusiasm would cause increased volatility, more so than bad news would cause – bad news would find such users still holding on to their precious – for the uses cited by Khairuddin (2016) - Bitcoins.

# References

Amihud, Y.: Illiquidity and stock returns: cross-section and time-series effects. J. Financ. Mark. 5(1), 31–56 (2002)

Amihud, Y., Mendelson, H.: Liquidity and stock returns. Financ. Anal. J. 42(3), 43–48 (1986)

Balcilar, M., Bouri, E., Gupta, R., Roubaud, D.: Can volume predict Bitcoin returns and volatility? A quantiles-based approach. Econ. Model. 64, 74–81 (2017)

Baur, D.G., Dimpfl, T.: Excess volatility as an impediment for a digital currency (2018)

Baur, D.G., Glover, K.: A gold bubble? (No. 175) (2012)

Bollerslev, T., Kretschmer, U., Pigorsch, C., Tauchen, G.: A discrete-time model for daily S and P500 returns and realized variations: jumps and leverage effects. J. Econ. **150**(2), 151–166 (2009)

Bouri, E., Azzi, G., Dyhrberg, A.H.: On the return-volatility relationship in the Bitcoin market around the price crash of 2013. Econ.-Open-Access Open-Assess. E-J. **11**, 1–16 (2017)

Carroll, R., Kearney, C.: Do trading volumes explain the persistence of GARCH effects? Appl. Financ. Econ. **22**, 1993–2008 (2012). https://doi.org/10.1080/09603107.2012.692871

Cermak, V.: Can Bitcoin become a viable alternative to fiat currencies? An empirical analysis of Bitcoin's volatility based on a GARCH model (2017)

European Central Bank (ECB): Virtual Schemes (2012). www.ecb.int/pub/pdf/other/virtualcurrencyschemes201210en.pdf

Gervais, S., Kaniel, R., Mingelgrin, D.H.: The high-volume return premium. J. Financ. **56**(3), 877–919 (2001)

Ghysels, E., Santa-Clara, P., Valkanov, R.: There is a risk-return trade- off after all. J. Financ. Econ. **76**(3), 509–548 (2005)

Glosten, L.R., Jagannathan, R., Runkle, D.E.: On the relation between the expected value and the volatility of the nominal excess return on stocks. J. Financ. **48**, 1779–1801 (1993)

Harrison, P., Zhang, H.H.: An investigation of the risk and return relation at long horizons. Rev. Econ. Stat. **81**(3), 399–408 (1999)

Judge, G.G., Griffiths, W.E., Hill, R.C., Lutkepohl, H., Lee, T.C.: The Theory and Practice of Econometrics, 2nd edn. Wiley, New York (1985)

Karpoff, J.M.: The relation between price changes and trading volume: a survey. J. Financ. Quant. Anal. **22**, 109–126 (1987). https://doi.org/10.2307/2330874

Kasper, D.: Evolution of Bitcoin-volatility comparisons with least developed countries' currencies (2017)

Khairuddin, I.E., Sas, C., Clinch, S., Davies, N.: Exploring motivations for Bitcoin technology usage. In: Proceedings of the 2016 CHI Conference Extended Abstracts on Human Factors in Computing Systems, pp. 2872–2878. ACM, May 2016

Koutmos, G., Booth, G.G.: Asymmetric volatility transmission in international stock markets. J. Int. Money Financ. **14**, 747–762 (1995)

Li, J., Wu, C.: Stochastic volatility, liquidity and intraday information flow. Appl. Econ. Lett. **18**(16), 1511–1515 (2011). https://doi.org/10.1080/13504851.2010.543077

Liu, W.: A liquidity-augmented capital asset pricing model. J. Financ. Econ. **82**, 631–671 (2006)

Ludvigson, S.C., Ng, S.: The empirical risk–return relation: a factor analysis approach. J. Financ. Econ. **83**(1), 171–222 (2007)

Miller, E.M.: Risk, uncertainty, and divergence of opinion. J. Financ. **32**(4), 1151–1168 (1977)

Nam, K., Pyun, C.S., Avard, S.L.: Asymmetric reverting behavior of short-horizon stock returns: an evidence of stock market overreaction. J. Bank. Financ. **25**(4), 807–824 (2001)

Nelson, D.B.: Conditional heteroskedasticity in asset returns: a new approach. Econometrica **59**, 347–370 (1991)

O'Hara, M.: Market Microstructure Theory. Blackwell, Cambridge (1995)

Parker, J.C., Li, C.H.: How Bad is Bad News; How Good is Good News? Bank of Canada (2006)

Schwert, G.W.: Stock market volatility. Financ. Anal. J. **46**(3), 23–34 (1990)

Wallace, B.: The rise and fall of Bitcoin. Wired, 23 November (2011)

Wu, L.: Reverse return-volatility asymmetry, and short sale constraints: evidence from the Chinese markets. Presented at the EFMA Annual Meeting 2017 (2017)

Yermack, D.: Is Bitcoin a real currency? An economic appraisal. In: Handbook of Digital Currency, pp. 31–43 (2015)

# Verify-Your-Vote: A Verifiable Blockchain-Based Online Voting Protocol

Marwa Chaieb[1]([✉]), Souheib Yousfi[2], Pascal Lafourcade[3],
and Riadh Robbana[2]

[1] Faculty of Sciences of Tunis, Tunis, Tunisia
chaiebmarwa.insat@gmail.com
[2] National Institute of Applied Science and Technology, Tunis, Tunisia
souheib.youssfi@gmail.com, riadh.robbana@gmail.com
[3] LIMOS, University Clermont Auvergne, Clermont-Ferrand, France
pascal.lafourcade@uca.fr

**Abstract.** Blockchain provides the possibility to design new types of applications and systems that allow their users to store data in a secure and transparent way. In this paper, we design a fully verifiable online electronic voting protocol using a blockchain. Our e-voting protocol, called VYV for Verify-Your-Vote, involves cryptographic primitives based on Elliptic-Curve Cryptography (ECC), pairings and Identity Based Encryption (IBE). It ensures the following privacy and security properties: only eligible voter can vote, authentication of the voter, vote privacy, receipt-freeness, fairness, individual and universal verifiability. Furthermore, we formally prove the security of our protocol, using ProVerif tool.

**Keywords:** Online e-voting · Blockchain · Elliptic Curve Cryptography
ProVerif · Verifiability

## 1 Introduction

Blockchain [1, 2] is a technology of storage of information. It can be seen as a digital, decentralized, public and large register where all exchanges made between its users are recorded in a public and secure way, without the control of a central entity. It was first introduced in 2008, by Nakamoto in his paper [3], where he described a peer to-peer payment system that allows e-cash transactions directly, without relying on financial institutions. In 2014, Buterin proposed a Blockchain called *Ethereum* [4]. Ethereum helps us to achieve verifiability, and also to ensure the non-malleability of exchanges in our e-voting systems.

Online e-voting systems aim at providing better level of security than traditional voting systems. Modern cryptography helps us to increase the security comparing to traditional voting systems. We recall the security properties for e-voting systems presented in [5, 6]:

© Springer Nature Switzerland AG 2019
M. Themistocleous and P. Rupino da Cunha (Eds.): EMCIS 2018, LNBIP 341, pp. 16–30, 2019.
https://doi.org/10.1007/978-3-030-11395-7_2

- **Eligibility:** Only the registered voters can vote, and nobody can submit more votes than allowed (typically only one vote per voter is counted, even if several ballots can be casted).
- **Fairness:** No preliminary results that could influence other voters' decisions are made available.
- **Robustness:** The protocol can tolerate a certain number of misbehaving voters.
- **Integrity:** Is the assurance of the accuracy and consistency of votes.
- **Verifiability:** It is usually split into 2 properties: *Individual Verifiability*: Each voter can check whether his vote was counted correctly. *Universal Verifiability*: Anybody can verify that the announced result corresponds to the sum of all votes.
- **Vote-Privacy:** The votes are kept private. This can also be modeled as an unlinkability between the voter and his vote.
- **Receipt-Freeness:** A voter cannot construct a receipt which allows him to prove to a third party that he voted for a certain candidate. This is to prevent vote-buying.
- **Coercion-Resistance:** Even when a voter interacts with a coercer during the entire voting process, the coercer cannot be sure whether he followed his instructions or actually voted for another candidate.

In [5, 6] the authors proposed a more fine grain hierarchy for privacy notions. We consider simple versions of such properties and use them to prove the security of our protocol in Proverif. In most of cases, online voting systems that vouch for verifiability, use a trusted web server as a public *bulletin board* to display all public values. We take advantage from Blockchain technology to ensure secure and verifiable elections.

**Our Contributions:** We design a secure online electronic voting protocol called Verify-Your-Vote (VYV for short). We use Blockchain technology as a bulletin board which allows us to have a verifiable election. The use of Blockchain ensures election integrity thanks to its property of immutability. Moreover, our protocol ensures the following properties: only eligible voter can vote, authentication of the voter, vote privacy, receipt-freeness, fairness, individual and universal verifiability. We also use Proverif in order to formally prove the security of VYV.

## 2   Related Work

We describe several e-voting systems that claim to provide online elections based on Blockchain, which are used or were supposed to be used for elections in the last years. In Table 1, we summarize the security properties of these voting system.

*TIVI* [7]: is designed by the company Smartmatic. It is an online voting solution based on biometric authentication. It checks the elector's identity via a selfie. An elector only needs to upload a picture of his face to the system before the vote, and then facial recognition technology compares his facial biometry to the image downloaded during the registration phase. Tivi ensures several security properties such as eligibility since it provides different authentication techniques, votes secrecy thanks to the encryption mechanism and taking advantage from Blockchain technology, universal verifiability and votes integrity are guaranteed. This system provides also voters' anonymity since it includes a mixing phase and individual verifiability by the mean of a

QR code stored during voting phase and checked later via a smartphone application. However, this system has some weaknesses. In fact, it does not provide any mechanism to protect voters from coercion. Moreover, voters have the right to vote only once.

Our protocol VYV meets all the properties guaranteed by TIVI. In addition, it provides mechanisms to ensure receipt-freeness and make it possible to an indecisive voter to access to the voting system and change his vote before the end of the voting phase.

*Follow My Vote* [8]: each voter needs a web cam and a government-issued ID to authenticate himself. A trusted authority verifies the identity of each voter, authorizes only eligible voters to cast their ballots and provides them with pass-phrases needed in case of changing their votes in the future. After voting and casting his ballot to the election Blockchain, each voter is able to see his vote counted in the ballot box. Additionally, voters can watch the election progress in real time as votes are cast. Follow My vote online voting system respects a limited number of security properties. In fact, it includes an authentication phase which ensures voter's eligibility. It allows voters to locate their votes, and check that they are both present and correct using their unique voter ID. Nevertheless, this voting system does not meet several security properties. Indeed, it requires a trusted authority to ensure voter confidentiality and hide the correspondence between the voters' real identity and their voting key. If this authority is corrupted, votes are no longer anonymous. This authority has also the possibility to change votes since it has all voters' pass-phrases so votes integrity is compromised. Votes secrecy is not verified by this system because votes are casted without being encrypted. Moreover, the ability to change votes, coupled with the ability to observe the election in real time compromise fairness property. This system is not coercion resistant and it does not ensure universal verifiability.

Compared to Follow My Vote voting system, Verify-Your-Vote ensures more privacy and security properties. In fact, our protocol provides votes privacy without relying on trusted authorities since it is based on Blockchain and cryptographic primitives (ECC and IBE). We also ensure fairness thanks to the definition of a list of timers that delimit each phase, votes integrity thanks to Blockchain and universal verifiability thanks to ECC.

*Open Vote Network* [9]: it is a boardroom scale online voting system written as a smart contract on Ethereum. This smart contract is owned by an administrator who is in charge of the election set up and voters authentication. This voting system guarantees diverse security properties. It ensures votes confidentiality since they are encrypted before being cast. It is a self tallying protocol so it warrants universal verifiability. Thanks to the commit phase, it ensures that no partial result can be calculated. Finally, each voter can check that his vote has been recorded as cast and cast as intended by inspecting the Blockchain. Open Vote Network is not coercion resistant. It supports only elections with two options (yes or no) and with a maximum of 50 voters due to the mathematical tools that they used. Finally, it needs to trust the election administrator to ensure that only eligible voters have the right to vote.

Unlike this protocol, Verify-Your-Vote protocol ensures eligibility of voters even if the administrator is corrupted because the list of all eligible voters is published and can be verified by everyone. Additionally, our protocol is designed to support large scale elections with multiple options.

*Agora Voting System* [10]: Composed of four technology layers: the Bulletin Board blockchain (based on skipchain architecture [11]), Cotena (a tamper-resistant logging mechanism built on top of the Bitcoin blockchain), the Bitcoin blockchain and Votapp (the application layer of the Agora network). Agora's voting system proceeds in 6 stages. It starts with a configuration phase. During this phase, the election administrator creates a configuration file that contains election parameters. The second step is the casting phase in which voters fill out, review, encrypt and submit their ballots. Ballots are sealed by the Agora's software using the threshold ElGamal cryptosystem. The voter casts her encrypted ballot to the Bulletin Board and signs the transaction with her digital identity credentials. Before casting the vote, a locator (a snapshot of the encrypted ballot) is delivered to the voter. This locator is used for individual verifiability. Next, we move to the anonymization phase in which election authority runs all ballots through a mixing network to anonymize the encrypted ballots cast on the Bulletin Board using the Neff shuffling. Once ballots have been anonymized, all the authorities have to collectively decrypt them and publish them with decryption correctness proof. Votes are then calculated. The final result is published on the Bulletin Board. The final step is the auditing phase. Agora's voting system offer the possibility to audit election results at every stage of the voting process. If the election process is successfully verified, a final attestation is signed with the auditors' private key. Our propounded protocol VYV guarantees the same security properties that are respected by Agora voting system. However, we use different cryptographic primitives. In fact, we exploit the Elliptic Curve Cryptography (ECC), pairings and Identity Based Encryption (IBE). An other difference between VYV protocol and Agora voting system is that Agora is a platform that provides, for each stage, different alternatives (for example it supports different modalities of authentication), however our approach is much more precise since it includes specific phases and technologies.

**Table 1.** Security properties of TIVI, Follow My Vote and Open Vote Network.

|  | TIVI | Follow My Vote | Open Vote Network | Agora |
|---|---|---|---|---|
| Eligibility | ✓ | ✓ | Trusted administrator | ✓ |
| Fairness | ✓ | ✗ | ✓ | ✓ |
| Integrity | ✓ | ✗ | ✓ | ✓ |
| Individual verifiability | ✓ | ✓ | ✓ | ✓ |
| Universal verifiability | ✓ | ✗ | ✓ | ✓ |
| Vote-Privacy | ✓ | ✗ | ✓ | ✓ |
| Receipt-freeness | ✗ | ✗ | ✗ | ✓ |
| Coercion resistance | ✗ | ✗ | ✗ | ✗ |
| Voting policy | Single vote | Multiple vote | Single vote | No available information |

**Outline:** In next section, we briefly introduce Ethereum and present an overview of cryptographic primitives used in our protocol. Then in Sect. 4, we present the structure of the ballots, we also detail the different steps and entities of our protocol. In Sect. 5, we prove the security of VYV using ProVerif, a verification tool. Finally we conclude in the last section.

# 3  Preliminaries

This section presents succinctly the basic notions associated to Ethereum and cryptographic primitives used in our approach.

**Ethereum:** Is a global computer, which anyone can program and use as he wishes. This computer is always on, it is secure, and everything that is done using this computer is public. It allows to develop a new category of applications called decentralized applications [4] (DApps). These applications run on the Ethereum network, which is made up of several thousand computers that constantly communicate. They share the same data which are stored on the Blockchain. Ethereum includes within its blocks executable programs that trigger actions based on information received or conditions reached. We are talking here about smart contracts. A smart contract is an autonomous program that, once started and deployed in the Blockchain, executes predefined conditions. Ethereum can be seen as a transaction based state machine, where transactions can change the state. This latter keeps track of interactions and is composed of "accounts". Usually, there are two types of accounts:

- **Externally Owned Account (EOA):** it is a user-controlled account, serves to identify external agents. It is characterized by a public/private key pair. An EOA can send transactions to transfer ether or trigger a contract code. It is controlled by its private key and has no associated code, this private key is used to sign transactions and prove the sender's identity.
- **Contract account:** is a set of code and data that is located at a definite address. It has only a public key. Its execution is activated by transactions received from other accounts.

Ethereum accounts are identified by their addresses which are constructed from the public key by taking the last 20 bytes.

**Elliptic Curve Cryptography:** Elliptic curves are used for asymmetric operations such as key exchanges on a non-secure channel, which is called cryptography on elliptic curves or ECC (Elliptic Curve Cryptography). ECC is more efficient than discrete logarithm systems such as DSA [12], ElGamal [13] and also RSA [14]. ECC offers equal security for a far smaller key size.

**Pairings** [15, 16]: Another advantage of elliptic curve cryptography is that a bilinear operator can be defined between groups. The pairings are obtained from the Weil and the Tate pairing [17, 18] on special kinds of elliptic curves. Let $G_1$ be an additive cyclic group of order a prime number q and $G_2$ a multiplicative group of the same order q. A function $e : G_1 \times G_1 \rightarrow G_2$ is called a bilinear cryptographic coupling (also called pairing) if it satisfies the following properties:

1. Bilinearity: for all $P, Q \in G_1$ and $a, b \in Z; e(aP, bQ) = e(P, Q)^{ab}$,
2. Non-degeneration: $e(P, P)$ is a generator of $G_2$ and so $e(P, P) \neq 1$,
3. Computability: there is an efficient algorithm to compute $e(P, Q)$ for all $P, Q \in G_1$.

**Identity-Based Encryption** [19]: Pairings were introduced into many crypto-graphic primitives such as signatures or encryption. But the application that remains the most important is Identity-Based Encryption (IBE). Indeed, one of the big problems of public key cryptosystems is the management of keys. There are certification authorities but these are not recognized everywhere and the implementation of a public key infrastructure (PKI) is very expensive. It was Shamir [20], who in 1984 suggested using people's identities as public keys. He proposed to no longer resort to expensive PKI: the key of an individual is directly related to his identity: for example, his e-mail address. The first IBE protocol was proposed in 2001 by Boneh and Franklin [21]. Its main blemish is that the Private Key Generator (PKG) knows the private key. This defect can be corrected by using a distributed PKG like that of Pedersen [22] or Gennaro et al. [23]. In these protocols, a master key is generated in a distributed manner. Each of the m PKGs randomly constructs a fragment. All that is required is that part of these PKGs be online in order to retrieve the private key.

## 4    Verify-Your-Vote Protocol

We design an online e-voting system that uses Blockchain technology, called Verify-Your-Vote (VYV). It is an online voting systems that provides verifiability, uses a *public bulletin board*[1] to display all public values and offers a persistent view to all voters. In VYV, we take advantage from Blockchain technology and explore the feasibility of using this technology as a public bulletin board. We present now the different entities involved in VYV, the ballot structure and the different phases that constitute VYV protocol.

### 4.1    Protocol Entities

Our system is composed of the following entities:

- **Registration Server (RS):** It is a trusted server, its role is to register eligible voters and provide them with their authentication parameters.
- **Election Administrator (A):** It is an externally owned account that manages the election. This includes defining a list of timers to ensure that the election takes place in a timely manner, setting the election parameters, authenticating voters and constructing ballots in cooperation with tallying authority.
- **Eligible Voters (V):** Each voter has an externally owned account. He has the right to vote and casts his choice several times before the end of the voting phase and only his last vote is finally counted.

---

[1] It is a public board where everyone can read and append only information. The written data cannot be deleted.

- **Tallying Authority (TA):** It is an externally owned account. We have as many tallying authorities as candidates. They participate in the construction of ballots, decrypt votes, calculate the election final result and publish the different values that allow voters to check the accuracy of the count.

## 4.2   Ballot Structure of VYV

The main idea of our ballots design is inspired from [24]. We describe the structure of the ballots of VYV in Table 2. Each blank ballot contains four pieces of information: its number "$B_N$", candidates' names "$name_j$", candidates' pseudo ID "$C_j$" and the counter-values "$C_{Vj}$" that are used as a receipt by voters. The ballot number is unique. The pseudo ID is the position of the candidate in the ballot, it is calculated from an initial order and an offset value. Counter-values are used for verification. They are calculated for each candidate and depend on the ballot number and the name of the candidate. All these informations are obtained by using cryptography primitives. We detail the construction of ballots in the setup phase.

**Table 2.** Ballot structure.

| Ballot number $B_N$ | | | |
| --- | --- | --- | --- |
| Pseudo ID "$C_j$" | Candidate "$name_j$" | Choice | Counter-value "$C_{Vj}$" |
| 0 | Paul | ☐ | $C_{V1}$ |
| 1 | Nico | ☐ | $C_{V2}$ |
| 2 | Joel | ☐ | $C_{V3}$ |

## 4.3   Election Stage

Here is how the election process works in six steps.

**Setup:** This phase is described in Fig. 1.

1. The election administrator starts by generating the following election parameters and publishes them on the bulletin board:

   - $G_1$ an additive cyclic group of order a prime number q,
   - $G_2$ a multiplicative group of the same order q,
   - Hash function: $H_1 : \{0, 1\}^* \rightarrow G_1$.

   The administrator defines some timers to respect the phases of the election:

   - $T_{beginElection}$: The election administrator starts the election process and constructs ballots,
   - $T_{beginVote}$: The tallying authority sends ballots to voters. Each voter encrypts his choice and casts it,
   - $T_{finishVote}$: Each voter must vote before this time,
   - $T_{beginTally}$: The tallying authority decrypts votes and proceeds to the tally,
   - $T_{finishTally}$: The tallying authority must finish tallying by this time and begin the verification,

- $T_{finishElection}$: All voters must verify election result before this time.

2. Ballots are constructed in this phase. For each ballot, the election administrator generates a germ $g_1$ and a random number $D_1$, encrypts them with his public key $PK_A$, the obtained cipher is denoted by $\{g_1, D_1\}_{PK_A}$. This value is called the ballot number and is denoted by $B_N$. He also calculates the offset value using this formula: offset = $H(g_1)$ mod m, where $m$ is candidates' number.
3. The administrator sends the bulletin number $B_N$ and the offset value to the tallying authorities to complete the bulletin construction.
4. Tallying authorities calculate the different counter-values using the following formula: $C_{Vj} = e(Q_{name\,j}, S_j.Q_{Bn})$, where e() is the pairing function, $S_j$ is the secret key of the tallying authority j, $Q_{namej} = H_1(name\,_j)$ and $Q_{Bn} = H_1(B_N)$ are two points of the elliptic curve $E$.

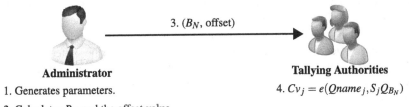

**Administrator**
1. Generates parameters.
2. Calculates $B_N$ and the offset value.

3. $(B_N, \text{offset})$

**Tallying Authorities**
4. $Cv_j = e(Qname_j, S_jQ_{B_N})$

**Fig. 1.** Setup phase.

**Registration Phase:** This phase takes place offline. The voter registers at a polling station. After verifying his legitimacy by a face to face meeting, the voter accesses a server called "Registration Server". The registration process is described in Fig. 2.

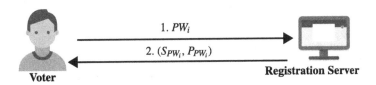

**Voter**

1. $PW_i$
2. $(S_{PW_i}, P_{PW_i})$

**Registration Server**

**Fig. 2.** Registration phase.

1. Every eligible voter enters a password $PW_i$.
2. The registration server returns to the voter its authentication parameters $S_{PWi}$ and $P_{PWi}$ where: $S_{PWi} = S_{RS\_A}.H_1(PW_i)$ and $P_{PWi} = H_1(PW_i)$. Where $S_{RS\_A}$ is a secret value shared between the registration server and the administrator.

**Authentication Phase:** We give an overview of this phase in Fig. 3.

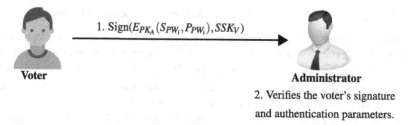

**Voter**

1. $Sign(E_{PK_A}(S_{PW_i}, P_{PW_i}), SSK_V)$

**Administrator**

2. Verifies the voter's signature
and authentication parameters.

**Fig. 3.** Authentication phase.

1. The voter encrypts his authentication parameters $(S_{PWi}, P_{PWi})$ with the administrator public key "$PK_A$", signs them with his signature secret key "$SSK_V$" and sends them to the administrator. To encrypt voter's authentication parameters with $PK_A$ we use Paillier cryptosystem [25], which outlines an asymmetric non-deterministic encryption algorithm with homomorphic additive properties. The security of the Paillier scheme is based on the problem of computing n-th residues in $\mathbb{Z}_{n^2}^*$. To sign voter's authentication parameters we use RSA signature scheme [14].
2. To verify voter's legitimacy, the administrator verifies the voter's signature, decrypts the authentication parameters, calculates $S_{RS\_A}.P_{PWi}$ and compares it with the value of $S_{PWi}$, if he finds the same value then the voter is registered and has the right to vote.

After being successfully authenticated, each eligible voter has access to an interface that allows him to create his own externally owned account on the election Blockchain and publish his public key as well as his address (which is derived from the public key by taking the last 20 bytes of the hash of the public key).

**Voting:** This step is illustrated in Fig. 4.

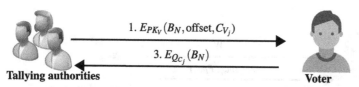

**Tallying authorities**

1. $E_{PK_V}(B_N, \text{offset}, C_{V_j})$

3. $E_{Q_{C_j}}(B_N)$

**Voter**

2. Decrypts ballot, chooses a candidate
and encrypts his choice.

**Fig. 4.** Voting phase.

1. The tallying authority randomly chooses a ballot for each voter, encrypts it with the voter's public key $PK_v$ (that has been published on the bulletin board during authentication phase) and sends it to the voter in a transaction on our Blockchain.
2. The voter decrypts his ballot using his secret key, chooses a candidate with pseudo ID $C_j$ and encrypts his bulletin number $B_N$ with $Q_{Cj} = H_I(C_j)$,
3. He casts his vote to the tallying authority via the blockchain.

Each voter should memorize the counter-value corresponding to the chosen candidate and casts its vote before $T_{finishVote}$.

**Tallying:** Each tallying authority is dedicated to calculate the number of votes of a specific pseudo ID ($C_j$): for example the first tallying authority "$TA_1$" decrypts, with its secret key $S_1.Q_{C1}$, all bulletins that was encrypted with the public key $Q_{C1}$ (certainly these ballots contain votes for candidates with $C_j = 0$). Votes decryption reveals numbers of ballots. Each authority consults the exchange history with the administrator stored in the Blockchain to derive the value of the offset corresponding to each bulletin number. From each bulletin number and its corresponding offset, tallying authorities reconstruct ballots, identify chosen candidates and increment counters. The final result of the election must be published before $T_{f\,inishTally}$.

**Verification:** To verify that the tallying authorities take into account all voters' ballots, the verification phase is organized around two sub-phases: It consists first of all in the reconstruction of counter-values associated with the ballot and the name of the candidate. From the bulletin number and the name of the associated candidate, each tallying authority calculates the corresponding counter-value. Counter-values are published during this phase in the bulletin board. They must be identical to the receipts of the voters. Thus, each voter should access to the Blockchain and check the existence of his counter-value in the list of reconstructed counter-values. The second sub-phase uses the homomorphism property of pairings to check the accuracy of the count. In fact, at the end of tallying phase, each tallying authority "$TA_k$" publishes on the bulletin board the count of each candidate: $\sigma_{k,name_j} = \sum_{i=1}^{l_j} S_k Q_{B_{Ni}}(name_j)$; Where $lj$ is the number of votes received by the candidate j, $S_k$ is the private key of the tallying authority k and $B_{Ni}(name_j)$ is the ballot number of the vote i that corresponds to the candidate with name "$name_j$".

Using these values and public counter-values, voters can check on the Blockchain the count of each candidate and the accuracy of the final result. In fact, we have:

$$\prod_{i=1}^{l} C_{V_i} = \prod_{j=1}^{m}\prod_{i=1}^{l_j} C_{V_i}(name_j) = \prod_{k=1}^{m}\prod_{j=1}^{m}\prod_{i=1}^{l_j} e\left(Q_{name_j}, S_k Q_{B_{Ni}}(name_j)\right)$$
$$= \prod_{k=1}^{m}\prod_{j=1}^{m} e\left(Q_{name_j}, \sum_{i=1}^{l_j} S_k Q_{B_{Ni}}(name_j)\right) = \prod_{k=1}^{m}\prod_{j=1}^{m} e\left(Q_{name_j}, \sigma_{k,name_j}\right) \tag{1}$$

These equalities use the bilinear property of $e$:

$$\prod_{i=1}^{l_j} e\left(Q_{name_j}, S_k Q_{B_{Ni}}(name_j)\right) = e\left(Q_{name_j}, \sum_{i=1}^{l_j} S_k Q_{B_{Ni}}(name_j)\right)$$

# 5 Security of VYV

We first informally analyze the following security properties for our protocol.

- **Eligible voter:** VYV ensures that only eligible voters join the election Blockchain and participate to the voting process thanks to both registration and authentication phases. During the registration phase, we verify each voter identity via a face to face meeting and only eligible voters are provided with authentication parameters. At the end of this phase, the RS publishes the list of registered voters in the Blockchain. Hence everybody can check the validity of this list. The authentication phase ensures that only registered voters have access to our election Blockchain, create their externally owned account and publish their public keys and addresses. Another advantage of VYV is the linear complexity of the authentication phase. In most cases, online e-voting systems verify the eligibility of each voter by comparing his authentication parameters with a list of registered voters' authentication parameters. Thus, if an election include n voters we have $n^2$ operations of comparison. Whereas, in our case, we verify for each voter if $P_{PWi} = S_{RS\_A}.S_{PWi}$ so if we have an election with $n$ voters, we execute only $n$ verification operations.
- **Fairness:** Votes are encrypted before being casted so we can not get partial results.
- **Integrity:** The fact of casting and storing votes in the Blockchain safeguard them from being altered or deleted thanks to the immutability property of the Blockchain.
- **Individual verifiability:** This property is respected by our protocol thanks to our ballots structure that includes counter-values $C_{Vj}$. These values serve as receipts to voters and make it possible to verify that their votes have been cast an intended without disclosing who they voted for.
- **Universal verifiability:** Each tallying authority publishes on the bulletin board the count of each candidate and counter-values. From these parameters, everybody can verify the accuracy of the final result by checking the Eq. (1). This equation checks the equality between the product of $C_{Vj}$ and the sum of the counts displayed by tallying authorities. If every voter finds his receipt in the list of all counter-values and no claim has been detected and if the equality is verified, then we are sure that the election final result is correct. Thus tallying authorities can not modify, delete or add counter-values since voter's number is public. If one or more tallying authorities try to change the count of one or more candidates, the equation will not be checked and therefore any cheating attempt is detected.
- **Vote-Privacy:** This property is ensured thanks to the use of Blockchain which is characterized by the anonymity of its transactions. In fact every voter is identified in the election Blockchain by a public key and address that have no relationship with his real identity. Votes privacy is ensured even if all authorities present in our approach collaborate. In fact, they cannot establish the relationship between a voter and his vote: the registration server can make the correspondence between the voter's real identity and his authentication parameters, the tallying authorities can make the correspondence between a vote and the public address that sends this vote but no one, except the voter himself, can make the connection between a voter's public address and his authentication parameters since the creation of the Blockchain account is performed by the voter.

- **Receipt-freeness:** In our case, voter cannot find his vote from the counter-value $C_{Vj}$ and the other public parameters. He cannot therefore prove that he voted for a given candidate.
- **Coercion resistance:** Our protocol is not resistant to coercion. A coercer can force a voter to vote for a certain candidate and check his submission later using the counter-value.

Table 3 resumes the security properties of VYV.

**Table 3.** Security properties of Verify-Your-Vote.

| Verify-Your-Vote | |
| --- | --- |
| Eligibility | ✓ |
| Fairness | ✓ |
| Integrity | ✓ |
| Individual verifiability | ✓ |
| Universal verifiability | ✓ |
| Vote-Privacy | ✓ |
| Receipt-freeness | ✓ |
| Coercion resistance | ✗ |
| Voting policy | Multiple |

**Formal Verification:** We perform an automated security analysis using the verification tool ProVerif [26]. It analyzes secrecy, privacy and authentication properties of a given protocol described in Applied Pi Calculus. The Applied Pi calculus is a variant of the Pi Calculus extended with equational theory over terms and functions. It is a language for describing concurrent processes and their interactions on named channels. To describe processes with the Applied Pi calculus, one needs to define a set of names, a set of variables and a signature that consists of the function symbols which will be used in order to define terms. These function symbols have arities and types. In addition, the function symbols come with an equational theory.

To model our protocol in the Applied Pi Calculus, we define a set of types and functions. To represent the encryption, decryption, signature and hash operations, we use the following function symbols: `aenc(x,pkey)`, `adec(x,skey)`, `pk(skey)`, `sign(x,sskey)`, `checksign(x,spkey)`, `spk(sskey)`, `H1(x)`.

Intuitively, `aenc` and `adec` stand respectively for asymmetric encryption and asymmetric decryption, `aenc` and `adec` follow this equation: `adec(aenc(x,y), pk(y)) = x`. The `pk` function generates the corresponding public key of a given secret key. We also assume the hash operation which is denoted with the function `H1`.

The two functions `sign` and `checksign` provide, respectively, the signature of a given message and the verification of the signature. They respect the following equation: `checksign(sign(x,y),spk(y)) = x`.

We model our protocol as a single process. All our Proverif codes are available on the following website:

http://sancy.univ-bpclermont.fr/ ~ lafourcade/VYVCodeProVerif/

We also define the following queries to prove votes secrecy, voters' authentication and votes privacy.

- **Verification of votes secrecy:** To capture the value of a given vote, an attacker has to intercept the values of two parameters: the ballot number Bn and the pseudo ID of the chosen candidate Cj. Thus we use the following queries: query attacker (Bn) and query attacker(C1).

  When executing the code, ProVerif proves the votes secrecy in few seconds.
- **Verification of voters' authentication:** Authentication is captured using correspondence assertions. The protocol is intended to ensure that the administrator authenticates all voters. Therefore, we define the following events:
- **event acceptedAuthentication(bitstring, bitstring):** used by the voter to record the fact that it has been successfully authenticated,
- **event VerifiesParameters(bitstring, bitstring):** used by the administrator to record that he verified voter's authentication parameters.

  We also define the following query:

  query a: bitstring, b: bitstring;

  event acceptedAuth (a,b) == > event VerifyParameters (a,b).

  ProVerif proves authentication of voters immediately.
- **Verification of votes privacy:** To express votes privacy we prove the observational equivalence property between two instances of our process that differ only in the choice of votes. To do that, we use choice[V1,V2] to represent the terms that differ between the two instances. Likewise, we use the keyword sync to express synchronization which help proving equivalences with choice since they allow swapping data between processes at the synchronization points.

  We also succeed to prove votes privacy with Proverif.


# 6  Conclusion

We have proposed a new Blockchain-based e-voting system. Our propounded solution, VYV, refers to the ECC, IBE and pairings. Through our solution several security properties such as eligibility, fairness, verifiability and receipt-freeness are ensured. Like-wise, we modeled the protocol with ProVerif tool and proved that it guarantees votes privacy, secrecy and voters' authentication. Differently from some previous schemes, the recipient of the voter can be used to check his vote while still providing privacy. To provide a higher security level, other properties have to be adopted. Thus, future work will be devoted to guarantee coercion resistance. Finally, the implementation of this protocol constitutes interesting future areas of work.

# References

1. Aradhya, P.: Distributed ledger visible to all? Ready for blockchain? In: Huffington Post, April 2016
2. Garay, J.A., Kiayias, A., Panagiotakos, G.: Proofs of work for blockchain protocols. IACR Cryptology ePrint Archive 2017/775 (2017)
3. Nakamoto, S.: Bitcoin: a peer-to-peer electronic cash system, November 2008
4. Buterin, V.: A next generation smart contract and decentralized application platform (2014)
5. Dreier, J., Lafourcade, P., Lakhnech, Y.: A formal taxonomy of privacy in voting protocols. In: Proceedings of IEEE International Conference on Communications, ICC 2012, pp. 6710–6715. IEEE (2012)
6. Dreier, J., Lafourcade, P., Lakhnech, Y.: Vote-independence: a powerful privacy notion for voting protocols. In: Garcia-Alfaro, J., Lafourcade, P. (eds.) FPS 2011. LNCS, vol. 6888, pp. 164–180. Springer, Heidelberg (2012). https://doi.org/10.1007/978-3-642-27901-0_13
7. smartmatic: Tivi (2016). http://www.smartmatic.com/voting/online-voting-tivi/
8. Followmyvote: Follow my vote (2012). https://followmyvote.com/
9. McCorry, P., Shahandashti, Siamak F., Hao, F.: A smart contract for boardroom voting with maximum voter privacy. In: Kiayias, A. (ed.) FC 2017. LNCS, vol. 10322, pp. 357–375. Springer, Cham (2017). https://doi.org/10.1007/978-3-319-70972-7_20
10. Gailly, N., Jovanovic, P., Ford, B., Lukasiewicz, J., Gammar, L.: Agora: bringing our voting systems into the 21st century (2018)
11. Nikitin, K., et al.: CHAINIAC: proactive software-update transparency via collectively signed skipchains and verified builds. In: 26th USENIX Security Symposium, Vancouver, BC, Canada, 16–18 August 2017, pp. 1271–1287 (2017)
12. National Institute of Standards and Technology: FIPS PUB 186-2: Digital Signature Standard (DSS). National Institute for Standards and Technology, Gaithersburg, MD, USA, January 2000
13. ElGamal, T.: A public key cryptosystem and a signature scheme based on discrete logarithms. IEEE Trans. Inf. Theory 31(4), 469–472 (1985)
14. Rivest, R.L., Shamir, A., Adleman, L.: A method for obtaining digital signatures and public-key cryptosystems. Commun. ACM 21(2), 120–126 (1978)
15. Boneh, D.: Pairing-based cryptography: past, present, and future. In: Wang, X., Sako, K. (eds.) ASIACRYPT 2012. LNCS, vol. 7658, p. 1. Springer, Heidelberg (2012). https://doi.org/10.1007/978-3-642-34961-4_1
16. Rossi, F., Schmid, G.: Identity-based secure group communications using pairings. Comput. Netw. 89, 32–43 (2015)
17. Barreto, P.S.L.M., Kim, H.Y., Lynn, B., Scott, M.: Efficient algorithms for pairing-based cryptosystems. In: Yung, M. (ed.) CRYPTO 2002. LNCS, vol. 2442, pp. 354–369. Springer, Heidelberg (2002). https://doi.org/10.1007/3-540-45708-9_23
18. Aranha, D.F., Knapp, E., Menezes, A., Rodríguez-Henríquez, F.: Parallelizing the Weil and Tate pairings. In: Chen, L. (ed.) IMACC 2011. LNCS, vol. 7089, pp. 275–295. Springer, Heidelberg (2011). https://doi.org/10.1007/978-3-642-25516-8_17
19. Boneh, D., Franklin, M.: Identity-based encryption from the weil pairing. SIAM J. Comput. 32(3), 586–615 (2003)
20. Shamir, A.: Identity-based cryptosystems and signature schemes. In: Blakley, G.R., Chaum, D. (eds.) CRYPTO 1984. LNCS, vol. 196, pp. 47–53. Springer, Heidelberg (1985). https://doi.org/10.1007/3-540-39568-7_5

21. Boneh, D., Franklin, M.: Identity-based encryption from the Weil pairing. In: Kilian, J. (ed.) CRYPTO 2001. LNCS, vol. 2139, pp. 213–229. Springer, Heidelberg (2001). https://doi.org/10.1007/3-540-44647-8_13

22. Pedersen, T.P.: A threshold cryptosystem without a trusted party. In: Davies, D.W. (ed.) EUROCRYPT 1991. LNCS, vol. 547, pp. 522–526. Springer, Heidelberg (1991). https://doi.org/10.1007/3-540-46416-6_47

23. Gennaro, R., Jarecki, S., Krawczyk, H., Rabin, T.: Secure distributed key generation for discrete-log based cryptosystems. J. Cryptol. **20**(1), 51–83 (2007)

24. Chaum, D., Ryan, P.Y.A., Schneider, S.: A practical voter-verifiable election scheme. In: di Vimercati, S., Syverson, P., Gollmann, D. (eds.) ESORICS 2005. LNCS, vol. 3679, pp. 118–139. Springer, Heidelberg (2005). https://doi.org/10.1007/11555827_8

25. Paillier, P.: Public-key cryptosystems based on composite degree residuosity classes. In: Stern, J. (ed.) EUROCRYPT 1999. LNCS, vol. 1592, pp. 223–238. Springer, Heidelberg (1999). https://doi.org/10.1007/3-540-48910-X_16

26. Blanchet, B., Smyth, B., Cheval, V., Sylvestre, M.: Proverif 1.98pl1: Automatic cryptographic protocol verifier, user manual and tutorial (2017)

# To Chain or Not to Chain? A Case from Energy Sector

Marinos Themistocleous[1,2(✉)] ⓘ, Kypros Stefanou[1,2],
Christos Megapanos[2], and Elias Iosif[1]

[1] University of Nicosia, Nicosia, Cyprus
{Themistocleous.m, Stefanou.k, Iosif.E}@unic.ac.cy
[2] University of Piraeus, Piraeus, Greece

**Abstract.** During the last decade, Blockchain technology has attracted a lot of attention as it has the potential to disrupt the existing ecosystem and transform the way we do business. In this paper we investigate the energy supply chain and we examine the impact of the development of a blockchain solution in the area of solar energy. Our findings illustrate that blockchain technology can disrupt many areas of this sector including disruptions in the product, process, position and paradigm.

**Keywords:** Blockchain technology · Smart contracts · Solar energy
Action research · Disruptive innovation

## 1 Introduction

The blockchain disruptive innovation effect, was probably not clearly realized and understood by Nakamoto when he published his famous Bitcoin paper back in 2008 (Nakamoto 2008). During the last decade we have seen so many applications of blockchain and cryptocurrencies, that have revolutionized existing practices and introduced new disruptive ways of doing business (Delgado et al. 2017; O'Dair and Beaven 2017). The examples are endless ranging from academic certificates published on a blockchain to land registry solutions, healthcare applications, fintech and supply chain management implementations to name a few (Cocco et al. 2017; Cuccuru 2017; Dai and Vasarhelyi 2017; Gomber et al. 2018; Lei et al. 2017; Lemiex 2016).

In this paper we concentrate on the energy sector to describe the current way of doing business as well as its limitations. Then we propose a disruptive way of selling and buying energy through a solution that combines blockchain technology, Internet of Things (IoT) and smart energy grids (Christidis and Devetsikiotis, 2016, Kshetri 2017; Li et al. 2018; Novo 2018). Such an application leads to radical changes to the existing business models and ecosystem and brings new challenges for the existing energy players and the new entrants.

The remaining of this paper is organized as follows: In Sect. 2 a review of the blockchain technology is presented, followed by the conceptualization and the research question of this paper. Section 4 describes the research methodology adopted in this article where Sect. 5 reports the empirical data and it is followed by the Analysis and Discussion section. Conclusions are drawn in the last section of this paper.

© Springer Nature Switzerland AG 2019
M. Themistocleous and P. Rupino da Cunha (Eds.): EMCIS 2018, LNBIP 341, pp. 31–37, 2019.
https://doi.org/10.1007/978-3-030-11395-7_3

## 2  Background Review

Blockchain technology is like Internet in a sense that it cannot be manipulated or switched off by anybody. It was initially introduced in late 2008 and its first application was the well-known Bitcoin crypto-data. A Blockchain is a list of blocks with each block containing a number of transactions. Each block consists off (a) a pointer to the previous block using a cryptographic hash, (b) a timestamp and (c) transactions data. Blockchain technology decentralizes trust and enables value flow without intermediaries. As a result, it reduces cost and complexity and increases trust. It is based on distributed ledger which means that all members of the blockchain share an identical ledger (system of records) instead of maintaining their own proprietary view of it (Dorri et al. 2017; Shermin 2017).

   The main characteristics of the Blockchain technology are consensus, provenance, immutability and finality:

- **Consensus:** the blockchain uses consensus mechanisms to verify that each new block that is appended to the chain is a valid one. Even though consensus mechanisms have a critical role in the functionality of the blockchain they have some limitations too. For instance, consensus mechanisms like Proof Of Work (PoW) are expensive in terms of the energy they consume or the computational workload.
- **Provenance:** All participants of a Blockchain, know the history of changes of an asset (e.g. they know where the asset came from as well as all the details about the changes in the ownership of this asset over time). This means that information and cryptocurrencies are traceable. For instance, with blockchain technology we know where a bitcoin was mined and its whole journey from the miner's wallet to our wallet. In other words, we can know whether or not a specific bitcoin was used for illegal purposes.
- **Immutability:** A blockchain (or distributed) ledger is an append only ledger which means that transactions cannot be amended once they are recorded on a ledger. In case of an error, a new transaction can be used to reverse the error Bloomberg (2018).
- **Finality:** In blockchain there is only one way to study a specific transaction or to find out who owns what, as we only need to visit the ledger. The blockchain ledger is the only source of truth and it is trusted by all participants.

## 3  Conceptualization

The current landscape of the energy supply chain, involves multiple stages and participants. As it is illustrated in the Fig. 1, the supply chain begins with the production of energy in the power stations and it is followed by the transmission and the distribution of the power for consumption by the commercial and industrial business consumers and residential clients.

   In such a supply chain, various actors do participate like the energy producers, intermediaries (e.g. energy grid owners), business and residential consumers. The underlying business model used in most of the cases is that of producer-consumer. The current landscape and business model are associated with numerous limitations that have an impact on the participants. In this paper, we focus more on the limitations of the existing landscape in solar energy sharing as our empirical data come from that area (Pop et al. 2018).

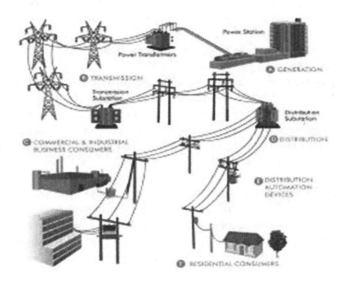

**Fig. 1.** Current landscape of energy supply chain

Solar energy companies tend to install and manufacture thousands of solar units for the residential market, while some of them are also providing leasing services. A basic limitation is related to the fact that energy derived from the company's farm is sold at a specific price to consumers. The price is predefined, and it is fixed which is not "fair" for the participants. There are periods that solar energy production costs less compared to other times and this is not reflected in the bills.

In addition to this, solar energy production may look better and more efficient than fossil fuels, but such a process is generally not transparent and trustworthy, as it is centralized. Consumers should trust these companies that they actually produce the volume of renewable energy they claim. Another limitation of the current landscape is the absence of a peer-to-peer local marketplace. The last but not least limitation is that electricity producers do not get paid immediately but usually after 2 months.

Based on the abovementioned limitations and the existing landscape we formulate the following research question which we are investigating in the next sections:

*RQ1: How does the implementation of blockchain applications in energy sector disrupt the current ecosystem and models?*

# 4   Research Methodology

To test the abovementioned research question, we adopted a qualitative methodology and employed action research approach. We chose action research as we participated in an applied research project that focused on the development of a blockchain solution in solar energy. According to Rapoport (1970), *"action research aims to contribute both to the practical concerns of people in an immediate problematic situation and to the goals of social science by joint collaboration within a mutually acceptable ethical framework"* (Rapoport 1970, p. 499). Action research focuses on the collaboration of practitioners and researchers (Avison et al. 2007) and it is an appropriate methodology for our case as we had an active role in the whole project and we took decisions related to the analysis, architectural design, implementation and testing of the blockchain solution.

For the purpose of this research we collaborated with a solar energy firm with presence in European Union (EU) and the United States of America (USA). Due to confidentiality reasons we will refer to this organization using the coded name Solar ENergy CORPoration (SenCorp). The project started in June 2017 and ended a year later on and the main participants where SenCorp and the authors. During the whole duration of the project we spent 2 days a week working with the company in its premises and the remaining time we worked from our laboratory at the University. Data was collected thru observation, artifacts (e.g. memos, white papers, internal documents), semi-structured and unstructured interviews that took place during coffee and lunch breaks or face-to-face meetings with key employees. Overall, we had interviews with 14 key players from SenCorp. Data were triangulated using various triangulation methods such as data, investigator and theory triangulation.

## 5  Empirical Data

For the purpose of this project we employed Ethereum as a blockchain platform to exchange data and cryptos. We also used Hierarchical Deterministic (HD) wallet as this is an advanced and secure type of wallet that works better with Ethereum. Since Ethereum is based on the use of tokens that can be sold, bought, or traded we employed Ethereum Request for Comment 20 (ERC20). ERC20 defines a common list of rules that Ethereum based tokens should follow. ERC20 specifies six functions (total supply, balanced of, allowance, transfer, approve, transfer from) and two events (transfer, approval) that an Ethereum token contract should implement. We also implemented smart contracts to automate and speed up transactions. Smart contracts are programmable contracts stored in a blockchain and executed by computers that eliminate the middlemen. In doing so, smart contracts can manage agreements between different parties-users, save data about an application, provide utility to other contracts and automate the transfer of tokens between users, based on an agreement. To implement our solution, we used Remix-IDE, solidity and testRPC as well as proof of work as consensus algorithm. The outcome of this implementation is a blockchain application that exchanges information between Ethereum and our smart contracts. The application facilitates the communication and support the transactions among users and smart energy batteries installed at home level.

The solution automates the following basic scenario:

- Solar panels are installed on the roof of home users to produce energy.
- The amount of the solar energy produced is stored locally using smart batteries.

- The owner of the battery, sets the price and the quantity of the energy (s/)he wants to sell, based on the competition and the weather conditions.
- In case (s/)he reaches an agreement with a potential buyer, (s/)he discharge the electricity from the battery to the energy grid.
- Smart meters are used to calculate the quantity of the electricity sold and the transaction is completed through the use of smart contracts and the financial compensation through the use of cryptocurrencies. All relevant transactions are put in a block that is sent for validation.
- Proof of work is used as a consensus mechanism to validate the block, and the block is finally attached to the blockchain.
- Using the smart grid the buyer receives the energy he bought and consumes it at home or to charge his/her electric car.

Currently the following improvements are in progress:

- A specialized team of experts is enhancing the features and functionality of the smart batteries by incorporating sensors-Internet of Things (IoT).
- In collaboration with SenCorp we design Artificial Intelligence (AI) algorithms to improve the performance and enhance decision making.

Upon completion of the above improvements the smart battery will automatically be able to:

- decide whether to sell or buy energy
- analyze existing and historical data to define the selling price
- operate on a machine to machine (M2M) mode with no or limited human intervention.

# 6 Analysis and Discussion

In order to test our research question, we use the 4Ps framework proposed by Tidd and Bessant (2013) that investigates innovation at Product, Process, Position and Paradigm levels.

**Product Innovation** refers to the changes in the things (products/services) which an organization offers; (e.g. a new car design, a new insurance package). In our case, the proposed solution supports the creation of new applications, such as smart contracts, decentralized trust services, etc. In addition to this, private keys that store transferable ownership rights can be used to control physical objects (keys, operation control, etc.), thereby connecting blockchains to IoT and the physical world. Another type of product innovation we have in our case is thru the application tokens which are the fuel of decentralized value networks and crowd-sourced distributed ventures.

**Process Innovation** denotes changes in the ways in which they are created and delivered; (e.g. Amazon's logistics and vertical/horizontal integration). From the empirical data it appears that we observe changes in the process due to the use of cryptocurrency which relies on novel forms of labor and consensus (computational power, proof-of-stake or other issuance/verification mechanism). Moreover, we notice changes as now governance is based on consensus, instead of a single point of control (both at the network level (majority consensus) and at the transaction level (e.g. multi-sig)). A third process innovation comes from blockchain application; while elements of the transaction verification and currency issuance mechanism are innovative in themselves (such as PoW/PoS/etc.), when used in the context of the blockchain, they implement a novel process of establishing the veracity of any transaction/record in a shared ledger.

**Position Innovation** states changes in the context in which the products/services are introduced like for example the Coca Cola's journey from a patent medicine to a world-leader in soft drinks. Through our use case we can see changes in position innovation in terms of decentralized governance, Initial Coin Offerings (ICOs) and autonomous economic agents.

**Paradigm Innovation** refers to the changes in the underlying mental and business models (e.g. digital currencies, blockchain, ICOs, DAOs.). In our case we notice a real business model transformation as through the proposed application we can alter the business model from producer-consumer to prosumer. It is clear that with such an application transforms the commercial, industrial business and residential clients to entities that are able to produce, sell, buy and consume energy.

## 7  Conclusion

The introduction of blockchain technology brings tremendous changes and challenges to our business environment. Through this work we study the potential impact of the implementation of blockchain applications in the energy sector. In doing so, we developed a blockchain solution for an industrial partner from a solar energy sector and we investigate its impact on the disruption of the current ecosystem and models. We used an action research approach to test our research question and we worked with our industrial collaborator for about one year. The empirical data reveal that the application of blockchain in energy may cause significant disruption at different innovation levels such as product, process, position and paradigm. One of our main findings is the transformation of the underlying business model from producer-consumer to prosumer or to peer to peer. Clearly there is ground for further research as there are many issues and challenges in this area. For example, the implementation of peer to peer energy applications requires legal and regulatory changes in many countries. Since we are still in the early stages of blockchain adoption there are many open issues that need to be examined and addressed with regulatory issues being among the most important.

## References

Avison, D., Baskerville, R., Myers, M.D.: The structure of power in action research projects. In: Kock, N. (ed.) Information Systems Action Research. ISIS, vol. 13, pp. 19–41. Springer, Boston (2007). https://doi.org/10.1007/978-0-387-36060-7_2

Bloomberg, J.: Eight reasons to be skeptical about blockchain (2018). https://www.forbes.com/sites/jasonbloomberg/2017/05/31/eight-reasons-to-be-skeptical-about-blockchain/#7ef65f125eb1. Accessed 21 Jan 2018

Christidis, K., Devetsikiotis, M.: Blockchains and smart contracts for the internet of things. IEEE Access **4**, 2292–2303 (2016). https://doi.org/10.1109/ACCESS.2016.2566339

Cocco, L., Pinna, A., Marchesi, M.: Banking on blockchain: costs savings thanks to the blockchain technology. Futur. Internet **9**(3), 1–20 (2017). https://doi.org/10.3390/fi9030025

Cuccuru, P.: Beyond Bitcoin: an early overview on smart contracts. Int. J. Law Inf. Technol. **25**(3), 179–195 (2017). https://doi.org/10.1093/ijlit/eax003

Dai, J., Vasarhelyi, M.A.: Toward blockchain-based accounting and assurance. J. Inf. Syst. **31**(3), 5–21 (2017)

Delgado-Segura, S., Pιrez-Solδ, C., Navarro-Arribas, G., Herrera-Joancomartv, J.: A fair protocol for data trading based on Bitcoin transactions. Futur. Gener. Comput. Syst. (2017). https://doi.org/10.1016/j.future.2017.08.021

Dorri, A., Steger, M., Kanhere, S.S., Jurdak, R.: BlockChain: a distributed solution to automotive security and privacy. IEEE Commun. Mag. **55**(12), 119–125 (2017). https://doi.org/10.1109/MCOM.2017.1700879

Gomber, P., Kauffman, R.J., Parker, C., Weber, B.W.: On the Fintech revolution: interpreting the forces of innovation, disruption, and transformation in financial services. J. Manag. Inf. Syst. **35**(1), 220–265 (2018)

Kshetri, N.: Can blockchain strengthen the internet of things? IT Prof. **19**(4), 68–72 (2017)

Lei, A., Cruickshank, H., Cao, Y., Asuquo, P., Ogah, C.P.A., Sun, Z.: Blockchain-based dynamic key management for heterogeneous intelligent transportation systems. IEEE IoT J. **4662**, 1–12 (2017)

Lemieux, V.L.: Trusting records: is blockchain technology the answer? Rec. Manag. J. **26**(2), 110–139 (2016)

Li, G., Meng, H., Zhou, G., Gao, Y.: Energy management analysis and scheme design of microgrid based on blockchain. Dianli Jianshe/Electr. Power Constr. **39**(2), 43–49 (2018)

Nakamoto, S.: Bitcoin: a peer-to-peer electronic cash system (2008). http://www.bitcoin.org

Novo, O.: Blockchain meets IoT: an architecture for scalable access management in IoT. IEEE IoT J. **5**(2), 1184–1195 (2018)

Tidd, J., Bessant, J.: Managing Innovation: Integrating Technological, Market and Organizational Change, 5th edn. Wiley, Chichester (2013). ISBN: 978-1-118-36063-7

O'Dair, M., Beaven, Z.: The networked record industry: how blockchain technology could transform the record industry. Strat. Chang. **26**(5), 471–480 (2017)

Pop, C., Cioara, T., Antal, M., Anghel, I., Salomie, I., Bertoncini, M.: Blockchain based decentralized management of demand response programs in smart energy grids. Sensors (Switzerland) **18**(1), 162 (2018)

Shermin, V.: Disrupting governance with blockchains and smart contracts. Strat. Chang. **26**(5), 499–509 (2017)

Rapoport, R.: Three dilemmas of action research. Hum. Relat. **23**(6), 499–513 (1970)

# Continuance Intention in Blockchain-Enabled Supply Chain Applications: Modelling the Moderating Effect of Supply Chain Stakeholders Trust

Samuel Fosso Wamba[(✉)]

Toulouse Business School, Toulouse, France
s.fosso-wamba@tbs-education.fr

**Abstract.** If blockchain technologies are emerging as important game changers in the supply chain, this is largely attributed to their high operational and strategic business value. While this high potential is acknowledged by the practitioner's literature, very few empirical studies have been conducted on the factors explaining the adoption, use and continuance of blockchain-enabled supply chain applications. To fill this knowledge gap, this study extended the expectation-confirmation model (ECM) by integrating the supply chain stakeholders trust to analyze to the continuance intention in blockchain-enabled supply chain applications. The proposed model was tested and supported by the data collected among 344 supply chain professionals in India. The paper ends up with the formulation of important implications for practice and research.

**Keywords:** Blockchain · Continuance intention · Supply chain
India · Supply chain trust

## 1 Introduction

Blockchain technologies are emerging as important game changer in the supply chain, especially because of their high potential benefits and capabilities. These technologies could transform almost all supply chain-related processes, including by reducing supply chain errors and by enabling supply chain automation [1] and end-to-end supply chain security.

While the benefits related to blockchain technologies-enabled supply chain applications have been discussed by media, very few empirical studies have conducted to assess their real business value. For example, a systematic review conducted by [2] on bitcoin, blockchain and FinTech in the supply chain found that the survey method approach was used for only 8% of the recorded cases. Consequently, this study aims to bridge the knowledge gap identified in the literature by developing an extended version of the ECM that integrates the supply chain stakeholders trust to analyze the continuance intention in blockchain-enabled supply chain applications.

We draw on the literature on blockchain, studies using the ECM as well as studies on supply chain stakeholders risk to address our research objective. After the

© Springer Nature Switzerland AG 2019
M. Themistocleous and P. Rupino da Cunha (Eds.): EMCIS 2018, LNBIP 341, pp. 38–43, 2019.
https://doi.org/10.1007/978-3-030-11395-7_4

introduction, the firsts section of this study describes the theoretical development. The next sections deal with our research methodology and the discussion of the results.

The paper ends with a conclusion, research implications, and the limitations and future research perspectives of the study.

## 2 Theoretical Development

The model developed in this study (Fig. 1) is an extension of the expectation-confirmation model [3, 4] with supply chain stakeholders trust. The expectation-confirmation model (ECM) was proposed by [3] to assess cognitive beliefs that influence the user's intention to continue using information systems (p. 351). The author argued that "users' continuance intention is determined by their satisfaction with IS use and perceived usefulness of continued IS use. User satisfaction, in turn, is influenced by their confirmation of expectation from prior IS use and perceived usefulness" (p. 351).

The ECM has been used by various scholars in different settings. For example, [5] extended the ECM by incorporating the theory of planned behavior to examine the mobile data service continuance. [6] used an extended version of the ECM to investigate the continuance use of mobile instant messaging in South Korea. [7] developed and tested several adoption and continuance models. [8] incorporated the perceived risk into the ECM to assess the continuance intentions of physicians using electronic medical records.

Drawing on this stream of research, we propose the subsequent hypotheses in the context of blockchain-enabled supply chain applications:

**H1**: Perceived usefulness has a significant positive effect on satisfaction.
**H2**: Confirmation has a significant positive effect on satisfaction.
**H3**: Confirmation has a significant positive effect on perceived usefulness.
**H4**: Satisfaction has a significant positive effect on the user's intention to keep using blockchain technologies-enabled supply chain applications.

Moreover, we argued that in the context of supply chain, trust among supply chain stakeholders will play an important role in the adoption, use and continued use of blockchain technologies-enabled supply chain applications. Indeed, prior studies found that trust plays an important role during the IS adoption and use process [9, 10].

[11] argued that inter-organization trust is an important decision factor during the adoption process of electronic procurement. We draw on these prior studies and propose that in the context of blockchain technologies-enabled supply chain applications, trust among all supply chain stakeholders will play a critical role not only during the adoption, use and continuance process, but also for satisfaction. Therefore, we propose the following hypotheses:

**H5**: Supply chain stakeholders trust has a significant positive effect on the user's intention to continue to use blockchain technologies-enabled supply chain applications.
**H6**: Supply chain stakeholders trust will moderate the relationship between satisfaction and the user's intention to continue to use blockchain technologies-enabled supply chain applications.

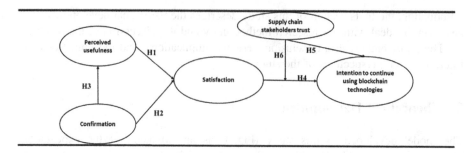

**Fig. 1.** Proposed research model

**Table 1.** Loadings, composite reliability (CR) and average variance extracted (AVE) values of our constructs

| Constructs | Item | Loadings | CR | AVE |
|---|---|---|---|---|
| Confirmation (CONF) | CONFI1 | 0.866 | 0.906 | 0.763 |
| | CONFI2 | 0.893 | | |
| | CONFI3 | 0.861 | | |
| Intention to continue to use blockchain technologies (CONT) | CONT1 | 0.871 | 0.881 | 0.711 |
| | CONT2 | 0.872 | | |
| | CONT3 | 0.783 | | |
| Perceived usefulness (PU) | PU1 | 0.821 | 0.897 | 0.686 |
| | PU2 | 0.820 | | |
| | PU3 | 0.851 | | |
| | PU4 | 0.819 | | |
| Satisfaction (SAT) | SAT1 | 0.833 | 0.916 | 0.731 |
| | SAT2 | 0.869 | | |
| | SAT3 | 0.865 | | |
| | SAT4 | 0.852 | | |
| Supply chain stakeholders trust (SCTRU) | SCTRU1 | 0.864 | 0.903 | 0.700 |
| | SCTRU2 | 0.807 | | |
| | SCTRU3 | 0.854 | | |
| | SCTRU4 | 0.821 | | |

## 3  Methodology

The study uses a web-based survey to collect data from 344 (70.1% males and 29.9% females) supply chain professionals who have at least three years of experience with blockchain in India. The data collection process was handled by a market research firm called ResearchNow (https://www.researchnow.com/?lang=gb). Our items were adapted from prior studies [3, 12]. They were all measured using a seven (7)-point Likert scale. The data analysis was realized using **SmartPLS**, version 3.0 [13], which is a partial least squares (PLS) structural equation modeling (SEM) tool. It is a relevant tool to evaluate the SEM measurement and structural model. In addition, it has various useful data analysis approaches embedded into the tool, including the two-stage approach proposed by [14] to assess the moderating effect.

## 4 Results and Discussion

Table 1 displays all information related to the reliability and validity of our constructs. We can see that all the values of the loadings, CR and AVE are respectively higher than 0.7, 0.7 and 0.5, all of which are the acceptable threshold values suggested in the literature [15, 16]. Therefore, we can include all constructs in the proposed research model.

The discriminant validity was tested by comparing the correlation matrix values with the square root of the AVEs in the diagonals. As we can see in Table 2, all the values of the square root of the AVEs in the diagonals are higher than the inter-correlation with other constructs, thus confirming the discriminant validity [17–19].

Table 3 describes the results of the structural model, including the moderation effect analysis. It clearly indicates that all the standardized path coefficients of all our proposed hypotheses are significant at the levels of 0.001 (for CONF → PU, CONF → SAT, SAT → CONT and SCTRU → CONT) and 0.05 (for PU → SAT and the moderating relationship). Consequently, all our proposed hypotheses (H1–H6) are supported (Table 4).

**Table 2.** Correlation and AVEs

|        | 1      | 2      | 3      | 4      | 5      |
|--------|--------|--------|--------|--------|--------|
| CONF   | 0.874* |        |        |        |        |
| CONT   | 0.795  | 0.843* |        |        |        |
| PU     | 0.605  | 0.591  | 0.828* |        |        |
| SAT    | 0.746  | 0.734  | 0.551  | 0.855* |        |
| SCTRU  | 0.609  | 0.574  | 0.717  | 0.625  | 0.837* |

*Square root of AVEs on the diagonal

**Table 3.** Results of the structural model, including the moderation effect analysis.

|               | Beta(sig.) | T Statistics (|O/STDEV|) |
|---------------|------------|--------------------------|
| CONF → PU     | 0.605****  | 11.249                   |
| CONF → SAT    | 0.651****  | 8.957                    |
| PU → SAT      | 0.158**    | 2.131                    |
| SAT → CONT    | 0.646****  | 9.599                    |
| Moderator     | 0.081**    | 2.382                    |
| SCTRU → CONT  | 0.236****  | 3.862                    |

****P < 0.001; ***P < 0.01; **P < 0.05; *P < 0.1

**Table 4.** Results of hypothesis tests.

| Hypothesis | Results |
|---|---|
| H1: Perceived usefulness has a significant positive effect on satisfaction | Supported |
| H2: Confirmation has a significant positive effect on satisfaction | Supported |
| H3: Confirmation has a significant positive effect on perceived usefulness | Supported |
| H4: Satisfaction has a significant positive effect on the intention to keep using blockchain technologies-enabled supply chain applications | Supported |
| H5: Supply chain stakeholders trust has a significant positive effect on the intention to continue to use blockchain technologies-enabled supply chain applications | Supported |
| H6: Supply chain stakeholders trust will moderate the relationship between satisfaction and the intention to continue to use blockchain technologies-enabled supply chain applications | Supported |

## 5 Conclusion and Future Research Directions

The main objective of this work was to apply an extended version of the ECM [3] that integrates the supply chain stakeholders trust to assess the continuance intention to use blockchain technologies-enabled supply chain applications. Data were collected from supply chain professionals in India and were analyzed using version 3.0 of SmartPLS in order to test the proposed research model. The study's results provided a strong empirical validation of all our proposed hypotheses when using the ECM in the context of blockchain technologies-enabled supply chain applications.

The study also highlighted the importance of trust among supply chain stakeholders in supporting a continued use of blockchain technologies-enabled supply chain applications. However, further research may be needed to solve further issues related to the use of survey; longitudinal case studies could well be used in this regard. In addition, it would be interesting to study unobserved heterogeneity in the use of SEM to study blockchain-enabled applications [20].

## References

1. PWC: Shifting patterns: the future of the logistics industry, p. 20. PWC (2016)
2. Wamba, S.F., et al.: Bitcoin, Blockchain, and FinTech: a systematic review and case studies in the supply chain. Working Paper, Toulouse Business School (2018)
3. Bhattacherjee, A.: Understanding information systems continuance: an expectation-confirmation model. MIS Q. **25**(3), 351–370 (2001)
4. Oliver, R.L.: A cognitive model of the antecedents and consequences of satisfaction decisions. J. Mark. Res. **17**(4), 460–469 (1980)
5. Kim, B.: An empirical investigation of mobile data service continuance incorporating the theory of planned behavior into the expectation – confirmation model. Expert Syst. Appl. **37**(10), 7033–7039 (2010)
6. Oghuma, A.P., et al.: An expectation-confirmation model of continuance intention to use mobile instant messaging. Telematics Inform. **33**(1), 34–47 (2016)

7. Sun, Y., Jeyaraj, A.: Information technology adoption and continuance: a longitudinal study of individuals' behavioral intentions. Inf. Manag. **50**(7), 457–465 (2013)
8. Ayanso, A., Herath, T.C., O'Brien, N.: Understanding continuance intentions of physicians with electronic medical records (EMR): an expectancy-confirmation perspective. Decis. Support Syst. **77**, 112–122 (2015)
9. Gong, X., et al.: Examining the role of tie strength in users' continuance intention of second-generation mobile instant messaging services. Information Systems Frontiers (2018)
10. Sharma, S.K.: Integrating cognitive antecedents into TAM to explain mobile banking behavioral intention: a SEM-neural network modeling. Information Systems Frontiers (2017)
11. Al-Hakim, L., Abdullah, N.A.H.N., Ng, E.: The effect of inter-organization trust and dependency on e-procurement adoption: a case of Malaysian manufacturers. J. Electron. Commer. Organ. **10**(2), 40–60 (2012)
12. Carter, L., Bélanger, F.: The utilization of e-government services: citizen trust, innovation and acceptance factors. Inf. Syst. J. **15**(1), 5–25 (2005)
13. Ringle, C.M., Wende, S., Becker J.-M.: SmartPLS 3 (2014). www.smartpls.com
14. Chin, W.W., Marcolin, B.L., Newsted, P.N.: A partial least squares latent variable modeling approach for measuring interaction effects: results from a monte carlo simulation study and an electronic-mail emotion/adoption study. Inf. Syst. Res. **14**(2), 189–217 (2003)
15. Hair, J.F., Sarstedt, M., Ringle, C.M., Mena, J.A.: An assessment of the use of partial least squares structural equation modeling in marketing research. J. Acad. Mark. Sci. **40**, 414–433 (2012)
16. Sun, H., Zhang, P.: An exploration of affective factors and their roles in user technology acceptance: mediation and causality. J. Am. Soc. Inform. Sci. Technol. (JASIST) **59**, 1252–1263 (2008)
17. Chin, W.W.: The partial least squares approach for structural equation modeling (1998)
18. Chin, W.W.: How to write up and report PLS analyses. In: Handbook of Partial Least Squares, pp. 655–690 (2010)
19. Fornell, C., Larcker, D.F.: Evaluating structural equation models with unobservable variables and measurement error. J. Mark. Res. **18**, 39–50 (1981)
20. Becker, J.-M., et al.: Discovering unobserved heterogeneity in structural equation models to avert validity threats. MIS Q. **37**(3), 665–694 (2013)

# Big Data and Analytics

# Big Data Analysis in UAV Surveillance for Wildfire Prevention and Management

Nikos Athanasis[1,3], Marinos Themistocleous[1,2(✉)] (iD),
Kostas Kalabokidis[3], and Christos Chatzitheodorou[3]

[1] University of Piraeus, Piraeus, Greece
mthemist@unipi.gr
[2] University of Nicosia, Nicosia, Cyprus
Themistocleous.m@unic.ac.cy
[3] University of Aegean, Mytilene, Greece
{athanasis,kalabokidis,geoml7029}@geo.aegean.gr

**Abstract.** While wildfires continue to ravage our world, big data analysis aspires to provide solutions to complex problems such as the prevention and management of natural disasters. In this study, we illustrate a state-of-the-art approach towards an enhancement of UAV (Unmanned Aerial Vehicle) surveillance for wildfire prevention and management through big data analysis. Its novelty lies in the instant delivery of images taken from UAVs and the (near) real-time big-data oriented image analysis. Instead of relying on stand-alone computers and time-consuming post-processing of the images, a big data cluster is used and a MapReduce algorithm is applied to identify images from wildfire burning areas. Experiments identified a significant gain regarding the time needed to analyze the data, while the execution time of the image analysis is not affected by the size of the pictures gathered by the UAVs. The integration of UAVs, Big Data components and image analysis provides the means for wildfire prevention and management authorities to follow the proposed methodology to organize their wildfire management plan in a reliable and timely manner. The proposed methodology highlights the role of Geospatial Big Data and is expected to contribute towards a more state-of-the-art knowledge transfer between wildfire confrontation operation centers and firefighting units in the field.

**Keywords:** Geospatial Big Data · Wildfire prevention · UAV surveillance

## 1 Introduction

Climate change trends and anthropogenic reasons have severely increased the number of wildfires worldwide over the last years. Approximately 50,000 fires per year have occurred during the past three decades in the Euro-Mediterranean region (Portugal, Spain, France, Italy and Greece) that resulted in about half a million hectares of burnt area each year [1].

Advances in control engineering and IT science made possible to develop Unmanned Aerial Vehicles (UAVs) that enable to obtain a "bird's-eye-view" of the environment. UAVs provide an easy and cost-efficient way for collecting a large

© Springer Nature Switzerland AG 2019
M. Themistocleous and P. Rupino da Cunha (Eds.): EMCIS 2018, LNBIP 341, pp. 47–58, 2019.
https://doi.org/10.1007/978-3-030-11395-7_5

amount of high-resolution spatial data. Unlike satellite imagery, aerial imagery with UAVs can be captured and processed within hours rather than days.

Despite the intensive research activities regarding the contribution of UAVs in wildfire management [2–5], many challenges are still open. Images and sensor data gathered from UAVs require heavy analysis before to be delivered to the end users. However, in emergency situations of a fire ignition, the gathered data should be processed and presented instantaneously. Image processing is too time-consuming and costly for heavy computation tasks such as to rectify and mosaic the UAV photography for large areas. The volume of the aerial imagery digital data is so large and is growing at such a pace that its management with conventional storage and analysis methods is becoming increasingly difficult [6]. Not only an enormous volume of geographic data is required and produced, but also such data change with high frequency. In many cases, the data processing and spatial analysis over the acquired data set require expensive investments in terms of hardware, software and personnel training among other overhead costs. Extracting the valuable information from the huge amount of image data by detecting and analyzing the various entities in these images is challenging.

This article presents a state-of-the-art approach towards an enhancement of UAV surveillance for wildfire prevention and management. Its novelty lies in the instant delivery of images captured by the UAVs and a big-data oriented image analysis. Instead of relying on stand-alone computers and time-consuming post-processing of the images, a computer cluster is used that exploits the principles of parallel programming. As a result, the amount of processing time is radically reduced and the wildfire prevention and management authorities can be immediately alerted in a reliable and timely manner in case of a wildfire occurrence. Furthermore, the proposed scalable approach can be used independently of the number of the available UAVs and the area that has to be covered. This is due to the big data cluster that provides the means for scalable calculations and (near) real-time response.

The rest of this paper is structured as follows. In the next Section, we review several approaches for UAV surveillance for wildfire prevention and management and we highlight the necessity to develop a big data-oriented approach. In Sect. 3 we analyze the methodology followed and we explain how the images captured from the UAVs are transferred in (near) real-time to a big data cluster where an image analysis algorithm is executed to extract the pictures showing flames of fires. Experiments and results are presented in Sect. 4, while concluding remarks are discussed in Sect. 5.

## 2 UAVs in Wildfire Prevention and Management

A survey on technologies for automatic forest fire monitoring, detection and suppression using unmanned aerial vehicles and remote sensing techniques can be found in [7]. UAVs have already been deployed after several disasters in the recent past such as Hurricane Katrina [8] and Hurricane Wilma [9]. Nardi (2009) concluded that UAVs were potentially useful and could provide a new source of information to initial attack/response.

Quaritsch [11] described how microdrones (called *cDrones*) were used to provide to the first responders a quick and accurate overview of the affected area and augment the overview image with additional information, such as detected objects or the trajectory of moving objects. More specifically for wildfire management, [12] exploited UAV technology for the characterization of Mediterranean riparian forests. An unmanned aircraft system for automatic forest fire monitoring and measurement had also been introduced in [13].

Both the United States Federal Emergency Management Agency (FEMA)[1] and the European Commission's Joint Research Center (JRC)[2] have noted that aerial imagery inevitably presents a big data challenge [14]. In [15], a theoretical approach for exploring the connection between surveillance and big data was described, while [16] showcased the EarthServer Big Earth Data Analytics engine as an integrated solution for big data challenges in Earth Sciences. Nguyen [17] used machine learning techniques to perform extensive experiments of damage assessment using images from major natural disasters. Athanasis [18, 19] described the integration of Geographic Information Systems (GIS) modeling outputs with real-time information from Twitter for wildfire risk management and real-time earthquake monitoring.

Image analysis for large-scale land-cover recognition had been explored among others by [20] and [21]. Image analysis for object detection and pixel classification in fire detection systems had also been analyzed in [22], while [23] used fuzzy logic to separate fire and non-fire pixels. UAV-based forest fire detection using image analysis had been analyzed in [24] and [25].

Despite the aforementioned research activities, there is a significant research gap of the contribution of big data analysis in UAV surveillance for wildfire prevention and management since it is a relatively new area of investigation. This article tries to fill in this research gap by describing a methodology for analyzing images from UAVs in a big data cluster. The goal is the immediate alert of the firefighting agencies in case of a fire emergency. The integration of UAVs, Big Data components and image analysis provides the means to create state-of-the-art fire management services.

## 3  Methodology

Our approach relies on instant copying of the images captured by the UAVs into a Hadoop big data cluster, where the Hadoop image processing library HIPI [26] is utilized. The HIPI image processing library is utilized to take advantage of parallel execution through the MapReduce framework [27] for the calculation of the average pixel color of the images captured by the UAVs. Afterwards, the color distance between the average pixel color of the images captured by the UAV and the average pixel color of a pre-defined picture showing flames of fire is calculated. If the color distance is less than a pre-calculated maximum allowed value, the picture is considered to be "highly dangerous" and is overlaid on top of a prototype web-based system where the fire authorities can take the necessary wildfire management actions immediately.

---

[1] https://www.fema.gov/.

[2] https://ec.europa.eu/info/departments/joint-research-centre_en.

### 3.1 Transferring Images to the Cluster

During the flight of the UAVs (Fig. 1a), images in high quality are saved in a micro SD Card. However, since our goal is to transfer the pictures captured by the UAV to the big data cluster in real-time, we use low-quality cached pictures and a handheld device (tablet/smartphone) with 4G connection connected to the UAV through the corresponding remote controller (Fig. 1b). It is very important to have an optimal quality of the transmission link between the UAVs and the handheld device to achieve a fast and stable data transmission and avoid any data loss. For this purpose, the UAVs are connected to a remote controller through a Wi-Fi 5.8 GHz frequency channel. The remote controller is connected to the UAVs with the ability to receive and transmit information constantly. The UAVs and the controller use an FM-FM signal modulation/demodulation scheme for their communication. One of the advantages of the frequency modulation is that it does not suffer from audio amplitude variations as the signal level varies when the UAV travels further away or the signal noise exists; and it makes FM ideal for use in the current application where signal levels constantly vary.

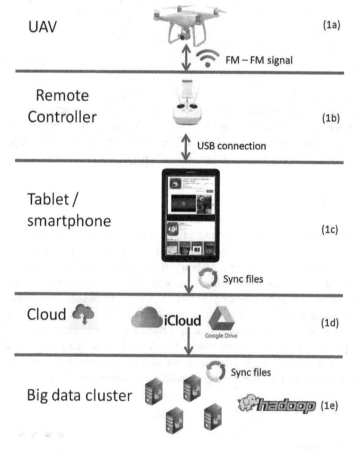

**Fig. 1.** Transferring images from the UAV to the big data cluster in (near) real-time

The controller acts as a bridge between the drone and the tablet. The controller and the tablet are connected through a USB cable to download all the necessary data, such as the status of the flight or the camera adjustments as well as the low-quality cached photo from the drone.

At the tablet/smartphone (Fig. 1c), a corresponding flight controlling application is used (such as the DJI GO 4–For drones[3] or the Litchi for DJI Mavic/Phantom/Inspire/Spark[4]) that controls the UAV during the flight and provides access to the low-quality pictures sent by drone to the tablet through the remote controller. Each cached photo sent from the UAV through the remote controller is saved at the tablet in a specific storage area, called *photo album*. The album is uploaded in the Cloud with an application such as the iCloud Drive[5] and the Google Drive[6] (Fig. 1d). The synchronization with the Cloud is done automatically when the cloud application notices any change at the album, like adding of a photo or removal of a photo. Thus, when a new photo is added to the photo album in the tablet, the cloud application uploads it into the internet. The cloud application also requires a stable internet connection to upload fast the new photos; this is accomplished with the connection to a 4G network or to a WI-FI network through a 4G card mounted to the tablet. Once the data are uploaded, the cloud application synchronizes the data and transfers them into the big data cluster (Fig. 1e).

### 3.2   Calculation of the Average Pixel Color

We utilize the HIPI (Hadoop Image Processing Interface) as an image processing library designed to be used with the Apache Hadoop MapReduce parallel programming framework. By using the Hadoop MapReduce software framework, software applications can be easily developed that process vast amounts of data in parallel on large clusters in a reliable, fault-tolerant manner. HIPI facilitates the MapReduce style of parallel programs by providing a solution for storing large collections of images on the Hadoop Distributed File System (HDFS) and make them available for efficient distributed processing. The input of any HIPI program is a collection of images represented as a single file on the HDFS, called HipiImageBundle (HIB). The images inside a HIB are assigned to individual *map* tasks in a way that attempts to maximize data locality, a cornerstone of the Hadoop MapReduce programming model. The records emitted by the *map* task are collected and transmitted to the *reduce* task according to the built-in MapReduce shuffle algorithm that attempts to minimize network traffic. The *reduce* tasks are executed in parallel and their output is aggregated and written to the HDFS. In our approach, the *map* task computes the average pixel color over a single image and the *reduce* task adds these averages together and divide by their count to compute the total average pixel color. Because the map tasks are executed in parallel, the entire operation for calculating the average pixel color is performed much faster than if we were using a single machine.

---

[3] https://play.google.com/store/apps/details?id=dji.go.v4&hl=en.

[4] https://play.google.com/store/apps/details?id=com.aryuthere.visionplus&hl=en.

[5] https://www.apple.com/lae/icloud/.

[6] https://www.google.com/drive/.

### 3.3    Calculation of the Color Distance

Based on the calculated average pixel color of the images, the next step in our methodology is to calculate how "close" the average pixel color is to a pre-defined picture showing flames of fire. Given the RGB (Red, Green, Blue) values of two colors $R_1B_1G_1$ and $R_2B_2G_2$, the Euclidian distance for calculating the color distance between two colors is defined by the following formulae [28]:

$$distance = \sqrt{(R_2 - R1)^2 + (G_2 - G_1)^2 + (B_2 - B_1)^2} \qquad (1)$$

However, the calculation of the color proximity based on the formulae (1) does not take into consideration differences in human color perception. A solution to this

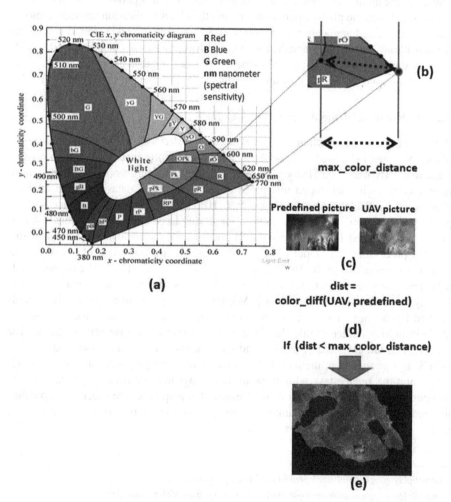

**Fig. 2.** Finding pictures "close" to a pre-defined picture showing flames of fire based on the CIELAB color space (Color figure online)

problem is to transform the RGB representations into the CIELAB color space that is designed to be perceptually uniform with respect to human color vision, meaning that the same amount of numerical change in these values corresponds to about the same amount of visually perceived change [29]. The CIELAB color space system characterizes colors by a luminance parameter Y and two color coordinates X and Y which specify the point on the chromaticity diagram (Fig. 2a). Once the color in the CIELAB color space is represented, the Delta-E distance metric using Euclidean Distance can be calculated. Based on the calculated distance, the maximum allowable color distance in the Red color space can be evaluated (Fig. 2b). Furthermore, the color distance between the average pixel color of the images from the UAV and a pre-defined picture showing flames of fire can also be calculated (Fig. 2c). If the distance is less than the pre-calculated maximum "permitted" color, an alert is sent to the fire headquarters with the geo-location of the picture for immediate wildfire management actions (Fig. 2d). The alert is created by overlaying the picture captured by the UAV on top of a corresponding Web GIS user interface (Fig. 2e).

## 4   Results

In order to test the proposed approach, several flights with UAVs have been conducted in the study area of Lesvos Island, Greece, during April of 2018. An initial test flight took place near the southern part of the island in a forest area. For the specific flight, we used the Phantom 4 UAV by DJI and the Litchi_app as the flight controlling application. Due to battery constraints, the UAV was able to fly only for 22 min so we had to take under consideration the flight time to create a proper and sufficient flight plan,

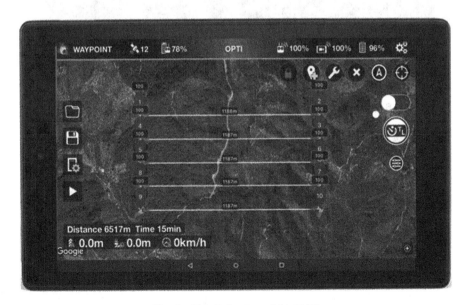

**Fig. 3.** The flight plan of the UAV

i.e. the one with the biggest area coverage. We placed 10 waypoints in a distance of 1.2 km from North to South and 147 m from West to East. The waypoints created a line that the UAV could travel on within a distance of 6.5 km. The created flight plan (Fig. 3) covers an area of 704,160 m². The drone started executing the mission from waypoint number one and ended to waypoint 10. The flight speed of the drone was set to 30 km/h and the flight altitude was at 100 m, leading to a flight with a total duration of 18 min.

**Welcome to the Big Data Wildfire System**

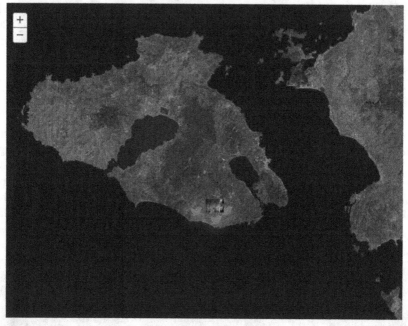

**Tweets @ Big Data Wildfire System**

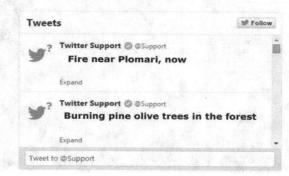

**Fig. 4.** The graphical user interface of the system

This flight altitude gave the ability to take photos with a ground sampling distance of 2.6 cm per pixel and a scale of 1:410. Totally, 296 images were captured in a sequence of two pictures per sec, transmitted and synced to the cloud with a total size of 176,328 MB.

We also used a cluster of 4 VMS with OS Ubuntu 11.04 64 bits, where the Hortonworks Data Platform (HDP) has been utilized. HDP is a massively scalable open source platform for storing, processing and analyzing large volumes of data. It consists of the Core Hadoop platform (Hadoop HDFS and Hadoop MapReduce), as well as other big data components such as Apache Pig, Apache Hive, Apache Spark etc. The first node has a CPU of Intel Core i7 3.6 GHz and 12 GB DDR4 of memory and acts as the JobTracker (master node) of the cluster, while the other has a CPU of Intel Core i5 2.6 GHz and 4 GB DDR3 of memory and act as the TaskTracker (slave nodes). Inside the big data cluster, the algorithms for the calculation of the average pixel color and the calculation of the color distance are executed in a parallel manner. Based on the color distance results, pictures from wildland fire areas are overlaid on the graphical user interface of a corresponding web-based system. For our purposes, the Geosocial Tweet System - GATES system was used [20]. Initially, the GATES system had been used for the integration of geo-referenced Twitter messages into a Web GIS for wildfire risk management. However, in the current approach, an extended GATES version has been developed as a graphical user interface of the proposed system. Figure 4 shows the extended graphical user interface of the system. In the upper part, the locations of the wildfire-related tweets, as well as the pictures captured by the UAV, are shown overlaid over a web map. In the bottom part of interface, the system shows the content of each related tweet.

For measuring the performance of our approach, we conducted several test flights for gathering a variable size of pictures. Figure 5 shows in x-axis the total size of data

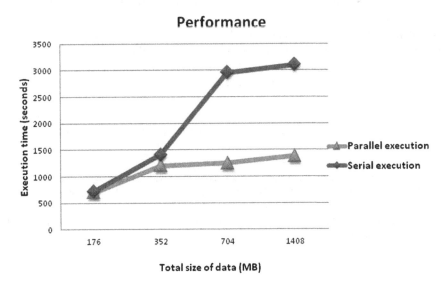

**Fig. 5.** Measuring the performance of the proposed methodology

and in y-axis the total execution time (in sec). We measured the time of parallel execution in the cluster consisting of the 4 VMs where the number of map tasks was equal to 4, while we also measured the execution time if only one VM was used and the number of map tasks was equal to 1, in order to evaluate the time for serial execution. From this diagram, it is clear to conclude that the processing time is not increased when the amount of data is increased. Thus, the proposed approach is a highly scalable solution and can be used independently of the total size of the data gathered. As a consequence, the approach can be used independently of the number of the available UAVs and the area that has to be covered.

## 5  Discussion and Conclusion

The integration of UAVs, Big Data components and image analysis is an important and valuable contribution to the overall disaster management effort. To the best of our knowledge, our approach is the first attempt that blends big data technology with image analysis for UAV surveillance. Our methodology provides the means to create state-of-the-art fire management services, where the civil protection authorities can promptly coordinate the emergency response crews and the affected population during a fire ignition.

A first prototype of the proposed approach has been tested by the local civil authorities in Lesvos Island, Greece, in the early 2018 wildfire season. Initial results show that there is a major improvement regarding the time needed to analyze the images retrieved by the UAVs, while the execution time of the image analysis is not affected from the area covered during the flights. Thus, wildfire prevention and management authorities can follow the proposed methodology to organize wildfire management plans in a reliable and timely manner. The instant and prompt delivery of images from areas affected by wildfires are the main advantages of the proposed methodology. The proposed methodology is expected to highlight the role of Geospatial Big Data and contribute towards a more state-of-the-art knowledge transfer between wildfire confrontation operation centers and firefighting units.

An obstacle to the proposed methodology is that even though the volume of images collected from the UAVs can be large, the level of noise in the resulting datasets is also extremely high. We are planning to cope with this disadvantage with the utilization of deep learning techniques such as Convolutional Neural Networks (CNN) techniques to classify images based on their content instead of relying on the results of the color distance.

**Acknowledgments.** This work has been partially conducted within the framework of the Greek State Scholarship Foundation (IKY) Scholarship Programs funded by the "Strengthening Post-Doctoral Research" Act from the resources of the OP "Human Resources Development and Lifelong Learning" priority axes 6, 8, 9, and co-financed by the European Social Fund (ESF) and the Greek Government.

# References

1. Kalabokidis, K., Athanasis, N., Vasilakos, C., Palaiologou, P.: Porting of a wildfire risk and fire spread application into a cloud computing environment. Int. J. Geogr. Inf. Sci. **28**(3), 541–552 (2014)
2. Hinkley, E.A., Zajkowski, T.: USDA forest service–NASA: unmanned aerial systems demonstrations–pushing the leading edge in fire mapping. Geocarto Int. **26**(2), 103–111 (2011)
3. Allison, R.S., Johnston, J.M., Craig, G., Jennings, S.: Airborne optical and thermal remote sensing for wildfire detection and monitoring. Sensors **16**(8), 1310 (2016)
4. Gambella, F., et al.: Forest and UAV: a bibliometric review. Contemp. Eng. Sci. **9**, 1359–1370 (2016)
5. Tang, L., Shao, G.: Drone remote sensing for forestry research and practices. J. Forest. Res. **26**(4), 791–797 (2015)
6. Villars, R.L., Olofson, C.W., Eastwood, M.: Big data: what it is and why you should care. White Paper, IDC, 14 (2011)
7. Yuan, C., Zhang, Y., Liu, Z.: A survey on technologies for automatic forest fire monitoring, detection, and fighting using unmanned aerial vehicles and remote sensing techniques. Can. J. For. Res. **45**(7), 783–792 (2015)
8. Pratt, K.S., Murphy, R., Stover, S., Griffin, C.: CONOPS and autonomy recommendations for VTOL small unmanned aerial system based on Hurricane Katrina operations. J. Field Robot. **26**(8), 636–650 (2009)
9. Murphy, R.R., Steimle, E., Griffin, C., Cullins, C., Hall, M., Pratt, K.: Cooperative use of unmanned sea surface and micro aerial vehicles at Hurricane Wilma. J. Field Robot. **25**(3), 164–180 (2008)
10. Nardi, D.: Intelligent systems for emergency response (invited talk). In: Fourth International Workshop on Synthetic Simulation and Robotics to Mitigate Earthquake Disaster (SRMED 2009) (2009)
11. Quaritsch, M., Kruggl, K., Wischounig-Strucl, D., Bhattacharya, S., Shah, M., Rinner, B.: Networked UAVs as aerial sensor network for disaster management applications. e & i Elektrotechnik und Informationstechnik **127**(3), 56–63 (2010)
12. Dunford, R., Michel, K., Gagnage, M., Piégay, H., Trémelo, M.L.: Potential and constraints of unmanned aerial vehicle technology for the characterization of mediterranean riparian forest. Int. J. Remote Sens. **30**(19), 4915–4935 (2009)
13. Merino, L., Caballero, F., Martínez-de-Dios, J.R., Maza, I., Ollero, A.: An unmanned aircraft system for automatic forest fire monitoring and measurement. J. Intell. Rob. Syst. **65**(1–4), 533–548 (2012)
14. Ofli, F., et al.: Combining human computing and machine learning to make sense of big (aerial) data for disaster response. Big Data **4**(1), 47–59 (2016)
15. Andrejevic, M., Kelly, G.: Big data surveillance: introduction. Surveill. Soc. **12**(2), 185–196 (2014)
16. Baumann, P., et al.: Big data analytics for earth sciences: the earthserver approach. Int. J. Digit. Earth **9**(1), 3–29 (2016)
17. Nguyen, D.T., Ofli, F., Imran, M., Mitra, P.: Damage assessment from social media imagery data during disasters. In: Proceedings of the 2017 IEEE/ACM International Conference on Advances in Social Networks Analysis and Mining, pp. 569–576. ACM (2017)
18. Athanasis, N., Themistocleous, M., Kalabokidis, K.: Wildfire prevention in the era of big data. In: Themistocleous, M., Morabito, V. (eds.) EMCIS 2017. LNBIP, vol. 299, pp. 111–118. Springer, Cham (2017). https://doi.org/10.1007/978-3-319-65930-5_9

19. Athanasis, N., Themistocleous, M., Kalabokidis, K., Papakonstantinou, A., Soulakellis, N., Palaiologou, P.: The emergence of social media for natural disasters management: a big data perspective. Int. Arch. Photogramm. Remote Sens. Spatial Inf. Sci. **XLII-3/W4**, 75–82 (2018). https://doi.org/10.5194/isprs-archives-XLII-3-W4-75-2018

20. Codella, N.C., Hua, G., Natsev, A., Smith, J.R.: Towards large scale land-cover recognition of satellite images. In: 2011 8th International Conference on Information, Communications and Signal Processing (ICICS), pp. 1–5. IEEE (2011)

21. Zhang, W., et al.: Towards building a multi datacenter infrastructure for massive remote sensing image processing. Concurr. Comput.: Pract. Exp. **25**(12), 1798–1812 (2013)

22. Hadjisophocleous, G.V., Fu, Z.: Literature review of fire risk assessment methodologies. Int. J. Eng. Perform.-Based Fire Codes **6**(1), 28–45 (2004)

23. Çelik, T., Ozkaramanlt, H., Demirel, H.: Fire pixel classification using fuzzy logic and statistical color model. In: 2007 IEEE International Conference on Acoustics, Speech and Signal Processing. ICASSP 2007, vol. 1, pp. I–1205. IEEE (2007)

24. Yuan, C., Liu, Z., Zhang, Y.: UAV-based forest fire detection and tracking using image processing techniques. In: 2015 International Conference on Unmanned Aircraft Systems (ICUAS), pp. 639–643. IEEE (2015)

25. Yuan, C., Liu, Z., Zhang, Y.: Vision-based forest fire detection in aerial images for firefighting using UAVs. In: 2016 International Conference on Unmanned Aircraft Systems (ICUAS), pp. 1200–1205. IEEE (2016)

26. Sweeney, C., Liu, L., Arietta, S., Lawrence, J.: HIPI: a Hadoop image processing interface for image-based mapreduce tasks. University of Virginia, Chris (2011)

27. Dean, J., Ghemawat, S.: MapReduce: simplified data processing on large clusters. Commun. ACM **51**(1), 107–113 (2008)

28. Agarwal, V., Abidi, B.R., Koshan, A., Abidi, M.A.: An overview of color constancy algorithms. J. Pattern Recogn. Res. **1**, 42–54 (2006)

29. Connolly, C., Fleiss, T.: A study of efficiency and accuracy in the transformation from RGB to CIELAB color space. IEEE Trans. Image Process. **6**(7), 1046–1048 (1997)

# Harnessing Cloud Scalability to Hadoop Clusters

Arne Koschel[1(✉)], Felix Heine[1], and Irina Astrova[2]

[1] Faculty IV, Department of Computer Science,
Hannover University of Applied Sciences and Arts,
Ricklinger Stadtweg 120, 30459 Hannover, Germany
akoschel@acm.org, felix.heine@hs-hannover.de
[2] Department of Software Science, School of IT,
Tallinn University of Technology, Akadeemia,
tee 21, 12618 Tallinn, Estonia
irina@cs.ioc.ee

**Abstract.** Apache Hadoop is a popular technology that proved itself as an effective and powerful framework for Big Data analytics. It broke from many of its predecessors in the "computing at scale" space by being designed to run in a distributed fashion across large amounts of commodity hardware instead of a few expensive computers. Many organizations have come to rely on Hadoop for dealing with the ever-increasing quantities of Big Data that they gather. "Harnessing cloud scalability to Hadoop clusters" means running Hadoop clusters on resources offered by a cloud provider on demand.

**Keywords:** Big Data · Cloud computing · Hadoop

## 1 Introduction

Big Data are big in two different senses. They are big in the quantity and variety of data that are available to be stored and processed. They are also big in the scale of analysis (or analytics) that can be applied to those data. Both kinds of "big" depend on the existence of supportive infrastructure. Such an infrastructure is increasingly being provided by the cloud like OpenStack or Amazon EC2.

Cloud architectures are being used increasingly to support Big Data analytics by organizations that make ad hoc or routine use of the cloud in lieu of acquiring their own infrastructure. On the other hand, Hadoop [1] has become the de-facto standard for storing and processing Big Data. It is hard to overstate how many advantages come with moving Hadoop into the cloud. The most important is scalability, meaning that the underlying infrastructure can be expanded or contracted according to the actual demand on resources. This paper presents a scalable Hadoop-based infrastructure for Big Data analytics, one that gets automatically adjusted if more computing power or storage capacity is needed. Adjustments are transparent to the users – the users seem to have nearly unlimited computation and storage resources.

© Springer Nature Switzerland AG 2019
M. Themistocleous and P. Rupino da Cunha (Eds.): EMCIS 2018, LNBIP 341, pp. 59–71, 2019.
https://doi.org/10.1007/978-3-030-11395-7_6

## 2 Challenges

The cloud computing technology is based on the concept of virtualization. However, the virtualization of a Hadoop cluster or more specifically HDFS (Hadoop Distributed File System) cluster is a challenging task. Unlike most common server applications, Hadoop has some special requirements for a cloud architecture. In particular, Hadoop requires for topology information about the utilized infrastructure. Hadoop then uses this information to manage replications in HDFS. If the infrastructure consists of more than one cluster, Hadoop ensures that at least one replication is stored in a different hardware cluster than the other replications to allow for data access even when the whole cluster is unavailable. Moreover, Hadoop tries to perform computing tasks near the required data to avoid network transfers, which are often slower than local data access.

A cloud architecture abstracts the physical hardware to hide the infrastructure details from the hosted instances. Furthermore, shared storage pools are often used to store instances instead of having a dedicated storage in every computing node. Shared storage pools and missing topology information of the Hadoop instances might lead to multiple HDFS replications onto the same physical storage pool. Also Hadoop's paradigm to avoid network traffic by allocating computing tasks near the data storage would be broken, since shared storage pools are often connected via a network. As a consequence, the performance of cluster would probably be massively decreased due to unnecessary replications and increased network traffic.

## 3 Related Work

Cloud providers have started to offer prepackaged services that use Hadoop under the hood, but do most of the cluster management work themselves. The users simply point the services to data and provide the services with jobs to run, and the services handle the rest, delivering results back to the users. The users still pay for the resources used, as well as the use of the services, but save on all of the management work [5].

Examples of prepackaged services include:

- **Elastic MapReduce:** This is Amazon Web Services' solution for managing Hadoop clusters through an API. Data are usually stored in Amazon S3 or Amazon DynamoDB. The normal mode of operation for Elastic MapReduce is to define the parameters for a Hadoop cluster like its size, location, Hadoop version and variety of services, point to where data should be read from and written to, and define steps to run jobs. Elastic MapReduce launches a Hadoop cluster, performs the steps to generate the output data and then tears the cluster down. However, the users can leave the cluster running for further use and even resize it for greater capacity.
- **Google Cloud Dataproc:** It is similar to Elastic MapReduce, but runs within Google Cloud Platform. Data are usually stored in Google Cloud Storage.
- **HDInsight:** This is Microsoft Azure's solution, which is built on top of Horton-works Data Platform. HDInsight works with Azure Blob Storage and Azure Data Lake Store for reading and writing data used in jobs. Ambari is included as well for cluster management through its API.

Despite their advantages like ready availability and ease of use, prepackaged services only work on the cloud providers offering them. Organizations can be worried about being "locked in" to a single cloud provider, unable to take advantage of competition between the providers. Moreover, it may not be possible to satisfy data security or tracking requirements with the services due to a lack of direct control over the resources [5].

In addition to prepackaged services, cloud providers offer Hadoop-as-a-Service (HaaS) for Big Data analytics [6]. However, HaaS offerings share the same disadvantages as prepackaged services in terms of moving further away from the open source world and jeopardizing interoperability. Moreover, since unlike to prepackaged services they are not explicitly based on Hadoop, there is a separate learning curve for them, and the effort could be wasted if they are ever discarded in favor of an application that works on Hadoop or on a different cloud provider [5].

In contrast, this paper presents open source software that is able to support multiple cloud providers.

## 4   Architecture

Figure 1 gives an overview of the architecture of a Hadoop-based infrastructure for Big Data analytics. This architecture is multilayered – different layers allocate the different responsibilities of Big Data software. An upper layer uses a lower layer as a service.

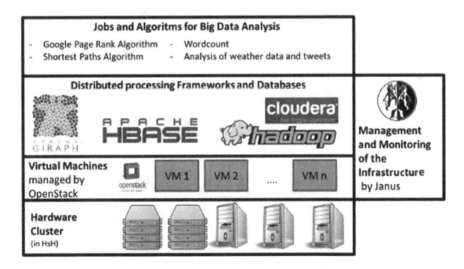

**Fig. 1.** Architecture of Hadoop-based infrastructure for Big Data analytics [7].

The architecture comprises the following layers:

- **Hardware (or physical) clusters:** This is the bottom layer. It is composed of all physical machines that are wired together either by the Internet or by a direct network connection. A physical cluster is abstracted by means of virtualization.
- **Virtual machines:** On top of the hardware clusters, we installed virtual machines to form a hardware abstraction layer. A virtual machine acts like a physical computer except that software running on the virtual machine is separated from the underlying hardware resources. This layer is managed by OpenStack, which eases the management of virtual machines by a standardized API.
- **Distributed processing frameworks and databases:** This layer is composed of Hadoop, HDFS, HBase, MapReduce, Giraph Pregel and Cloudera. Cloudera is a distribution, which delivers many Apache products, including Hadoop and HBase.
- **Jobs and algorithms for Big Data analytics:** This is the application layer that is responsible for Big Data analytics. Here we implemented many algorithms like Google's PageRank, Shortest Paths and Word Count. The algorithms are parallelized using programming models like MapReduce [2] and Giraph Pregel [3].
- **Management and monitoring of the infrastructure:** This layer is responsible for managing both the physical and virtual clusters using an API. Here we implemented Janus, our own written software, which provides an API to automate the launching, management and resizing of Hadoop clusters. Figure 2 shows an overview of architecture of Janus that can be viewed as a link between the OpenStack's cloud manager and the Cloudera Manager. Janus connects both sides by utilizing classes, which implement two abstract interfaces: iCloud and Hadoop-Mgr. This is done to ensure that the core logic of Janus will not be changed even if another cloud provider like Amazon is added. On the cloud management side, these are classes of OpenStack or Amazon EC2, which implement the iCloud interface. On the Hadoop cluster management side, these could be the Hortonworks Ambari Manager Wrapper or the Cloudera Manager Wrapper classes, which implement the Hadoop-Mgr interface.

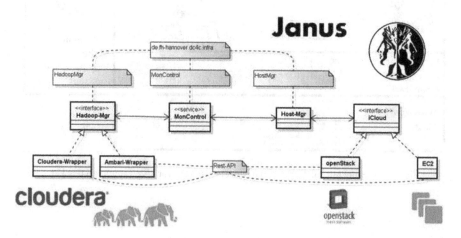

**Fig. 2.** Architecture of Janus [7].

# 5  Application Scenarios

We identified two major application scenarios for the architecture. One was about the storage capacity offered to the users. If the storage capacity becomes scarce, the infrastructure will automatically increase the size of the HDFS. If the physical limits of the hardware get reached, the infrastructure will automatically contact another cloud provider. This could be a private cloud provider like another university or partner organization or a public cloud provider like Amazon. The users get the possibility to define prioritization of external clouds to minimize the expenses, which arise when commercial public clouds are used. Whenever a Hadoop cluster needs to be extended, Janus searches for a new suitable host system in all managed the OpenStack clouds. Thereby currently used clouds are preferred, so that a Hadoop cluster will only be extended into a new cloud as a last resort. Within each managed cloud, Janus searches for hosts, which are currently not used by the Hadoop cluster that should be expanded. If more than one host system could run a new instance, the host with the lowest count of running instances is selected. In either case, such expansion should be considered as a temporal and rapid solution to prevent data loss, which would occur if the cloud could not store any further data. In the long term, it would be necessary to buy additional hardware to offer more storage capacity within the cloud to release expensive public cloud instances.

We had two separate OpenStack installations, each having one OpenStack master and several OpenStack computing nodes. The first cloud consisted of five servers with a quad-core processor and 16 GB RAM. The second cloud consisted of three servers with a quad-core processor and 128 GB RAM. All the servers were utilizing a local RAID-0 array as their data storage to ensure highest storage performance. Redundancy was achieved by the internal replication mechanisms of HDFS. To simulate the scaling mechanism into a public cloud, we configured Janus to treat the second cloud as the public cloud. Janus broke with the anti-affinity of instances in a Hadoop cluster in the simulated public cloud and launched new instances wherever resources were available.

Another application scenario concerned the computation power of the cloud. As more and more different users would use the cloud for their Big Data analytics, a single job could get really slow if the virtual computing nodes reach their limits. The solution for this scenario is to start further virtual computing nodes in the cloud to take over additional analysis jobs. If the physical limits of the hardware also get reached, additional computation power will be obtained from an external cloud. An important point, which has to be taken into consideration when expanding into a public cloud, is the storage location of sensitive data. The users may want not to offer those data to a public cloud provider just because the infrastructure is running out of storage. In this case, the users are given the possibility to mark their data as sensitive so that the infrastructure can avoid the exposure of those data. To realize this scenario, the cloud solution has to move other non-sensitive data to the public cloud to free storage for the sensitive data.

Based on the application scenarios, we created two rules to react to storage capacity or computing power bottlenecks. Both rules are checked in a cyclic interval. If a rule gets violated, the defined action will be started and no further checks of any other rule are done until the violation is fixed. One rule is `HdfsCapacityRule`. This rule is used to monitor the free disk space in HDFS; it creates a new Hadoop node if a given threshold is violated for a given timeframe. Another rule is MapRedSlotsRule. It is triggered when a given percentage of the available MapReduce slots have already been in use. When this rule is violated for a given timeframe, a new Hadoop node is created too.

## 6   Evaluation

To evaluate the architecture, we used it to find out a correlation between the weather conditions and the mood of Twitter users. For this purpose, we collected weather and Twitter data. The weather data were classified into different categories, each representing different weather conditions, from very good to very bad weather depending on how Twitter users perceived the weather. The Twitter data were also divided into categories, depending on whether the Twitter users were in a good or bad mood when they wrote their tweets. Finally, both data sets were correlated to see if there is a relationship between the weather category and the positive or negative sentiment of tweets.

### 6.1   Test Data

To collect the tweets, we used the twitter4j library that returned the Twitter data as a stream. Since Twitter limited the stream bandwidth, we collected the tweets that were emitted in a certain location. Each tweet was saved as a JSON object in HBASE.

We collected the weather data from a website www.openweathermap.org. More specifically, we used the REST API to retrieve the weather data depending on a longitude and latitude. To collect the weather data, a Java program (WeatherCollector.java) was used, which queried the data in the desired area and stored the data in HBase. The geographical position was used as a key for the corresponding database record (see Fig. 3). To ensure an equal distribution of keys, each key was hashed with the md5 hashing algorithm.

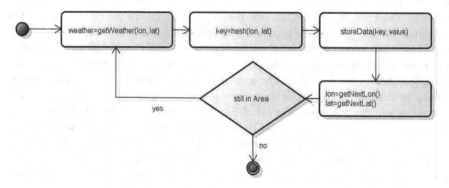

**Fig. 3.** Programming flow of the weather data procurement.

Before the weather data were correlated with the Twitter data, the two corresponding tables were joined by a MapReduce job. In the Map phase the longitude, latitude and the date were extracted from the weather and Twitter data. The longitude and latitude of a tweet were round up. These values (the longitude, latitude and date) were concatenated. This resulted in the output key by which the data could be aggregated in the Shuffle phase and distributed to a Reducer. In the Reduce phase, the weather-dataset was found, which had the slightest deviation in respect to the time of the tweet. These two data sets (weather and Twitter data) were stored in a text file on which the `TwitterWeatherCorrelation` job ran ultimately.

To correlate a tweet and the associated weather data, another MapReduce job was run. In the Map phase, the evaluation of the tweets and the weather conditions (as Twitter users perceived) was determined. Then the output key was generated by concatenating these two values. The output value was simply 1, so that the Reducer could count how often a weather condition and a related tweet sentiment were matched. In the Reduce phase, the values of the input list were summed up to generate the count.

## 6.2    Test Process

Figure 4 shows data flow. The crawler programs for weather conditions and tweets stored their data in HBase. The database was then copied to a HDFS file representation. All the following jobs ran on both HBase and HDFS. The `TwitterWeatherJoin` job joined the related weather and tweet data records. The `TwitterWeatherCorrelation` and `TwitterWeatherCorrelationCoefficient` jobs analyzed the correlation between the weather condition and the mood of Twitter user. The `TweetsPerGeoLocation` job counted the amount of tweets in the desired area for a given date and time interval, which needed the tweets as a data source.

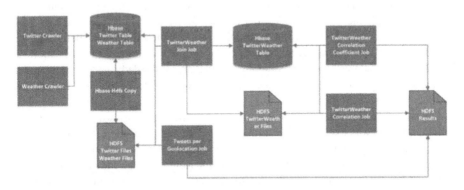

**Fig. 4.** Data flow during test process.

The comparison of HBase and HDFS started with the `TwitterWeatherJoin` job, which created a new table in HBase and a new file in HDFS. Beforehand the crawler was stopped, the amount of data for the comparison was the same. After the `TwitterWeatherJoin` job had finished, the other jobs ran on those data for both HDFS and HBase.

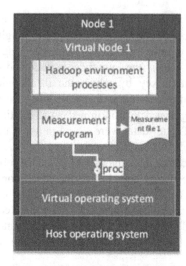
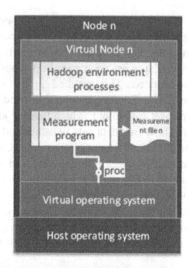
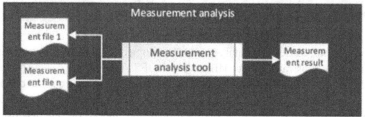

**Fig. 5.** Architecture of measurement program.

Figure 5 shows the architecture of a measurement program. All measurements were collected through the program, which used the UNIX proc interfaces like `/proc/stat` or `/proc/meminfo` inside a virtual machine. These interfaces delivered the current status of the infrastructure for a specific property like the CPU utilization or disk I/O. All virtual machines were running exclusively on the dedicated physical node. Therefore, possible differences in the measurements inside or outside the virtual machine could be negligible.

On every virtual node, an instance of the measurement program was started, when a computation job was executed. The program queried the proc interfaces at a configurable interval, e.g., every 10 s and wrote the measured values as one record in a measurement file. As a result, at the end of the measurement, the file contained many records. After the measurement, all files from every node were transferred to a measurement analysis tool. The values from all files were summed up and the final result was calculated with the tool (in our case, Excel).

The Cloudera cluster consisted of four virtual machines each with 14 GByte main memory. The memory size was very important to ensure a smoothly execution of the jobs. The memory configuration was based on a recommendation of the Ambari project for nodes with 16 GByte main memory including HBase. Due to a higher memory demand of the single Mapper and Reducer tasks, the Mapper slot quantity was reduced to two for each node. Each job started a configurable number of Mapper-Reducer tasks and allocates the Mapper-Reducer slots on the cluster. During the first comparison tests, problems with HBase in the `TwitterWeatherJoin` job on the Reducer phase occurred. These problems were timeout errors. Because of that we reduced the starting Reducers to four and increased the remote procedure handler for `TwitterWeatherJoin` job in HBase. As a result, in this job for HBase only four of the eight Reducer slots were occupied. All following HBase and HDFS jobs had the same Reducer and Mapper quantity.

## 6.3  Test Results

Figures 6, 7, 8, 9, 10 and 11 summarize the results of our evaluation. A large difference in the runtimes can be seen on the example of the `TwitterWeatherJoin` (TWJoin) job, where HBase was three times slower than HDFS. This was due to the HBase's ability to filter or query data prior to the Mapper phase based on the data timestamp. Such a filter was also tested on HBase. In particular, the filter test was repeated three times, but it always showed the same runtime. That is, in the case of HBase, the filter did not have any effect on the runtime. As expected, all other jobs had similar runtimes on both HBase and HDFS.

The disk I/O measurements showed that HBase usually had a much higher number of write requests than HDFS. Noticeable was the high number of writes on the `TwitterWeatherCorrelation` (TWCorrelation) and `TwitterWeather Correlation` (TWCorrelationCoefficient) jobs, although those jobs did not produce much data.

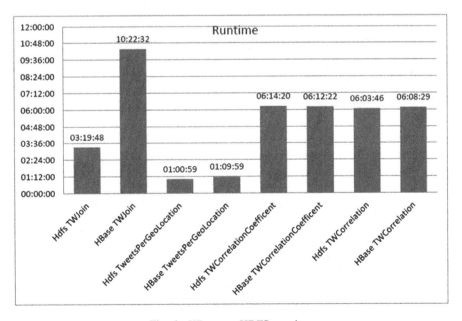

**Fig. 6.** HBase vs. HDFS: runtime.

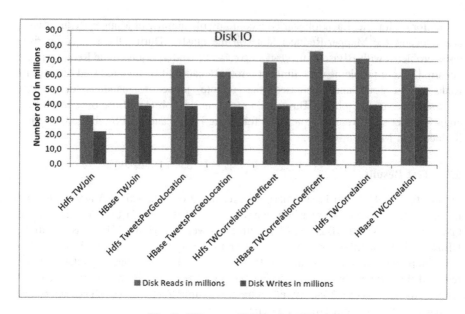

**Fig. 7.** HBase vs. HDFS: disk I/O.

The network I/O measurements showed a very big difference between HBase and HDFS. For example, in the case of the `TweetsPerGeoLocation` job, this difference exceeded 100 times. Generally, the Hadoop framework is based on the principle "move computation to the data." However, the measurements showed that HBase transmitted all data over the network and thus, did not follow that principle.

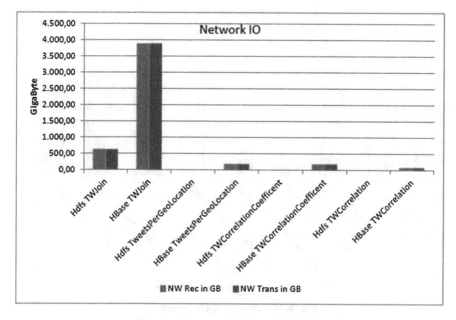

**Fig. 8.** HBase vs. HDFS: network I/O.

The measurements of CPU utilization showed that the jobs did not use all CPU resources. The CPU utilization was calculated based on a system-CPU and a user-CPU and was deducted with a stolen-CPU. A stolen-CPU described a situation where a virtual machine requested the CPU resources, but the virtual machine manager was servicing another process outside the virtual machine. The CPU utilization on HDFS was between 50–60% for all the jobs. HBase had a CPU utilization of 25% on the

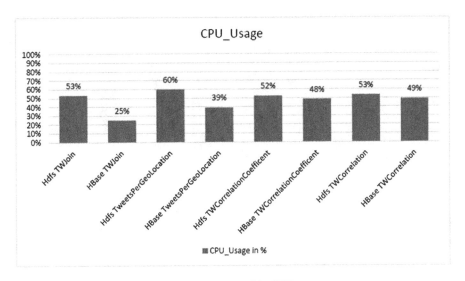

**Fig. 9.** HBase vs. HDFS: CPU usage.

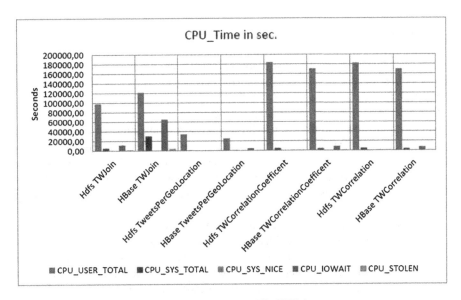

**Fig. 10.** HBase vs. HDFS: CPU time.

`TwitterWeatherJoin` (TWJoin) job and around 40–50% on the rest jobs. The measurements of CPU time showed that HBase has a high CPU I/O wait time on the `TwitterWeatherJoin` (TWJoin) job, which was according to the network I/O and disk I/O.

The measurements of RAM utilization showed that it was over 90% on all jobs on both HBase and HDFS. This result was due to the fact that the memory cache belonged to the used memory. The measurements gathered only free and used memory.

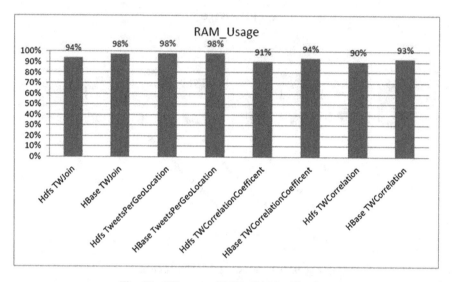

**Fig. 11.** HBase vs. HDFS: RAM utilization.

## 7 Conclusion

Big Data analytics requires not just algorithms and data, but also physical platforms where the data are stored and processed. This class of infrastructure is now available through the cloud.

Our work was aimed at developing a Hadoop-based infrastructure for Big Data analytics, which gets automatically adjusted if more computing power or storage capacity is needed. One of the main challenges in the development of such an infrastructure was the integration of Big Data software framework like Hadoop into a cloud architecture as both are designed for contrary purposes. Moreover, a Big Data software framework is usually complex and its usage requires a lot of practice, knowledge and experience.

The main result of our work was the implementation of an architecture for the infrastructure. That architecture enabled to run Hadoop clusters in the OpenStack cloud and thus, made them scalable on demand. Finally, the architecture had been used to evaluate the performance of different persistence layers and computational models for processing Big Data. More specifically, the persistence layers were evaluated by comparing the storage of Big Data onto HDFS and HBase. The computational models were compared by executing the PageRank algorithm on Big Data with two different programming models: MapReduce and Giraph Pregel [4].

## 8  Future Work

In the current version of Janus, rules monitor only a single property of Hadoop cluster and check if that property violates a certain threshold. These rules were primarily used to prove that a Hadoop cluster can be automatically adjusted when the CPU usage per node increases or the HDFS capacity gets too low. A future work could be to extend the existing rule engine to support rules, which monitor multiple properties. Another enhancement could be to monitor complex events occurred in a Hadoop cluster, e.g., when every Friday night a weekly computation is started and from week to week the performance gets lower. For this purpose, historical measurements have to be stored and evaluated.

**Acknowledgement.** Irina Astrova's work was supported by the Estonian Ministry of Education and Research institutional research grant IUT33-13.

## References

1. White, T.: Hadoop: The Definitive Guide 3. O'Reilly Media, Sebastopol (2012)
2. Shook, A.: MapReduce Design Patterns. O'Reilly Media, Sebastopol (2013)
3. Malewicz, G., et al.: Pregel: a system for large-scale graph processing. In: Proceedings of the 2010 ACM SIGMOD International Conference on Management of Data, New York, USA (2010)
4. Koschel, A., Heine, F., Astrova, I., Korte, F., Rossow, T., Stipkovic, S.: Efficiency experiments on Hadoop and Giraph with PageRank. In: Proceedings of 24th Euromicro International Conference on Parallel, Distributed, and Network-Based Processing, Heraklion Crete, Greece, pp. 328–331. IEEE (2016)
5. Havanki, B.: Moving Hadoop to the Cloud: Harnessing Cloud Features and Flexibility for Hadoop Clusters. O'Reilly Media, Sebastopol (2017)
6. Astrova, I., Koschel, A., Lennart, M.H., Nahle, H.: Offering Hadoop as a cloud service. In: Proceedings of the 2016 SAI Computing Conference, London, UK, pp. 589–595. IEEE (2016)
7. Astrova, I., Koschel, A., Heine, F., Kalja, A.: Scalable Hadoop-based infrastructure for big data analytics. In: Proceedings of the 13th International Baltic Conference on Data-Bases and Information Systems, Trakai, Lithuania. IEEE (2018)

# For What It's Worth: A Multi-industry Survey on Current and Expected Use of Big Data Technologies

Elisa Rossi[1], Cinzia Rubattino[1], and Gianluigi Viscusi[2(✉)]

[1] GFT Italia S.r.l., Genoa, Italy
{elisa.rossi,cinzia.rubattino}@gft.com
[2] École Polytechnique Fédérale de Lausanne (EPFL-CDM-MTEI-CSI),
Lausanne, Switzerland
gianluigi.viscusi@epfl.ch

**Abstract.** This article discusses the results of a multi-industry and multi-country survey carried out to understand the needs, requirements, and use of big data and analytics by public and private organizations in decision-making, business processes and emerging business models. In particular, these issues are analyzed in specific industries where big data exploitation may have not only an economic value but also and an impact on social value dimensions such as, e.g., public and personal safety. Furthermore, the survey aims at questioning the characteristics of big data ecosystems in different and specific domains, thus identifying existing or potential barriers to the development of new data-driven industrial sectors along the big data information value chain. Finally, the authors have identified three key challenges (big data efficiency, effectiveness, and accessibility) to classify the survey results that showed low utilization rate of the data collected, lack of right tools and capabilities, the low rate of digital transformation of the companies as the key concerns for the respondents.

**Keywords:** Big data · Big data technologies · Survey · Big data use

## 1 Introduction

Big data represents the typical case of a technical issue and subject that succeeded in entering the everyday life of lay people. These latter are usually informed by general magazines and newspapers not always working at the right level of granularity or abstraction - exception made for the report by journals such as, e.g., the Economist [1, 2] - rather than academia. The consequence is a diffuse general understanding of big data as mainly a substitute for "very large amount of data" that can tell everything a person can (actually) know about a topic and predict nearly exactly what to do then; thus, sometimes - when not often - big data are quite wrongly overlapped with the concept of artificial intelligence. Taking these issues into account, without mentioning the debate about how many "V"s are worth defining big data [3, 4], we can take as a proxy to common understanding of big data the following definition appeared in 2013 in the first issue of Big Data, one of the first journals on the topic published by Mary Ann Liebert, Inc: *Big data is data that exceeds the processing capacity of conventional*

© Springer Nature Switzerland AG 2019
M. Themistocleous and P. Rupino da Cunha (Eds.): EMCIS 2018, LNBIP 341, pp. 72–79, 2019.
https://doi.org/10.1007/978-3-030-11395-7_7

*database systems. The data is too big, moves too fast, or doesn't fit the structures of your database architectures. To gain value from this data, you must choose an alternative way to process it* [5]. However the clarity and appeal of the above definition as well as the number of resources made available for improving data science skills and big or open data policies, one of the main barriers for laypersons and businesses is related to the understanding of the types of data and the capacity [6] of current technological infrastructure, business process and business models to maintain, produce, and use big data [7], especially considering not only their economic value but their potential public and social value [8–12].

In this article we discuss the results of a multi-industry survey carried out to understand the needs, requirements, and use of big data and analytics by public and private organizations in decision-making, business processes and emerging business models having economic value and an impact on social value dimensions such as, e.g., public and personal safety. Furthermore, the survey aims at questioning the characteristics of big data ecosystems in different and specific domains, thus identifying existing or potential barriers to the development of new data-driven industrial sectors along the big data information value chain [13]. The paper is structured as follows. First, we discuss the related work and the research method adopted in this paper and the main results of the survey, before the conclusive remarks end the paper.

## 2 Related Work

The research presented in this article refers to two main topics of information systems (IS) research. The first one is acceptance and adoption of technology (in our case big data and the technology to use them, e.g. analytics) [14–16]. The technology acceptance model (TAM) [17] and its further developments [18] represent the most diffused and applied in terms of domains, where the main constructs are the 'perceived usefulness' and 'perceived ease of use' of a technology, integrated over the years by other dimensions, such as, e.g., performance expectancy, effort expectancy, social influence, and facilitating conditions as determinants of information systems' usage intention and usage behavior [19]. Considering the evaluation of IS success, the main reference is the DeLone and McLean (D&M) model and its evolution [20–22], where the original variables (system quality, information quality, use, user satisfaction, individual impact, and organizational impact) has been integrated, e.g., with service quality and intention to use, while adding net benefits as main impact. Furthermore, as for the evaluation of IS "success" and effectiveness, it is worth mentioning also the User Information Satisfaction (UIS) [23–25], and the effort by Wixom and Todd [26] to propose an integrated model of user satisfaction and technology acceptance.

However relevant the literature on IS adoption, acceptance, and success, the second topic, information value, is really at the core of the understanding of for what they are worth big data and analytics. As to this issue, Ahituv [27] identified three utility attributes (*timeliness*, *contents*, and *format*) to assess the value of an Information System (IS), considering them as arguments for information value as a function, adding *cost* as further attribute. Then, Ahituv [28] identified at theoretical level three types of value of information (see Fig. 1): the *normative value* (purely analytical,); the *realistic value* (based on the measurement of performances) the *perceived value* (subjective).

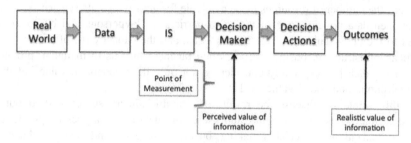

**Fig. 1.** Point of measurement of perceived and realistic value of information, adapted from [28], pp. 320–321.

Finally, Viscusi and Batini [29] have developed a model for digital information asset evaluation (see Fig. 2) based on an analysis of the literature on information value. The model considers information value as determined by costs and information utility. This latter is influenced by the information diffusion and by the information capacity of an organization or a user mediated by its/his/her set of information capabilities.

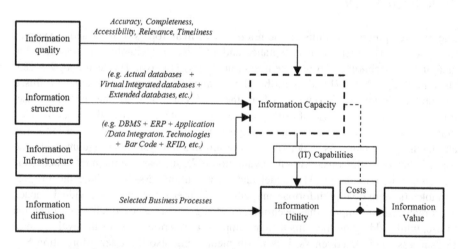

**Fig. 2.** A model for digital information asset evaluation, source [6].

As for the model, it is worth noting the elaboration there and further development by Viscusi and Batini [29] of the concept of *information capacity* as influenced by information quality, information structure, information infrastructure and defined as *"the current stock of understandings informed by a given installed base"* representing *"the potential of a digital information asset that can be defined and evaluated independently from the usage"* (p. 81).

## 3   Research Method

The exploratory research presented in this paper has been carried out through a survey method [30, 31] The survey was conducted online on a sample of industries and sectors including finance and insurance, automotive, information technology (IT), healthcare, smart home, public sector (municipalities and public authorities), public safety and law enforcement (police, emergency medical service fire service, search and rescue, army), research and education, and smart city (electronics, smart city technology providers, smart City planners). The different groups have been selected with a specific focus on the use of big data for creating and capturing not only economic value but also providing social value in terms of public safety and security for the final users or customers. Thus, the interest was on organizations that may have an impact on these issues while developing new business models driven or enabled by the use of big data and related technologies. Consequently, in order to have subjects potentially representing a potential big data ecosystem, we included citizens as end users, likewise.

**Table 1.**  Respondents groups and number of replies

| Respondents groups | Number of replies |
|---|---|
| Consultant | 6 |
| Executive | 22 |
| Scientist | 15 |
| Senior manager | 34 |
| Total | 77 |

The considered sample of industries and users covered a set of countries related to the researchers involved in the AEGIS project focused on big data for public safety and personal security [32], then extended to respondents from other countries for the above-mentioned categories. The survey has been carried out from January to March 2017, using multiple channels such as an online form, face to face, and telephone interviews. The invitations were sent by the AEGIS partners to direct links and contacts. The AEGIS researchers in charge of the surveys also conducted in-depth interviews for a specific sample among the ones above-mentioned, covering different roles and focus areas. The sample was made up of companies from finance and IT industry, due to the state of the art relevance of the latter for the big data technological infrastructure [33, 34] and the former for being traditionally characterized by the degree of information content of their product and information intensity of the value chain [35], thus being an example of data-driven industry [36]. Finally, we received 77 replies to the questionnaire out of 110 invitations (a response rate of 70%). In the following Section we discuss the main results both from the survey and the interviews. The respondents had different positions (e.g., product manager, project manager, research manager, chief executive officer, chief operation officer, head of IT, IT manager, research and development manager, academic or industry researchers, consultants, etc.) that have been clustered in the groups shown in Table 1.

## 4   Discussion of the Results

The respondents covered all the target groups (academia, automotive, aviation, aerospace, consulting, defense, energy, entertainment, financial services, healthcare, industry association, insurance, internet and social media, logistics, manufacturing, marketing and advertising, public sector, research, retail, smart home, telecommunications, transport), yet most of them coming from the information technology (IT) plies industry ($\sim$50%). Considering, the geographical distribution, all the countries of the partners of the project were covered (Austria, Cyprus, Germany, Greece, Italy, Sweden, Switzerland) with additional replies from Portugal, France, Belgium, Bulgaria, Luxembourg, the Netherlands, United Kingdom, Spain and, outside Europe, Mexico, Argentina, United States. The majority of the companies ($\sim$91%) has business activities in Europe.

Furthermore, there was also a regular distribution of respondents from small and medium-sized enterprises ($\sim$75%) and large entities with more than 1000 employees ($\sim$25%). Overall, while more than half of respondents (55.3%) has already a strategy in place for using big data and related technologies, only 34.2% among the respondents are effectively using big data and related technologies, 35.5% are starting using them, 13.2% are on a planning phase, and only 17.1% have no experience. Concerning the data sources, the most exploited sources are log ($\sim$45%), transactions ($\sim$32%), events (40%), sensors (32%), and open Data (30%). The latter are the ones with the higher rate of willingness for exploitation in the next 5 years together with Social Media and Free-Form Text. Quite surprisingly, the sample has shown little interest in data coming from phone usage, reports to authorities, radio-frequency identification (RFIDs) scans or point of sale (POS), selected by only $\sim$5% of the respondents, and geospatial data (10%). In general, $\sim$72.6% of data sources are multilingual, namely the language of the country of origin of the respondent; whereas only $\sim$50% of the sample declared to have the needed tools to handle different languages.

As for data sources considered relevant yet not fully exploited we count log, social media and open data, where the main obstacles preventing their use are related to security, privacy and legal issues, availability and discoverability of data, lack of a common data model and lack of the necessary skills or strategy within the organization. Actually, most of respondents (40%) stated that less than 10% of data collected is further processed for activities connected to value creation and capture, although they also foreseen an increase in the next five years. The limited exploitation of big data seems associated to a reduced information capacity of organizations and analytics capabilities [37, 38], where $\sim$one organization out of four has the right analytics to handle big data and $\sim$one organization out of six has the right tools to handle unstructured data expressed in natural language. However, the majority of respondents stated the willingness to have them in five years, the weakness could be related to the fact that more than 60% of respondents have both data collection and data analytics are in-house, while only a few are outsourced; thus, requiring an IT transformation rather than a simple reconfiguration or renew of the IT portfolio.

At present, the tools main technologies in use for big data analytics among the respondents are Hadoop (Apache) 21% and Microsoft Power BI (17%). Furthermore,

50% of the respondents answered they have tools to translate data between languages, from the survey no general tool(s) emerge as used for this purpose. Finally, only 36.5% of respondents declared that they share data with other subjects (especially, customers, public administration or governmental bodies and authorities, but also suppliers or partner companies) having an accountable added value in terms of development of new services, branding, and better decision-making.

## 5 Conclusion

The paper presented the results from a multi-industry and multi-country survey aimed to understand the needs and requirements as well the actual use of big data and analytics by public and private organizations, with a specific focus on social value impacts. Notwithstanding the descriptive nature of the survey and analysis of the results, the picture that emerges may provide an early understanding and outline further research on the following points, some of them partially resonating state of the art challenges in the management information systems literature, that we categorize in terms of *big data efficiency* (the capacity to simply elaborate big data), *effectiveness* (the capacity to elaborate big data and use it to create value), and *accessibility* of a given organization (the capacity to elaborate big data and use it to create value and capture value from their sharing):

- *Big data efficiency*: the survey showed a challenge in the *low utilization rate* at company level (IT is the main user, according to ~89% of the respondents) of the data collected including the ones pointed out as most relevant, due to data heterogeneity (i.e. structured and unstructured, and different languages) as well as privacy and security issues.
- *Big data effectiveness*: the survey showed a challenge in the *lack of right tools and capabilities* (~27% say not having them, and ~14% not knowing it) with the available tools considered difficult to use, especially for what concerns multilingual data.
- *Big data accessibility*: the survey showed a challenge in the *low rate of digital transformation of the company* (~40% says that less than 10% of the overall data collected by their organization are used for value generation activities), which could improve the data collection (~63%) and analysis (~67%), still mainly in-house, and data sharing with other entities (only ~38% of the respondents currently share their data).

Taking these issues into account, the survey and related results have limitations, related among other issues to the high percentage of the participants belonging to the IT industry and the number of respondents, which would require further sampling at country level for each industry among the ones considered as well as a granular consideration of demographic data. Nevertheless, we believe that the preliminary results discussed in this paper have at least the point of strength of highlighting some small traces of what could be the needs of organizations and the symptoms worth investigating for the under exploitation of big data by companies that are not "digital natives".

**Acknowledgements.** This work was supported by the AEGIS project, which has received funding from the European Union's Horizon 2020 research and innovation program under grant agreement No. 732189. The document reflects only the author's views and the Commission is not responsible for any use that may be made of information contained therein.

# References

1. The Economist: Big Data (2011)
2. The Economist: Data, data everywhere (2010)
3. IBM: What is big data? http://www-01.ibm.com/software/data/bigdata/
4. Kitchin, R., McArdle, G.: What makes big data, big data? Exploring the ontological characteristics of 26 datasets. Big Data Soc. **3**, 2053951716631130 (2016)
5. Dumbill, E.: Making sense of big data (editorial). Big Data **1**, 1–2 (2013)
6. Viscusi, G., Batini, C.: Digital information asset evaluation: characteristics and dimensions. In: Caporarello, L., Di Martino, B., Martinez, M. (eds.) Smart Organizations and Smart Artifacts. LNISO, vol. 7, pp. 77–86. Springer, Cham (2014). https://doi.org/10.1007/978-3-319-07040-7_9
7. Buhl, H.U., Röglinger, M., Moser, F., Heidemann, J.: big data - a fashionable topic with(out) sustainable relevance for research and practice? Bus. Inf. Syst. Eng. **5**, 65–69 (2013)
8. Benington, J., Moore, M.H.: Public Value - Theory and Practice. Palgrave Macmillan, Basingstoke (2011)
9. Cordella, A., Bonina, C.M.: A public value perspective for ICT enabled public sector reforms: a theoretical reflection. Gov. Inf. Q. **29**, 512–520 (2012)
10. Morris, S., Shin, H.: Social value of public information. Am. Econ. Rev. **92**, 1521–1534 (2002)
11. Batini, C., Rula, A., Scannapieco, M., Viscusi, G.: From data quality to big data quality. J. Database Manag. **26**, 60–82 (2015)
12. Viscusi, G., Castelli, M., Batini, C.: Assessing social value in open data initiatives: a framework. Futur. Internet **6**, 498–517 (2014)
13. Abbasi, A., Sarker, S., Chiang, R.H.L.: Big data research in information systems: toward an inclusive research agenda. J. Assoc. Inf. Syst. **17**, 3 (2016)
14. Oliveira, T., Martins, M.: Literature review of information technology adoption models at firm level. Electron. J. Inf. **14**, 110–121 (2011)
15. Thong, J.Y.L.: An integrated model of information systems adoption in small businesses. J. Manag. Inf. Syst. **15**, 187–214 (1999)
16. Oliveira, T., Thomas, M., Espadanal, M.: Assessing the determinants of cloud computing adoption: an analysis of the manufacturing and services sectors. Inf. Manag. **51**, 497–510 (2014)
17. Davis, F.: Perceived usefulness, perceived ease of use, and user acceptance of information technology. MIS Q. **13**, 319–340 (1989)
18. Venkatesh, V., Bala, H.: Technology acceptance model 3 and a research agenda on interventions. Decis. Sci. **39**, 273–315 (2008)
19. Venkatesh, V., Morris, M.G., Davis, G.B., Davis, F.D.: User acceptance of information technology: toward a unified view. MIS Q. **27**, 425–478 (2003)
20. DeLone, W.H., McLean, E.R.: Information system success: the quest for the dependent variable. Inf. Syst. Res. **3**, 60–95 (1992)
21. DeLone, W.H., McLean, E.R.: The DeLone and McLean model of information systems success: a ten-year update. J. Manag. Inf. Syst. **19**, 9–30 (2003)

22. Petter, S., DeLone, W., McLean, E.: Measuring information systems success: models, dimensions, measures, and interrelationships. Eur. J. Inf. Syst. **17**, 236–263 (2008)
23. Ives, B., Olson, M.H., Baroudi, J.J.: The measurement of user information satisfaction. Commun. ACM **26**, 785–793 (1983)
24. Baroudi, J., Orlikowski, W.: A short-form measure of user information satisfaction: a psychometric evaluation and notes on use. J. Manag. Inf. Syst. **4**, 44–59 (1988)
25. Iivari, J., Ervasti, I.: User information satisfaction: IS implementability and effectiveness. Inf. Manag. **27**, 205–220 (1994)
26. Wixom, B.H., Todd, P.A.: A theoretical integration of user satisfaction and technology acceptance. Inf. Syst. Res. **16**, 85–102 (2005)
27. Ahituv, N.: A systematic approach towards assessing the value of an information system. MIS Q. **4**, 61–75 (1980)
28. Ahituv, N.: Assessing the value of information: problems and approaches. In: DeGross, J.I., Henderson, J.C., Konsynski, B.R. (eds.) International Conference on Information Systems (ICIS 1989), pp. 315–325. Massachusetts, Boston (1989)
29. Viscusi, G., Spahiu, B., Maurino, A., Batini, C.: Compliance with open government data policies: an empirical assessment of Italian local public administrations. Inf. Polity. **19**, 263–275 (2014)
30. Newsted, P.R., Huff, S.L., Munro, M.C.: Survey instruments in information systems. MIS Q. **22**, 553 (1998)
31. Dillman, D.A., Smyth, J.D., Christian, L.M.: Internet, Mail, and Mixed-Mode Surveys: The Tailored Design Method. Wiley, Hoboken (2008)
32. AEGIS: Project At a Glance. https://www.aegis-bigdata.eu
33. Tsai, C.-W., Lai, C.-F., Chao, H.-C., Vasilakos, A.V.: Big data analytics: a survey. J. Big Data **2**, 21 (2015)
34. Chen, M., Mao, S., Liu, Y.: Big data: a survey. Mob. Netw. Appl. **19**, 171–209 (2014)
35. Porter, M.E., Millar, V.E.: How information gives you competitive advantage. Harv. Bus. Rev. **63**, 149–162 (1985)
36. Zillner, S., et al.: Big data-driven innovation in industrial sectors. In: Cavanillas, J.M., Curry, E., Wahlster, W. (eds.) New Horizons for a Data-Driven Economy, pp. 169–178. Springer, Cham (2016). https://doi.org/10.1007/978-3-319-21569-3_9
37. Sambamurthy, V., Bharadwaj, A., Grover, V.: Shaping agility through digital options: reconceptualizing the role of information technology in contemporary firms. MIS Q. **27**, 237–263 (2003)
38. Chen, D.Q., Preston, D.S., Swink, M.: How the use of big data analytics affects value creation in supply chain management. J. Manag. Inf. Syst. **32**, 4–39 (2015)

# A Step Foreword Historical Data Governance in Information Systems

José Pedro Simão and Orlando Belo[✉]

ALGORITMI R&D Centre, Department of Informatics, School of Engineering,
University of Minho, Campus de Gualtar, 4710-057 Braga, Portugal
obelo@di.uminho.pt

**Abstract.** From major companies and organizations to smaller ones around the world, databases are now one of the leading technologies for supporting most of organizational information assets. Their evolution allows us to store almost anything often without determining if it is in fact relevant to be saved or not. Hence, it is predictable that most information systems sooner or later will face some data management problems and consequently the performance problems that are unavoidably linked to. In this paper we tackle the data management problem with a proposal for a solution using machine-learning techniques, trying to understand in an intelligent manner the data in a database, according to its relevance for their users. Thus, identifying what is really important to who uses the system and being able to distinguish it from the rest of the data is a great way for creating new and efficient measures for managing data in an information system.

**Keywords:** Information systems management · Databases systems
Data governance · Data quality · Machine learning

## 1 Introduction

One of the most valuable business elements in an organization is an Enterprise Resource Planning (ERP) system. An ERP system serves as a cross - functional enterprise backbone that integrates and automates many internal business processes and information systems [1]. Generally, every ERP system has a huge database system beneath it, depending on the business scale of the organization. But, typically, they are pretty large and complex systems that are constantly transacting data and, consequently, they are continuously growing in terms of data. Usually, the information that is kept in an ERP system is very sensible. However, usually there are some parts of the global data that are not so important. Possibly, due to the fact that those parts are not so frequently used, are becoming historical throughout the lifetime of the system, or simply because that data does not represent any worthy value for system users. Assuming that an ERP system may support a business for years, it is predictable that in most cases there is some information that will lose value along its lifetime. Consequently, an enormous quantity of disposable information will be generated on the long run, being possible to identify and separate it from the rest, as already concluded. Nonetheless, this may also be a problem in any database regardless of its size [2, 3]. The question is how to do that?

© Springer Nature Switzerland AG 2019
M. Themistocleous and P. Rupino da Cunha (Eds.): EMCIS 2018, LNBIP 341, pp. 80–90, 2019.
https://doi.org/10.1007/978-3-030-11395-7_8

By classifying existent data, it is possible to know what is important and what is not, which is extremely valuable for an organization. For instance, for each and any case, it is possible to discover and create new governance policies for acting upon the classified data based on the fact of what is important for users and for business processes. For example, if the data dimension is the main concern of a particular entity, then it is probably better to remove the useless data, or store it somewhere else. Nevertheless, if the dimension is not so important, another good method for increasing system performance could be caching the most important data into a secondary memory structure with faster access. This could be very interesting if there is a huge volume of data in a database that cannot be removed, but only parts of it are used frequently. With the acquired knowledge, it is possible to act accordingly to system struggles, and establish a valid approach for enterprise data governance [4, 5]. However, the main concept to retain here is that it is only possible to have this range of new possibilities if there is a way to retrieve those conclusions from any database table dataset. User behaviour analysis [6] could be very helpful to determine what are his main tasks and duties on each session and making possible to translate and transform those conclusions into actions that are going to be applied to the data itself. Heuristic methods, like determining the most queried or frequent attribute of a table, or the most common value of an attribute, also provide information about what is important in a system.

In this paper we will expose and discuss the need for reducing the dimension of useless data and improve the quality of a database by knowing what is really important to a user, in order to propose an alternative data governance approach for information systems, tackling the data management problem using machine-learning techniques for dealing with data according to its relevance for users. In the following sections we will expose and discuss some related work (Sect. 2), present the data governance approach we designed for historical data in information systems (Sect. 3), and finally a brief set of conclusions and future working lines (Sect. 4).

## 2   Background

Relational databases were designed and built in an era completely different from this one and, consequently, they are not very adequate to this new age of information [7]. A database has to fit a certain purpose and to guarantee the requirements that have to be taken into consideration, often imposing database management policies redefinition to administrators. This why is so crucial to establish an effective approach for data governance. A strict plan and measures for ruling data is certainly going to be a major improvement in the way administrators control their systems and create solutions to oppose the eventual problems. Data management is not a single task or something that may be singularly identified. It can be seen as a collection of procedures and definitions that are related to the governance of the information in any database system. Basically, it is related with every aspect of systems' data, involving duties and procedures that have to be defined and executed for ensuring the quality of the systems. More specifically, some of the tasks that are included in data management are data reduction and inconsistency detection, the data strategy definition, which are a new and very interesting topic, data monitoring, business understanding and many others.

The development of Database Management Systems (DBMS) was probably the most influential improvement in database systems optimization. Still, these systems were unable to cope with the current state of the dimension of the data and business demands. Systems needed other kind of performance upgrades. Nevertheless, it is important emphasizing the relevance of DBMS and their evolution in this subject, which played the most crucial role. Given the current state of the information systems and DBMS, database designers struggled with the relational database tuning to be able to create sustainable ways for maintaining their systems. At the same time, we also assisted to the emergence of techniques for tuning databases, data storage and data management [8]. Disk striping and distributed techniques are also available for parallel processing and I/O access [9]. For some cases, caching is also an awesome optimization as well as some other more exquisite techniques, like query planners, query cost estimation or other strategies for improving querying performance were also key factors in the optimization subject [10, 11].

Other interesting ideas for data management came from data warehousing systems, which were concepts out of the box for the standards in any database system. Despite that, some of them really offered significant improvements in the performance, such as table denormalization or aggregation techniques, which are crucial for ensuring database performance. For example, a very interesting technique is the integrating usage analysis on cube view selection technique [12]. In brief, the optimization revolution is still a subject of huge relevance for investigation - new techniques are constantly being developed. The crucial idea to retain is that every information system has its own requirements and flaws and one must be able to identify them for develop better and adequate optimizations. If we changed our research view to the machine-learning domain we can realize the enormous breakthrough in the way humans analyse data, especially in the data-mining field. Machine learning techniques allow for learning from data and other sources of information, in order to build models that can be used to predict, score and classify data properties in a much easier way than before [13–15].

## 3   An Alternative Approach for Data Governance

### 3.1   The Relevance of the Data

The purpose of this research work was to formulate a solution for using machine learning methods for classifying data according to the relevance for users. With this capability it is possible to discover problems in a system as well as what evaluate its data quality. This kind of insights is truly valuable for improving data management and having a proactive behaviour towards this matter. Being aware of the problems that could affect the systems and where the value stands, the basic idea for a data governance solution is to identify and classify data according to their usage. The methodological approach we have follow (Fig. 1) was to develop a solution based on machine learning techniques for classifying data extracted from a database according to its relevance to users. Having every table instance classified, users or system administrators will have the ability to decide accurately about how to proceed and manage the information based on those results and conclusions. Basically, one can adapt data governance measures by having access to the relevance factor for each piece of information. The process acts as a low-level procedure, which analysis data on the operational level that unlocks new high-level measures for improving system performance and quality.

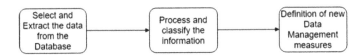

**Fig. 1.** A sketch of the main stages of the data governance approach.

Since the most adequate algorithms for classifying information are supervised methods, there must be a way to gather knowledge about system usage, and a translation into insights that may help the information classification process, according to the system's user relevance. One way this could be achieved is using database operational logs analysis, with the help of user behaviour detection systems, or simply by asking users what is preferable. Usually, databases operation registry is full of worthy information about the relevance of the data that may be explored. The behaviour detection may also provide more knowledge that could be induced on the training sets. As for the auxiliary systems, these represent further alternatives that must be explored in order to capture more information and tune the one that is already available. The coordination of all this ensures the consistency of the implementation process and provides expected results we expect. Finally, one more requirement that must be considered is the fact that it must be conducted a supervision through some follow-up tasks for ensuring the correctness of the solution and results.

## 3.2 Processing the Data

All the procedures we created were related with how data has to be extracted from a database, pre-processed and scaled before applying the machine learning process. Therefore, it is safe to say that the system we designed is composed by a main core and set of secondary systems for ensuring its efficiency and performance. The program and most of the auxiliary systems were built in Java [16], and as way to facilitate data processing and compatibility issues, we also select the machine-learning engine Weka platform [17], which offers a complete data mining module composed by machine learning algorithms for different mining processes [18]. Finally, for increasing the accuracy and explore further available algorithms, it was also implemented a deep learning algorithm offered by the H2O platform [19].

To better understand the data processing procedure and its application, we organized the architecture procedures in four major phases. The first one is the table selection or scope definition phase, which happens when the tables from the database system are selected before the data extraction, and therefore it is being defined the scope of analysis. Right after that, it is imperative to build the training and testing

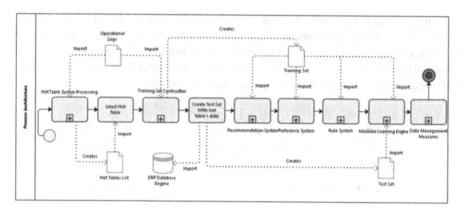

**Fig. 2.** A schematic view of the data processing system.

datasets. This is the second phase. Having access to the datasets, the next phase is to submit them into the machine- learning module so that they can be classified. Finally, we reach the fourth and final stage, where we adequate the management measures based on the analysis over the labelled data. In Fig. 2 we can see a schematic view of the data processing system and its auxiliary functional components, using a BPMN (Business Process Model and Notation) conceptual schema. In all the four distinct phases, the system starts for selecting the most adequate tables to be taken into further analysis through the observation of the database operational logs. The training set construction is next task to be performed. It uses the operational logs as well for performing the first scoring phase. Basically, it consists in defining an initial relevance grade for each logged instance from the table in analysis, according to its operation for building the first training dataset. The database operational logs were used to create the training set and to add general knowledge about the system. Building the testing set is a simple task, as it is only required to extract the database raw data and create an intermediate readable file by the machine-learning module. The procedures after the dataset construction tasks compose the training set second scoring phase, which is executed by the auxiliary system components. Each one of these systems adjusts and refines the training set initial relevance scoring differently, but are all based in knowledge about user preferences over data. The preference and rule systems act as a kind of filters based on user criteria about certain data aspects. However, rules perform a stronger influence than preferences. The "Recommendation System" component was designed to generate automatically suited user preferences over data by mining the initial association rules of the training set. It spares the hard work of having to define numerous preferences and rules for each data object. After having the training set scored, the machine learning engine processing composes the third phase.

In the "Machine-Learning Engine" component we incorporate the implementation of two supervised classifiers, namely the Naive Bayes classifier and a Deep Learning algorithm, along with some auxiliary tools for supporting the machine learning process. The choice on what is the best algorithm to perform the classifications was a hard one, since there is a fair amount of options and some perform better than others do, depending on each particular dataset and purpose. Another development issue was related to the data preparation of each different set, which demands specific data preparation procedures. Hence, from the analysis performed, the Naive Bayes algorithm seemed to offer the best performance with the minimum data preparation, which is ideal for the majority of the cases found.

## 3.3 Application Scenarios

In order to evaluate the data governance approach, we designed and conducted a set of tests over two distinct ERP databases (a university department ERP and a retail company ERP), analyzing both results to comprehend the usefulness of the solution proposed. For each application scenario we conducted a general execution over the entire database, and other specific test for analysing the effect of the process in the most impactful table of each information system, with the purpose to measure the total processing time, and have a broad idea of the feasibility of the approach in that matter. In both cases, the percentage of data classified with a new meaning was also analysed, since it is relevant to determine the potential usefulness of the procedure. The user behaviour detection system was also evaluated, having the purpose to compare the results of the procedure with the auxiliary system and study its impact and viability for other solutions based in the proposed process. Finally, for comparing the implemented machine learning algorithms, it was conducted a final evaluation, a single table test run in which both of the algorithms make the classification of the same dataset. Through this evaluation, it was possible to compare both algorithms in terms of performance, and acknowledge the real differences between both implementations. Single table tests were repeated three times for each application scenario, which allowed for getting an average of the measured results in the analysis phase.

| Table | University Department dbo.Movimentos | Retail Company dbo.Movimentos | | University Department | Retail Company |
|---|---|---|---|---|---|
| No. of attributes | 91 | 91 | Total no. of distinct tables with logs | 133 | 20 |
| No. of instances | 1,071,727 | 363,002 | No. of selected tables | 20 | 19 |
| No. of operational logs | 102,607 | 93,262 | Average no. of instances per selected table | 24,326 | 57,553 |
| No. of test executions | 3 | 3 | Average no. of operational logs per table | 13,007 | 76,331 |
| No. of preferences | 3 | 3 | Total no. of operational logs | 1,729,906 | 1,526,636 |
| No. of rules | 2 | 2 | | | |
| a) Application scenarios | | | b) General system | | |

**Fig. 3.** Execution tests results.

In Fig. 3(a) it is presented the specifications of the tests for each evaluated scenario. Note that rules and preferences were defined with additional analytical software. The strategy defined for performing the general system execution was similar to the one for single table tests. As for the number of tables to be analysed, it was only considered to be valid the ones that had operational logs registered. This way, it was ensured that only the tables that were used are selected. The "Hot Table System" component performs the selection process, and it has certain criteria that need to be defined. The first one to be defined is the minimum usage factor, 5% of the total logs, and its weight, 60% of the total assigned to define the colour for each table later in a coloured graph (Fig. 4). As for the space criteria, the minimum and maximum space factors weight the same (20% each) in the colour definition decision and their percentages were defined to be of 5% and 70%, respectively. From this, we selected 20 (15%) tables from the first ERP and 19 (95%) from the second one. These criteria values were equal for both scenarios for simplifying analysis, and the preferences and the rules were generated by a utility based on the most frequent attributes and values of each table. In Fig. 3(b) it is presented the details of the specifications for each case. Finally, we did a last test using the Deep Learning and Naive Bayes algorithms. The deep learner was implement to cope with the main algorithm's flaws, hence, it is seen as more powerful already. However, the purpose of this evaluation is to compare the actual difference between both of them and study the performance of the deep learning algorithm in particular. As for the actual specification of the test, it is the same as the single table test for the university department. The only change is the data preparation of the training set, which was adapted to fit each algorithm.

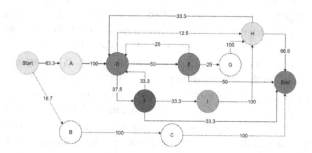

**Fig. 4.** An example of a coloured graph generated by the system. (Color figure online)

### 3.4   Evaluating the Process

We start the evaluation process with the university department ERP application scenario. Therefore, as for the general execution test, the prepared operational logs have more than 1,700,000 entries. From that total was possible to distinguish 133 different tables. The number of records reveals a small volume of system usage data due to the portion of tables that was possible to identify. This reveals that there is not enough information on most of the structures of the system in these logs. However, this is not a problem, because the remaining tables are not used. Thus, they are not relevant for analysis. From the available operational records, it was possible to build a structure with the queried tables for each user session, in order to create the corresponding coloured graph (Fig. 4). After the colouring phase of the graph it is possible to select the most adequate tables to be processed. From the resulting selection, about 15% (20) of the tables with records were selected, which greatly reduced the analysis process. Each table was processed after the selection process, by the machine-learning engine of the prototype to achieve the actual predictions. Once the procedure was finished, the average time measured was approximately 2 h and 3 min, which is an average of 6.15 min for each selected table. The average number of instances distinguished with a new meaning was of 74%, which means that it is possible to create new measures for a huge chunk of the total data. The instances classified as non-relevant were of 9.43% on average. This last percentage represents a more realistic portion of the data that could be removed, since it is given as little relevant. The average accuracy of the model measured was of about 83% from the cross-validation evaluation, which is a very acceptable result, since the data preparation was based on the generic approach defended. The execution time is believed also to be good, since the database has a dimension of about 4 GB of data to be classified, and the average of logs per table is 12,782 entries for preparing and training the models.

Next, we evaluated the retail company application scenario for comparing its results with the previously application case. In this case, the database is a kind of a small snapshot of the information held in one of the company store's information system. Nevertheless, the dimension of the data is quite similar to the first application scenario. In this second case, the time of general execution of the test on average for the three runs was 4 h, 10 min and 12 s, which represents an average of about 13 min for each processed table. This result was quite satisfying and at the same time expected, since the average number of operational records for each table (76,331) and the average of instances per table (57,553) were higher than in the previous scenario. This leads to an increased demand of the machine-learning engine, which leads to a lower performance when classifying data. The database only had 20 distinct tables in the operational logs, but the percentage of tables selected was much higher than in the previous case, which was of 95% (19) of the tables. This reveals that those tables represent the critical data for this scenario and a great majority of it was processed by the prototype. As for the classifications results and evaluation of the general execution tests, the average correctness accuracy for the predictions measured was of 97%, using cross-validation. This confirms the efficiency of the Naive Bayes algorithm, since the alternative was never used in this case. Besides, this excellent result also highlights the efficient data preparation arranged to construct the datasets that trained the models.

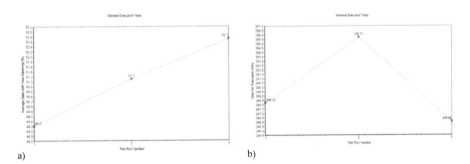

a)                                                    b)

**Fig. 5.** General execution tests analysis.

From this analysis it is also possible to conclude, that the evaluation conducted confers an elevate grade of confidence of the results created. From the classification analysis, it was possible to unveil that about 51% of the total data analysed was given a new meaning. This result is quite lower than the one registered in the previous case.

Nonetheless, it still reveals a good amount of data that could be treated to improve the system performance. Besides, the percentage of data classified as little relevant was of about 27%. This result is explained with the amount of historical data that is held in this second database – a large number of old purchases and sales records. In Fig. 5 we have two charts representing, respectively, the average data classified with a new meaning (a) as well as the average time for the three total executions of this test (b).

### 3.5    User Behaviour Detection

After the evaluation process we conducted a comparison of the general execution tests for the first application scenario against the same test specification, but now including the user behaviour system as an auxiliary scoring system. This way, the analysis focused on the same perspectives as in the previous tests. As for the results, the average execution time was quite similar to the analogue general execution tests, since the average duration measured was of 2 h and 23 min. The duration equivalence between this test and the general execution can be explained by the fact that there was only one modification between the two test specifications - the auxiliary scoring systems. The processing time from of scoring system is quite low in comparison with the machine-learning engine. Therefore, the performance was not affected significantly. With that comes another interesting fact, which is the good performance of the implemented scoring systems. Another factor that influenced the total duration was the request of the deep learner one more time (3 times on average) than in the general test execution. The average accuracy of the models measured by cross-validation evaluation was of 87%, which reveals the same efficiency as the one measured before. This also indicates that the auxiliary systems did not affect the machine-learning methods performance on building robust models.

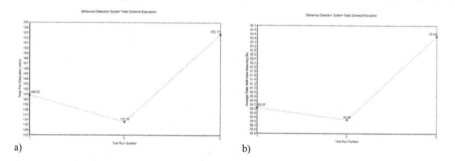

a)                                                                b)

**Fig. 6.** A schematic view of the data processing system.

However, the total percentage of data that was classified with a new meaning decreased a little. This time, the average value measured was of 61%, which reveals that the knowledge induced by the behaviour was not decisive enough. The reason for this was that behaviour was simulated and did not provide conclusive user preferences for refining the training sets of the models. To improve these results, it is required to capture real user behaviour for reflecting real usage knowledge and increase user preferences by combining this auxiliary system with the others. Nevertheless, the results achieved are quite enlightening for realising the feasibility of the system and its capability for improving the knowledge gathering that supports the defended the approach we did in this case. As for the duration of the procedure and average accuracy of the model, they demonstrate that the designed architecture for the process for building the predictive models is efficient and light in terms of performance. In Fig. 6 we present two charts showing the execution time (a) and the average data (b), respectively, with new meaning found in the three total executions of this test.

## 4    Conclusions and Future Work

Data management problems are a reality for many years to come, especially the ones related with data governance. It is quite important to discover new ways for handling data and improve governance measures for databases systems. An approach like the one we presented here could be a helpful way to attenuate such problems. It may not be the most effective solution since it has an error percentage associated with the results. Nonetheless, it is definitely a robust and different solution that could bring significant improvements in a large diversity of information systems. We believe that the data governance approach presented here is a valuable proposal due to the perceptions that it provides, in order to create and adapt management measures for implementing in an information system. Having data classified according to the relevance given by system users is a very effective way for discovering new insights about data, which can be used to refine data management processes of an information system. Additionally, the way we explored the problem of data governance is also a proper way for determining the quality of the data of a particular information system - what matters to system users matters to the system. This way, it is also believed that discovering the meaningful data to a user, implicitly is being defined what data quality is in a given system. Therefore, it is safe to say that the proposed data management process may serve as an example of a great tool for supporting data management in most information systems. The study of the impact of the application of this data management process in a long - term analysis will sustain some future research work. Understanding the impact in data quality and management will be a valuable validation of the approach we presented and discussed in this paper.

**Acknowledgments.** This work has been supported by COMPETE: POCI-01-0145-FEDER-007043 and FCT – Fundação para a Ciência e Tecnologia within the Project Scope: UID/CEC/00319/2013.

## References

1. George Marakas, G., O'Brien, J.: Management Information Systems. McGraw-Hill Education, New York City (2010)
2. Marr, B.: Big data overload: why most companies can't deal with the data explosion. Forbes (2016). https://www.forbes.com/sites/bernardmarr/2016/04/28/big-data-overload-most-comp anies-cant-deal-with-the-data-explosion/#70cbd9506b0d. Accessed 25 May 2018

3. Marr, B.: Big data: 20 mind-boggling facts everyone must read. Forbes (2015). https://www.forbes.com/sites/bernardmarr/2015/09/30/big-data-20-mind-boggling-facts-everyone-must-read/#618e985417b1. Accessed 25 May 25 2018
4. Russom, P.: Data governance strategies. Bus. Intell. J. 13(2), 13–15 (2008)
5. Newman, D., Logan, D.: Governance is an essential building block for enterprise information management. Gartner Research, pp. 1–9, May 2006
6. Angeletou, S., Rowe, M., Alani, H.: Modelling and analysis of user behaviour in online communities. In: Aroyo, L., et al. (eds.) ISWC 2011. LNCS, vol. 7031, pp. 35–50. Springer, Heidelberg (2011). https://doi.org/10.1007/978-3-642-25073-6_3
7. Grolinger, K., Higashino, W., Tiwari, A., Capretz, M.: Data management in cloud environments: NoSQL and NewSQL data stores. J. Cloud Comput. 2(1), 49:1–49:24 (2013)
8. Sakr, S., Liu, A., Batista, D., Alomari, M.: Survey of large scale data management approaches in cloud environments. IEEE Commun. Surv. Tutorials 13(3), 311–336 (2011)
9. LaBrie, R., Ye, L.: A paradigm shift in database optimization: from indices to aggregates, p. 5 (2002)
10. Jarke, M., Koch, J.: Query optimization in database systems. ACM Comput. Surv. 16(2), 111–152 (1984)
11. Ioannidis, Y.: Query optimization. ACM Comput. Surv. 28(1), 121–123 (1996)
12. Rocha, D., Belo, O.: Integrating usage analysis on cube view selection - an alternative method. Int. J. Decis. Support Syst. 1(2), 228 (2015)
13. Najafabadi, M.M., Villanustre, F., Khoshgoftaar, T.M., Seliya, N., Wald, R., Muharemagic, E.: Deep learning applications and challenges in big data analytics. J. Big Data 2(1), 1–21 (2015)
14. Qiu, J., Wu, Q., Ding, G., Xu, Y., Feng, S.: A survey of machine learning for big data processing. EURASIP J. Adv. Signal Process. (2016)
15. Al-Jarrah, O.Y., Yoo, P.D., Muhaidat, S., Karagiannidis, G.K., Taha, K.: Efficient machine learning for big data: a review. Big Data Res. 2, 87–93 (2015)
16. Arnold, K., Gosling, J., Holmes, D.: The Java Programming Language, 4th edn. Addison - Wesley, Upper Saddle River (2006)
17. Witten, I., Frank, E.: Data Mining: Practical Machine Learning Tools and Techniques. Morgan Kaufmann Series in Data Management Systems, 2nd edn. Morgan Kaufman, Amsterdam, Boston (2005)
18. Hall, M., Frank, E., Holmes, G., Pfahringer, B., Reutemann, P., Witten, I.: The WEKA data mining software: an update. ACM SIGKDD Explor. Newslett. 11(1), 10 (2009)
19. Candel, A., LeDell, E., Parmar, V., Arora, A.: Deep Learning with H2O - Booklet, 5th edn. H2O.ai, Inc., Mountain View (2017)

# Parliamentary Open Big Data: A Case Study of the Norwegian Parliament's Open Data Platform

Lasse Berntzen[✉], Rania El-Gazzar, and Marius Rohde Johannessen

University of South-Eastern Norway, Kongsberg, Norway
{lasse.berntzen,rania.el-gazzar,
marius.johannessen}@usn.no

**Abstract.** The paper presents a case study on the use of open big data in the Norwegian Parliament. A set of policy documents was examined to find motivation for publishing open data. The case study was based on an examination of the parliament website, combined with document studies and interviews. The paper concludes that third parties have used open data to create new applications that generate value for their users. Applying our findings to the open government benchmarking framework, we identify some national barriers and possible solutions to further promote the use and publication of open data.

**Keywords:** Open data · Big data · Parliament · Case study

## 1 Introduction

According to Open Knowledge International [1], open data is "data that can be freely used, modified and shared by anyone for any purpose". During the last decade, governments have promoted the use of open data by making data available in open data repositories. By making data available, it is possible for third parties to generate value by analyzing, visualizing and combining with data from other sources.

Laney [2] defines big data as data having high volume, high velocity and/or high variety. High volume refers to large amounts of data demanding both specialized storage and processing. High velocity refers to streams of real-time data, e.g., from sensor networks or large-scale transaction systems. Finally, high variety is about dealing with data from different sources having different formats.

Marr [3] finds the real value of big data is not in the large volumes of data itself but in the ability to analyze vast and complex data sets beyond anything we could ever do before. The introduction of new analysis techniques combined with new database technology has lowered the threshold of utilizing big data.

According to the Norwegian government's Digital Agenda [4], there are more than 1000 open datasets currently available in Norway. Most of them are found in the centralized data.norge.no repository, but several major organizations keep their own open data repositories, such as Statistics Norway, the weather service Yr.no, the Norwegian Central Bank, the Norwegian Labour and Welfare Administration, the Norwegian Mapping and Cadastre Authority, the Norwegian Public Roads Administration,

M. Themistocleous and P. Rupino da Cunha (Eds.): EMCIS 2018, LNBIP 341, pp. 91–105, 2019.
https://doi.org/10.1007/978-3-030-11395-7_9

the national Brønnøysund Register Centre, the Norwegian Parliament and many municipalities and county municipalities. There is no central registry over all available open data, which makes it difficult to get a complete overview. The various open data portals have links to applications and use cases, and many of them also have tutorials and guidelines for use.

The Norwegian Parliament has been actively using information and communication technology to increase transparency [5]. The website of the parliament provides access to documents used for decision making, minutes of meetings, and even webcasts of the meetings. The expansion to also provide access to the underlying data through application program interfaces and standard data formats shows the continuing commitment of the Norwegian Parliament to contribute to a transparent society.

The rest of the paper is organized as follows: Sect. 2 provides background, followed by Sect. 3 discussing theoretical perspectives on open government data. Section 4 discusses the methodology, and Sect. 5 presents our findings. The findings are discussed in Sect. 6, and finally, Sect. 7 provides a conclusion with a discussion of limitations and proposals for future work.

## 2  Background

Governments strive to reach acceptable levels of mutual government–citizen understanding by innovating with emerging computing technologies, such as open data and big data [6] to make a significant impact on societies through promoting government transparency and accountability, empowering citizens, and improving participation and public services [7, 8]. The emergence of open data and big data has received increasing interest from governments, which has been interpreted as a set of perceived potential benefits for governments and the whole society towards further democracy [9]. However, governments also experience barriers to widely adopt open data.

Benefits of open data for governments are categorized into political and social, economic, and operational and technical [10]. Political and social benefits of open data for governments include transparency and trust, democratic accountability, public engagement, self-empowerment of citizens, equal access to data, enabling the creation of new governmental and social services for citizens, improving citizen services, and improving policy-making processes. Economic benefits of open data for governments include stimulation of innovation by enabling the development of new products or services, contributing to the creation of a new sector adding value to the economy, and availability of information for companies and investors. The operational and technical benefits of open data for governments include enabling reuse of data instead of collecting it again; thus, removing duplicate efforts and costs. Furthermore, open data contribute to optimizing administrative processes, supporting decision-making by enabling comparisons, making it easy to discover and access the data, creation of new data based on combining several data items, ensured integrity and external quality of data, and the ability to merge and integrate public and private data.

The barriers to adopting open data for governments are categorized into institutional, task complexity, and technical [10]. The institutional barriers include the focus on barriers and neglect of opportunities, conflict between public values (transparency vs. privacy values), lack of uniform policy for publicizing data, no clear process for dealing with user input, and debatable quality of information. The transparency offered by open government data platforms makes it possible for the public to have a clear sight over the government's activities and decisions; however, excessive use of linked open data (discoverable open data) with big data analytics may put governments in a problematic privacy situation (e.g., surveillance) [11]. Task complexity barriers include the meaning of data is not explained, duplication of data and that data is available in various forms or before/after processing making question marks around the sources, and users might not be aware of its potential uses. Another complexity barrier to adopting open government data is that the heterogeneity of the government agencies' infrastructure makes it difficult to implement a large-scale open data infrastructure [12]. The technical barriers include not having the data in a well-defined format that is easily accessible, lack of standards, no central portal or architecture, and no standard software for processing open data.

Apparently, the majority of the barriers are related to the concept of open data per se; perhaps the concept is blurry and raises complexity and privacy issues. According to the European Open Data Portal (EODP)[1], open data is data that anyone (i.e., governments, businesses, and individuals) can access, use and share to create social, economic and environmental benefits. The openness of open data lies in its format and license; open data should be made available in a standard machine-readable format, and people are permitted unlimitedly to make different uses of it (i.e., transforming, combining and sharing it with others, or using it for commercial purposes). The EODP related the openness of open data to cost where open data must be free to use, but not necessarily free to access. For entities implementing government open data platforms, they incur costs for creating, maintaining and publishing useful open data, as well as the provisioning of real-time big data.

The World Wide Web Foundation (W3F) asserted that the open government data initiatives build on the involvement of government, civil society, and private sector [13]. The potential impacts of open government data depend on the choice and implementation of open government data policy [13]. In the US, the policies for creating, managing, disseminating and preserving digital government information were too complex and existed before the emergence of open data and big data technologies; thus, these policies failed to address the use of government open and big data [14]. As a result, it was recommended to develop a "Big and Open Data governance model" to address related issues, such as privacy, data accuracy and reuse, archiving and preservation, resources for data curation (accumulation, modification, integration, and manipulation), and developing data standards and sustainable data platforms [14]. In Australia, the government had an ambition and a plan to establish a policy for open

---

[1] www.europeandataportal.eu.

data, but the Australian government faced technical, legal and cultural barriers [8]. The Australian government lacked the consistency of how the open data would be formatted, had no clear sight to ensure sufficient de-identification of data about individuals in a manner that does not violate the Australian Privacy Act requirements [8]. The cultural barrier to open and big government data in Australia is manifested in the public service culture of favoring secrecy of information as a default position [8]. In the UK, the open government data implementation faced significant issues related to data sharing policy, standardization of open government data and systems, lack of awareness about open government data, and government responsibility in providing the resources needed for open government data implementation [15].

## 3   Theoretical Perspectives on Open Government Data

Due to the newness of the open data phenomenon, few seminal articles contribute to understanding the different elements of open data policies and factors that influence their impact. Through a comparative approach, a study by Zuiderwijk and Janssen [16] developed a framework arguing that policy environment and context (i.e., levels of government organizations, motivations and objectives, legislation, and political and cultural contexts) influence the policy content (i.e., amount of open data, type and quality of open data, and requirement for accessing open data). As a result, the policy content influences the extent to which performance indicators of open government data are met (i.e., usages, risks, and benefits). The performance indicators can tell which public value is created and its impact on society. The framework was used to compare seven Dutch governmental policies for open data, and the takeaways from this comparison were that policies should have both internal and external focus, focusing on the impact and stimulating the use of open data, and creating a culture of open data. The framework is argued to help to implement open government data policies and to improve existing open government data policies.

Another seminal study by Veljković, Bogdanović, and Stoimenov [17] argue that the problem with comparing (or benchmarking) open government initiatives is the lack of open government conceptual clarity. Based on this argument, the authors of the paper developed a conceptual model of open government based on a set of indicators related to five pillars of open government: Collaboration, open data, data transparency, government transparency, and participation. The indicators related to each pillar are demonstrated in Table 1.

An earlier study by Zuiderwijk and Janssen [18] relies on "coordination theory" to identify coordination needs and challenges for open data and uses a set of coordination mechanisms to address those challenges and needs towards improving policy-making and decision-making. The principal argument of Zuiderwijk and Janssen is that the activities of the open data community are to a large extent uncoordinated. This stems from a number of factors. These factors are:

(1) various stakeholders are involved in the open data process (i.e., open data publishers, open data facilitators, users of open data, and open data legislators);

**Table 1.** Components of open government conceptual model (adapted from [17])

| Open government pillars | Open government indicators |
|---|---|
| Collaboration | Collaborative solutions for: |
| | - Government-to-Government |
| | - Government-to-Citizen |
| | - Government-to-Business |
| Open data | Open data characteristics: |
| | - Complete |
| | - Primary |
| | - Timely |
| | - Accessible |
| | - Machine processable |
| | - Non-discriminatory |
| | - Non-proprietary |
| | - License-free |
| Data transparency | - Authenticity |
| | - Understandability |
| | - Reusability |
| Government transparency | - Procedures |
| | - Tasks |
| | - Operations |
| | - Regulations |
| Participation | - Open dialog |

(2) open data publishers often lack a clear sight over what is done with the data, which value they can create and how they can be used for improving their own policies and decisions; and

(3) the fact that open data publishers and users are often not aware of each other's needs and activities (i.e., the format of data preferred by users and how to stimulate the use of open data).

Thus, coordination is argued to be important, as it leads to a better understanding of the open data process and results in integrated actions, improved performance, and improved policies. Zuiderwijk and Janssen identified six specific coordination challenges:

(1) inappropriate regulatory environment;
(2) fragmentation of open data;
(3) unclear boundaries of responsibilities;
(4) lack of feedback on open data use;
(5) lack of interconnected processes; and
(6) lack of standardized and planned processes.

They argue that the coordination challenges may be solved, not guaranteed though, by a mix of three coordination mechanisms:

(1)  coordination by standardization;
(2)  coordination by the plan; and
(3)  coordination by feedback.

# 4    Methodology

Our study is exploratory; an exploratory case study is a suitable method to address the "how" research questions [19] and understand the phenomenon in its natural context [20]. Our study started with: (1) a review of general benefits of and barriers to open and big government data; (2) a review of open and big government data initiatives in the US, UK, and Australia and the barriers experienced by those initiatives; and (3) a review of theoretical perspectives on open government data. Our study is also interpretive, as the data collection was not guided by pre-assumptions from literature or theory, and the theory-guided our analysis of the empirical findings [21]. The empirical inputs to our study relate to the context of Norway and involved: (1) document analysis by looking into on document studies found on the Norwegian Parliament's website and snowballed websites via Google describing services created using the Norwegian Parliament's open data, in addition to published Norwegian policy documents describing the need for open data; and (2) two e-mail interviews; one with an officer at the Norwegian Parliament and one with an informant at the communication department in the Parliament. The communication department is responsible for the open data platform and management of "Holder de ord", the largest user of Parliament open data. The use of e-mail interview method is appropriate in occasions when the informants are busy to be interviewed synchronously and it gives the informants the opportunity to have enough time to think and answer the interviewer's questions at their convenience [22–24]. The purpose of analyzing the documents was to get an overview of available data, and the interviews provided evidence about the motivation and intended results of using open and big government data. The findings from the case study were analyzed using the benchmark conceptual model for open government [17].

## 4.1    Policy Documents as Driver for Open Data

Searching for open data at the government website revealed seven reports to the parliament (white papers), three official Norwegian reports and two planning and strategy documents. Thematically, the documents are tagged in the following areas: business, the EU, research and education, health and welfare, immigration, climate, municipalities, culture, crisis management, and transportation. The first document appeared in 2012. Table 2 provides an overview of the policy documents mentioning open data. The policy documents cover a wide range of areas and discuss how open data can be helpful in different ways. While the individual mentions might not be large sections of each document, this range shows that open data is seen as an essential part of digitizing the public sector, when it comes to facilitating public sector efficiency, innovation and business development, information dissemination/availability/accessibility, transparency and crisis management/crime prevention. Several of the documents describe hackathons as essential for promoting the use of open data.

**Table 2.** Overview of Norwegian policy documents mentioning open data

|  | Document | Content | Objectives for open data |
|---|---|---|---|
| Reports to the Parliament (Whitepapers) | Digital Agenda [4] | Goals and objectives for digitizing the public sector, open data as an enabler, use cases | Transparency, smart cities, information, business development |
|  | White Paper on Medicinal Products - Correct use – better health [25] | Open pharmaceutical information to facilitate user-centric health services, and also improve the quality of medicinal information | Information, business development, transparency, quality |
|  | Collaboration in the Nordic countries [26] | Collaboration on open data-driven applications in the Nordic countries through a Nordic hackaton | Innovation, business development |
|  | Norway and the United Nations: Common Future, Common Solutions [27] | Describes UN projects on open data and social media | Information, crisis management |
|  | Visual art [28] | Describes open data's potential for visual arts and museums, using digital catalogs and indexes | Availability, accessibility |
|  | National plan for transport [29] | Potential of open data to improve transport solutions | Efficiency |
|  | Between Heaven and Earth - Norwegian space policy for business and public benefit [30] | Potential of open data from space projects | Business development |
| Official Norwegian Reports (NOU's) | NOU 2013:2 Barriers to digital value creation [31] | Open data as an enabler for value creation through new and improved applications | Business development, efficiency, transparency democratization |
|  | NOU 2016:7 Norway in transition [32] | Open data as a source for work and business statistics | Business development, employment |
|  | NOU 2017:11 Future organization of the Police force [33] | Develop open data solutions for crime prevention and investigation | Crime prevention |
| Planning and strategy reports | Ministry of Culture: Strategy for Open Data [34] | Strategy for creating and publishing open data from cultural institutions | Transparency, information, business development |
|  | Strategy for Open Research [35] | Principles and guidelines for secure sharing of research data | Quality of research, access to data, business development |

The primary policy document for open data in Norway is the 2016 "Digital Agenda for Norway" [4], which outlines the goals, objectives and overall strategy for digitization of the Norwegian public sector. The digital agenda follows up on earlier digitization plans, and provides a brief historical overview: In 2011, government agencies were asked to publish data in machine-readable formats, and in 2012 all-new digital services should have built-in mechanisms for exporting data sets to machine-readable formats, and to facilitate access through APIs. To facilitate access to open data, the Agency for Public Management and eGovernment (DIFI) have established data.norge. no as host for open data, for those who are not running their own. The digital agenda also discusses guidelines and regulations for open data publishing, as well as the Norwegian Open Data License for the use of open data.

## 5  Findings on Open Data in the Norwegian Parliament

The Norwegian parliament's open data platform is run as a companion website to the main www.stortinget.no site. Data is accessed through an application program interface (API). The open data platform was developed as part of a major overhaul of the website, where data on voting in parliament was made accessible. The first version of the platform had voting data and data on the cases that were being voted on, as well as questions from members of parliament. Since the launch, there has been continuous development.

In 2014, the platform was expanded to include information about the individual members of parliament and XML versions of documents and meeting referendums dating back to 2008. Early 2015 another extension was implemented, this time with data on Parliament meetings, meeting agendas and data on public hearing processes, as well as meeting minutes dating back to 1998. The biography section for members of parliament was also expanded. The latest update came in 2017 when the platform received an overhaul including user registration, and all documents and publications from the Norwegian Parliament was published. In total, more than 20.000 documents were made available.

The current platform contains the following data: Parliament sessions and years, counties (members of parliament are elected from their county), topics, political parties represented in parliament (past and present), committees, members of parliament bio (past and present), members of government, questions raised, cases, voting sessions and decisions, meetings, agendas, hearings, list of speakers, publications. Data can be combined using API calls so that users can e.g., list all speakers from a party on a specific topic or case, data on how representatives vote on specific issues, etc. There are plans for further expansion, and the respondent reports that the next step is to make data available as downloads as well as through the API. This is because journalists and other non-technical users find the API challenging to use and have asked for downloadable formats and a more straightforward user interface, so they can access the data without having to hire programmers to do the work. The need for technical competence is reported as a significant obstacle to increased use. There are also plans for including even more datasets.

## 5.1   Parliament's Motivation and Drivers for Open Data

According to the interview respondent from the parliament, the motivation for the open data platform was both external and internal. There was much pressure for opening up data on voting in parliament, especially from the people behind the service "Holder de ord?" ("Do they keep their words?") (see section on use for details), as well as from journalists making freedom of information requests and wanting easier access to data. Internally, motivation was driven by the need to become more efficient. Before the launch of data.stortinget.no, a lot of data had to be manually filed, hard-copied and sent to the institutions using it.

Both internal and external motivation should be seen in the context of the open data movement that emerged a decade ago. Several key people from industry, IT, news and academia pushed for more openness and freely accessible data both from the government, government institutions, agencies, and research institutions. The main argument was that data is valuable, can lead to innovative services as well as increased transparency, and that taxpayers had already paid for the data to be made, so they should not have to pay again to access it. As a result, the Norwegian Mapping and Cadastre Authority made all their geographical data available in 2013, the national Meteorological Institute publishes open weather data, and research institutions are pushing towards open access publishing of both data and research publications.

## 5.2   Use Cases of Data from Parliament

Several organizations make frequent use of data from the Norwegian parliament:

**Holder de ord** (Keeping promises) is an independent organization made up of volunteers and funded by freedom of speech organizations and the open source community. Their volunteers combine voting data with the programs of political parties to examine if they vote in accordance with their programs, as well as other related issues. Data published at "Holder de ord" is used by citizens and media alike to examine how parties and individual members of parliament vote. As the organization is closely related to the Norwegian open source movement, all the code for the service is available on Github[2]. The service started in 2012 to monitor climate policy, but as the Parliament released more data the service soon expanded to cover all political topics.

The interview respondent says they have around 40.000 annual visits. While many are from media, researchers, and organizations, they also have a large user base of regular citizens interested in politics. In recent years, statistics from the site have been on the front page of major national newspapers and featured in several radio broadcasts from the national Norwegian Broadcasting Corporation (NRK).

**Samstemmer.net** is another example. The application won the hackathon *apps4Norway* by making a database of how questions and voting by members of the parliament. While the project is no longer active, the source code is available on Github[3].

---

[2] https://github.com/holderdeord.

[3] https://github.com/eiriks/samstemmer.

**Briatte.org**[4] was made by Francois Briatte and is a network visualization of the ties between members of parliament, based on the bills they sponsor. The visualization mostly shows that natural allies sponsor the same bills but a closer examination reveals some surprising ties between parties that rarely agree on anything in the media.

**Talk of Norway** is a research project conducted by the University of Oslo experimenting with various machine learning techniques applied to data from the Parliament to explore how parliament sessions work. The project is a collaboration between language technology and political science scholars.

**Hackathons:** Several hackathons initiated by the Agency for Public Management and eGovernment (Difi) have used data from parliament. More recently, the hackathon *Hack4.no*, a collaboration between the Norwegian Mapping and Cadastre Authority and the University of South-Eastern Norway, has used parliamentary data on several occasions. The 2017 second runner-up used data from the Parliament to create an app in collaboration with the Office of the Auditor General of Norway.

**Media Use:** While some media outlets, such as the Guardian's data journalism team, have become proficient users of open data, Norwegian media are falling somewhat behind. A couple of the major newspapers and the national Norwegian Broadcasting Corporation (NRK) use open data in some stories, but the potential is far more significant. One example where data from parliament contributed is the website krisepakke.no, where the newspaper Klassekampen worked with several local newspapers to track where funding allocated to companies suffering from the 2015 fall in oil prices finally ended up. While this is an excellent example of data journalism, most of the collection processes were based on manual freedom of information queries, indicating that the potential for open data is far higher than what is currently realized when it comes to the media's role as watchdog.

## 6  Discussion

The Norwegian Parliament has made an effort to make its data open despite few limitations. We revisit the benchmark conceptual model for open government [17] presented in Table 1 and rely on it to assess how well the open data from the Norwegian Parliament fulfill the goals of open government. Table 3 builds on Table 1 and is based on observations from the Parliament open data website. The evidence from our study indicates that the open data from the Parliament meets the open government indicators, except being discriminatory (i.e., difficult to access by non-technical users). Furthermore, there are no interactive means of interactive communication (e.g., social media, blogging, photo and video sharing, etc.), where people can share their ideas, give their feedback on various matters of concern, and be involved in the policy-making process.

While the Norwegian Parliament in isolation does well on the open government indicators, there are several coordination challenges were evident if we look at open data at the national level (see Table 4). These challenges have been identified by [18]

---

[4] http://briatte.org/parlviz/stortinget/.

**Table 3.** Open government indicators revisited

| Open government pillars | Open government indicators (mapped to our case) | Evidence found |
|---|---|---|
| Collaboration | Collaborative solutions for: Government-to-Government | Allowing collaboration with Nordic countries, solving transport problems, supporting crime prevention and investigation |
| | Collaborative solutions for: Government-to-Consumer | Supporting researchers |
| | Collaborative solutions for: Government-to-Business | Support for work and business statistics, and providing open data hosting platforms for businesses |
| Open data | Open data characteristics: complete | Yes, within boundaries of the open data initiative |
| | Primary data | Yes, open data platform is connected to archival systems, so data is the same |
| | Timely publication of data | Data is published as soon as it becomes available |
| | Accessible | Accessible through API |
| | Machine processable | Format is XML |
| | Non-discriminatory | No, non-technical users still cannot download and make use of the data. Planned updates will make data more accessible |
| | Non-proprietary | Yes: Published under Norwegian open data license[a] |
| | License-free | Yes: Published under Norwegian open data license |
| Data transparency | Authenticity | Yes, parliament is verified publisher and in control of repository |
| | Understandability | Partially: Data requires some technical competence for use, making it challenging to for example journalists with no technical background |
| | Reusability | Yes, handled by Norwegian open data license |
| Government transparency | Procedures Tasks Operations Regulations | The framework for transparency is in place through open data license and guidelines for open data found in the digital agenda. In the parliament transparency is satisfactory |
| Participation | Open dialogue? | No explicit feedback mechanism except contact information to people responsible for repository. Heavy users ("Holder de ord," some journalists) have an on-going dialogue with data owners, and suggestions are implemented at regular intervals |

[a]http://data.norge.no/nlod/en/2.0

and are said to be addressed, not guaranteed though, by three coordination mechanisms: standardization, plan, and feedback as discussed earlier in this paper. However,
these mechanisms require in-depth coordination-related knowledge [18].

Furthermore, the identified challenges are mostly related to a lack of central
organization. While there has been a push towards publishing open data, as shown in
the examination of policy documents, there is still no central organization with the
mandate to force agencies to publish their data despite the infrastructure, regulation and
resources/support are in place. Explanations from the literature were that motivations to
develop open data policies are diverse across the government organizations, some are
willing to create an open data policy, and some others are skeptic and concerned about
the risks associated with open data [16]. This requires promoting a culture of openness
based on recognizing the fundamental principle of institutionalizing public ownership
of open data [16]. The institutionalization of the openness culture should not happen by
the legal pressures only, but also by social and political pressures as well as by having
entrepreneurs within the government organizations [16]. Thus, we propose that the next
step for open data in Norway should be creating and institutionalizing a culture of
openness at a national level to push more agencies, municipalities and counties to
publish their data. Cases such as the Norwegian Parliament could be used to demonstrate the potential outcomes of open data sets.

**Table 4.** Coordination challenges at the national level

| Coordination challenge | Examples from Norwegian open government |
|---|---|
| Inappropriate regulatory environment | The regulatory environment is in place to some extent. What is lacking is a stronger push to make government agencies publish open data sets |
| Fragmentation of open data | Norwegian open data is scattered across a wide range of repositories, there is no published central register of open data, and while a standard for publication is suggested, it is not necessarily followed by everyone |
| Unclear boundaries of responsibilities | In the government, there is no central responsibility for open data. Agencies are free to decide what and whether to publish anything |
| Lack of feedback on, and discussion of, data use | |
| Lack of interconnected processes | |
| Lack of standardized and planned processes | |

## 7 Conclusion and Future Work

This paper discusses the use of big and open data in a parliamentary setting. In 2013 the
Norwegian Parliament decided to publish a number of data sets related to what is
happening in the Parliament. We have looked into the intentions behind the release of
these data sets and have also discussed if the release fulfilled the intentions of the

decision-makers. We have also provided some ideas for utilizing these data in a broader context. We present findings from Parliament and use policy documents to examine the motivation and push towards open data in Norway. Finally, we propose that government should orchestrate a national push to get more agencies to publish their data and that the national repository data.norge.no is given responsibility for mapping and linking to all open data repositories in Norway, in order to facilitate open data becoming big and open data. This recalls the need for Big and Open Linked Data (BOLD) while preserving the privacy and freedom of the citizens [11].

## 7.1    Limitations

The policy documents listed in Table 2 was obtained by searching for "big data" and "open data" on the national government website. The search was limited to policy documents (Official Norwegian Reports, government white papers and related documents). The authors know several public sector initiatives related to big and open data, and the number of policy documents discussing the use of big and open data will increase. Still, the policy documents shows the that big and open data is discussed within a wide range of policy areas.

The paper is limited to a study of the Norwegian Parliament, their open data efforts, and how the data is used by others. The study does not compare what other parliaments are doing, but the paper may provide some ideas for other researchers interested in their parliament policy and use of open data.

## 7.2    Future Work

The following presents some possibilities for further work, using the open data provided by the Norwegian Parliament.

(1) Providing more straightforward access to data, user-guides and analysis software. As one of the respondents says, many requests for data come from journalists and other with little or no technical knowledge. To expand on the use of open data, providers should work on developing simpler access to datasets, guides for how to use and combine data, as well as easy to use software that can help people to find usage areas for the data.

(2) Linking the data to other open data sources represents an opportunity to make applications that may deliver results beyond the aims of the decision makers. Data from parliament can be linked to statistical and economic data to provide a better understanding of the impact of policy decisions.

(3) Making better visualizations. Visualization is a powerful tool for making results of open data analysis more understandable for ordinary citizens.

(4) Promoting a culture of openness to be institutionalized through social, political, and entrepreneurial pressures.

Future work may also include a comparison of open data policies and practices of other parliaments, and also how open data policies and practices change over time.

# References

1. Open Knowledge International: The Open Definition. https://opendefinition.org. Accessed 31 May 2018
2. Laney, D.: 3D data management: controlling data, volume, velocity, and variety. Technical report. META Group (2001)
3. Marr, B.: Big Data – Using Smart Big Data Analytics and Metrics to Make Better Decisions and Improve Performance. Wiley, Hoboken (2015)
4. Ministry of Local Government and Modernisation: Meld. St. 27 (2015–2016) Digital agenda for Norway – ICT for a simpler everyday life and increased productivity (2016). https://www.regjeringen.no/en/dokumenter/digital-agenda-for-norway-in-brief/id2499897/. Accessed 31 May 2018
5. Berntzen, L., Healy, M., Hahamis, P., Dunville, D., Esteves, J.: Parliamentary web presence – a comparative review. In: Proceedings of the 2nd International Conference on e-Government (ICEG 2006), Pittsburgh, USA, 12–13 October 2006, pp. 17–25. Academic Conferences International (2006)
6. Clarke, A., Margetts, H.: Governments and citizens getting to know each other? Open, closed, and big data in public management reform. Policy & Internet 6(4), 393–417 (2014)
7. Chen, H., Chiang, R.H.L., Storey, V.C.: Business intelligence and analytics: from big data to big impact. MIS Q. 36(4), 1165–1188 (2012)
8. Hardy, K., Maurushat, A.: Opening up government data for big data analysis and public benefit. Comput. Law Secur. Rev. 33(1), 30–37 (2017)
9. Marton, A., et al.: Reframing open big data. In: The 21st European Conference on Information Systems, pp. 1–12 (2013)
10. Janssen, M., Charalabidis, Y., Zuiderwijk, A.: Benefits, adoption barriers and myths of open data and open government. Inf. Syst. Manag. 29(4), 258–268 (2012)
11. Janssen, M., van den Hoven, J.: Big and open linked data (BOLD) in government: a challenge to transparency and privacy? Gov. Inf. Q. 32(4), 363–368 (2015)
12. Conradie, P., Choenni, S.: On the barriers for local government releasing open data. Gov. Inf. Q. 31, 10–17 (2014)
13. World Wide Web Foundation: Open Data Barometer (2015). http://opendatabarometer.org/doc/3rdEdition/ODB-3rdEdition-Methodology.pdf. Accessed 31 May 2018
14. Bertot, J.C., et al.: Big data, open government and e-government: issues, policies and recommendations. Inf. Polity 19(1–2), 5–16 (2014)
15. Omar, A., Bass, J.M., Lowit, P.: A grounded theory of open government data: a case study. in the UK. In: UK Academy for Information Systems Conference Proceedings (2014)
16. Zuiderwijk, A., Janssen, M.: Open data policies, their implementation and impact: a framework for comparison. Gov. Inf. Q. 31(1), 17–29 (2014)
17. Veljković, N., Bogdanović-Dinić, S., Stoimenov, L.: Benchmarking open government: an open data perspective. Gov. Inf. Q. 31(2), 278–290 (2014)
18. Zuiderwijk, A., Janssen, M.: A coordination theory perspective to improve the use of open data in policy-making. In: Wimmer, Maria A., Janssen, M., Scholl, Hans J. (eds.) EGOV 2013. LNCS, vol. 8074, pp. 38–49. Springer, Heidelberg (2013). https://doi.org/10.1007/978-3-642-40358-3_4
19. Yin, R.K.: Designing case studies: identifying your case(s) and establishing the logic of your case study. In: Case Study Research: Design and Methods, 4th edn, pp. 25–66. SAGE Publications, London (2009)
20. Darke, P., Shanks, G., Broadbent, M.: Successfully completing case study research: combining rigour, relevance and pragmatism. Inf. Syst. J. 8(4), 273–289 (1998)

21. Walsham, G.: Interpretive case studies in is research: nature and method. Eur. J. Inf. Syst. **4**, 74–81 (1995)
22. James, N., Busher, H.: Credibility, authenticity and voice: dilemmas in online interviewing. Qual. Res. **6**(3), 403–420 (2006)
23. James, N.: The use of email interviewing as a qualitative method of inquiry in educational research. Br. Educ. Res. J. **33**(6), 963–976 (2007)
24. Meho, L.: E-mail interviewing in qualitative research: a methodological discussion. J. Am. Soc. Inf. Sci. Technol. **57**(10), 1284–1295 (2006)
25. Norwegian Ministry of Health and Care Services: Meld. St. 28 (2014–2015) White Paper on Medicinal Products – Correct use – better health (2015)
26. Norwegian Ministry of Foreign Affairs: Meld. St. 5 (2016–2017) Collaboration in the Nordic countries (white paper) (2016)
27. Norwegian Ministry of Foreign Affairs: Meld. St. 33 (2011–2012) Norway and the United Nations: Common Future, Common Solutions (white paper) (2012)
28. Norwegian Ministry of Culture: Meld. St. 23 (2011–2012) Visual art (white paper) (2012)
29. Norwegian Ministry of Transport and Communications: Meld. St. 33 (2016–2017) National Transport Plan 2018–2029 (white paper) (2017)
30. Norwegian Ministry of Trade, Industry and Fisheries: Meld. St. 32 (2012–2013) Between Heaven and Earth. Norwegian space policy for business and public benefit (2013)
31. NOU 2013:2 Barriers to digital value creation (Official Norwegian Reports) (2013)
32. NOU 2016:7 Norway in transition – Career guidance for individuals and society (Official Norwegian Reports) (2016)
33. NOU 2017:11 Better assistance Better preparedness. The future organisation of police specialist units (Official Norwegian Reports) (2017)
34. Ministry of Culture: Strategy for Open Data (2017)
35. Ministry of Education and Research: National strategy on access to and sharing of research data (2016). https://www.regjeringen.no/en/dokumenter/national-strategy-on-access-to-and-sharing-of-research-data/id2582412/. Accessed 31 May 2018

# Data Requirements Elicitation in Big Data Warehousing

António A. C. Vieira[1,2(✉)] [iD], Luís Pedro[2],
Maribel Yasmina Santos[1,3] [iD], João Miguel Fernandes[1,2] [iD],
and Luís S. Dias[1,2] [iD]

[1] ALGORITMI Research Centre, University of Minho, Braga, Portugal
{antonio.vieira,lsd}@dps.uminho.pt,
maribel@dsi.uminho.pt, jmf@di.uminho.pt
[2] University of Minho, Campus Gualtar, 4710-057 Braga, Portugal
a70415@alunos.uminho.pt
[3] University of Minho, Campus Azurém, 4800-058 Guimarães, Portugal

**Abstract.** Due to the complex and dynamic nature of Supply Chains (SCs), companies require solutions that integrate their Big Data sets and allow Big Data Analytics, ensuring that proactive measures are taken, instead of reactive ones. This paper proposes a proof-of-concept of a Big Data Warehouse (BDW) being developed at a company of the automotive industry and contributes to the state-of-the-art with the data requirements elicitation methodology that was applied, due to the lack of existing approaches in literature. The proposed methodology integrates goal-driven, user-driven and data-driven approaches in the data requirements elicitation of a BDW, complementing these different organizational views in the identification of the relevant data for supporting the decision-making process.

**Keywords:** Big Data · Big Data Warehouse · Analytics · Data Warehousing
Hive · Requirements · Industry 4.0

## 1 Introduction

Supply Chains (SCs) are complex and dynamic networks, wherein material and information exchanges occur, driven by demand and supply interactions between players [1]. Their goal is to fulfil customers' orders, at a minimum cost, by efficiently managing involved operations, such as: receipt materials, warehousing costs, production, transportation, among others. Companies try to efficiently manage their SC with different systems like SAP-ERP ("Systeme, Anwendungen und Produkte in der Datenverarbeitung" - German for "Systems, Applications & Products in Data Processing"), MRP (Material Requirements Planning) and other tailored-made solutions. Most of these allow companies to respond to specific problems of a given domain, producing large data sets in various formats, at increasingly higher rates. Yet, companies struggle with the extraction of additional knowledge from these data. Such a context is known as Big Data and is one of the pillars of Industry 4.0 [2].

© Springer Nature Switzerland AG 2019
M. Themistocleous and P. Rupino da Cunha (Eds.): EMCIS 2018, LNBIP 341, pp. 106–113, 2019.
https://doi.org/10.1007/978-3-030-11395-7_10

In alignment with Industry 4.0, and to face the needs of integrating, storing and processing data for decision-support in SCs, a Big Data Warehouse (BDW) system is being developed at a company of the automotive industry. For confidentiality reasons, its name cannot be disclosed. However, and to be possible to understand the complexity associated to this project, as well as the methodological approach proposed in this paper, some figures can be shared. The company in question is part of an international organization that is present in more than 60 countries. It incorporates around 3 000 associates with an estimated sales volume of 700 million euros. Regarding logistic figures, the company works with 600 suppliers spread around the world, which supply more than 8 000 different raw materials through around 230 000 inbound deliveries, per year. In its turn, this culminates in more than 1 200 different finished goods produced and shipped to around 250 customers around the world through more than 40 000 outbound deliveries per year.

Presently, a prototype of such system is finished and the purpose of this paper is to present the work conducted to identify its data needs. With such system, the company in question can accurately and timely perform data analytics methods and thus have a proactive approach, rather than a reactive one, due to the knowledge that is extracted from the integrated Big Data sets. At this point, the focus is not on the evaluation of the solution's performance, but rather in its feasibility deploying a proof-of-concept based on the integration of state-of-the-art contributions from different research areas.

The remaining of this paper is organized as follows. Section 2 discusses related literature. Section 3 describes the methodology applied to identify the data requirements of the BDW. Section 4 presents data sources and the data model used. Section 4.2 shows an example dashboard for data analytics tasks, supporting the decision-making process. Section 5 discusses conclusions and future research.

## 2  Related Work

The application of Big Data Analytics (BDA) in SCs is a recent and active research topic, engaged with the development of proactive mechanisms [3]. Kache et al. [4] consider that, despite the advantages of BDA, it is still in its early steps, regarding its application in SC management. In this regard, Tiwari et al. [5] characterized the available BDA techniques and provided a comprehensive review of BDA applications in SC contexts, between 2010 and 2016. Sanders [6] examined the use of BDA to extract knowledge and improve the performance of SCs of leading international companies. The author proposed a framework, based on lessons learned from experience. In their turn, Zhong et al. [7] analyzed several cases throughout the world and discussed their possible impacts on the decision-making process. The authors also reviewed currently used BDA technologies and identified some challenges, opportunities and future perspectives for BDA. Chen et al. [8] examined how the use of BDA can contribute to the added-value in a SC. Santos et al. [2] presented a BDA architecture, under an Industry 4.0 perspective, in a company of the Bosch Group. The presented architecture collects, stores, processes, analyzes and visualizes data related to quality complains and internal defect costs.

To the best of the authors' knowledge, less attention has been paid to the development of BDW systems, applied to SC of the automotive industry. More specifically, from the examples found in the literature, few are oriented towards SC management and no solution oriented towards SC problems of the automotive industry was found. This idea is also corroborated by Ivanov [9].

## 3    BDW Requirements Elicitation Methodology

The purpose of this section is to describe the methodology proposed for the data requirements elicitation. After the analysis of the available data sources, the dimensional modelling, a traditional approach for the development of Data Warehouses (DW) [10], was used. This approach is not mandatory for the development of a BDW, as usually, in Big Data contexts, NoSQL schema-free databases are used, with data models that may change over time. Notwithstanding, the authors opted to start with the dimensional modelling, due to some benefits that were identified. First, it allowed a better understanding of the data, culminating in a clearer view over the metrics, Key Performance Indicators (KPIs), organizational processes, and relevant dimensions of analysis. It also ensured the inclusion of the relevant data sources to the problem and the confidence that no relevant data is excluded. Furthermore, this approach also helped in the design phase, because it helped to define the structure of the used Hive tables. Whilst it is true that the dimensional model could have been ignored, the authors strongly believe that, as mentioned, it was helpful and was also the strategy followed by other authors [11–13].

To develop the multidimensional model, there are 2 main methods: (1) the Inmon's top-down [14] and (2) the Kimball's bottom-up [10]. The first consists in designing the DW as a centric system to respond to queries of all stakeholders. The Kimball method, also known as the multidimensional approach, starts by developing individual data marts and then combining them, using the bus matrix, into a single centric DW. In this work, the Kimball's method was followed. Thus, it was necessary to start the project with the business requirements definition phase [15, 16]. This phase, can, in its turn, be divided in three approaches: supply, user and goal-driven; the latter two can be considered as a single approach, known as demand-driven.

The supply-driven approach, also known as data-driven [15], is a bottom-up iterative approach, in which the user requirements are ignored in the first iteration. It consists in solely analyzing the operational data sources, assuming that it is possible to completely derive the DW conceptual model from the database schemas of the data sources. In the subsequent iterations, the user requirements are considered. This approach is simpler and cheaper (in time and money) than other approaches, because it only depends on the DW designer's skills and on the data complexity [15]. Yet, some barriers to implement this approach can be identified. For instance, if there are many data sources, deriving the DW conceptual model can become a very complex task. Furthermore, the lack of documentation, or domain experts, can also increase the complexity of interpreting the data schemas.

The user-driven approach is a bottom-up approach similar to the requirements definition phase in a software development project [15, 16]. In this approach, several types of sessions or interviews are conducted with specialists of different areas, to elicit their requirements. This is a complex task, because it demands that the views of individuals with different perspectives of the same problem and different sensibilities are combined. Thus, this approach can become time expensive, since business users rarely share a common and clear view over the goals and involved processes. One of the main benefits of this approach is that users are highly involved. According to Golfarelli [15], there are risks in only applying the user-driven approach, since users may leave their positions on a company, or even leave the company itself, increasing the difficulty in analyzing the data.

The goal-driven approach [16] consists in conducting a set of sessions with the top-management, to identify organizational goals. Thereafter, the different visions are merged, thus obtaining a consistent view of the global requirements. In comparison with the user-driven approach, in goal-driven approaches there is no risk of obsolete schemas, since the probability of identifying the most relevant indicators is maximized. Since this approach starts with obtaining a view of the global set of requirements for the central DW, it is often considered a top-down approach. Furthermore, due to its similarities with the user-driven approach, they are usually combined by DW designers and are referred as demand-driven. Combining the three approaches, the methodology depicted in Fig. 1 was adopted.

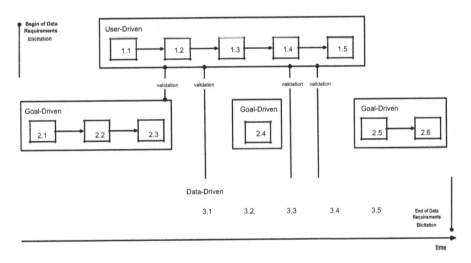

**Fig. 1.** Methodology for data requirements elicitation in Big Data Warehousing

As the figure suggests, both user-driven and goal-driven approaches were used in parallel, from the beginning of the data requirements definition. This was done by conducting workshops and interviews to: (1.1) obtain knowledge of the organization and problem domain; (1.2) clarification of relevant processes; (1.3) identify relevant data sources and tools to use; (1.4) get users' view of organizational needs; and (1.5) identify existing and new metrics (indicators). It was also important to complement the users' view with the top management's view to: (2.1) align with the organization strategy and business processes; (2.2) identify existing and new metrics and KPI; and, (2.3) gather managers' expectations.

At a given point, the goal and user driven approaches are complemented by the data-driven, to start analyzing the relevant data sources. Throughout this phase, new organizational contexts may arise in which new processes or users must be considered, leading to the need of adding or replacing data sources. These new findings (2.4) must be aligned with the top management and can lead to the identification of new business processes or users. As data is being analyzed, a set of validations is done, as depicted in Fig. 1. In the data-driven approach it is important to: (3.1) map the data sources (which data sources must be considered?); (3.2) conduct the proper data profiling, i.e., describe the data fields; (3.3) classify the available data sources and compare them; (3.4) select and reject data sources or fields (justifying each option); and (3.5) identify the relevant metrics. At the end of the requirements identification, it is important to (2.5) validate the conducted work, aligning all involved stakeholders. Furthermore, it may be necessary to (2.6) prioritize business processes implementation, due to time restrictions, for instance.

# 4    BDW Prototype Development

Section 4.1 describes part of the developed multidimensional data model, and Sect. 4.2 presents the environment for supporting the decision-making process.

## 4.1    Dimensional Modelling

For this prototype, 3 fact tables (FT) and 6 dimensions (DIM) were considered, as depicted in Fig. 2. This data is collected from different systems, one of them being SAP. This implied the inclusion of around 100 different attributes, from which, due to confidentiality reasons, only some of them are disclosed in this figure.

The "FT_SpecialFreights" stores records of facts about special freights that were ordered for materials. These are usually expensive and only ordered when material disruptions are imminent. "DIM_SpecialFreight" is a junk dimension of this fact table, integrating different descriptive attributes that give semantics to the stored facts. "FT_Deliveries" stores records of facts related to the arrivals of materials to the plant. These arrivals have a scheduled delivery date and an actual arrival date. This fact table, among other attributes, also stores the difference between these dates, given relevant information about the deviations between the planned and the verified. "FT_EarlyArrivals" stores records of facts concerned with the arrival of materials before the scheduled time. In these situations, the materials are kept on different warehouses than the used for the remaining stored materials. This ensures that suppliers send orders to arrive on the scheduled dates and reduces the warehouse occupation. "DIM_EarlyArrival" is a junk dimension of this fact table, storing a wide range of descriptive attributes. Finally, 4 shared dimensions between the 3 fact tables were considered: DIM_Date, DIM_Time, DIM_Material and DIM_Supplier.

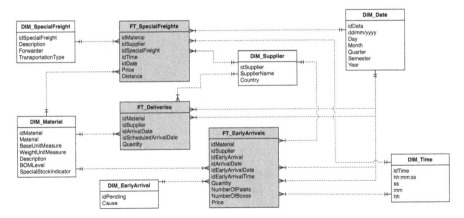

**Fig. 2.** Multidimensional data model

An evolution of this model is expected. In fact, up to this stage, other 7 data sources were considered and are currently being analyzed: around 250 more attributes were already analyzed and integrated in our data model and it is expected that many more be integrated in the following months.

### 4.2 Big Data Analytics

For the proof-of-concept of the BDW prototype presented in this paper, the Big Data Analytics component showed in this section only focuses on the total cost of special freights. In this sense, Fig. 3 shows an analytical dashboard created for this analysis.

The map graph shows the total cost of special freights of materials by countries of the respective suppliers. In its turn, at the bottom left, the Treemap depicts the number of special freights from a given supplier and the corresponding total cost of these freights, grouped by country, and using the same color scale of the map graph. The size of the boxes is proportional to the number of special freights, while the color is associated to the total cost of those special freights. At the bottom right, the bar graph gives more detail about the number and values associated to these special freights. Fictitious names were assigned to the suppliers, due to the confidentiality of this data.

As the graphs suggest, the country with more special freights (considering the cost) is Portugal (e.g., supplier s2), with a total cost of more than 600 K €. In its turn, Germany is the country with more suppliers, also presenting a total cost for special frights above the average. On another perspective, Netherlands and Hong Kong are examples of countries with total costs for special freights below the average.

Despite the conclusions withdrawn from the analysis of this data, the purpose of this section is to demonstrate the usefulness and potential benefits of using Big Data Analytics in logistic contexts.

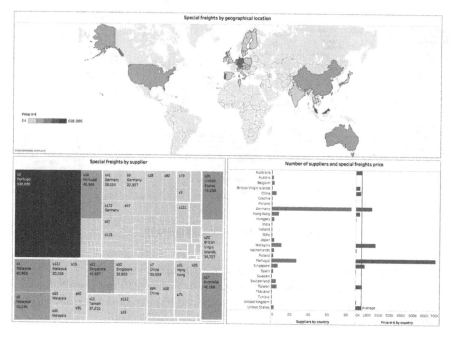

**Fig. 3.** Interactive dashboard for analyzing data related with special freights (Color figure online)

## 5   Conclusions

Companies that are part of dynamic SCs face themselves with the need of tools to aid in the decision-making process [1]. Most of these solutions respond to particular problems, producing huge amounts of operational data, generated in various formats at increasingly higher rates. Yet, there is still a lack of solutions to integrate this data, contributing to a better decision-making process. The purpose of this paper is to propose a methodology for the data requirements elicitation of a BDW, integrating data from different sources of a company that is part of an international organization of the automotive industry.

The development of the BDW started with the requirements elicitation phase, consisting in applying combined user, goal and data-driven approaches, to obtain the relevant attributes, data sources and KPIs. Despite not being necessary to create a multidimensional data model to develop a BDW, the authors chose this path, because: (1) it allowed a better understanding of the data, organizational processes and relevant KPI to include in the BDW; (2) it ensured the inclusion of the all relevant data, making sure that no important attributes were excluded; (3) it helped in the definition of Hive tables to use. The proposed proof-of-concept makes available interactive dashboards, contributing to a better analysis of the stored data. Next steps include the integration of more data sources. Ultimately, it is expected that the company will be able to perform data analytics methods and, thus, have a proactive approach, rather than a reactive one, when extracting knowledge from its Big Data sets.

**Acknowledgements.** This work is supported by COMPETE: POCI-01-0145- FEDER-007043 and FCT – *Fundação para a Ciência e Tecnologia* within the Project Scope: UID/CEC/00319/ 2013; by European Structural and Investment Funds in the FEDER component, through the Operational Competitiveness and Internationalization Programme (COMPETE 2020) [Project no 002814; Funding Reference: POCI-01-0247-FEDER-002814] and by the Doctoral scholarship PDE/BDE/114566/2016 funded by FCT, the Portuguese Ministry of Science, Technology and Higher Education, through national funds, and co-financed by the European Social Fund (ESF) through the Operational Programme for Human Capital (POCH).

# References

1. Levi, D.S., Kaminsky, P., Levi, E.S.: Designing and Managing the Supply Chain: Concepts, Strategies, and Case Studies. McGraw-Hill, New York City (2003)
2. Santos, M.Y., et al.: A Big Data system supporting Bosch Braga Industry 4.0 strategy. Int. J. Inf. Manag. **37**(6), 750–760 (2017)
3. Ponis, S.T., Ntalla, A.C.: Supply chain risk management frameworks and models: a review. Int. J. Supply Chain Manag. **5**(4), 1–11 (2016)
4. Kache, F., Seuring, S.: Challenges and opportunities of digital information at the intersection of Big Data Analytics and supply chain management. Int. J. Oper. Prod. Manag. **37**(1), 10–36 (2017)
5. Tiwari, S., Wee, H., Daryanto, Y.: Big data analytics in supply chain management between 2010 and 2016: insights to industries. Comput. Ind. Eng. **115**, 319–330 (2018)
6. Sanders, N.R.: How to use big data to drive your supply chain. Calif. Manag. Rev. **58**(3), 26–48 (2016)
7. Zhong, R.Y., Newman, S.T., Huang, G.Q., Lan, S.: Big Data for supply chain management in the service and manufacturing sectors: challenges, opportunities, and future perspectives. Comput. Ind. Eng. **101**, 572–591 (2016)
8. Chen, D.Q., Preston, D.S., Swink, M.: How the use of big data analytics affects value creation in supply chain management. J. Manag. Inf. Syst. **32**(4), 4–39 (2015)
9. Ivanov, D.: Simulation-based single vs. dual sourcing analysis in the supply chain with consideration of capacity disruptions, big data and demand patterns. Int. J. Integr. Supply Manag. **11**(1), 24–43 (2017)
10. Kimball, R.: The Data Warehouse Toolkit: Practical Techniques for Building Dimensional Data Warehouse, vol. 248, no. 4. Willey, New York (1996)
11. Santos, M.Y., Costa, C.: Data warehousing in big data: from multidimensional to tabular data models. In: Proceedings of the Ninth International C* Conference on Computer Science & Software Engineering, pp. 51–60 (2016)
12. Costa, E., Costa, C., Santos, M.Y.: Efficient Big Data modelling and organization for Hadoop hive-based data warehouses. In: Themistocleous, M., Morabito, V. (eds.) EMCIS 2017. LNBIP, vol. 299, pp. 3–16. Springer, Cham (2017). https://doi.org/10.1007/978-3-319-65930-5_1
13. Santos, M.Y., Costa, C.: Data models in NoSQL databases for big data contexts. In: Tan, Y., Shi, Y. (eds.) International Conference on Data Mining and Big Data, vol. 9714, pp. 475–485. Springer, Cham (2016). https://doi.org/10.1007/978-3-319-40973-3_48
14. Inmon, W.H.: Building the Data Warehouse. Wiley, Hoboken (2005)
15. Golfarelli, M.: From user requirements to conceptual design in data warehouse design. IGI Global (2010)
16. Abai, N.H.Z., Yahaya, J.H., Deraman, A.: User requirement analysis in data warehouse design: a review. Procedia Technol. **11**, 801–806 (2013)

# Towards Integrations of Big Data Technology Components

Kalinka Kaloyanova$^{(\boxtimes)}$ (iD)

Faculty of Mathematics and Informatics, Sofia University, Sofia, Bulgaria
kkaloyanova@fmi.uni-sofia.bg

**Abstract.** Addressing the increasing volumes of data requires specific technologies, sophisticated methods and tools. Recently, the Big data processing' challenge gave a strong impulse to the development of new data technologies. Considering that organizations still use their traditional database applications, reconciliation of both cases will be a more effective way to manage data functions in the organizations. In this paper we propose a framework for processing Big data based on technologies provided by Oracle. We also discuss some performance aspects of the proposed framework.

**Keywords:** Big data · Database (DB) · NoSQL · Hadoop · MapReduce
Oracle

## 1 Introduction

Recently, the volume, the rate of accumulation and the diversity of data in general have been steadily increasing, which leads to the rapid development of Big data and technological enhancements associated with it [6]. Saving and retrieving Big data is a challenge because of huge data volumes, the variety of information, and the dynamics of the sources [3].

To derive a real value from Big data companies need to combine their business principles with technologies that are able to efficiently retrieve and organize data from variety of sources with different structures in order to analyze it [18]. For these purposes a number of different platforms have been developed recently [17]. In this paper we discuss technologies implemented by Oracle to process Big data. We chose this specific Oracle implementation because of Oracle's big data strategy to extend the current enterprise information architecture to incorporate Big data [14]. In spite of many documents, guides, tutorials, etc. being published, the use of these technologies and tools is still not trivial. A lot of questions arise – where to start, which technologies should be implemented at the beginning, how to organize data, how to evaluate the results? Here we introduce a framework to facilitate the use of several core Big data technologies supported by Oracle. First, we briefly introduce the used technologies in Sect. 2, then we discuss some ways of their implementation in Sect. 3. Furthermore, we reveal some results concerning the data preparation and discus the methods choice.

© Springer Nature Switzerland AG 2019
M. Themistocleous and P. Rupino da Cunha (Eds.): EMCIS 2018, LNBIP 341, pp. 114–120, 2019.
https://doi.org/10.1007/978-3-030-11395-7_11

## 2   Background, Methodologies and Tools

Due to the volumes and the variety of the data that is being created, traditional applications cannot process them effectively. The vast amount of complex and mostly unstructured data requires new methods for organization and analysis in a high performance manner [4]. Traditional relational databases are based on transactions in order to guarantee data consistency and integrity [10]. When huge data volumes are processed, these databases cannot scale efficiently to match capacity and performance aspects.

### 2.1   Big Data Processing

There is no single solution for Big data processing and different companies offer a variety of approaches in this area. After introducing MapReduce as a framework for processing large data sets [5] a lot of technologies have been developed to manage Big data [7]. Hadoop, the most notable open source framework of MapReduce implementation, provides a distributed file system - Hadoop Distributed File System (HDFS) to store data and to scale and process intensive parallel computational tasks on this data [2].

The biggest providers of information management technologies apply different approaches to integrate Hadoop for Big data processing. Most of the solutions add extra components to this open source component. For example, IBM is following this approach as offering its Hadoop decision through Info Sphere Big Insights. Oracle also builds Big data platforms adding its own products to the Apache component. Microsoft integrated Hadoop with Windows Azure and MS SQL Server, and SAP integrated Hadoop with the SAP HANA real data platform [11].

### 2.2   Oracle Big Data Technology Solutions

To answer Big data requirements at enterprise level Oracle provides its own solutions, which extend the current enterprise information architecture to incorporate big data processing.

Oracle Big Data Appliance is a specific system that delivers Big data solutions, tightly integrated with the classical ones. Key elements in this infrastructure are Oracle NoSQL Database and Hive, used to capture and store data [12], and Hadoop Distributed File System to allow large data volumes to be organized and processed while keeping data on the original data storage cluster [14].

Oracle reveals its NoSQL solution as a scalable, distributed database where data is stored as "key-values" pairs. Unlike HDFS which use files to store unstructured data Oracle NoSQL DB support hash indexing for efficient data distribution [15].

As Hive is used to query data in HDFS, Oracle support several connectors to integrate Big data with classical Oracle solutions (Oracle Database, Oracle Exadata) and to increase the performance for data analysis [14].

Oracle Big Data SQL is a tool that simplifies SQL queries to data stored in both relational databases and Hadoop/NoSQL stores [1].

# 3  A Framework for Data and Tools Integration

A satisfactory solution for Big data processing should provide an easy access to data stored in new configurations, and should facilitate the integration of Big data storage platforms with the classical Oracle solutions. Therefore, we will look at different ways of integrating "Big data" solutions with Oracle Database.

We propose a framework that uses a set of technologies to facilitate Big data processing and to provide an environment to enable different types of data processing. The core components we integrate in the framework are:

- Apache Hadoop - Hive, HDFS, MapReduce and Yarn Manager
- Oracle NoSQL Database
- Oracle Database 12c
- Oracle Big Data SQL
- Oracle Big Data Connectors.

Oracle Big Data Connectors are required due to the integration of Hadoop frame data and the Oracle Database [12]. The capabilities provided by Oracle Big Data SQL are used to execute queries on the data stored on the Big Data storage platforms. Using this approach, a direct access is achieved to HDFS via an Oracle Database external table. After that a classical SQL tool could be used to access the data set, providing unified queries [1].

After setting the test environment (installing, configuring and loading data in HDFS and Hive), different cases could be explored to demonstrate and compare the data integration capabilities of Big Data storage platforms with Oracle Database. We explored a set of scenarios to investigate opportunities to:

- Access and load a Hive table with Oracle SQL Connector for HDFS
- Access and load HDFS files with Oracle SQL Connector for HDFS
- Load HDFS files into Oracle Database with Oracle Loader for Hadoop in Online Mode
- Generate Data Pump files with Oracle Loader for Hadoop in Offline Mode that can be accessed and managed with Oracle SQL Connector for HDFS.

Based on the experiments, we compared the work of Oracle SQL Connector for HDFS and Oracle Loader for Hadoop in order to determine how they can be used effectively.

## 3.1  Initial Data Loading

Several initial steps are needed to prepare the framework to provide different options. First, data should be loaded into different structures. For this purpose, data should be loaded into HDFS as a file, loaded into a new Hive DB and loaded into an external table. Also an Oracle DB 12c scheme should be created to hold the data in the classical way.

Several options could be implemented for loading data into Oracle DB:

- Using Oracle SQL Connector for HDFS to access hive table
- Using Oracle SQL Connector for HDFS to access the HDFS files
- Using Oracle Loader for Hadoop (in Online and Offline mode).

We performed several tests using Oracle internal table, Oracle Hive, HDFS text file, and Oracle Data pump. The external tables were created using different Big Data Connectors configurations. We made a set of experiments in order to compare the capabilities of Oracle SQL Connector for HDFS and Oracle Loader for Hadoop and to determine where one of them or a combination of both to be used in the case of integrating Hadoop data.

All experiments were realized on a data set of 13,932,633 "log" entries.

The main considerations of the implementation of the above methods are presented in Table 1.

**Table 1.** Data load methods.

| Method | Description |
|---|---|
| Oracle Database directly accesses HDFS text files using Oracle SQL Connector for HDFS (OSCH) | The fastest way to upload data: <br> - Good to use when there is no resources for Hadoop to transform data before charging <br> - Only text files can be used as input data (any other data format must be transformed) <br> - Text data may remain on the HDFS server <br> - Uses the most processing time on the Database Server |
| Oracle Loader for Hadoop creates a direct path link for each reduce task | The best Online Method: <br> - Database Server processor time is minimal <br> - Data is loaded after preprocessing <br> - The need of files administration at the intermediate steps is eliminated |
| Oracle Loader for Hadoop (OLH) creates Oracle Data Pump files and access or load them from HDFS with Oracle SQL Connector for HDFS | The fastest way to load files using Oracle Loader for Hadoop: <br> - Low CPU time on the Database Server <br> - Data load can be scheduled for the hours of low database server load <br> - Data may remain on the HDFS server. It could be accessed via OSCH for HDFS without loading into the Oracle Database |

More information about the implementation of the discussed methods is shown below.

Figure 1 illustrates the load times for HDFS data in Oracle Database. The measured times are "end-to-end": from the start of MapReduce job with OLH, until the data is stored into the Oracle Database.

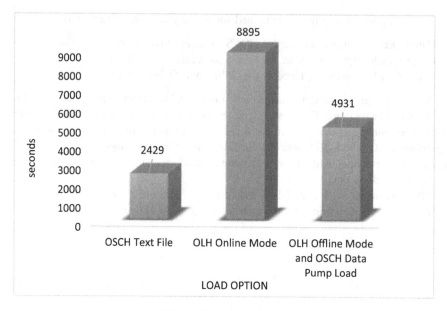

**Fig. 1.** "End-to-end" load

The results shown on Fig. 1 indicate that the fastest way to load data "end-to-end" is to use Oracle SQL Connector for HDFS with a text file located on HDFS. On the other hand, it spends the most processing time on the Database Server.

If count only the data load time itself, loading the Data Pump files with OLH in Offline Mode gives the best results and significantly less CPU usage (see Fig. 2).

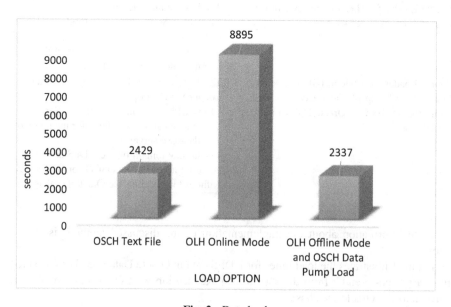

**Fig. 2.** Data load

Working with OLH in Online Mode is considerably slower than others, but the use of the processor time is the minimal one. This is particularly important for the online data load, as it allows applications to continue to work normally (without reducing performance due to data load).

The choice of a method for data loading depends on the priority: the rate of the load time or the minimization of the processing time used on the Database Server. Creating Oracle Data Pump files in Hadoop usually offers the best balance for quick boot and less load on the database server.

### 3.2  Exploring Data

Furthermore, different scenarios could be performed on this framework. We provided a variety of tests to compare the execution times of SQL queries over data stored in Oracle Database as well as in the Big Data storage platform. The experiments were separated into several categories: analytical queries, queries for specific data, join queries including Oracle internal tables, etc. Some results of these tests were discussed in [9].

## 4  Conclusion

Big Data processing has recently become a fundamental part of the work of most companies. The application of the right set of technologies to manage this data is the key step in the Big data processing. To address this problem, we proposed a specific frame-work that uses several Big data solutions implemented by Oracle. We discussed briefly these methodologies and tools supported by Oracle, then we proposed a decision to integrate them into a specific framework. We reviewed some data processing issues and based on our experience we provided useful recommendations for data preparation in order to enable different options for the use of the framework.

The proposed framework could be further extended to new scenarios for exploring Big data like incorporating advanced analytics in connection with the results discussed in [8] and integrating Data Mining techniques, based on some conclusions from [16].

**Acknowledgments.** This work was sponsored by the University of Sofia "St. Kliment Ohridski" SRF under the contract 80-10-143/2018.

## References

1. An Enterprise Architect's Guide to Big Data, Oracle Enterprise, White Paper. http://www.oracle.com/technetwork/topics/entarch/articles/oea-big-data-guide-1522052.pdf.   Accessed 16 May 2018
2. Apache Hadoop: What is Apache Hadoop. http://hadoop.apache.org. Accessed 16 May 2018
3. Beyer, M., Laney, D.: The Importance of 'Big data': A Definition. Gartner, ID G00235055 (2012)
4. Chen, P.C.L., Zhang, C.: Data-intensive applications, challenges, techniques and technologies: a survey on big data. Inf. Sci. **275**, 314–347 (2014)

5. Dean, J., Ghemawat, S.: MapReduce: simplified data processing on large clusters. Commun. ACM **51**(1), 107–113 (2008)
6. De Mauro, A., Greco, M., Grimaldi, M.: What is big data? A consensual definition and a review of key research topics. In: AIP Conference Proceedings, vol. 1644, p. 97 (2015). https://doi.org/10.1063/1.4907823
7. Gandomi, A., Haider, M.: Beyond the hype: big data concepts, methods, and analytics. Int. J. Inf. Manage. **35**(2), 137–144 (2015)
8. Kovacheva, Z., Naydenova, I., Kaloyanova, K., Markov, K.: Big data mining: in-database Oracle data mining over hadoop. In: AIP Conference Proceedings, vol. 1863, p. 040003 (2017)
9. Kaloyanova, K.: An educational environment for studying traditional and big data approaches. In: Proceedings of INTED2018 Conference, Valencia, Spain, pp. 4270–4274 (2018)
10. Molina, H., Ullman, J., Widom, J.: Database Systems: The Complete Book, 3rd edn. Pearson Education Inc., London (2009)
11. OECD: Data-Driven Innovation: Big Data for Growth and Well-Being. OECD Publishing, Paris. https://books.google.bg/books?isbn=9264229353. Accessed 28 May 2018
12. Oracle® Big Data Appliance Software User's Guide, rel. 2. https://docs.ora-cle.com/cd/E37231_01/doc.20/e36963.pdf. Accessed 16 May 2018
13. Oracle Big Data Connectors. http://www.oracle.com/technetwork/bdc/big-data-connect-ors/overview/ds-bigdata-connectors-1453601.pdf. Accessed 16 May 2018
14. Oracle: Big data for Enterprise, An Oracle White paper, June 2013. http://www.ora-cle.com/us/products/database/big-data-for-enterprise-519135.pdf. Accessed 17 Apr 2018
15. Oracle NoSQL Database Concepts Manual, 12c Release 2. https://docs.ora-cle.com/cd/NOSQL/html/ConceptsManual/Oracle-NoSQLDB-Concepts.pdf. Accessed 08 May 2018
16. Orozova, D., Todorova, M.: How to follow modern trends in courses in "databases" - introduction of data mining techniques by example. In: Proceedings of the 11th Annual International Technology, Education and Development Conference, Valencia, Spain, pp. 8186–8194 (2017)
17. Watson, H.J.: Tutorial: big data analytics: concepts, technologies, and applications. Commun. Assoc. Inf. Syst. **34**, Article no. 65 (2014). http://aisel.aisnet.org/cais/vol34/iss1/65
18. Zschech, P., Heinrich, K., Pfitzner, M., Andreas, H.: Are you up for the challenge? Towards the development of a big data capability assessment model. In: Proceedings of the 25th European Conference on Information Systems (ECIS), Portugal, pp. 2613–2624 (2017)

# Experimental Evaluation of Big Data Analytical Tools

Mário Rodrigues[1] , Maribel Yasmina Santos[2] ,
and Jorge Bernardino[1,3(✉)]

[1] Polytechnic of Coimbra - ISEC (Coimbra Institute of Engineering),
Coimbra, Portugal
a21190357@alunos.isec.pt, jorge@isec.pt
[2] ALGORITMI Research Centre, University of Minho, Guimarães, Portugal
maribel@dsi.uminho.pt
[3] CISUC – Centre of Informatics of University of Coimbra, Coimbra, Portugal

**Abstract.** Due to the extensive use of SQL, the number of SQL-on-Hadoop systems has significantly increased, transforming Big Data Analytics in a more accessible practice and allowing users to perform ad-hoc querying and interactive analysis. Therefore, it is of upmost importance to understand these querying tools and the specific contexts in which each one of them can be used to accomplish specific analytical needs. Due to the high number of available tools, this work performs a performance evaluation, using the well-known TPC-DS benchmark, of some of the most popular Big Data Analytical tools, analyzing in more detail the behavior of Drill, Hive, HAWQ, Impala, Presto, and Spark.

**Keywords:** Big Data · SQL-on-Hadoop · Query processing
Big Data Analytics

## 1 Introduction

Big Data as a research topic is still in an early stage, although in recent years Big Data has been an emergent topic across several business areas, being supported by a considerable number of technologies and tools. One of the main challenges is how to handle the massive volume and variety of data efficiently.

In the Big Data scope, Structured Query Language (SQL) or SQL-based processing tools have gained significant attention, as many enterprise data management tools rely on SQL, and, also, because many users are familiar and comfortable with the underlying language. For an organization, this opens up Big Data to a much larger audience, increasing the return of investment in this field. In the technological point of view, this potentiated the development of a wide number of SQL-on-Hadoop systems. However, not all SQL-based querying tools are suited for the same scenarios, being a challenge to understand their characteristics, supporting the selection of the most appropriate one for a particular analytical scenario. As diverse descriptive information about these tools and their architectures is available, this work selected a set of the most representative ones, based on the available literature, and performs a benchmark aimed to understand

© Springer Nature Switzerland AG 2019
M. Themistocleous and P. Rupino da Cunha (Eds.): EMCIS 2018, LNBIP 341, pp. 121–127, 2019.
https://doi.org/10.1007/978-3-030-11395-7_12

the contexts in which each tool shows its main advantages and drawbacks. The experimental evaluation is based on the well-known TPC-DS Benchmark [1] for analyzing Drill, HAWQ, Hive, Impala, Presto and Spark.

The remaining of this paper is organized as follows. Section 2 presents the related work. Section 3 describes the testing environment. Section 4 presents the obtained results and performs a performance evaluation of the analyzed tools. Finally, Sect. 5 concludes discussing the main findings and presenting some future work.

## 2 Related Work

As Big Data is identified as one of the biggest IT trends of the last few years, several technological developments address querying and processing tools. With this growth, SQL processing, namely SQL-on-Hadoop, has been widely studied, analyzing and evaluating the performance of several processing tools. The work performed on [2] provides a performance comparison of Hive and Impala using the TPC-H benchmark and a TPC-DS inspired workload, analyzing the I/O efficiency of their columnar storage formats. The results show that Impala is faster than Hive, either on MapReduce and on Tez for the overall TPC-H and TPC-DS benchmarks. In [3, 4], the motivation for using Hadoop is presented, along with the strengths and limitations of tools like Impala Hive, BigSQL, HAWQ, and Presto. The work of [5] presents the results using the TPC-DS queries, comparing response times for a single user and for 10 concurrent users, using Impala, Hive, and Spark, showing that Impala was the only engine that provided interactive query response on both user scenarios.

The work of [6] presents an overview of the reasons for using SQL access on Hadoop, also giving an overview of IBM Big SQL and comparing it with Hive, Impala, and HAWQ. This work shows that HAWQ and Impala can provide good performance in different scenarios. In [7], the authors present Impala giving an overview of its architecture and main components, also demonstrating its performance when compared against other popular SQL-on-Hadoop systems like Spark, Presto, and Hive. The authors also present and compare the compression of data that can be achieved using file formats like Avro, Parquet and Text. For comparison, the authors use the file format that performs best on each tool and show that Impala has faster response time executing queries in single and multi-user query execution.

Another benchmark of SQL-like Big Data technologies is presented in [8], using queries that involve table scans, aggregations and joins. When comparing Hive, Presto, Drill and Spark, the authors conclude that Presto has an outstanding runtime on performance over other big data solutions and that Spark has an edge for analytics/machine learning. In [9], characteristics like latency and ANSI SQL completeness are used to evaluate Drill, Hive, Impala, and Spark. It is highlighted that Hive requires low maintenance and that is simple to learn, but not suited for real-time queries; Impala has lower query latency, but out-of-memory errors are very frequent if available memory is not enough to process data. In [10], the authors use a denormalized TPC-H schema for testing Hive, Spark, Presto, and Drill in a low cost cluster. The results show that it is possible to achieve adequate query execution times on modest hardware.

As can be seen, a comprehensive set of works in this field is available, many of them based on theoretical analysis of the tools, some others based on benchmarks, demonstrating tools performance. None of these works performs the analysis, in the same experimental evaluation, of the six selected tools, Drill, HAWQ, Hive, Presto, Spark and Impala (for detailed information about these tools and their architectures, please refer to their specific documentation or to [11]). Another motivation to compare these tools is the opportunity that they bring, making available SQL to the Hadoop ecosystem and extending Big Data query processing and analysis to a wider public. In this work, each tool was deployed using the most performant optimized file format, with Impala storing data using Parquet files and the remaining tools using the Stinger initiative with the Optimized Row Columnar (ORC) file format [7]. The objective is to identify the most appropriate scenarios for using each tool.

## 3   Experimental Environment and Available Data

This work uses a Hadoop with 4 nodes, where the hardware configuration of each node includes one octa-core CPU 1.80 GHz, 16 GB of RAM, connected through a gigabit Ethernet, with 64-bit CentOS Linux 7 as the operating system. For deploying the tools, the Hortonworks HDP 2.5 distribution was used, except for Cloudera Impala, as this tool requires a Cloudera's distribution, in this work the CDH 5. Regarding data, it can be stored in Hadoop in several formats, but the ones that perform best are Parquet and ORC, providing lightweight and fast access to compressed data with columnar layout, boosting IO performance. All tools were tested using the ORC format, except Impala that used the Parquet file format. In terms of data, the TPC-DS benchmark was used, generating three different datasets of different Scale Factors (SF), namely 10, 30 and 100 GB. This benchmark includes a total 99 queries (59 *ad hoc*, 41 reporting, 4 iterative online analytical processing and 23 data mining). From this set, and to evaluate the tools' interactive querying capabilities, 16 *ad hoc* queries were used (Fig. 1).

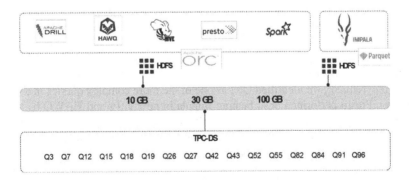

**Fig. 1.**  Experimental context

# 4 Results

This section presents the results obtained from performing part of the TPC-DS benchmark on the 10, 30 and 100 GB datasets. All queries were run 5 times each and special attention was given to eliminate time variations by cleaning the file system cache before running each query. The final execution time is the average of the 5 runs.

Interactive or *ad hoc* queries capture the dynamic nature of a Decision Support System. The TPC-DS is a complex benchmark, comprising 99 queries performed over a data warehouse schema. The schema is composed by several snowflakes with shared dimensions, consisting in 17 dimensions and 7 fact tables, with a total of 24 tables. As already mentioned, we performed a subset of the TPC-DS *ad hoc* queries. Regarding the 10 GB dataset, Fig. 2, we can observe overall reasonable executions times. Spark is the slowest tool in this SF, being slower than Hive in all queries. We were surprised by this fact since Spark has been documented to perform much better than Hadoop-based solutions like Hive. The fastest tools for this SF were Impala and HAWQ, where Impala surpasses HAWQ in all queries except for Q43. Although Presto was always behind Impala and HAWQ with significant differences, it was able to perform all the queries with quick response times (most of the queries ran under 10 s). We can see that these tools achieved nearly instant execution times, specially Impala reaching times below 1 s in some queries like Q12, Q42, Q55 and Q96. Impala and HAWQ take an above average execution time (comparing with the other queries) when executing Q82. This query is also the longest query on Hive and Spark, taking nearly 3x more than Drill, HAWQ and Presto. This can be explained as the query uses the two biggest fact tables present in the data model, Inventory and Store_sales, processing a high volume of data. For the 30 GB SF, the execution times do not increase linearly. Similar to the 10 GB workload, HAWQ and Impala are the fastest tools, with HAWQ the fastest one in the total processing time, obtaining better times in Q7, Q18, Q19, Q27, Q43 (in this case nearly 50% faster) and Q84. Hive kept surpassing Spark in all queries while Presto was the third quickest tool, being about 2x slower than HAWQ and Impala.

Like in the previous SF, Q3 has the longest execution time, comparing the average times. Q7 also keeps running on above average query execution time on Presto and specially on Drill (only 4 s faster than Hive) due to the heavy aggregates, ordering and grouping functions. Another case where this kind of operations affect performance can be observed when we perform Q18, having the longest running time on Spark and the second slowest query on Hive. This query joins data from fact table Catalog_sales and 4 dimension tables, performing 7 average functions over Catalog_Sales columns. Also, as in the previous SF, we identified Q82 as one of the more complex queries in terms of processing. Presto performed best, beating Impala in nearly 9 s and HAWQ by almost 14 s, respectively, and being followed by Drill, performing the query in 15 s. For Q43, Q52 and Q55, although with a small difference, Drill managed to surpass Presto. For Q52 and Q55, Presto had almost the same performance as Hive, calling our attention to the behavior of the tools in the following SF.

In TPC-DS, we were able to run almost all queries, except Q82 for Presto due to intensive IO motivated by complex joins. Impala was the fastest tool, considering the overall time needed to run all the queries, with significant time differences to the other

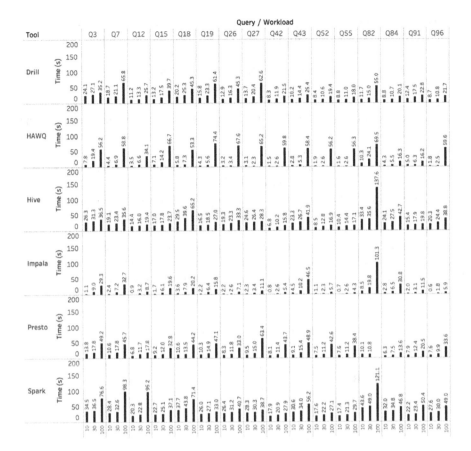

**Fig. 2.** TPC-DS results for the three workloads (10, 30 and 100 GB)

tools. After analyzing the obtained results, we find that Hive is less suitable for querying in a low data volume, due to the long coordination time of jobs, but if we look at the different SF, as the data volume grows, Hive substantially improves its performance, surpassing HAWQ in most of the queries. Evaluating the total time needed to execute all the queries, Hive also surpassed Presto, being faster in ten out of the sixteen queries. In the previous SF, we saw that HAWQ was the fastest tool, followed by Impala. Now, this volume of data has a huge negative effect on HAWQ, being now the slowest tool.

## 5 Discussion and Conclusions

Big Data processing tools can deal with the massive quantity of data that exists nowadays, allowing users to perform ad-hoc querying [11, 12]. Analyzing the presented results, we can consider that there is no one-size fits all SQL-on-Hadoop tool. From the results presented above, we can now summarize the main findings in terms of the overall performance of the in-memory processing tools with the different workloads: 10 GB, 30 GB and 100 GB. For this, Table 1 includes six columns, ranged from 1 to 6, classifying each tool attending to its overall performance in each workload. Presto, Impala and HAWQ started as the fastest tools, providing very fast response times. In the 10 GB and 30 GB SF, relatively small datasets that our cluster resources can manage, we see that these three in-memory tools provide excellent times compared with the ones provided by Hive, Drill and Spark, being adequate tools for supporting interactive/*ad hoc* querying capabilities. When the data volume increases, in this benchmark with the 100 GB workload, some of these tools start to struggle with the available RAM memory, as considerable amounts of intermediate data are processed. In those cases, some of the tools automatically activate the "Spill to Disk" functionality, increasing query execution times. For Hive, although taking more time to process, Hive showed its robustness, being able to perform all the queries. Although being more adequate for batch data processing, it was able to show better performance than tools like HAWQ or Presto with increased data volumes. Therefore, we have to acknowledge Hive's robustness, being an adequate tool when it is critical to perform all the queries. When real-time interactive data processing is needed, the best tools can be Impala, Presto and HAWQ, depending on the data volume, with the fastest response times.

**Table 1.** Performance classification

| TPC-DS | | 1 | 2 | 3 | 4 | 5 | 6 |
|---|---|---|---|---|---|---|---|
| | 10 GB | IMPALA | HAWQ | presto | DRILL | HIVE | Spark |
| | 30 GB | HAWQ | IMPALA | presto | DRILL | HIVE | Spark |
| | 100 GB | IMPALA | HIVE | DRILL | presto | Spark | HAWQ |

In this benchmark, the "Spill to Disk" option was disable in Presto (as this is its by default configuration), which can be critical for finishing some queries. Regarding Impala, certain memory-intensive operations write temporary data to disk (the "Spill to Disk") when Impala is close to exceed its memory limit on a particular host. This feature ensured successfully query completeness, rather than failing with an out-of-memory error. The tradeoff is decreased performance due to the extra disk I/O to write the temporary data and read it back. Thus, this feature improves reliability, but the slowdown its significant. Both Impala and Presto have good performance and are very popular between users, showing best or worst performance depending on the query and the operators/functions it includes. Presto has the advantage of being fully ANSI SQL compliant and Impala only supports HiveQL. For Spark, we were surprised by the times obtained in the benchmark, being in many cases the slowest tool, even though it operates with in-memory processing like the top performers HAWQ, Impala and Presto, leading us to believe that it is more suited when the objective is not just querying data, but performing advanced analytics, Machine Learning and streaming processing. Regarding Drill, we consider it as the best performing tool after the referenced in-memory options, since in most cases provided better performances than Hive and Spark.

As future work, we propose to use the TPC-H and TPC-DS benchmarks with increased data volumes, in a cluster with more RAM memory. Also, since Hive is in constant development and was able to catch up in some scenarios the fastest tools, we should be aware of major current developments like the recent LLAP (Live Long and Process). We consider that Hive's performance can do more than batch processing, and with these constant developments, may address real-time interactive analysis.

**Acknowledgements.** This work is supported by COMPETE: POCI-01-0145- FEDER-007043 and FCT – *Fundação para a Ciência e Tecnologia* within the Project Scope: UID/CEC/00319/2013 and by European Structural and Investment Funds in the FEDER component, through the Operational Competitiveness and Internationalization Programme (COMPETE 2020) [Project no 002814; Funding Reference: POCI-01-0247-FEDER-002814]. The hardware resources used were provided by INCD – *In-fraestrutura Nacional de Computação Distribuída*, an unit of FCT.

# References

1. Transaction Processing Performance Council: TPC BenchmarkTM H Standard Specification Revision 2.17.2 (2017)
2. Floratou, A., Minhas, U.F., Ozcan, F.: SQL-on-Hadoop: full circle back to shared-nothing database architectures. Proc. VLDB Endow. **7**(12), 1295–1306 (2014)
3. Owl, C.: The SQL on Hadoop landscape: an overview (Part I) (2015). http://cleverowl.uk/2015/11/19/the-sql-on-hadoop-landscape-an-overview-part-i/
4. Owl, C.: The SQL on Hadoop landscape: an overview (Part II) (2015). http://cleverowl.uk/2015/12/25/the-sql-on-hadoop-landscape-an-overview-part-ii/
5. Devadutta Ghat, D.K., Rorke, D.: New SQL Benchmarks: Apache Impala (Incubating) Uniquely Delivers Analytic Database Performance (2016). https://blog.cloudera.com/blog/2016/02/new-sql-benchmarks-apache-impala-incubating-2-3-uniquely-delivers-analytic-database-performance/
6. Sakr, S.: A brief comparative perspective on SQL access for Hadoop. In: Recent Advances in Information Systems and Technologies, vol. 1, pp. 1–9 (2014)
7. Kornacker, M., et al.: Impala: A Modern, Open-Source SQL Engine for Hadoop. In: CIDR (Conference on Innovative Data Systems Research) (2015)
8. Grover, A., et al.: SQL-like big data environments: case study in clinical trial analytics. In: 2015 IEEE International Conference on Big Data (Big Data), pp. 2680–2689 (2015)
9. MapR: SQL on Hadoop Details (2017). https://mapr.com/why-hadoop/sql-hadoop/sql-hadoop-details/
10. Santos, M.Y., et al.: Evaluating SQL-on-Hadoop for big data warehousing on not-so-good hardware. In: Proceedings of the 21st International Database Engineering and Applications Symposium - IDEAS 2017, pp. 242–252 (2017)
11. Rodrigues, M., Santos, M.Y., Bernardino, J.: Describing and comparing big data querying tools. In: Rocha, Á., Correia, A.M., Adeli, H., Reis, L.P., Costanzo, S. (eds.) WorldCIST 2017. AISC, vol. 569, pp. 115–124. Springer, Cham (2017). https://doi.org/10.1007/978-3-319-56535-4_12

# Cloud Computing

# Model for Improved Load Balancing in Volunteer Computing Platforms

Levente Filep[(⊠)]

Faculty of Mathematics and Computer Science,
Babeş-Bolyai University, Cluj-Napoca, Romania
f.levi@cs.ubbcluj.ro

**Abstract.** Distributed computational platforms, especially volunteer based ones, become popular over the past decades due to the cheap access to resources. The majority of these Volunteer Computing (VC) platforms are based on client-server architecture, therefore susceptible to server-side bottlenecks and delays in project completion due to lost Workload Units (WU). This paper presents a new model for a computing platform that offloads the tasks of WU creation from centralized servers to the network nodes and with the use of a remote checkpoint system, it can re-create lost WUs from failed or unavailable nodes. With these improvements, it can achieve better scaling and load balancing, and due to the checkpoints, only a limited amount of computation is lost due to node failure. Simulation results of the model's behavior are also present and interpreted.

**Keywords:** Volunteer computing · Load balancing · Scalability
Workload unit recovery

## 1 Introduction

Over the past decades, several volunteer-based distributed computational projects have been deployed as a collaboration between scientists and the public in the role of volunteers who donate their idle computing resources. By analyzing these platforms, we conclude that the majority of these are based on client-server architecture, which offers easy deployment and maintainability. Nonetheless, improvements can be made to how they harness the resources offered by volunteers, handle lost workload units and on reducing the bottleneck on their centralized servers.

This paper proposes a computational platform model with a P2P network architecture based on the super-peer concept that offloads the workload related tasks from centralized servers to the network nodes, and in combination with a remote checkpoint system aims at more efficient load balancing and better resource harnessing with a reduced computational loss in case of node failure.

© Springer Nature Switzerland AG 2019
M. Themistocleous and P. Rupino da Cunha (Eds.): EMCIS 2018, LNBIP 341, pp. 131–143, 2019.
https://doi.org/10.1007/978-3-030-11395-7_13

## 2  Background

Some of the earliest, long-lived and most popular frameworks aimed at volunteer computing [13] are distributed.net, The COSM Project, and BOINC. These are the basis of some of the most successful volunteer-based projects like GENOME@home, Folding@home, SETI@home, Atlas@home, etc. Besides these, there were a number of other framework proposals, but these never gain mainstream popularity like the previously mentioned ones. By far the most popular framework is BOINC whose combined projects performance exceeds $20PetaFLOPS$ with an average of over 300.000 active contributors and over 1.2 million total participants.

The applications deployed on these platforms are massively parallel in nature, which are often described as "embarrassingly parallel problems" in the literature. In short, these problems can be easily broken down to WUs which then can be computed without any interaction between them. For such applications, the client-server architecture suits well, however, it can be a limiting factor for other types of applications. The COSM framework features peer-to-peer support, but without a native sub-task identification on the underlying protocol to keep track of parallel branches, this falls in the hand of the project developers requiring supplemental development effort.

The main operating principle for the majority of these systems is the distribution of WUs to volunteer machines where these are processed, and the results submitted back to the project servers. To ensure a project finishes in a timely manner, WUs are assigned a deadline for completion. If one is not completed before this deadline expires, the server redistributes the WU to another volunteer. Missing the deadline is often caused by nodes exiting the network and never returning or excessive downtime. Further limitations regarding the network nodes can be mentioned:

- starvation: when all WUs are distributed and some volunteers remain idle.
- overload: a node gets a WU that cannot compute before deadline expiration.

"Starving" nodes and WUs missing the deadline can be perceived as lost computation. Furthermore, a few WUs missing the deadline delay the project completion. This limitation is due to lack of a remote checkpoint system to preserve partial computation.

Another weakness of this type of architecture is the communication bottleneck at the servers, mainly I/O, in case of intense WU transfers or bandwidth saturation when dealing with a massive amount of messages. Most popular projects on BOINC suffer from server bottleneck. A series of enchantments ware implemented aimed at decreasing the server load and improve volunteer resource harnessing, such as on-demand WU creation and WUs distribution the volunteer nodes based on their hardware performance.

Several papers in the literature focused on eliminating the server bottleneck by improving WU distribution. Such a proposal made Muratat et al. [10] as an extension for the BOINC middleware [2] involves WU download by a group of nodes and distribution between themselves. In the particular paper, the authors also proposed the migration of the extra WUs when a node is leaving the network. Alonso-Monsalve et al. [1] suggested the use of specially designated data-nodes for WU distribution.

Peer-to-Peer techniques and extensions for BOINC like systems ware proposed by Costa et al. [5], Elwaer et al. [8], Bruno and Ferreira [4]. The authors aimed at using P2P transfer protocols for more efficient WU distribution.

In recent years, volunteer computing platforms for the web have also emerged. These eliminate the need for client-side software by using the volunteer's browser instead. Such an example is COMCUTE [6] developed by Czarnul et al.

Nonetheless, all these frameworks are still client-server based. With the given propositions the server bottleneck can be eased, however, neither the limitations on the types of distributed applications nor the problem of project delay caused by WUs missing the deadline is addressed. Further improvements with significant impact seem limited by the inability of the client-side middleware to dynamically create, split or merge the WUs after application deployment. Arguably, this limitation arises because not all data-sets can be "cut" at arbitrary points and still maintaining the integrity of the resulting chunks. Since each distributed application is different, the middleware-application cooperation is required to overcome this limitation. Such cooperation requires a different kind of framework that provides specialized API facilitating this, thus allowing easier application development. In this paper, such a framework model is proposed, presented and analyzed.

## 3  Proposed Model

The model presented here aims at offloading the creation and distribution of WUs from centralized servers directly to the network nodes, thus eliminating centralized server bottleneck and using a remote checkpoint system for lost WUs recovery, thus reducing lost computation. In short, the goals of the proposed model are:

- dynamic workload creation and reassignment: when nodes become available either by finishing existing computation or by joining the network.
- workload merging: recombination of computed child workload results with it's parent on arbitrary network node, instead of centralized servers.
- workload re-creation: in case of a failed node, the assigned WU is re-created when the child WUs are finished or the overall project is nearing completion.
- remote workload checkpoints: periodic or upon graceful exit of nodes.

Nonetheless, some form of supervision is required to maintain network balance. Due to the volatile behavior of nodes in VC networks, these roles are fulfilled by nodes with high availability and network bandwidth, which will be referred to as supervisor nodes. Thus, the proposed model uses a decentralized P2P architecture with super-peer concept [3]. With the majority of tasks being offloaded from the centralized servers, these only act as network gateways through which applications can be deployed and data collected.

A persistent issue in VC is that the nodes behind a NAT cannot be directly contacted; therefore these maintain an open connection with the supervisor which acts as a proxy through which communication can be initiated.

Since supervisor nodes also participate in the computation, ensuring their fast response time requires that the supervising tasks be executed on higher priority threads compared to those that run the computation.

## 3.1 Internal Ranking System

In the proposed model, an internal ranking system is used for supervisor node selection. This ranking is made available to the applications to facilitate custom overlay creation for special purposes. The ranking consists of the following values:

- average measured uptime
- average measured available performance (since only harnessing volunteer idle resources, this does not equal the overall hardware performance)
- average measured bandwidth between nodes

Since different ranking systems may require only a single or a unique combination of these value, for better flexibility and expansibility, the middleware broadcast these, as separate values so these values can be used according to specific requirements.

## 3.2 Workload Objects

To achieve the goals of the model, WUs require an extension with an additional set of vital information. This collection of data, referred to in the following as Workload Object (WOB), contains, but not limited to the following fields:

- ID (unique identification of WOB); Application ID.
- Identifier id of parent: required for WU result recombination.
- List of child identifiers: required for parallel branch tracking and WOB recombination and recovery.
- Checkpoint data: minimal set of information from which computation can be resumed at any given time and on arbitrary participating node.
- Boundary identification: identifies which part of the problem or the overall data-set is being processed.
- Estimated computational effort: total and left (in *FLOPS*).
- State of computation: i.e. in progress, suspended or waiting for child (for handling by the middleware).
- Result data: contains partial or full result of computation.
- Metadata: application specific uses.

JSON representation of the WOB is ideal, as its a wide-spread, easy to integrate and open standard format.

Handling large datasets and still maintain a small size for the WOB is achievable using the boundary information which identifies the part from the dataset that is required by the WOB. The part (chunk) of data can be pulled from the database server or shared among the nodes as needed. Resource transfers techniques have already been well researched in the literature [5, 8] and will not be further discussed in this paper.

### 3.3   Load Balancing

The basis of load balancing in the presented model is creation, migration or reassignment, and merging of WOBS. A project always starts with an initial WOB injected into the network through the gateway which then gets split into child WOBs as the computation progresses. Finally, as the whole computation nears completion, all WOBs are merged back together into the original parent.

**WOB Requests.** The workload is distributed on-demand as participant nodes in the given project broadcast WOB request messages. First, the supervisor nodes are queried for any stored WOBs. If they have any stored, a WOB offering message will be generated as a reply to the query. Otherwise, the supervisor node will forward the requesting message to all its connected nodes. The WOB request process at the requester node is presented in Algorithm 1, while Algorithm 2 describe the request handling at the supervisor node.

---

**Algorithm 1** WOB request process at requester node

---

1: Broadcast WOB request message to supervisor
2: **while** waiting $R_T$ time for response **do**
3:     For each response $R$ received store in $RList$
4: **end while**
5: **if** $RList$ is empty **then**
6:     Notify supervisor of idle state
7:     Request middleware to suspend application
8: **else**
9:     Select workload $W_{Sel}$ with $max(W.EffortLeft)$ from $RList$
10:     **for all** $W_R$ in $RList$ **and** $W_R \neq W_{Sel}$ **do**
11:         Send **reject** message to $W_R.OriginNode$        ▷ reject notification
12:     **end for**
13:     Send **Accept** workload message $W_{Sel}.OriginNode$
14:     Wait for WOB transfer from $W_{Sel}.OriginNode$
15:     **if** response is Error **then**
16:         Restart algorithm
17:     **else**
18:         Accept WOB
19:         Notify supervisor of WOB location, node state
20:         Begin computing WOB
21:     **end if**
22: **end if**

---

---

**Algorithm 2** WOB request handling at the supervisor node

---

1: Received WOB request message
2: **if** Stored $WOB$ exists **then**
3:     Select the appropriate WOB based on the requester ranking (1)
4:     Transfer WOB to requester
5: **else**
6:     Forwards WOB request message to connected nodes (2)
7: **end if**

---

**Notes:**

1. When storing multiple WOBs, the selection will take into consideration both the uptime of the node as well as its performance
2. The broadcast includes the WOB requesting node's ranking and identification. The supervisor also acts as a proxy between the requester and nodes behind a NAT. There is a significant place for improvements on how to select the nodes to which WOB request is forwarded to; if we choose all of them or a limited number based on their remaining workload size.

**WOB Creation.** If a node can split its workload, then based on the requester ranking, it will generate an appropriate response message containing the size of the workload offered. For optimal balancing, the offering should contain an appropriate amount of data so that the two nodes will finish their computation at about the same time. If the data-set computational effort is linear (i.e. data-set analysis), then a $W_R$ sized offering can be created using the following formula:

$$W_R = \frac{W_C}{1 + \frac{P_C}{P_R}} \tag{1}$$

where $W_C$ is the amount of workload left on the current node, while $P_C$ and $P_R$ are the performance values of the present, respectively the requester node. The values of $W_R$, $W_C$, $P_C$ and $P_R$ are expressed in *FLOPS*. The workload interval that is split, as illustrated in Fig. 1, is identified by the boundary cursor position (where the computation is at the moment) and the right position of the assigned interval from the overall workload.

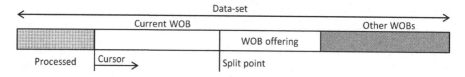

**Fig. 1.** Workload interval splitting

In other cases, since the ranking values are transmitted separately, any required combination of these can be used in concordance with specific requirements.

To minimize the number of messaging in a large-scale network, only nodes that can offer workload answer requests. In this case, the requester node has to wait a certain amount of time before assuming all workload offerings have arrived.

From multiple offerings received by the requester node, this selects one depending on its needs and ranking. Workload fragmentation can be minimized if the largest workload offering is accepted.

If the requester node doesn't receive any reply within the "wait" period, it notifies the supervisor of its idle state and requests the middleware to be suspended, allowing other applications to harness the node's resources. However, if a late offering message arrives the application will be resumed to handle this and possibly accept the offering. The supervisor will also keep a list of its idle nodes available to all connected nodes, which can send notification of workload if such becomes available. This method facilitates load balancing when data is created at run-time.

The following two procedures describes the handling of WOB offering (Algorithm 3) and the WOB acceptance procedure (Algorithm 4).

---

**Algorithm 3** WOB offering process

1: Received WOB request message from $RNode$
2: **if** WOB present **then**
3:     **if** current WOB can be split **then**
4:         Create offering based on $RNode.Rank$
5:         Lock offered workload part (1)                    ▷ Prevent overlapping offerings
6:         Send offering to $RNode$
7:     **end if**
8: **end if**

---

**Note:**

1. the lock remains active until acceptance/rejection message is received or lock timeout occurs.

---

**Algorithm 4** WOB creation and transfer process

1: Received WOB acceptance message from $RNode$
2: **if** offered WOB still available **then**          ▷ Computation might have started
3:     Split current WOB and create new $WOB_{Resp}$
4:     Send $WOB_{Resp}$ to $RNode$
5: **else**
6:     Reply failure message
7: **end if**

---

**WOB Storage.** Excess WOB can occur if the requester node fails after acceptance message is sent, resulting in a newly created WOB, or a node leaves the project and its unfinished WOB is transferred off. In such cases, the connected supervisor node will store the WOBs for later redistribution when nodes become available. Handling lost WOBs due to failed nodes is described in Sects. 3.5 and 3.6.

**Additional Balancing Techniques.** Section 3.6 describes the use of checkpoints to resume the computation of the WOB on a different node. In traditional frameworks, a few WUs can delay the project completion and potentially leave the rest of the participating nodes idle while these WUs are redeployed and computed again. In contrast, the proposed model can improve on this. Anticipating project completion can be done without a full network query about the state of each WOB and counting the remaining work. When a node enters an idle state (not receiving any WOB offerings) we can assume the project nears its completion. In this case further balancing can be done, namely, existing WOBs suspended and migrated to faster machines or WOBs from exited nodes re-created using the stored checkpoints and reassigned to idle nodes to ensure faster project completion.

### 3.4 WOB Location and Query

Without centralized servers, we rely on the messaging between the network nodes to find a specific WU and query its status. Traditional message flooding algorithms like Gossip [7], Gnutella [12], etc., in the current model are unsuitable to handle large-scale networks due to the number of messages involved and the amount of time required for query message propagation to all participating nodes.

The query time can be significantly improved by decreasing the number of nodes that we query. If each supervisor node keeps a list of the WOBs located in their sub-set or cluster of nodes, then the query effort can be reduced solely to these supervisors. A similar technique was proposed by Ye et al. [14] as an improvement to Gnutella search, while a number of other search algorithms for P2P networks have been analyzed and compared in the literature [9, 11].

For optimal network operation, the sub-set size must be dynamically adjusting, using splitting and merging operations, based on the available resources on the supervisor nodes at any given moment. Due to space limitations, this will be further discussed in a future paper.

Keeping an updated list of the WOB locations and status, WOB information is always updated when it involves a transfer or status change. In case of transfer, the accepting node notifies its supervisor about the new location of the WOB in question. The footprint of this operation is relatively low as it only requires one notification and one acknowledge message pairs to be exchanged.

### 3.5 Fault Tolerance

Use of supervisor nodes introduces a one-point failure in the model, especially when relying on volunteer nodes. As a solution, supervisor node replication is proposed. As discussed in the previous chapter, the supervising nodes maintain several critical lists and data for the operation of the network, such as WOB location list, idle nodes, WOB and checkpoint storage. With these data replicated among them, the network can tolerate multiple supervisor failures.

Failure of supervisor nodes can be detected either by a regular heartbeat among the replicates or by a connected node. Connected nodes must be aware of multiple supervisors to avoid reconnecting to the network if one fails. After a failure detection, an election can take place to select a new supervisor from the local cluster.

Replication also comes with an unexpected benefit. Since the number of connections a supervisor can handle at a given moment limits the size of the subset, having multiple supervisors, the connected nodes can be divided among them, especially after a supervisor election, thus allowing an increased sub-set size.

### 3.6  WOB Recovery

WOB recovery is an essential step to avoid WOB redeployment and restarting the entire computation of this. Loss of a WOB can be detected in the following cases:

- child WOB is computed and ready to be merged with its parent WOB
- parent WOB queries the status of child WOBs
- network heartbeat (regular queries about project status)

WOB recovery is achieved through a global checkpoint system. Checkpoints are created in most frameworks for crash recovery and resuming computation. In the presented model the checkpoint data is part of the WOB, however, this alone is not enough to properly restore a WOB, therefore, the entire WOB is used as a checkpoint.

Checkpoint storage is automatically handled by the middleware. A copy is also stored on the supervisor nodes for possible use in recovery processes. With the checkpoint system, the maximum computation loss that can occur is equal to the difference between two checkpoints. Algorithm 5 presents the steps for WOB recovery.

A checkpoint is created with the WOB, when suspended (i.e. the node gracefully exits the network) or at regular intervals. The size of these is greatly application (problem) dependent, therefore, the checkpoint interval must be set in accordance to prevent network congestion at the supervisor node. Depending on the node connection, the middleware can transfer the checkpoint either directly to the supervisor node or indirectly.

---

**Algorithm 5** WOB Recovery

---

 1: Query status and location of WOB
 2: **if** WOB is unavailable **then**
 3:     Trigger **WOB request process**                    ▷ Request other workload
 4:     **if** no WOB Offerings **then**                    ▷ Begin recovery
 5:         Request last checkpoint from supervisor
 6:         Re-create WOB
 7:         **if** WOB workload can be split **then**
 8:             Notify supervisor of available workload    ▷ Idle nodes get notified
 9:         **end if**
10:         Resume computation of WOB
11:     **end if**
12: **end if**

---

## 3.7   Application Development

The presented model requires application-middleware cooperation which can be achieved with a minimal number of messages to which the application registers through the message handlers provided by the middleware. This minimal set of these messages are the following:

- MSG_CHECKPOINT_AND_TERMINATE: create and transfer checkpoint to middleware and terminate computation.
- MSG_CHECKPOINT_AND_RESUME: get checkpoint from middleware and resume computation.
- MSG_WOB_REQUEST: receives requester ranking. If possible to split own workload, estimate workload offering size, respond with appropriate message.
- MSG_WOB_OFFERING: receives a WOB offering.
- MSG_WOB_ACCEPTED: receives requester ranking. Split the workload, create new WOB and transfer. Store child identification for result merger.
- MSG_WOB_RECEIVED: handling a received WOB
- MSG_APP: receives application specific message

For easy application development, the middleware provides an appropriate API facilitating the integration with the specific functions of the model. These include:

- WOB status query, status update, location update, create and transfer, receive WOB
- WOB request, send offer
- Peer message functions

Utilizing the API provided by the middleware, the underlying network structure is hidden from the application. Since WOB query results contain the location and host identification of this, with the middleware's API, communication can be established between parallel branches of an application, facilitating the development of other types of applications besides the common, massively parallel ones.

# 4   Simulation and Results

Model behavior was evaluated using simulation as it provides a controlled environment and the possibility to conduct experiments with an arbitrary number of nodes, node performance, network connection quality between nodes and workload size. The simulation was run on custom build software that replicates the model, middleware and application behavior. Simulation time is counted from zero seconds up until the project completion.

For simplicity, the presented experiment involves a small project consisting of a workload with 10.000 chunks and $20.000 GFLOPS$ computational effort per chunk ($Chunk_{CT} = \sim 6$ min:40 s), which puts the overall project size to $200 PetaFLOPS$. A number of 20 nodes with equal speeds of $50 GFLOPS$ is used with a constant latency of 50 ms between them. An additional 1 to 10 ms is used for simulating the answering the different types of messages. Workload splitting was done using Eq. 1. Amount of downloaded data is not discussed here.

Two scenarios ware tested here, one with and one without any node failures involved. The first one was to examine the load balancing by measuring node idle times, while the second to test the WOB recovery and the difference in the project completion time between the two. In the second scenario, five nodes ware removed simultaneously 21 h into the simulation representing five nodes permanently exiting the network. To obtain the project completion delay caused by the "failed" nodes an additional five nodes ware added immediately after their removal. Workloads size on the removed nodes was between 6.240.000 and 25.000.000*GFLOPS*. In BOINC like systems such considerable size workloads are not assigned to a single node. However, this size is due to the boundary identification values, while the actual data is to be downloaded on a per-chunk basis as the computation progresses. As WOB splitting is done at the network nodes, large workloads will exist early on, but as the project progresses, they will be further segmented into smaller pieces.

**Table 1.** Simulation results of both scenarios

|  | Scenario #1 | Scenario #2 |
|---|---|---|
| Project completion | 02d 07 h:36 m:00 s:300 ms | 02d 07 h 47 m:00 s:150 ms |
| WOBs | 69 | 102 |
| WOB queries | 123 | 148 |
| WOB transfers | 69 | 102 |
| Number of checkpoints | 1126 | 1132 |
| Number of messages | 6745 | 7837 |
| Average node idle time | 03 m:59 s:397 ms | 02 m:35 s:560 ms |
| Worst idle time | 07 m:12 s:072 ms | 06 m:45 s:885 ms |
| Failed nodes | 0 | 5 |
| Computational effort lost | 0 | 600, 192*GFLOPS* |

Due to the load balancing, the expected worst idle times should not exceed the chunk compute time. The small excess in Table 1 is caused by rounding in Eq. 1, while no values over $1.5 \times Chunk_{CT}$ ware observed.

Due to the remote checkpoint system, the actual lost computation amount is between 119.921 and 120.019, meaning approximately 6 computed chunks per node, giving a total of 200 min of lost computation. The fairly similar amounts are due to the equal computing power of the nodes, while the small differences are due to the delays in WOB distribution and communication delays.

Interpreting the results from Table 1, the lost 40 min of computation per node only delayed the project completion by 11 min. In the best case scenario, the total of 200 min loss distributed evenly among the 20 nodes delays the project completion by 10 min. On a client-server architecture and without WU recovery, the five lost WUs would delay the project by the WU deadline expiration plus 40 min. Furthermore, after the WUs redeployed and without an on-demand WU creation and distribution, the rest of the participating nodes are "starved". In the presented model, the recovered WOBs are further split into smaller, thus balancing the remaining workload. The use of WU deadline is also not required.

# 5 Conclusions

This paper presented a new computational framework model aimed at better harnessing the resources offered by volunteers through a new method of load balancing and offloading the workload related tasks from centralized servers to the network nodes themselves, thus eliminating potential bottlenecks on these. A workload recovery using remote checkpoints was also presented. The combination of the above methods also increases project completion.

From a distributed application point of view, the presented model offers several benefits, such as control of workload splitting and dynamic workload creation at any given time into the computation. The possibility of sub-branches tracking using WOB location queries can be viewed as a basis for developing other types of application besides the familiar massively parallel ones.

However, besides the presented benefits, the disadvantage of the model is a complex middleware and increased difficulty in application development.

**Acknowledgements.** This work was supported by the Collegium Talentum 2017 Programme of Hungary.

# References

1. Alonso-Monsalve, S., Garcia-Carballeira, F., Calderón, A.: A new volunteer computing model for data-intensive applications. Concurrency Comput.: Pract. Exp. **29**(24) (2017). https://doi.org/10.1002/cpe.4198
2. Anderson, D.P.: Boinc: a system for public-resource computing and storage. In: Proceedings of the 5th IEEE/ACM International Workshop, Pittsburgh, USA, pp. 4–10. IEEE Computer Society (2004)
3. Beverly Yang, B., Garcia-Molina, H.: Designing a super-peer network. In: Proceedings 19th International Conference on Data Engineering, Bangalore, India, pp. 49–60. IEEE (2003). https://doi.org/10.1109/ICDE.2003.1260781
4. Bruno, R., Ferreira, P.: Freecycles: efficient data distribution for volunteer computing. In: Proceedings of the Fourth International Workshop on Cloud Data and Platforms, Amsterdam, Netherlands, pp. 1–6. ACM (2014)
5. Costa, F., Silva, L., Kelley, I., Taylor, I.: Peer-to-peer techniques for data distribution in desktop grid computing platforms. In: Danelutto, M., Fragopoulou, P., Getov, V. (eds.) Making Grids Work, pp. 377–391. Springer, Boston (2008). https://doi.org/10.1007/978-0-387-78448-9_30
6. Czarnul, P., Kuchta, J., Matuszek, M.: Parallel computations in the volunteer–based comcute system. In: Wyrzykowski, R., Dongarra, J., Karczewski, K., Waśniewski, J. (eds.) PPAM 2013. LNCS, vol. 8384, pp. 261–271. Springer, Heidelberg (2014). https://doi.org/10.1007/978-3-642-55224-3_25
7. Demers, A., et al.: Epidemic algorithms for replicated database maintenance. In: Proceedings of the Sixth Annual ACM Symposium on Principles of Distributed Computing, pp. 1–12. ACM, New York (1987) https://doi.org/10.1145/41840.41841
8. Elwaer, A., Taylor, I., Rana, O.: Optimizing data distribution in volunteer computing systems using resources of participants. Scalable Comput.: Pract. Exp. **12**, 193–208 (2011)

9. Kapoor, H., Mehta, K., Puri, D., Saxena, S.: Survey of various search mechanisms in unstructured peer-to-peer networks. Int. J. Comput. Appl. **68**(6), 21–25 (2013). https://doi.org/10.5120/11584-6917

10. Muratat, Y., Inabatt, T., Takizawat, H., Kobayashi, H.: Implementation and evaluation of a distributed and cooperative load-balancing mechanism for dependable volunteer computing. In: International Conference on Dependable Systems & Networks: Anchorage, Alaska, USA, pp. 316–325. IEEE (2008)

11. Priyanka, C., Deeba, K.: A comparative study on optimization of search in overlay networks. Int. J. Comput. Sci. Mob. Appl. **1**(4), 34–38 (2013)

12. Ripeanu, M.: Peer-to-peer architecture case study: Gnutella network. In: Proceedings First International Conference on Peer-to-Peer Computing, Linkoping, Sweden, pp. 99–100. IEEE (2001)

13. Sarmenta, L.F.: Volunteer computing. Ph.D. thesis, Massachusetts Institute of Technology (2001)

14. Ye, F., Zuo, F., Zhang, S.: Routing Algorithm Based on Gnutella Model. In: Cai, Z., Li, Z., Kang, Z., Liu, Y. (eds.) ISICA 2009. CCIS, vol. 51, pp. 9–15. Springer, Heidelberg (2009). https://doi.org/10.1007/978-3-642-04962-0_2

# Towards a Formal Approach for Verifying Dynamic Workflows in the Cloud

Fairouz Fakhfakh[(✉)], Hatem Hadj Kacem, and Ahmed Hadj Kacem

ReDCAD Laboratory, University of Sfax, Sfax, Tunisia
{fairouz.fakhfakh,Hatem.Hadjkacem}@redcad.org,
Ahmed.Hadjkacem@fsegs.rnu.tn

**Abstract.** Dynamic workflow applications are increasingly used in many enterprises to satisfy the variable enterprise requirements. Cloud computing has gained a particular attention to run these applications. However, due to lack of formal description of the resource perspective, the behavior of Cloud resource allocation cannot be correctly managed. This paper fills this gap by proposing a formal model which verifies the correctness of dynamic workflow changes in a Cloud environment using the Event-B method. Our model considers properties related to control flow, data flow and resource perspectives. It aims to preserve the correctness of workflow properties at both design time and runtime.

**Keywords:** Dynamic workflow · Cloud resources · Formal model
Data flow

## 1 Introduction

Today's enterprises are faced with a dynamic environment that is characterized by fierce competition and high customer demands. Therefore, the capability to dynamically adapt their workflows (e.g. add, replace or remove tasks) has become a major requirement. Workflow adaptation is necessary, for example, in case of strategy shifts, changes in the customer behavior and the occurrence of unexpected situations. Generally, changes can take place at two levels: model level and instance level. In this context, one of the most difficult challenge is to ensure that change operations are applied correctly and do not cause any inconsistencies. So, it is necessary to find the adequate properties which guarantee the correctness of dynamic workflow changes.

Several approaches have been proposed to ensure the correctness of workflow changes [1–5]. However, they are mainly interested in control flow perspective. The description of resource perspective in dynamic workflows has not been sufficiently studied yet. Some previous researches have considered constraints related to resources [6]. Nevertheless, they have been limited to human resources and have neglected other types of resources particularly Cloud computing resources. In fact, Cloud computing is being increasingly used for deploying and executing workflow applications [7]. It offers different types of resources on demand. The main characteristics of Cloud such as elasticity and shareability bring many verification issues which influence the system performance. Boubaker et al. [8] have presented a formal specification to validate the consistency of resource allocation for workflow applications. However, they consider

M. Themistocleous and P. Rupino da Cunha (Eds.): EMCIS 2018, LNBIP 341, pp. 144–157, 2019.
https://doi.org/10.1007/978-3-030-11395-7_14

static workflows and don't take into account the dynamic adaptation which consists in changing workflows during execution. Also, the existing works do not take into account the data flow correctness during workflow adaptation.

Basically, our aim in this paper is to ensure the correctness of dynamic workflow changes while considering control flow, data flow and resource perspectives. To do so, we introduce a set of constraints which must be respected. Particularly, we define properties related to (i) structural and behavioral correctness which refer to the control of structural inconsistency at model and instance levels such as isolated tasks, deadlock, (ii) semantic correctness which refers to domain constraint requirements, (iii) data flow correctness which consists in preserving the correctness of the data inputs and outputs of tasks and (iv) resource behavior correctness which consists in verifying some constraints (i.e. sharebility and elasticity) and ensuring a correct allocation at design time and runtime. Concretely, we propose a formal model based on Event-B method [9, 10] which focuses on the refinement technique to deal with the complexity of a system. In fact, this technique consists in introducing the different properties in a step-by-step fashion. It is the foundation of the correct-by-construction approach.

The remainder of this paper is organized as follows: In Sect. 2, we introduce our motivating example. Section 3 details our proposed formalization of dynamic workflows in a Cloud environment. In Sect. 4, we illustrate the verification of our Event-B specification. The related work is presented in Sect. 5. Finally, the last Section concludes and provides insights for future work.

## 2  Motivating Example

To illustrate our approach, we consider an order processing scenario of an online store. We use BPMN[1] modeling language to describe our process (see Fig. 1). The latter is triggered when a consumer logins in the shop's website (T1). Then, it can check whether the ordered articles are available or not (T2). Next, the total cost is calculated (T3). Afterwards, the payment is carried out according to the customer preferences: using bank transfer (T4) and credit card (T5). If the customer approves the order (T6), the tasks T7 and T8 can be performed. After that, an invoice is generated (T9) and an email is sent to the customer (T10). Finally, the order will be delivered to the customer (T11).

Non-human resources are required to execute most of these tasks. For example, the first task is performed in a virtual machine, T1 and T2 share a database service hosted in the Cloud, etc. Workflow applications continuously evolve to respond to certain requirements. We cite, for example, market evolution, policies shift and changes in the customer behavior. Thus, the support of dynamic changes has become crucial for the success of many enterprises. The changes can take place at two levels: the model level and the instance level. For instance, a new requirement to compute the total cost has become necessary.

---

[1] Business Process Modeling Notation: http://www.bpmn.org/.

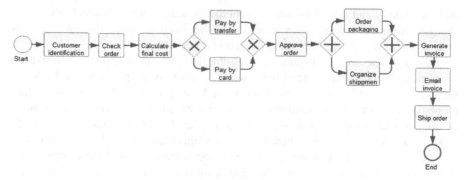

**Fig. 1.** Motivating example

It consists in substituting the task (T3) by a block of tasks which consists in waiving the shipping fee if the total amount exceeds 80$. Otherwise, a shipping cost will be added. This cost depends on the customer's address. Then, two new tasks "Get shipment address" and "Include shipment fee" are introduced before T3. Also, a new option that allows the customer to subscribe to loyal customer is added after approving the order (T6). After subscription, the customer profile will be updated and on the next connection, the discount rates will be applied. In addition, there is the case of some commercial events organized by large companies such as Black Friday and Cyber-Monday. These events are intended to encourage online shopping by applying significant discount rates. So, the number of users becomes higher which may cause server overload and some unforeseen exceptions.

In order to cope with these situations, changing workflow application during execution has become an important requirement. However, without control, these changes can lead to some errors such as infinite execution and deadlock situations. Also, they can cause problems at the resource management level. For instance, an inserted task must be assigned to a resource. In addition, substitution or deletion of tasks require a new resource assignment. Moreover, a non-shareable resource cannot be affected to more than one task instance. So, in order to ensure the correctness of a dynamic workflow application in the Cloud, we propose using formal techniques. We focus on constraints related to control flow and resource perspective. These constraints cover both the design and the execution requirements. Our goal is to avoid inconsistencies before deploying the application or even purchasing the needed resources from a Cloud provider.

## 3  Formal Modeling of a Dynamic Workflow in the Cloud

In this section, we present our Event-B model of dynamic workflows highlighting the behavior of resource allocation. As illustrated in Fig. 2, six abstraction levels are defined:

(1) The machine WfM0 models the coordination between tasks and the adaptation actions at the workflow model level. This machine uses the context WfC0 which defines the different elements of a workflow.
(2) The machine WfM1 refines WfM0 and integrates some semantic constraints while preserving the workflow correctness.
(3) The machine WfM2 refines WfM1 and introduces the execution instances of a workflow and its tasks. In addition, it considers the adaptation actions at the instance level. This machine sees the context WfC2 which extends WfC0.
(4) In the machine WfM3, the properties related to data flow perspective are considered.
(5) The resource assigned to workflow tasks are added to the machine WfM4. We take into account the shareability property of Cloud resources. WfM4 sees the context WfC4 which extends WfC3.
(6) In the machine WfM5, we specify the behavior of the resource instances as well as the elasticity property to manage the workflow changes at runtime. This machine uses the context WfC5 which extends WfC4.

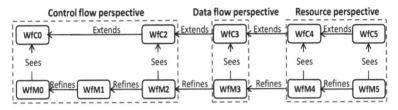

**Fig. 2.** Event-B model

In the following parts, we describe these abstraction levels in detail.

## 3.1 Formalizing the Control Flow Perspective

In this subsection, we introduce the first part of our model which is spread over three abstraction levels. It models the control flow perspective that presents the workflow tasks and their execution order.

### 3.1.1 Abstract Specification

In the abstract model, we describe the first level of our specification which holds the workflow nodes and their relations. We begin by presenting the first context WfC0 which contains a finite set (*NODES*) to define the node of a workflow. We distinguish three types of nodes: tasks (TASKS), split connectors (*ND_SPLIT*) and join connectors (*ND_JOIN*). *ND_SPLIT* and *ND_JOIN* have three types of connectors: AND, XOR and OR.

The goal of the initial machine WfM0 is to define coordination between tasks. WfM0 sees the context WfC0 described above. We define the variable *ND* to store the nodes of a workflow application. *ND* is a subset of *NODES* that includes tasks, *split* connectors, and *join* connectors of a workflow (inv1, inv2 and inv3). In BPMN, each connector (*split* or *join*) has a type. This is specified using the total function *CON_Type* (inv4). The execution order of the nodes is modeled using the variable *Seq* specified in the invariant (inv5). Also, we define two sets *Initial_Tasks* and *Final_Tasks* which store, respectively, the initial and final tasks of a workflow (inv6).

$$
\begin{aligned}
&\mathbf{inv1}: ND \subseteq NODES \\
&\mathbf{inv2}: Tasks \subseteq TASKS \wedge ND\_split \subseteq ND\_SPLIT \wedge \\
&ND\_join \subseteq ND\_JOIN \\
&\mathbf{inv3}: ND = Tasks \cup ND\_split \cup ND\_join \\
&\mathbf{inv4}: CON\_Type \in ND \rightarrow (ND\_SPLIT \cup ND\_JOIN) \\
&\mathbf{inv5}: Seq \in ND \leftrightarrow ND \\
&\mathbf{inv6}: Final\_Tasks \subseteq Tasks \wedge Initial\_Tasks \subseteq Tasks
\end{aligned}
$$

– **Structural constraints:** To ensure the structural correctness of a workflow, we introduce some constraints. To specify these constraints, we define the variable *closure*. The latter expresses the transitive closure[2] which determines all the nodes accessible from a given node of the workflow. It takes as input the sequential relations between nodes. The invariants that characterize a transitive closure according to Abrial [9] are presented in inv10, inv11, inv12 and inv13.

$$
\begin{aligned}
&\mathbf{inv7}: \forall x1, x2, T \cdot T \in Tasks \setminus Initial\_Tasks \wedge x1 \mapsto T \in Seq \wedge x1 \neq x2 \Rightarrow x2 \mapsto T \notin Seq \\
&\mathbf{inv8}: \forall x1, x2, T \cdot T \in Tasks \setminus Final\_Tasks \wedge T \mapsto x1 \in Seq \wedge x1 \neq x2 \Rightarrow T \mapsto x2 \notin Seq \\
&\mathbf{inv9}: \forall nds \cdot nds \in ND\_split \wedge nds \in ran(Seq) \Rightarrow card(Seq^{-1}[\{nds\}]) = 1 \\
&\mathbf{inv10}: closure \in (ND \leftrightarrow ND) \rightarrow (ND \leftrightarrow ND) \\
&\mathbf{inv11}: \forall r \cdot r \subseteq closure(r) \\
&\mathbf{inv12}: \forall r \cdot closure(r); r \subseteq closure(r) \\
&\mathbf{inv13}: \forall r, s \cdot r \subseteq s \wedge s; r \subseteq s \Rightarrow closure(r) \subseteq s \\
&\mathbf{inv14}: \forall node, T0 \cdot node \in ND \wedge T0 \in Initial\_Tasks \wedge node \neq T0 \Rightarrow \\
&node \in (closure(Seq)[\{T0\}]) \\
&\mathbf{inv15}: \forall node, Tf \cdot node \in ND \wedge Tf \in Final\_Tasks \wedge node \neq Tf \Rightarrow (closure(Seq)[\{node\}]) \\
&\cap \{Tf\} \neq \varnothing
\end{aligned}
$$

There are some constraints intended for each workflow element. For example, each task (except the initial ones) has exactly one incoming arc (inv7), each task (except the final ones) has exactly one outgoing arc (inv8), each split connector has exactly one incoming arc (inv9), etc. Moreover, a workflow is considered to be sound if it can satisfy two conditions which ensure that each workflow node has a path from the initial task to the final task. Firstly, all workflow nodes can be activated, i.e. every node can be reached from the initial task (inv14). Secondly, for each task in the workflow, there is at least one possible path leading from this task to a final task (inv15).

– **Behavioral constraints:** The soundness of a workflow can be affected by two types of errors: deadlock and lack of synchronization [11]. These errors are caused by a mismatch between joins and splits connectors. In order to prevent these situations during workflow adaptation, we introduce some invariants. These invariants must be preserved by all the defined events. In Fig. 3, we show an example of a lack of synchronization.

---

[2] The transitive closure of a simple oriented graph is the graph obtained by keeping the nodes and adding the arcs (*x*, *y*) for which there is a path from *x* to *y* in the initial graph.

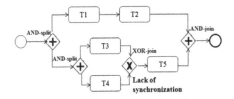

**Fig. 3.** Lack of synchronization situation

In fact, the task T5 can never be activated. This situation is not allowed by defining an invariant which guarantees that an AND-split should not be followed by an XOR-join or an OR-join.

- **Adaptation patterns:** The adaptation patterns (or change operations) are actions taken to react to some events triggered at runtime. To allow the workflow dynamic change, a variety of adaptation patterns can be supported [12]. In this work, we define some primitive of atomic operations that can be used to modify a workflow model or instance:
  - Insert($T$, $a$, $b$): Insert task $T$ between $a$ and $b$
  - Replace($T_1$, $T_2$): Replace task $T_1$ by $T_2$
  - Remove($T$, $a$, $b$): Remove task $T$ from the workflow.

Each operation is associated with formal pre/post-conditions which are necessary to preserve the correctness of the respective model. It is specified by an event in Event-B. Due to lack of space, we illustrate in this paper only the event *Remove_Task* which aims to remove a task $T$ at the model level (see below). This event can be triggered if some conditions are met. Indeed, we have to check that the tasks $T$, its predecessor "$a$" and its successor "$b$" are different (grd1) and successive (grd2). The actions defined in the clause "THEN" consist in updating the nodes and the workflow tasks (act1 and act2), the *Seq* and *closure* variables containing the relations between the nodes (act3 and act4) as well as the variable *CON_Type* (act5).

```
EVENT      Remove_Task
ANY        T, a, b
WHERE
  grd1 : T ∈ Tasks ∧ a ∈ Tasks ∧ b ∈ Tasks ∧ a ≠ b
  grd2 : a ↦ T ∈ Seq ∧ T ↦ b ∈ Seq
THEN
  act1 : Tasks := Tasks \ {T}
  act2 : ND := ND \ {T}
  act3 : Seq := (Seq \ {a ↦ T, T ↦ b}) ∪ {a ↦ b}
  act4 : closure :∈ (ND \ {T} ↔ ND \ {T}) → (ND \ {T} ↔ ND \ {T})
  act5 : CON_Type :∈ (ND \ {T}) → (ND_SPLIT ∪ ND_JOIN)

END
```

### 3.1.2   First Level of Refinement
We define the semantic constraints as domain specific requirements that have to be respected during the workflow execution. We present in Table 1 the set of the semantic constraints that we have considered.

**Table 1.** Semantic constraints

| Constraint | Meaning |
|---|---|
| Mandatory ($T_i$) | Task $T_i$ must be executed |
| Dependency ($T_i$, $T_j$) | The presence of $T_i$ imposes the restriction that $T_j$ must be included |
| Obligation ($T_i \Rightarrow T_j$) | If $T_i$ is executed) $\Rightarrow T_j$ must be executed |
| Sequence ($T_i$, $T_j$) | $T_j$ must be executed after $T_i$ (if both $T_i$ and $T_j$ are present) |

According to the example shown in Fig. 1, we can define the following semantic constraints:

- Mandatory ($T1$): Task $T1$ is mandatory.
- Dependency ($T1$, $T2$): Task $T2$ is dependent on $T1$.
- Obligation ($T7 \Rightarrow T8$): If task $T7$ is performed, the task $T8$ should be executed.
- Sequence ($T8$, $T9$): Task $T9$ should be executed after $T8$.

Formally, to specify these constraints, we add four variables (*Mandatory, Dependency, Obligation* and *Sequence*), each of which is intended for a semantic constraint (see inv1, inv2, inv3 and inv4). The relation between the abstract variable *Seq* and the concrete variable *Sequence* is defined by the gluing invariant inv5. The latter proves that each two tasks having a sequence constraint are necessarily successive.

```
inv1 : Mandatory ⊆ Tasks
inv2 : Dependency ⊆ Tasks × Tasks
inv3 : Obligation ⊆ Tasks × ℙ(Tasks)
inv4 : Sequence ⊆ Tasks × Tasks
inv5 : ∀Ti, Tj·Ti ↦ Tj ∈ Sequence ⇒ Ti ↦ Tj ∈ Seq
```

The dynamic adaptation actions must preserve the correctness of the semantic constraints already defined. To do so, we reinforce the guard component of the events associated with the adaptation patterns by adding new conditions. For example, in the refinement of the event Insert_Task presented in WfM0, we add a new guard ($a \mapsto b \notin$ *Sequence*) which forbids the insertion of the task $T$ between two successive tasks ($a$ and $b$) that have a sequence constraint.

### 3.1.3    Second Level of Refinement

At this level, we specify the behavior of workflow instances as well as the changes at the instance level.

- **Behavior of the workflow instances:** In a new context WfC2 which extends the context WfC0, we define the sets *WF_INST* and *NODE_INST*. These latter represent respectively the possible workflow instances and all the node instances in the system. *NODE_INST* is composed of three sub-sets: task instances, "*split*" connectors and "*join*" connectors. Each task instance goes through different states during its lifetime. In our previous work [13], we have showed the task instance life cycle inspired from [14].

After its creation, a task instance takes the state "*Initiated*". It goes to the state "*Running*" if a resource is allocated to it. Then, it can be suspended during its running. In this case, it can resume its execution or restart again. If this task instance chooses to continue its running, two cases can be presented. It can successfully complete its execution by moving to the state "*Completed*", otherwise it passes to the state "*Failed*" if it fails.

In order to specify the behavior of workflow and task instances, we define in the machine WfM2 a subset of *WF_INST* called *WF_Inst* which stores all the created instances of a given workflow (inv1).

```
inv1 : WF_Inst ⊆ WF_INST
inv2 : Node_Inst ⊆ NODE_INST
inv3 : Task_Inst ⊆ TASK_INST
inv4 : TaskInst_State ∈ TaskInst → TASK_STATES
inv5 : NDInst_WFInst ∈ NodeInst → WFInst
inv6 : TaskInst_Model ∈ Task_Inst ⇸ Tasks
inv7 : SeqInst ∈ WFInst → (Node_Inst ↔ Node_Inst)
```

In the same way, we use *Node_Inst* and *Task_Inst* which represent respectively the node and the task instances of a workflow (inv2 and inv3). Also, we define the total function *TaskInst_State* (inv4) which gives the current state of a task instance and *NDInst_WFInst* which gives the workflow instance to which a node instance belongs (inv5). Furthermore, a partial function is used *TaskInst_Model* to associate each task instance with its corresponding model (inv6). To specify the execution order of node instances, we use the total function *SeqInst* defined in inv7. The behavior of a task instance is formally modeled by introducing some events.

Firstly, we define the event AddWFInst which can create a new workflow instance *wfi*. After that, the event AddTaskInst aims to create a new task instance *Ti* of a workflow task noted *T*. The event RunTaskInst is raised if the task instance *Ti* belongs to *Task_Inst* (grd1) and has the state "*Initiated*" or "*Suspended*". Once the event RunTaskInst is activated, the task instance *Ti* takes the state "*Running*" (act1). For each transition of task states, we define an event that allows the transition from one task instance state to another (SuspendTaskInst, CompleteTaskInst, etc.)

```
EVENT      RunTaskInst
ANY        Ti
WHERE
  grd1 : Ti ∈ Task_Inst
  grd4 : TaskInst_State(Ti) ∈ {Initiated, Suspended}
THEN
  act1 : TaskInst_State(Ti) := Running
END
```

- **Workflow changes at the instance level:** We consider three adaptation actions which aim to change a workflow instance (insertion, deletion and substitution of a task). Formally, each adaptation action is specified by an event. In what follows, We provide below the event Insert_Task_Instance which consists in inserting a task *T* between two task instances *a* and *b*. This event is guarded by some conditions which check whether the tasks instances *a* and *b* belong to the same workflow instance (grd4). Besides, these two instances are successive and do not have a sequence constraint (grd5 and grd6). Moreover, the successor task $b$ has the state "*Initiated*" (grd7). In the action component, we update the sets *Task_Inst*, *Node_Inst*, *Seq_Inst*, *NDInst_WFInst* and *TaskInst_State* to take into account the new task instance.

```
EVENT       Insert_Task_Instance
ANY         T, a, b, Wfi
WHERE
  grd1 : Wfi ∈ WF_Inst
  grd2 : T ∈ TASK_INST ∧ T ∉ Task_Inst
  grd3 : a ∈ dom(TaskInst_Model) ∧ b ∈ dom(TaskInst_Model)
  grd4 : NDInst_WFInst(b) = Wfi ∧ NDInst_WFInst(a) = Wfi
  grd5 : Wfi ↦ {a ↦ b} ∈ SeqInst ∧ a ≠ T ∧ b ≠ T
  grd6 : TaskInst_Model(a) ↦ TaskInst_Model(b) ∉ Sequence
  grd7 : TaskInst_State(b) = Initiated
THEN
  ...
END
```

## 3.2   Formalizing the Data Flow Perspective: Third Level of Refinement

We distinguish three types of data flow errors that can be introduced during workflow adaptation [15]:

- **Input missing:** An input missing error occurs if a task T has an input "*d*" and there is no task before T having "*d*" as output.
- **Output redundancy:** A task T has an output redundancy error if its output "*d*" is never used by workflow tasks after it. This means that there is no task after T having the input "*d*".
- **Output lost:** A task T has an output lost error if its output "*d*" is overridden (killed) by another task after it, which has also the output "*d*".

  To ensure the preservation of data flow correctness in case of workflow adaptation, we reinforce the guard component of the events allowing to change a workflow at instance and model levels. Due to space limitation, we illustrate only the event Remove_Task. When deleting a task $T$ between two successive tasks $a$ and $b$ from a workflow model, we distinguish two possible situations (see Fig. 4).

- **The deleted task has an input "*d*":** We consider a task T having an input "*d*" and another task Tk which produces this output. Removing the task T from the workflow can cause an output redundancy problem since the datum "*d*" created by Tk will not be used. Thus, we must guarantee the presence of a task Ti after Tk having "*d*" as input. Also, we verify the absence of a task Tr having an output "*d*" and located between Ti and T (or between T and Ti). Formally, we refine the event Remove_Task event and we add a new condition necessary for its triggering.
- **The deleted task has an output "*d*":** We consider a task T having an output "*d*" and another task Tj after T using this output. When removing the task T, it is necessary to make sure that it exists a task Ti before T having "*d*" as output. In addition, we check the presence of a task Tm between Ti and T having "*d*" as input in order to remedy the problem of output loss. Formally, this is modeled by adding a new condition to the event Remove_Task.

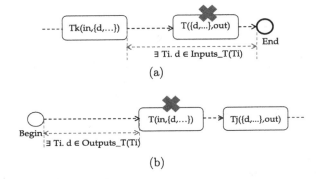

**Fig. 4.** Correctness criteria in case of task deletion

## 3.3 Formalizing the Resources Perspective

In this section, we take into account the resource perspective and some properties of Cloud resources. For this purpose, we introduce two levels of abstraction.

### 3.3.1 Fourth Level of Refinement

In this step, we extend the context WfC3 by adding Cloud resources to our model. For this reason, we introduce in the context WfC4, a new set named RES which represents all the available resources. In the fourth refinement (machine WfM4), we add the variable *WF_Resources* (a subset of RES) that represents the resources used to run a given workflow (inv1). In addition, we formally define the allocation dependency between a task and its resources through the variable AllocDep (inv2). A cloud resource can be shareable or non-shareable (inv3). Then, we introduce a new variable, named "*Shareable*", defined as a total function which determines whether the resource is shareable or not. According to inv4, each resource assigned to many tasks (*card* $(AllocDep[\{res\}]) > 1$) is necessarily shareable.

**inv1:** $WF\_Resources \subseteq RES$
**inv2:** $AllocDep \in WF\_Resources \rightarrow \mathbb{P}(Tasks)$
**inv3:** $Shareable \in WF\_Resources \rightarrow BOOL$
**inv4:** $\forall res \cdot res \in WF\_Resources \wedge (card(AllocDep[\{res\}]) > 1 \Rightarrow Shareable(res)$
$= TRUE)$

### 3.3.2 Fifth Refinement Level

In this level, we have attempted to formally specify the behavior of the resource instances and the elasticity of cloud resources. In order to model the resource instances created for a workflow, we add the context WfC5 which extends WfC4. WfC5 defines the set *RES_INST* which represents all possible resources instances. In addition, we introduce a subset of *RES_INST*, called *RES_Inst*, which contains the resource instances assigned to a workflow (inv1). Furthermore, the *RESInst_Model* function assigns each instance to its corresponding resource model (inv2). Each resource instance can take different states during its life cycle. This is ensured by the function *RESInst_State* (inv3).

**inv1:** $RES\_Inst \subseteq RES\_INST$
**inv2:** $RESInst\_Model \in RES\_Inst \rightarrow WF\_Resources$
**inv3:** $RESInst\_State \in RES\_Inst \rightarrow RES\_States$

This life cycle is independent of the Cloud resource type [13]. After its creation, a resource instance passes to the state *"Inactive"*. When it is assigned to a task instance, it goes to the state *"Allocated"*. Once the corresponding task instance begins its execution, the resource goes to the state *"Consumed"*. After the task instance completion, it takes the state *"Inactive"* for future reassignment, if it is shareable, otherwise it will be released.

Formally, to define the resource states, we add to the context WfC5 a set called *RES_States* which contains these states. For each transition, we introduce an event that describes the transition from one resource instance state to another (AddRESInst, AllocateRESInst, etc.).

At this level, we add other properties expressed by invariants to ensure the consistency of our model. These properties specify the relationship between the states of a resource instance and those of a task instance:

- Each resource instance (*ri*) which takes the state *"Allocated"* must have an allocation relation with a task instance (*Ti*) in the *"Initiated"* state.
- If a resource instance (*ri*) takes the state *"Consumed"*, it must have an allocation relation with a task instance (*Ti*) in the *"Running"* or *"Suspended"* state.
- If a task instance (*Ti*) is in the *"Completed"* state and it has an allocation relation with a non-shareable resource instance (*ri*), then *ri* must be in the state *"Released"*.

At this refinement level, we also specify the elasticity property of Cloud resources. This property allows to manage resources in order to respond to dynamic changes at the workflow level. Thus, we refine the events that consist in changing workflow at the instance level by adding some constraints. In what follows, we present the event Insert_Task_Inst which is refined in two events. In fact, we distinguish the case of shareable and non-shareable resource which is assigned to the inserted task instance:

- The first refinement is specified by the event Insert_Task_Instance_NonSh. This event introduces two new conditions to check if the inserted task *T* has an allocation relation with a non-shareable resource *ri* in the inactive state (grd8 et grd9). As a result, the resource *ri* takes the state *"Allocated"* (act6) and it will be added to the set *RES_Inst* (act7).

```
EVENT      Insert_Task_Instance_NonSh
REFINES    Insert_Task_Instance
ANY        T, a, b, Wfi, ri
WHERE
  ...
  grd8 : Shareable(RESInst_Model(ri)) = FALSE ∧ RESInst_State(ri) = Inactive
  grd9 : TaskInst_Model(T) ∈ AllocDep(RESInst_Model(ri))
THEN
  ...
  act6 : RESInst_State(ri) := Allocated
  act7 : RES_Inst := RES_Inst ∪ {ri}
END
```

– The second refinement is specified by Insert_Task_Instance_Sh event, by reinforcing the guard component. In fact, we add a new guard which verifies if the resource assigned to the task *T* is shareable. In the action component, we update the variable *RES_Inst*. The resource *ri* can take the state *"Allocated"* if the event AllocateRESInst is activated.

## 4 Verification of the Formal Development

In this section, we describe the verification of our formal development. We distinguish two types of properties that can be formally verified: the static and the dynamic properties. We prove the correctness of static properties, which are expressed in terms of invariants, using proof obligations. This consists in proving that the invariants hold in all states: they hold initially and must be maintained by each event. However, the dynamic properties depend on different states of the system taken at different times. We verify these properties using LTL [16] since they can not be expressed using invariants.

- **Verification of static properties:** To demonstrate the correctness of our formal specification, a number of POs should be discharged. There are 488 POs generated by the Rodin platform. 271 POs (56%) are automatically discharged, while the others (217 POs = 44%) which are more complex require the interaction with the provers. Formal definitions of all proof obligations are given in [9].
- **Verification of dynamic properties:** In order to verify dynamic properties, we used PROB plugin of Rodin. In fact, these properties cannot be specified as invariants since they refer to several states of the system taken at different moments. Due to lack of space, we only present two properties:
  - After its creation, a resource instance takes the state *Inactive*. We verified this property using an LTL formula involving the *Next*(X) operator:

$$G(\{ri \notin RES\_Instances\} \Rightarrow X\{ri \in RES\_Instances \Rightarrow (RES\_Instance\_State(ri) = Inactive)\})$$

  - If a resource instance *ri* is in the state *Consumed*, it will remain in this state until it passes to the state *Released* or the state *Inactive*:

$$G((\{T \in Task\_Instances \wedge Task\_Instance\_State(T) = Initiated\}) \Rightarrow (\{T \in Task\_Instances \wedge Task\_Instance\_State(T) = Initiated\}) \cup (\{T \in Task\_Instances \wedge Task\_Instance\_State(T) = Running\}))$$

## 5 Related Work

Several approaches have been proposed to verify the correctness of dynamic workflow changes [4, 17, 18]. Nevertheless, they have focused mainly on control flow perspective.

Song et al. [15] have introduced a preliminary study on the criteria ensuring the data flow correctness during workflow adaptation. However, they did not present any formal proofs to verify them. Also, some researches have considered the resources perspective. But, they have been limited to human resources such as [6]. To the best of our knowledge, the existing works do not formally model and verify the Cloud resource perspective for a dynamic workflow. Boubaker et al. [8] have tackled the problem of validating the consistency of resource allocation. However, their work is intended for static workflows. They do not consider dynamic structural changes during execution to deal with exception and evolution.

Thus, our approach intends to meet the defined criteria in Table 2. In fact, we aim, in this paper, at providing an Event-B model in order to preserve the correctness of dynamic changes for a workflow application. Our solution verifies properties related to control flow and data flow perspectives. Also, it checks the matching between tasks and Cloud resource according to some constraints.

**Table 2.** Evaluation of the approaches ensuring the correctness of workflow changes

| Ref | Modeling language | Control flow perspective | | | Data flow perspective | Resource perspective | Incremental verification | Formal verification |
|---|---|---|---|---|---|---|---|---|
| | | Structural | Behavioral | Semantic | | | | |
| [1] | − | − | − | + | − | − | − | − |
| [18] | − | − | − | + | − | − | − | − |
| [19] | − | + | + | − | − | − | − | − |
| [20] | EPCs | + | + | − | − | − | − | + |
| [3] | − | − | + | + | − | − | − | − |
| [6] | − | − | + | + | − | + | − | − |
| [4] | − | − | + | − | − | − | − | + |
| [17] | BPMN | + | + | + | − | − | + | + |
| Our approach | BPMN | + | + | + | + | + | + | + |

## 6  Conclusion

In this paper, a formal model which ensures the correctness of dynamic workflows in the Cloud is proposed, using the Event-B method. Our model specifies some constraints related to control flow and data flow perspectives. Also, it verifies the Cloud resource properties at design time and runtime. The correctness of our model is checked by discharging all proof obligations. In this work, we have considered change operations which consist in inserting, deleting and substituting a task. We plan, in our future work, to consider more complex change operations. We aim also to deal with workflow loop pattern. Finally, we intend to extend this work by taking into account the vertical elasticity which consists in changing the capacity of resources at runtime.

# References

1. Sadiq, S.W., Orlowska, M.E., Sadiq, W.: Specification and validation of process constraints for flexible workflows. Inf. Syst. **30**(5), 349–378 (2005)
2. Ly, L.T., Rinderle, S., Dadam, P.: Semantic correctness in adaptive process management systems. In: Dustdar, S., Fiadeiro, J.L., Sheth, A.P. (eds.) BPM 2006. LNCS, vol. 4102, pp. 193–208. Springer, Heidelberg (2006). https://doi.org/10.1007/11841760_14
3. Kumar, A., Yao, W., Chu, C.-H., Li, Z.: Ensuring compliance with semantic constraints in process adaptation with rule-based event processing. In: Dean, M., Hall, J., Rotolo, A., Tabet, S. (eds.) RuleML 2010. LNCS, vol. 6403, pp. 50–65. Springer, Heidelberg (2010). https://doi.org/10.1007/978-3-642-16289-3_6
4. Asadi, M., Mohabbati, B., Grner, G., Gasevic, D.: Development and validation of customized process models. Syst. Softw. **96**, 73–92 (2014)
5. Barron, M.A.Z., Ruiz-Vanoye, J.A., Díaz-Parra, O., Fuentes-Penna, A., Loranca, M.B.B.: A mathematical model for optimizing resources of scientific projects. Computación y Sistemas **20**(4) (2016)
6. Kumar, A., Yao, W., Chu, C.H.: Flexible process compliance with semantic constraints using mixed-integer programming. INFORMS J. Comput. **25**(3), 543–559 (2013)
7. Ahmed, E., Naveed, A., Hamid, S.H.A., Gani, A., Salah, K.: Formal analysis of seamless application execution in mobile cloud computing. Supercomputing **73**(10), 4466–4492 (2017)
8. Boubaker, S., Mammar, A., Graiet, M., Gaaloul, W.: Formal verification of cloud resource allocation in business processes using Event-B. In: Advanced Information Networking and Applications, pp. 746–753. IEEE (2016)
9. Abrial, J.R.: Modeling in Event-B: System and Software Engineering. Cambridge University Press, Cambridge (2010)
10. Rezaee, A., Rahmani, A.M., Movaghar, A., Teshnehlab, M.: Formal process algebraic modeling, verification, and analysis of an abstract fuzzy inference cloud service. Supercomputing **67**(2), 345–383 (2014)
11. Van Dongen, B., Mendling, J., Van Der Aalst, W.: Structural patterns for soundness of business process models. In: Enterprise Distributed Object Computing, pp. 116–128. IEEE (2006)
12. Weber, B., Reichert, M., Rinderle-Ma, S.: Change patterns and change support features-enhancing flexibility in process-aware information systems. Data Knowl. Eng. **66**(3), 438–466 (2008)
13. Fakhfakh, F., Kacem, H.H., Kacem, A.H., Fakhfakh, F.: Preserving the correctness of dynamic workflows within a cloud environment. In: Knowledge-Based and Intelligent Information & Engineering Systems (2018)
14. Hollingsworth, D., Hampshire, U.: Workflow management coalition: the workflow reference model. Document Number TC00-1003 19 (1995)
15. Song, W., Ma, X., Cheung, S.C., Hu, H., Lü, J.: Preserving data flow correctness in process adaptation. In: Services Computing, pp. 9–16. IEEE (2010)
16. Lamport, L.: The temporal logic of actions. ACM Trans. Program. Lang. Syst. **16**(3), 872–923 (1994)
17. Boubaker, S., Mammar, A., Graiet, M., Gaaloul, W.: An Event-B based approach for ensuring correct configurable business processes. In: Web Services, pp. 460–467 (2016)
18. Ly, L.T., Rinderle, S., Dadam, P.: Integration and verification of semantic constraints in adaptive process management systems. Data Knowl. Eng. **64**(1), 3–23 (2008)
19. Hallerbach, A., Bauer, T., Reichert, M.: Guaranteeing soundness of configurable process variants in provop. In: Commerce and Enterprise Computing, pp. 98–105. IEEE (2009)
20. van der Aalst, W.M., Dumas, M., Gottschalk, F., Ter Hofstede, A.H., Rosa, M.L., Mendling, J.: Preserving correctness during business process model configuration. Formal Aspects Comput. **22**(3), 459–482 (2010)

# Investigating the Factors Affecting the Adoption of Cloud Computing in SMEs: A Case Study of Saudi Arabia

Fahad Alghamdi[1(✉)], Dharmendra Sharma[1], and Milind Sathye[2]

[1] Faculty of Science and Technology, University of Canberra,
Canberra, ACT, Australia
{Fahad.alghamdi,Dharmendra.sharma}@canberra.edu.au
[2] Faculty of Business, Government, and Law, University of Canberra,
Canberra, ACT, Australia
Milind.sathye@canberra.edu.au

**Abstract.** Cloud computing technology offers promising business advantages for small and medium-sized enterprises. In Saudi Arabia, the adoption of cloud computing by SMEs has so far occurred relatively slowly. This study investigates the factors affecting the adoption of cloud computing by SMEs in Saudi Arabia. A sample of fourteen interviews conducted with IT experts provides a foundation for exploring new factors that affect this decision, as incorporated into a conceptual model developed for this study. This model draws on the Technology-Organisation-Environment framework but adjusted based on new contextual factors. Factors such as the duration of software implementation, software integration, and software customisation guided this study. Furthermore, experts were of the view that other factors such as culture and technology infrastructure also impacted the adoption of cloud computing among SMEs. This study bridges the gap in the literature on cloud computing adoption with new evidence from the unexplored context of Saudi Arabia.

**Keywords:** Cloud computing · Saudi Arabia · SME · Technology
TOE framework

## 1 Introduction

Since its beginnings as a recognisable concept in 2007, cloud computing has rapidly grown as a reliable alternative to an owner's use of in-house computing resources to supply necessary computational power [1]. The National Institute of Standards and Technology (NIST), a subsidiary agency of the Department of Commerce in the United States, refers to cloud computing as a "model" rather than the physical representation of that model [2]. NIST defines cloud computing as focusing on a "shared pool of configurable computing resources" that users are able to access with virtually no processing delay, as the intent of the model is to substitute local computing resources for distal ones (*i.e.*, on servers belonging to providers) with no perceptible difference in operational quality [2]. The delivery media of cloud computing consist of an integrated

M. Themistocleous and P. Rupino da Cunha (Eds.): EMCIS 2018, LNBIP 341, pp. 158–176, 2019.
https://doi.org/10.1007/978-3-030-11395-7_15

network of computer servers, storage capacity, software applications, and dedicated service processes in a provider organisation.

Prior literature found that cloud computing favourably impacts SMEs' performance and sustainability [3–5]. For example, cloud computing enables the SMEs to access features of advanced technology that entail lower costs and risk than previously available options [6]. Cost savings are the most significant benefit that SMEs can obtain from the adoption of cloud computing [7].

The motivation for this study stems from the following considerations: First, despite the advantages of cloud computing, the adoption rate by SMEs in Saudi Arabia is still very low [8]. Indeed, limited literature exists on the factors that affect the adoption of cloud computing by Saudi Arabian SMEs. Second, the present study brings to the fore several new factors that affect SMEs' decisions to adopt cloud computing, which prior literature has thus far overlooked. Specifically, current studies in cloud computing adoption by SMEs need to consider factors such as the duration of cloud implementation, the smoothness of both system integration and data synchronisation, and the customisability of the underlying software [9]. These factors therefore guide the present study, which additionally explores novel factors based on user input. Third, in addition to its purely theoretical contribution, this study highlights the practical implications of cloud computing adoption among Saudi Arabian SMEs in particular.

Currently, the contribution of SMEs to the Saudi gross domestic product (GDP) is lower and poorer than the contributions of other G20 members [10]. If SME contributions to GDP are to increase, the SMEs need to adopt cost-effective technologies such as cloud computing. However, few studies are currently available to specify the forces that are impeding the adoption of cloud computing by Saudi SMEs. In response to this gap in the literature, the present study aims to inform Saudi government policy to increase cloud computing uptake and ultimately to contribute to the growth of this important sector of the Saudi economy.

The structure of this paper begins with a literature review of the field of technology adoption as applied to cloud computing, followed by an explanation of the conceptual model based on current theory. The discussion then turns to an explanation of the data and method used for exploring the impediments of cloud computing adoption among Saudi Arabian SMEs. A display of the results follows in turn, with an analysis and conclusion to discuss implications for theory and practice.

## 2    Literature Review

### 2.1    Cloud Computing Adoption by SMEs

Several studies have acknowledged the factors influencing organisations' decisions to adopt cloud computing. Although SMEs represent most of businesses in any country [4, 11], the literature generally discusses the use of cloud computing in the context of large organisations [9]. Table 1 list exceptions to this rule across several countries. Aside from such exceptions, few studies explore cloud computing in the SMEs context [4]. A better understanding of issues related to SMEs' adoption of cloud computing is therefore urgently necessary [12]. The objects of analysis that the research should address include the duration of cloud implementation, data synchronisation, customisation of cloud solutions, and smooth integration of information between cloud solutions and other services [9]. To date, no study has yet explored these issues. Meanwhile, other research has encouraged the exploration of additional factors in other contexts [3, 4]. Accordingly, the purpose of this study is to build an enhanced model of those factors that affect the adoption of cloud computing in small and medium-sized enterprises to advance the research along the lines suggested by the noted authors.

**Table 1.** Recent advances of cloud computing adoption in SMEs

| Citation | Model | Type | Context | Key finding |
|---|---|---|---|---|
| Al Isma'ili et al. [13] | TOE, DOI | Quantitative empirical | Australia | Adoption drivers: Tech. (cost savings, relative advantages, compatibility, trialability), Org. (firm size, top mgt. support, firm innovativeness, IS knowledge), Env. (market scope, external computing support) |
| Al Isma'ili et al. [14] | TOE, DOI, ANT | Qualitative, interviews | Australia | Adoption influencers: security concerns, cost savings, privacy, geographical restrictions |
| Alshamaila et al. [4] | TOE | Qualitative, interviews | UK | Adoption drivers: relative advantage, risk, compatibility, reach, trialability, firm size, top mgt. support, innovation bias, prior experience, external computing support, industry, market scope, supplier efforts |
| Amini et al. [5] | TMR | Quantitative, empirical | Iran | Top manager behaviours (analyser, motivator, vision setter, task master) affect adoption decisions |
| Bharadwaj and Lal [15] | DOI, DCT, TAM | Qualitative, case study | India | Adoption influencers: perceived usefulness and ease of use, relative advantage, vendor credibility, org. technology orientation |
| Gupta et al. [9] | TOE | Quantitative | India | Adoption drivers: ease of use, convenience, data security, data privacy. Biases against collaborating through cloud. Perception of low reliability |
| Liu et al. [16] | FIU | Qualitative, four case studies | China | Value-creating potential of cloud computing comes mainly from flexibility of usage, ubiquity of customer access, and capacity for integration, which create organisational agility |
| Mahara [17] | ETP | Quantitative, empirical | India | Main adoption driver is economic. Main impediment is data security, backup capability, availability |
| Mikkonen and Khan [11] | TOE | Qualitative, interviews | Finland | Adoption drivers: cost savings, flexibility, scalability, risk reduction, data security, IT support |
| Seethamraju [18] | TOE, DOI, TAM | Qualitative, four case studies | India | Adoption drivers: vendor reputation, software fit, IT support, vendor involvement |
| Trinh et al. [19] | TOE, DOI, PMT | Conceptual | SaaS | Security risk is a predominant factor to consider in adoption decision |

Notes: ANT (actor network theory); CT (contingency theory); DCT (dynamic-capabilities theory); DOI (diffusion-of-innovation theory); ETP (economical–technological–people model); FIU (flexibility–integration–ubiquity model); PMT (protection motivation theory); TAM (technology adoption model); TOE (technology–organisation–environment framework); TMR (top management roles).

## 2.2    Cloud Computing Adoption by Saudi SMEs

Small and medium-sized businesses are defined in various ways. While in some countries the definition of small and medium firms is based on assets, in other countries the definition depends on the number of employees [20]. The General Authority for Small and Medium Enterprises in Saudi Arabia (SMEA) categorises SMEs as micro, small, and medium [21]. The characteristics for each category are set out in Table 2. This division is based on two factors, namely, the number of employees and annual revenue. The SMEA is an official government agent responsible for controlling, supporting, and managing the SMEs sector in Saudi Arabia. The present study will adopt the SMEA's definition because it is most relevant to the officially trackable system that the Saudi government uses.

**Table 2.**  SME types in Saudi Arabia.

| Firm size | Employees | Annual revenue | |
|---|---|---|---|
| | | SAR | USD |
| Micro firm | 1–5 | $\leq 3$ million | $\leq 810,000$ |
| Small firm | 6–49 | 3 to 40 million | 810,000 to 10.8 million |
| Medium firm | 50–249 | 40 to 200 million | 10.8 million to 54 million |

Note: The General Authority for Small and Medium Enterprises (SMEA) places a firm in the larger category based on employee and revenue criteria [22]. The SMEA categorises firms with at 250 or more employees or over SAR 200 million in annual revenue as large firms.

A study of the presence of cloud computing among SMEs in Saudi Arabia using a sample of 80 SMEs in Jeddah found that most respondent organisations had yet to adopt cloud computing [8]. Nevertheless, the study also found that the majority of SME managers admitted that cloud computing would help their organisations gain many advantages. They concluded that SMEs did not oppose cloud computing, but were simply unsure how to use it. Security and privacy issues were a relatively minor concern for SMEs in the decision over whether to use cloud computing [8]. In fact, the cloud computing adoption rate by SMEs in Saudi Arabia is still very low. Despite the low adoption rate, the study concluded that cloud computing was a promising technology with significant advantages for SMEs in Saudi Arabia. Moreover, the study stated that more studies are needed to explore the factors that drive the adoption of cloud computing usage in small and medium-sized enterprises in Saudi Arabia. Another study examined the decision of cloud computing adoption by small and medium-sized enterprises in Saudi Arabia, with similar findings [23]. The study investigated the factors affecting SMEs decisions to adopt cloud computing based on the BOCR (benefits–opportunities–cost–risk) framework. Using an analytical hierarch process (AHP) to construct their structural model, the authors collected data from a sample of 120 IT experts in SMEs in Riyadh. Benefits and opportunities were the first and second strongest factors in the results. SMEs in Saudi Arabia see the benefits of cloud computing and new business opportunities as more important than cost and risk assessments. The risk factors fell into third place in the analysis and featured security and privacy issues. Cost factors were the least important. This observation indicates that the priority of the benefits and opportunities for SMEs are exceeding the associated costs of moving from traditional IT systems to cloud computing [23]. However, the study was unable to generalise to all SMEs in Saudi Arabia, because it only took place in one city (Riyadh), where the conditions are significantly different from those of other cities.

In view of the foregoing findings from previous studies, the present study aims to provide a better understanding of the reasons for the slow adoption rate of cloud computing in the Saudi SME sector. This study thus seeks to contribute to existing research by exploring the influences of new technological factors such as the duration of cloud implementation, the availability of customisation of cloud solutions, and the capability of cloud solutions to integrate services with other systems inside and outside the firm. This study is also unique in that it has gathered the views of experts working with major technology providers in Saudi Arabia, rather than the views of SMEs managers.

# 3    Conceptual Model: Adoption of Cloud Computing

## 3.1    Theoretical Background

The theoretical framework used for this study is Tornatzky and Fleischer's three-factor model of technological, organisational, and environmental forces (TOE) [24]. The intent of this framework is to examine the key technology adoption factors at the organisation level of analysis [25]. Under this framework, an organisation's choice to adopt new technology is a product of interactions among three broad forces: (a) the nature of the organisation's current and immediately available technology [24]; (b) the organisation's resource needs, training needs, and change orientation [17]; and (c) the competitive and technological pressures and accommodations of the task environment [4, 26]. The primary strength of the TOE framework is its comprehensive nature. The framework is precise enough to provide predictive power for empirical analysis, while flexible enough to adapt to a variety of organisational and technological contexts. The model is also adaptable to new organisational situations [18, 27, 28].

The TOE concept quickly entered into the scholarly literature with Cooper and Zmud's study of technological diffusion, which the authors sought to explain from the perspective of a broader range of forces than merely that of technology *per se* [29]. The framework differed from prior efforts to explain technological diffusion by incorporating relevant aspects of organisational decision behaviour and the demands of the external task environment into a comprehensive explanatory apparatus. The TOE framework subsequently appeared in Iacovo, Benbasat, and Dexter's study on electronic data interchange [30]. It thus entered the more abstract literature where organisation theory overlaps with systems theory and thereby established itself as a dynamic model for linking theory to practice [31].

## 3.2    Technology Adoption: Social Impact

The social impact on new technology adoption has been perceptible by several studies [32, 33]. This field involves assessments into how people generally alter their social behaviour when confronted with technological media that partially or fully bridge the gap between individual and social action [34]. From the cultural perspective, certain cultures have higher degrees of resistance to risky situations than do other cultures. With respect to Saudi's culture, the prejudgment fear from using external servers impeded SMEs' decisions makers from taking a step toward adoption of cloud computing. The use of external servers invites a level of security risk that is more appreciable than the corresponding risk expected from the use of in-house servers. The logic behind this proposition is that external servers, owned by cloud providers, contain such large amounts of proprietary data as to render them attractive targets of hackers or data thieves [19].

### 3.3   Research Model

The model for this study maintains the core structure of the TOE framework, but it also incorporates additional variables. It includes the list of factors proposed by Gupta, Seetharaman, and Raj, which the authors suggested to be in need of methodical exploration to test their effects on the adoption of cloud computing by small and medium-sized enterprises [9]. The model also combines multiple sets of factors found in previous models and incorporates factors that were suggested in experts' interviews investigations. Figure 1 presents the proposed conceptual model for this study.

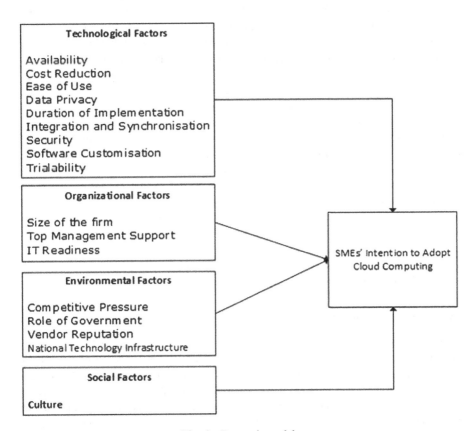

**Fig. 1.** Research model.

The model show in Fig. 1 presents the three generic categories of the TOE framework as antecedents of SMEs adoption of cloud computing, with reference to the Saudi context. The subsidiary elements within each category are products of the literature, which has addressed each element in some form over time. Given the qualitative, interview-based nature of this study, the content of the interview questions will therefore touch on these elements as far as possible. The additional category of social factors depicts culture, which has emerged during the experts' interviews as a main influencer on SMEs' decisions to adopt cloud computing. Therefore, this social context was added to the conceptual model of this study.

# 4   Methodology

## 4.1   Research Design

This research uses a qualitative approach to identify the factors that affect the adoption of cloud computing by SMEs in Saudi Arabia. This approach is suitable for gaining potentially new insights into aspects of experience that available surveys may overlook [13]. With similar justifications, other researchers have also used the qualitative approach to discover new factors of technology adoption that the extant literature might have overlooked [35, 36]. In this sense, the present study is exploratory in nature and anticipates potentially rendering its thematic findings into a quantifiable (*i.e.*, survey-based) form in future research. Accordingly, to clarify the factors hypothesised for inclusion in the initial research model, this study has collected samples of IT experts' knowledge through semi-structured interviews with experts in cloud computing who were working with major technology providers in Saudi Arabia.

The design of the interview content consisted of open-ended questions. The questions revolved around the central theme of asking experts to offer their views of factors that might affect SMEs adoption of cloud computing in Saudi Arabia. The interview questions also addressed the theme of expert expectations regarding the future of cloud computing in the Saudi Arabian SMEs sector. To ensure clarity of interview questions, the interview design included a careful step of validation, followed by several revisions. Academic personnel, including both researchers and doctoral students, provided the responsiveness necessary for the pilot phase of developing the interview structure. The pilot phase aimed to increase each question's reliability, clarity, and linkage with the research objectives. The University of Canberra's Human Research Ethics Committee approved this research project (HREC 17-31).

## 4.2   Data Collection and Analysis

The interviews took place from June to September 2017. Each interview lasted between 50 and 90 min. As a first step, the selection of interviewees consisted of first establishing a sampling frame consisting of identifying as many small to medium-sized technology providers in Saudi Arabia as possible. The result was a list of 253 firms. In this first phase of creating the sampling frame, the firms had to specialise in information technology, with or without cloud computing among their services. The request for participation, as fielded to all of the identified companies, screened first-wave responses to target those firms that offered cloud computing services exclusively. Responses arrived from 41.5% of the companies, whereof 25 offered cloud computing services. A follow-up request for participation to those 25 firms resulted in a list of 16 experts that were willing to participate in the interview process. Two respondents were unable to meet the remaining qualifications (as described below), so the final sample consisted of 14 IT experts. Table 3 shows the participants' profiles. To maintain anonymity, the table uses arbitrary acronyms to represent the participants.

**Table 3.** Participants' profiles.

| Participant | Education level | Experience | Main area of expertise |
|---|---|---|---|
| Expert AD | Master's degree | >19 years | Software development and sales |
| Expert FE | Bachelor's degree | >10 years | Business solutions development |
| Expert ST | Bachelor's degree | >10 years | IT security |
| Expert ND | Master's degree | >15 years | Solutions architecture |
| Expert AA | Bachelor's degree | ~12 years | Computer science and marketing |
| Expert MA | Bachelor's degree | ~8 years | Cloud computing |
| Expert TA | Bachelor's degree | >6 years | Market sizing, sales, and pre-sales cycle |
| Expert WA | Bachelor's degree | >20 years | IT and marketing |
| Expert SA | Bachelor's degree | >13 years | IT sales |
| Expert AT | Master's degree | >5 years | Cloud development |
| Expert RJ | Bachelor's degree | ~16 years | IT and marketing |
| Expert TB | Master's degree | ~18 years | IT and marketing |
| Expert OE | Bachelor's degree | >20 years | IT and marketing |
| Expert IS | Bachelor's degree | ~8 years | IT management and marketing |

The aforementioned process provided a foundation for data saturation, which occurs within the first 12 interviews, as long as the range of interviewees represents the true range of experiential types in the population [37]. The additional qualifications for participation included having more than five years of working experience in IT and working in an area of their respective SME in which they had some influence over marketing decisions. These criteria served to ensure that the participants possessed the correct type of expertise to answer the questions. The selection of participants created a mix that included certain international technology providers, such as Microsoft and Oracle, some major, local technology providers, such as Saudi Telecommunication Company STC, Mobily, and ELM, and some smaller, local technology providers as well. This mixture of participants from different technology providers in the country established a reasonable basis for obtaining a comprehensive view on the topic.

Each interview session was subject to audio recording with the participant's permission. After completing each interview session, the process entailed transcribing the data into a Microsoft Word™ document which enabled sufficient time for analysis. Two primary ways exist by which to analyse qualitative data [38]. The first approach is deductive, wherein researchers can use a predetermined framework or theory to analyse the data. The second approach is inductive, wherein the researchers make limited use of a predetermined theory or framework in analysing the data [38]. The present study uses a hybrid of both the inductive and the deductive approaches. This hybrid approach is useful if the researcher uses both data-driven codes and theory-driven codes in the same analysis [39]. This study therefore first employed an inductive analysis to explore new factors that derive from the data and to discover emergent themes.

The use of thematic analysis is dominant in qualitative analysis. This method involves analysing transcripts, identifying themes within the data, and supporting each theme with some evidence from the available text [38]. In this study, the researcher created a transcript document for each respondent's interview results. The analysis began with a reading of each transcribed interview, to create a summary. Each summary included the most frequently expressed themes within the participant's responses. Before moving to next step, the researcher reviewed the coding to ensure that it conformed to the original data, to avoid the risk of deviating from the participant's intent. After that step, the researcher derived new themes from the data according to the categories of the theoretical framework (TOE model) used in this study.

The final phase of the thematic analysis consisted of consolidating the themes and noting their percentage occurrence among the respondents. For example, 93% of the respondents mentioned cost reduction in some way, as one of the reasons to adopt cloud computing among SMEs. In plain terms, only one of the 14 experts failed to mention cost as a consideration, hence the 93% result (*i.e.*, 13 out of 14). Thus, the more commonly represented a theme proved to be, as a function of how many of the participants mentioned it, the greater is the level of importance that one may attribute to the idea behind the theme. In turn, insofar as a theme proves to be important to SMEs adoption in the collective view of the sample of experts represented in this study, later research will incorporate the theme into a quantitative survey to measure it more methodically in a future, larger sample. Moreover, testing the same themes, in this way, among users of cloud computing, in contrast to IT experts, may validate the perceptions of the experts featured in this study.

## 5    Findings and Discussion

As noted previously, the main objective of this study was to identify the factors that affect the adoption of cloud computing by SMEs in Saudi Arabia. Based on the TOE framework, which served as the guiding lens through which to identify relevant themes in this study, these factors fell into three contexts: (a) technological context; (b) organisational context; and (c) environmental context as per TOE model. In addition, this study found that certain sociol factors, such as Saudi's culture, are important factors affecting SMEs' decision to adopt cloud computing. Therefore, a new (d) social context was added to the research model for this study. The following sections present and discuss the findings within each context.

### 5.1    Technology Context

Technological context refers to the internal and external technologies related to the organisation [24]. These factors include the nature of the technology, its availability, and other considerations. In this context, the majority of the experts agreed with the validity of the factors incorporated into the research model of this study. Table 4 shows the percentage of experts' support of each technological factor in the research model.

**Table 4.** Experts' views of technological factors.

| Factor | Support | Non-support |
|---|---|---|
| Cost reduction | 93% | 7% |
| Ease of use | 85% | 15% |
| Security | 72% | 28% |
| Data privacy | 57% | 43% |
| Availability | 86% | 14% |
| Software package customisation | 71% | 29% |
| Duration of implementation | 93% | 7% |
| Smooth service integration and data synchronisation | 71% | 29% |
| Trialability | 71% | 29% |

**Cost Reduction.** As is visible in the above table, 93% of the experts support the notion that cloud computing will result in cost reduction. The SMEs must operate with limited resources, so the cost factor is important to them. Most interviewees indicated the cost factor as the first consideration when SMEs make their decisions about adopting cloud computing. For example, RJ stated, *"There is no question about this, total saving in the cloud might reach 60%–70%, absolutely, this saving will affect their decision".*

**Ease of Use.** The majority of experts agreed that ease of use of the cloud services was a significant factor in adopting cloud computing. The data showed that about 85% of the participants support the impact of this factor in SMEs decisions to move to cloud computing. For example, OE commented, *"Usability features in cloud computing are important for SMEs' decision makers".*

**Security.** This factor produced different views across the experts. However, all of the participants agreed that cloud computing is more secure than what the SMEs typically have in their environments. Concerning the security impact on SME decisions to adopt cloud computing, it was found that about 72% of the participants support the claim that security has a major impact in SMEs' decisions to adopt cloud adoption. Many of the experts noted this impact. For example, IS responded, *"The first question from SMEs is about security".*

**Data Privacy.** The nature of the data within SMEs determines the level of privacy concern in the firm. Of the respondents, about 57% of the experts cited data privacy as an issue for SMEs to adopt cloud computing. This is clearly visible in the quotes by experts such as *ST: "They are trying to get the benefits of the cloud without risking their data privacy".*

**Availability.** The responses showed the high importance of this factor in SME decisions to adopt cloud computing. The need to keep the system up and running is a vital issue for SMEs. In all, about 86% of the experts believe that SMEs decisions to adopt cloud computing are at least partially a function of the available time of the service. This finding is evident in the response of expert ST: *"Cloud offers high business continuity, always available"*.

**Software Customisation.** Many experts' views supported the importance of this factor to adoption decisions for SME cloud computing. Of the respondents, 71% of experts believed that SMEs are willing to move to the cloud if they can find a customised package that serves their specific needs. This finding is apparent in many experts' responses, such as *FE: "In Saudi Arabia market, organisations are looking for customised cloud solution as much as possible"*.

**Duration of Implementation.** This factor was important to 93% of the experts. Time to market is one of many reasons that experts think is driving SMEs to adopt cloud computing. The responses by many experts reflected this observation, such as *ND: "This is very important for SMEs, they need to get on the ground very quickly"*.

**Smooth Services Integration and Data Synchronisation.** This factor proved to be one of the major issues affecting SMEs decisions to adopt cloud computing. Of the participants, about 71% of the experts support the impact of this factor on SMEs adoption decisions. One of the reasons was the integration with government online services, which will save them considerable time and expense. This is visible in many responses by the experts, such as *OE: "If you have a solution that is not compatible or cannot be integrated with the cloud solution, for sure, this will hinder the adoption"*.

**Trialability.** Letting people interact more with the solution before actually using it proved to be a major concern for SMEs to adopt cloud computing. The data show that around 71% of the experts expect awareness and acceptance to increase after exposure to a trial version of the solution. Many experts' responses reflect the positive impact of a trial version on SME decisions to adopt cloud computing, such as *ST: "On cloud computing trial version is a free kit, this has positive impact"*.

## 5.2   Organisational Context

Organisational context addresses the organisation's resources and characteristics from the perspective of decision making [17]. In this context, all factors have shown validity as having a significant effect on SMEs decisions to adopt cloud computing by the majority of experts. Table 5 shows the percentage of support for each factor in the research model. Furthermore, selected experts' statements serve to establish the validity of each factor.

**Table 5.** Experts' views of organisational factors.

| Factor | Support | Non-support |
| --- | --- | --- |
| Top management support | 86% | 14% |
| Size of firm | 100% | 0% |
| Technology readiness | 76% | 24% |

**Top Management Support.** Top managers are the decision makers in any organisation. It is practically a universal axiom that top management support is necessary for any kind of major organisational change. This study shows the influence of this factor on SMEs decisions to adopt cloud computing, as 86% of the experts support the impact that top management has in these decisions, such as EF: *"Of course, their role in decisions is very effective"*.

**Size of Firm.** The size of the firm is a very influential force on the decision to adopt cloud computing. Larger firms have greater economies of scale than do smaller ones, so they can more easily dedicate resources to the adoption of new technologies. The data show 100% support from the experts, who think that smaller firms would be quicker than larger ones to take steps toward cloud computing. This claim was clearly stated by many experts, such as SH: *"Definitely, SMEs are quicker to adopt cloud"*.

**IT Readiness.** A firm's technology resources will affect its decision to adopt cloud services in various ways. This observation concords with the views of 76% of the experts in this study, who indicated that the greater the number of IT experts and resources in the firm, the lower will be the chance of adopting cloud computing in the firm. This finding can be seen in the answer by experts such MA: *"More technological resources will create more resistance to go for cloud"*. One reason for this resistance may be the life cycle of the technology resources in question, as TB stated, *"If they recently invested in on premise solution, this will limit their move to cloud"*.

## 5.3   Environmental Context

The environmental context refers to the arena in which a firm operates [3, 4]. In this context, government regulation is the main influencing factor, as supported by almost all of the experts. However, a majority of the experts also stated that competition in the market might encourage SMEs to adopt cloud computing technology. Moreover, the national technology infrastructure is added to this context, as stated by more than 50% of the experts. Table 6 below show the percentages of experts' views of each factor in this context, as supported by evidence from the interviews.

**Table 6.** Experts' views of environmental factors.

| Factor | Support | Non-support |
| --- | --- | --- |
| Competitive pressure | 57% | 43% |
| Government regulations | 93% | 7% |
| Vendor reputation | 71% | 29% |
| National technology infrastructure | 60% | 40% |

**Competitive Pressure.** Results showed that the competition in the market will impact SMEs' decisions to adopt cloud computing. Of the respondents, 57% of the experts indicated the impact of this factor on the decision makers in the firm. They mentioned that high competition in the market will drive the firm to look at new business opportunities, and cloud computing will be the vehicle to enable new business scenarios, as WA said, *"Another thing is the competition on the market, if a company doesn't enhance their way of doing the business, then there is a higher possibility of other company to win their position in the market by adopting and making faster changes"*.

**Government Regulations.** In terms of the impact of the government on SMEs decisions to adopt cloud computing, 93% of the experts confirmed this effect. They attributed the strong impact of government to several factors, such as government as the driver of the market in Saudi Arabia, as TB stated, *"A lot of SMEs will follow the government directions"*. Furthermore, the current grey area of government cloud policy is another factor, as ND said, *"Government do this grey area on purpose, they are not sure to allow cloud or not"*.

**Vendor Reputation.** The majority of the experts agreed that SMEs are very interested in the strength of vendors' names in the market. More than 71% of the experts support the validity of this impact in SME decisions to adopt cloud services. This support is shown in the responses by experts such as TA: *"Yes, here in Saudi SMEs care about names and brands of the providers"*.

**National Technology Infrastructure.** The availability of the latest technological infrastructure in the country will drive the adoption of cloud computing by SMEs in Saudi Arabia and *vice versa*. This factor emerged among many of the experts from the open-end questions in the environmental context. High speed and bandwidth of the Internet is a form of the technology infrastructure that 60% of the experts mentioned to have vital impact on SME decisions to adopt cloud computing, as stated by ST: *"The most important thing is the technology infrastructure in the country such as internet connectivity, high bandwidth, internet speed"*. Furthermore, the absence of local data centres with reasonable prices for SMEs slows the adoption of cloud services, as 57% of the experts supported the impact of this factor in SME decisions to adopt cloud computing, as MD stated: *"Data centre is one of the biggest problems here, we don't have many local data centre"*.

## 5.4   Social Context

Social factor also plays a role in technology adoption as drawn from the interviews outcomes. There is more disagreement on this among the experts surveyed. The disagreement appears to be in general with the fact that the TOE model does not include social factors. Rather, this category appeared to be important to the Saudi context based on the prior literature [4], which suggested that culture might play a role in attitudes toward technology adoption. Table 7 lays out the experts' views of Social factor.

**Table 7.** Experts' views of social factor.

| Factor | Support | Non-support |
|--------|---------|-------------|
| Culture | 57% | 43% |

**Culture.** Among the experts, 57% believed culture to play a role in technology adoption decisions among SMEs in Saudi Arabia. For example, AA stated, *"The problem is that you want to meet most people not all people and here comes an issue with the culture in Saudi Arabia that we do not study the stuff that people need. The market is not ready"*. Similarly, OE stated, *"The problem here is the word of mouth in Saudi, the word of mouth here is 'cloud is not safe and not secure', but when we have a look on these giant companies like Microsoft, Google, Amazon, do you think with all respect to our capabilities on EXCEED, do you think are there any comparison between us in the security environment? Of course not, they are more advance, highly advance more than anyone in the market"*. Lastly, WN stated, *"The public view of the cloud technology also affects the firm's decision to adopt cloud"*.

# 6    Limitation and Future Research Direction

The current study focused on investigating the current factors affecting the adoption of cloud computing by SMEs in Saudi Arabia. Therefore, its applicability is limited to that scope and context. Future research should investigate the factors affecting cloud computing by SMEs in the other Gulf countries (*viz.*, the Gulf Cooperation Council), which share many similarities with Saudi Arabia. Future studies should also compare and investigate the factors affecting the cloud computing in large private-sector *versus* public-sector organisations and compare those findings with the results revealed in this study.

Furthermore, the sample used to investigate the factors affecting cloud computing by SMEs in Saudi Arabia was limited to experts who were working with technology providers in the country. Future studies may therefore consider investigating another sample of views, such as technology policy makers in government or other cloud-computing-related samples from other sectors, in addition to non-technical company directors and entrepreneurs. These additional insights will stand to enrich the literature of cloud computing adoption. Due to the limited time, as well as the cost, to carry out this study, the method used to achieve the objectives was limited to a qualitative approach (semi-structured interviews). Other researchers may therefore see fit to use different methods, such as observations or case studies.

Lastly, the developed model in this study can be used by other researchers to investigate the factors that impact the adoption of other types of technology on SMEs decisions. Cloud computing is a special kind of technology, which many people see as removing an organisation's data resources and placing them within a distal structure that may be difficult to access, at least in the perceptions of many people. Other kinds of technology, which enable in-house adoption, will assuredly create different impressions, hence the need to study those other variants separately. In addition, future researchers may wish to extend the use of the model presented in this paper by adding new factors, such as the educational level of SMEs staffs.

# 7  Conclusion

This research focused on the factors affecting the adoption of cloud computing by SMEs in Saudi Arabia. Due to limited literature in the Saudi Arabia context, the present study employed in-depth semi-structured interviews of technology providers' cloud computing experts to investigate the factors affecting the adoption of cloud computing by SMEs in Saudi Arabia. The experts were asked to validate the impact of factors from the TOE model, as incorporated in the initial portion of the study. The findings derived from this research confirmed the impact of all factors in the initial model. Of the results, technology cost, ease of use, the duration of cloud implementation, integration and data synchronisation, and software functional customisation, size of firm, and government regulations proved to have a significant impact on SMEs decisions to adopt cloud computing. To date, the literature had not validated the impact of factors such as duration of cloud services implementation, customisation of cloud services, or integration between the new cloud services and other services in the firm on SMEs decisions to adopt cloud computing. This study has therefore taken the step to confirm, with evidence from experts, the impact of these factors on Saudi SMEs decisions. Moreover, a quantitative study is currently in progress to test the direct and indirect impact of each factor, the relationships among the factors, and the model's overall fit level. The results will be published soon.

## Appendix: Interview Questions

Section 1: Interview background

1. Can you tell us about yourself?
   Prompts:
   a. How old are you?
   b. How much working experiences do you have in IT field?
   c. what is your education level?

   Section 2: Background information and services provided by the firm to SMEs in Saudi Arabia

1. Can you tell us about your firm?
   Prompts:
   a. when did your frim established?
   b. What is your firm type of client based?
   c. What is the number of employees in your firm?
2. Can you describe the current situation of the cloud computing market in Saudi Arabia? prompts: what do you expect in the future in regard to this matter?
3. How do you describe the capability of the services you provide to enhance and develop SMEs?

4. What are the cloud products/services offered by your organisation to SMEs and why?
5. As a cloud services provider, could you describe the advantages gained by SMEs if they adopt cloud services?

Section 3: Factors affecting the adoption of cloud computing by SMEs (based on TOE)

In this section, questions will be divided into three categories: technology factors, organisational factors, environmental factors.

First: technological factors

6. What do you think about technology factors that affect the adoption of cloud computing by SMEs in Saudi Arabia?
7. Could you describe in detail the impact of each of the following factors on the SMEs' decision to adopt cloud computing?
   a. The cost reduction that the firm may achieve by using cloud services compared to the traditional IT model.
   b. The capability of cloud services to facilitate a flexible complementation, interaction, synchronisation and exchange of data with existing applications in the firm.
   c. The availability of cloud services that meet specific functional requirements needs of the firm.
   d. The duration between the implementation of cloud services and the benefiting of these services by the firm.
   e. The security measures utilised by the firm.
   f. The ability to smoothly utilise the implemented cloud services by the firm's staff.
   Prompts: are there any trial run before full implementation?
8. Are there any additional factors besides the ones discussed earlier that you would like to add?

Second: organisational factors

9. In your opinion, what are the most important internal organizational factors that affect the adoption of cloud computing by SMEs in Saudi Arabia?
10. How do you describe the effect of the following factors on the decision of SMEs to adopt cloud computing?
    Prompts:
    a. Top management support of cloud services?
    b. Size of firm?
    c. Technological resources that the firm has in relation to cloud services?
11. Are there any additional factors besides the ones discussed earlier that you would like to add?

Third: environmental factors

12. In your opinion, what are the most environmental factors that affect the adoption of cloud computing by SMEs in Saudi Arabia?
13. How do you describe the effect of the following factors on the decision of SMEs to adopt cloud computing?

Prompts:

a. The pressure faced by the firm due to competition in the market.

b. The government cloud regulations and policies.

c. The reputation of cloud services providers.

14. Are there any additional factors besides the ones discussed earlier that you would like to add?

15. Please feel free to discuss any other issues, concerns or opinions pertaining to this subject.

Thank you for your time.

# References

1. Vouk, M.A.: Cloud computing: issues, research, and implementations. J. Comput. Inf. Technol. **16**(4), 235–246 (2008)
2. Mell, P., Grance, T.: The NIST Definition of Cloud Computing. National Institute of Standards and Technology, Gaithersburg (2009)
3. Abdollahzadehgan, A., Hussin, A.R.C.: The organizational critical success factors for adopting cloud computing in SMEs. J. Inf. Syst. Res. Innov. **4**(1), 67–74 (2013)
4. Alshamaila, Y., Papagiannidis, S., Li, F.: Cloud computing adoption by SMEs in the North East of England. J. Enterp. Inf. Manag. **26**(3), 250–275 (2013)
5. Amini, M., Bakri, A., Sadat Safavi, N., Javadinia, S.A., Tolooei, A.: The role of top manager behaviours on adoption of cloud computing for small and medium enterprises. Aust. J. Basic Appl. Sci. **8**(1), 490–498 (2014)
6. Yeboah-Boateng, E.O., Essandoh, K.A.: Factors influencing the adoption of cloud computing by small and medium enterprises in developing economies. Int. J. Emerg. Sci. Eng. **2**(4), 13–20 (2014)
7. Miller, M.: Cloud Computing: Web-Based Applications That Change the Way You Work and Collaborate Online. Que, Indianapolis (2008)
8. Yamin, M., Al Makrami, A.A.: Cloud computing in SMEs: case of Saudi Arabia. Int. J. Inf. Technol. **7**(1), 853–860 (2015)
9. Gupta, P., Seetharaman, A., Raj, J.R.: The usage and adoption of cloud computing by small and medium businesses. Int. J. Inf. Manag. **33**(5), 861–874 (2013)
10. Kim, J.Y.: 2016 Growth Strategy, Saudi Arabia. G20, Hangzhou (2016)
11. Mikkonen, I., Khan, I.: Cloud computing: SME company point of view. In: Ferenčikova, S., Šestáková, M. (eds.) Management Challenges in the 21st Century, pp. 59–79. Vysoká Škola Manažmentu, Bratislava (2016)
12. Marston, S., Li, Z., Bandyopadhyay, S., Zhang, J., Ghalsasi, A.: Cloud computing: the business perspective. Decis. Support Syst. **51**(1), 176–189 (2011)
13. Al Isma'ili, S., Li, M.X., Shen, J., He, Q.: Cloud computing adoption determinants: an analysis of Australian SMEs. In: Proceedings of the Pac-Asia Conference on Information System, p. 5826 (2016)
14. Al Isma'ili, S., Li, M.X., Shen, J., He, Q.: Cloud computing services adoption in Australian SMEs: a firm-level investigation. In: Proceedings of the Pac-Asia Conference on Information System, p. 5824 (2016) [2016b]

15. Bharadwaj, S.S., Lal, P.: Exploring the impact of cloud computing adoption on organizational flexibility: a client perspective. In: Proceedings of the International Conference on Cloud Computing Technologies, Applications and Management, pp. 121–131 (2012)
16. Liu, S., Yang, Y., Ran, W.X.: The value of cloud computing to internet-based SMEs: a multiple case study from China. In: Proceedings of the Pac-Asia Conference on Information System, p. 5 (2016)
17. Mahara, T.N.: Indian SMEs perspective for election of ERP in cloud. J. Int. Technol. Inf. Manag. **22**(1), 5 (2013)
18. Seethamraju, R.: Adoption of software as a service (SaaS) enterprise resource planning (ERP) systems in small and medium sized enterprises (SMEs). Inf. Syst. Front. **17**(3), 475–492 (2015)
19. Trinh, T.P., Pham, C.H., Tran, D.: An adoption model of software as a service (SaaS) in SMEs. In: Proceedings of the Pac-Asia Conference on Information System, p. 18 (2015)
20. Al Saleh, A.: Exploring strategies for small and medium enterprises in Saudi Arabia. Paper presented at the Doctoral Symposium of the Research Institute for Business and Management. Manchester Municipal University, Manchester, UK (2012)
21. Alenzy, M.Z.: Strategic approach of saudi small and medium-sized enterprises: more of emergent or deliberate? Int. Bus. Res. **11**(3), 110–117 (2018)
22. Mansha'at. Know the Size of Your Business. Mansha'at. Riyadh: General Authority for Small and Medium Enterprises (2018). https://smea.gov.sa/en
23. Khan, S., Khan, M.S.A., Kumar, C.S.: Multi-criteria decision in the adoption of cloud computing services for SME's based on BOCR analysis. Asian J. Manag. Res. **5**(4), 621–634 (2015)
24. Baker, J.: The technology–organization–environment framework. In: Dwivedi, Y., Wade, M., Schneberger, S. (eds.) Information Systems Theory, vol. 28, pp. 231–245. Springer, New York (2012). https://doi.org/10.1007/978-1-4419-6108-2_12
25. Gangwar, H., Date, H., Ramaswamy, R.: Understanding determinants of cloud computing adoption using an integrated TAM-TOE model. J. Enterp. Inf. Manag. **28**(1), 107–130 (2015)
26. Alkhater, N., Wills, G., Walters, R.: Factors influencing an organisation's intention to adopt cloud computing in Saudi Arabia. In: Proceedings of the International Conference on Cloud Computing Technology and Science (CloudCom), pp. 1040–1044 (2014)
27. Aharony, N.: Cloud computing: information professionals' and educational technology experts' perspectives. Libr. Hi Tech **32**(4), 645–666 (2014)
28. Schlagwein, D., Thorogood, A., Willcocks, L.P.: How commonwealth bank of Australia gained benefits using a standards-based, multi-provider cloud model. MIS Q. Exec. **13**(4), 209–222 (2014)
29. Cooper, R.B., Zmud, R.W.: Information technology implementation research: a technological diffusion approach. Manag. Sci. **36**(2), 123–139 (1990)
30. Iacovou, C.L., Benbasat, I., Dexter, A.S.: Electronic data interchange and small organizations: adoption and impact of technology. MIS Q. **19**(4), 465–485 (1995)
31. Chau, P.Y., Tam, K.Y.: Factors affecting the adoption of open systems: an exploratory study. MIS Q. **21**(1), 1–24 (1997)
32. AlAwadhi, S., Morris, A.: The use of the UTAUT model in the adoption of E-government services in Kuwait. In: Proceedings of the 41st Annual Hawaii International Conference on System Sciences, p. 219. IEEE (2008)
33. Alkhater, N., Walters, R., Wills, G.: An empirical study of factors influencing cloud adoption among private sector organisations. Telematics Inform. **35**(1), 38–54 (2017)

34. Siddharthan, N.S., Narayanan, K.: Technology: Corporate and Social Dimensions. Springer, New York (2016). https://doi.org/10.1007/978-981-10-1684-4
35. Alharthi, A., Alassafi, M.O., Walters, R.J., Wills, G.B.: An exploratory study for investigating the critical success factors for cloud migration in the Saudi Arabian higher education context. Telematics Inform. **34**(2), 664–678 (2017)
36. Alkhater, N., Wills, G., Walters, R.: Factors affecting an organisation's decision to adopt cloud services in Saudi Arabia. In: Proceedings of the International Conference on Future Internet of Things and Cloud (FiCloud), pp. 553–557 (2015)
37. Guest, G., Bunce, A., Johnson, L.: How many interviews are enough? An experiment with data saturation and variability. Field Methods **18**(1), 59–82 (2006)
38. Burnard, P., Gill, P., Stewart, K., Treasure, E., Chadwick, B.: Analysing and presenting qualitative data. Br. Dent. J. **204**(8), 429–432 (2008)
39. Fereday, J., Muir-Cochrane, E.: Demonstrating rigor using thematic analysis: a hybrid approach of inductive and deductive coding and theme development. J Qual. Methods **5**(1), 80–92 (2008)

# CSCCRA: A Novel Quantitative Risk Assessment Model for Cloud Service Providers

Olusola Akinrolabu[1(✉)], Steve New[2], and Andrew Martin[1]

[1] Department of Computer Science, University of Oxford,
Oxford OX1 3PR, UK
{olusola.akinrolabu, andrew.martin}@cs.ox.ac.uk
[2] Said Business School, University of Oxford, Oxford OX1 1HP, UK
steve.new@sbs.ox.ac.uk

**Abstract.** Assessing and managing cloud risks can be a challenge, even for the cloud service providers (CSPs), due to the increased numbers of parties, devices and applications involved in cloud service delivery. The limited visibility of security controls down the supply chain, further exacerbates this risk assessment challenge. As such, we propose the Cloud Supply Chain Cyber Risk Assessment (CSCCRA) model, a quantitative risk assessment model which is supported by cloud supplier security assessment (CSSA) and cloud supply chain mapping (CSCM). Using the CSCCRA model, we assess the risk of a Customer Relationship Management (CRM) application, mapping its supply chain to identify weak links, evaluating its security risks and presenting the risk value in dollar terms, with this, promoting cost-effective risk mitigation and optimal risk prioritisation.

**Keywords:** Cloud computing · Quantitative risk assessment · Supply chain Transparency · Security Rating Service

## 1 Introduction

The use of cloud resources has changed the way data is stored, shared, and accessed. The use of public cloud typically means that organisation's data and applications are managed outside their *trust boundary* and often require a complex and dynamic supply chain which lacks clearly defined boundaries. This new approach to IT service delivery introduces a new set of risks. While we argue that cloud is often more secure, compared to many enterprise networks, the extent of this security is hard to verify, seeing that CSPs who should be more aware of cloud risks, find it difficult to audit or assess risks due to limited visibility of security controls and lack of supplier transparency down the supply chain [14].

The multi-tenancy characteristics of the cloud, coupled with its dynamic supply chain have been identified as two areas of challenge to cloud risk assessment. This challenge is further exacerbated by the predominant use of qualitative or weak quantitative, traditional IT risk assessment methods in assessing cloud risks [2]. Studies into the supply chain of cloud services have shown that at least 80% of a typical software-as-a-service (SaaS) application is made up of assembled parts, with each component

M. Themistocleous and P. Rupino da Cunha (Eds.): EMCIS 2018, LNBIP 341, pp. 177–184, 2019.
https://doi.org/10.1007/978-3-030-11395-7_16

representing a different level of risk [17]. As such, IT risk assessment methods, e.g. ISO 27005, which were developed in the days of end-to-end service delivery, are now unable to cope with the inherent risks within the dynamic cloud supply chain [16].

This study presents CSCCRA, a quantitative risk assessment model which adopts the systems thinking approach to solving complex system problems [8]. The CSCCRA model is built out to empower CSPs to make reliable inferences about the risk of their cloud service after careful analysis of its interconnected supply chain and an assessment of the security posture of component suppliers. It builds on existing risk assessment standards and guidance documents such as ISO/IEC 27005:2011, ISO/IEC 31010:2009, NIST 800-30v1, and the Factor Analysis of Information Risks (FAIR) methodology. Using the CSCCRA model, we conceptualise and analyse the security risk of a CRM cloud application.

The structure of the paper is as follows we present the literature on cloud risk assessment and supply chain risks in Sect. 2. Then we articulate the CSCCRA model in Sect. 3. The CSCCRA is used to assess the risk of a CRM application in Sect. 4, followed by conclusions and future work in Sect. 5.

## 2 Literature Review

This section focuses on a review of existing risk assessment models, the cloud supply chain, and identifies a gap in cloud risk assessment.

### 2.1 Cloud Risk Assessment

Cloud risk assessment is defined as a step by step, repeatable process used to produce an understanding of cloud risks associated with relinquishing control of data or management of services to an external service provider [11]. Currently, and despite the very many discourses about cloud computing risks, there is no structured framework for identifying, assessing and managing cloud risks [10]. The lack of a systematic approach and expert subjectivity synonymous with risk assessments, particularly qualitative, has led to inconsistencies in cloud risk assessment.

Seeing that cloud deployments are rapidly evolving due to new service provider offerings and changing compliance and regulatory landscape, risk assessment solutions would seem not to be keeping pace with cloud growth. In Table 1, we present a cross-section of proposed cloud risk assessment methods which like CSCCRA, are quantitative and can be used by CSPs to assess the risk of cloud service provision.

### 2.2 Cloud Supply Chain Risks

The supply chain of a cloud service can be defined as a complex system of two or more parties that work together to provide, develop, host, manage, monitor or use cloud services [1]. We define cloud supply chain risk as the probability of an internal or external event targeted at a cloud service or its extended network of suppliers, causing a disruption or failure to cloud operation and leading to reductions in service levels and security posture, with a possible increased cost of remediation. The cloud supply chain

**Table 1.** Existing cloud risk assessment models

| Author/Year | Cloud risk assessment description | Method | Implementation | Risk value | Use of experts | Supply chain |
|---|---|---|---|---|---|---|
| Djemame et al. [5] | Risk assessment framework with methodologies for the identification, evaluation, mitigation & monitoring of cloud risks during the various stages of cloud provision | Semiquantitative | No | Risk score | No | Yes |
| Fito et al. [6] | A cloud risk assessment model for analysing the data security risks of confidential data. It prioritises cloud risks according to their impact on Business Level Objectives (BLO) | Semiquantitative | Yes | Risk score | No | No |
| Saripalli and Walters [15] | A quantitative risk and impact assessment of cloud risk events based on six key security objectives | Semiquantitative | No | Risk score | Yes | No |
| Sendi and Cheriet [16] | The model uses fuzzy multi-criteria decision-making technique to assess cloud risks | Quantitative | Yes | Risk score | No | No |
| Sivasubramanian et al. [18] | The model measures cloud risks in terms of impact, occurrence and disclosure, to arrive at a Risk Priority Number (RPN) | Semiquantitative | No | Risk score | No | No |

employs "aggressive sourcing" based on free-market principles rather than collaboration, which increases cloud risks. Furthermore, the risks associated with the processes, procedures, and practices used to assure the integrity, security, resilience, and quality of cloud services increases with the on-demand, automated, and multi-tenanted cloud, down the supply chain [3].

## 2.3 Research Gap and Proposal

As shown in Table 1, only one of the risk assessment models used by CSPs considered the inherent risks in the supply chain. With the cloud supply chain made up of small and medium businesses (SMBs), whose vulnerability to cyber attacks magnifies into the supply chains, there is a need to assess cloud risks from a supply chain perspective, identifying the sub-providers involved in service delivery and evaluating their security controls.

As such, we propose the CSCCRA model, which we argue, addresses the problem of supply chain risks in the cloud. Currently, no in-depth study has been conducted to address this problem, and since information security is all about decision-making, we believe that our quantitative and iterative approach to cloud risk assessment, will provide organisations with an objective result, that is consistent, easy to understand, and encourages continuous mitigation of cloud risks.

## 3  The CSCCRA Model

The CSCCRA model (see Fig. 1) considers the dynamism of the cloud supply chain and looks to address the gap on cloud supply chain transparency, and how the lack of visibility of supplier's security controls have contributed to the inadequate level of cloud risk assessment. Given the scarcity of initiatives for the practical implementation of a quantitative cloud risk assessment, the development of the CSCCRA model aims to contribute towards improving the state-of-the-art in cloud risk assessment. It hopes to achieve this by showing how a holistic quantitative risk assessment and decision analysis model provides a unique capability for capturing the dynamic behaviour of risks within a cloud supply chain and measuring the overall risk behaviour. While numerous scholars have openly questioned the subjectivity of expert's estimate in quantitative analysis, our implementation of CSCCRA aims to prove that despite the lack of historical data, cloud risk assessments can achieve increased objectivity through the use of controlled experimentation, clearly defined model, peer reviews, and calibration of the expert judges [7].

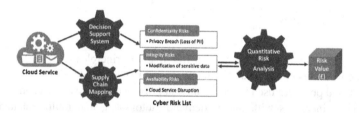

**Fig. 1.** Overview of CSCCRA model

The three components of the CSCCRA model are as follows [1]:

1. **Quantitative Risk Assessment:** The CSCCRA model goes beyond the IT industry norm to apply a quantitative assessment method to cloud risks. It expresses risk as the combination of the probability of an event and its consequences as per ISO Guide 73:2009, and follows a rigorous process in the identification and evaluation of security risk factors. With uncertainty being the primary factor in risk analysis, the CSCCRA model makes use of a probabilistic estimate of risk factors, e.g. threat frequency, vulnerability and loss magnitude, representing the forecast as a distribution (e.g. PERT, Poisson).

2. **Cloud Supplier Security Assessment:** The CSSA is a decision support system and a novel addition to cloud risk assessment. It functions as a Security Rating Service (SRS) for the suppliers involved in the delivery of the cloud service [12]. The CSCCRA model requires cloud providers to be aware of their supply chain and have sufficient information about the processes and capabilities of their vendors. Being a Multi-criteria security assessment tool, the CSSA follows a formal and rigorous process which involves decomposing the cloud service into its component objects and using an improper linear model to rate suppliers based on identified security criteria, resulting in the identification of suppliers with poor security postures.

3. **Cloud Supply Chain Mapping:** Providing end-to-end supply chain visualisation while assessing cloud risk makes it amenable to analyse and explore areas of weakness, strengths and the potential risks to a cloud service while also supporting collaboration and decision-making within the chain [19]. The benefit of a graphical representation of the inherent risk in the supply chain helps to counter any documented biases in risk estimation and decision- making and is thought to have an impact in reducing the cognitive load involved in the estimation of risk factors [9].

## 4   Scenario of a SaaS Provider Using CSCCRA Model

In this section, we describe the steps involved in the risk assessment of a CRM SaaS application using the CSCCRA model (see Fig. 2). The CRM application is built using the services of Platform-as-a-Service (PaaS-A) provider, whose function is hosted on Infrastructure-as-a-Service-A (IaaS-A) and uses a Structured Query Language (SQL) database hosted by IaaS-B. Furthermore, the CRM application makes use of four API providers for services such as customer billing, custom 'social search', monitoring, and identity & access management (IAM). To further complicate the relationship, the IAM and monitoring API providers built their applications using the same platform provider, PaaS-B, who also runs on the IaaS-A infrastructure.

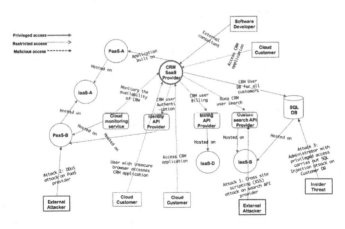

**Fig. 2.** The supply chain map of the CRM cloud service

### 4.1   Cloud Supplier Security Assessment

The CSCCRA model is designed in such a way that both CSSA and CSCM processes take place before cloud risk identification, to enable the CSP to acquire a sound knowledge of the underlying factors contributing to their security risks (see Fig. 1). Using the details contained in the supply chain map, stakeholders within the CSP rate the suppliers on security capabilities, process, reliability and compliance factors. According to Robyn Dawes, human judges are good at picking out the right predictor variables (risk factors) and coding them, but poor at integrating information from diverse and incomparable sources [4].

As part of overcoming the human subjectivity challenge, the CSSA tool is implemented based on an improper linear model, known as Dawes model, which employs the z-score method of unit-weighted regression. Figure 3 shows the rating of the Five Tier-1 suppliers based on six predictive attributes: estimated outage, supplier criticality, past Service Level Agreement (SLA), security practice, security certification, and process maturity.

| CSP's list of suppliers | Estimated outage duration (hrs) | Criticality of the supplier (1 for critical, 0 for commodity) | Past SLA performance (0 for didn't meet SLA, 1 for achieved | General security practice (with 1 being very poor, 5- moderate, 10- | Industry security certification and standard processes) (1-10 compliance (0 for non certified, 1 for industry certified) | Process Maturity (1-5, with 1 being initial, 2- Repeatable, 3- Defined, 4- Measured, 5- Optimised) | Weighted z-scores | z-score Estimated outage | z-score Criticalit y of the supplier | z-score Past SLA performance | z-score General security practice | z-score Industry certificati on | z-score Maturity | Total Weighted z-scores. In this case, a negative z-score means the risk is lower than average. A positive z-score means it is higher |
|---|---|---|---|---|---|---|---|---|---|---|---|---|---|---|
| PaaS-A Hosting | 3 | 1 | 1 | 9 | 1 | 4 | | -1.33 | 0.45 | -0.45 | -1.23 | -0.45 | -0.73 | -0.62 |
| Identity CSP | 5 | 1 | 1 | 8 | 1 | 4 | | -0.59 | 0.45 | -0.45 | -0.35 | -0.45 | -0.73 | -0.35 |
| Billing CSP | 8 | 0 | 1 | 8 | 1 | 4 | | 0.52 | -1.79 | -0.45 | -0.35 | -0.45 | -0.73 | -0.54 |
| Custom API CSP | 10 | 1 | 0 | 7 | 0 | 3 | | 1.26 | 0.45 | 1.79 | 0.53 | 1.79 | 1.10 | 1.15 |
| Database CSP | 7 | 1 | 1 | 6 | 1 | 3 | | 0.15 | 0.45 | -0.45 | 1.40 | -0.45 | 1.10 | 0.37 |

**Fig. 3.** Security assessment of the CRM suppliers

## 4.2 Risk Identification and Analysis

From the vantage point of the just concluded supplier assessment, the CSP stakeholders can visualise their areas of weakness. With the Search API vendor being a critical supplier, who has missed SLA in the last year and has the highest estimated outage, the focal CSP will be paying close attention to this supplier when drawing up their comprehensive list of security risks. A potential risk identified by the CSP is the compromise of confidential customer data due to a Cross-Site Scripting (XSS) attack on the custom search vendor.

For this scenario, the stakeholders assess the confidentiality risk using the available information about the custom search supplier, its criticality, security assessment rating etc. This information assists them in making estimates on the impact, probability, and frequency of the risk. These estimates are presented as a probability distribution, including lower bound, most likely, and upper bound values, made to a 90% confidence interval. The risk factor estimates are then used as input into the Monte Carlo simulation tool, see Table 2. The use of Monte Carlo helps to build models of possible risk results, reducing the impact of inherent uncertainty involved in the risk estimation. It calculates the risk result over a specific number of iterations, each time using a different set of random values from the probability functions and at the end producing a distribution of possible risk values for a risk item [13].

**Table 2.** Risk calculation of custom search API attack using @RISK software for Monte Carlo simulation (10,000 iterations & 5 simulations)

| Uncertain Inputs | Parameter of Distribution | | | |
|---|---|---|---|---|
| | Distri-bution | Lower Bound | Most Likely | Upper Bound |
| Probability of risk (without controls) (PWC) | PERT | 5% | 7% | 10% |
| Control Efficiency (CE) | PERT | 2% | 3% | 4% |
| Impact cost (IC) | PERT | $5,000 | $14,500 | $70,000 |
| Frequency of occurrence per year (Fr) | Poisson | 1 | | |
| | | | | |
| Estimated Risk Value (ERV) | Without Controls | With Controls | | |
| 5% Percentile | $0 | $0 | | |
| Mean | $3,177.30 | $1,828.40 | | |
| 95% Percentile | $9,105.86 | $5,452.16 | | |

# 5    Conclusion and Future Work

This study set out to identify the supply chain gap in cloud risk assessment and propose the CSCCRA model as a way of bridging this gap. Using the proposed model, we showed how the decomposition of risk items into its various risk factors, allows decision makers to investigate cloud risks, avoiding extreme subjectivity in their evaluation. Although targeted at CSPs, a distinctive contribution of this study is that it caters for the complexities involved in cloud delivery and adapts to the dynamic nature of the cloud, enabling CSPs to conduct risk assessments at a higher frequency, in response to a change in the supply chain. The CSCCRA is a rigorous and dynamic risk assessment model, which combines aspects of various disciplines and can be applied to the risk assessment of many composite services.

Future work will see us integrate the security factors achieved during our recently completed Delphi study into the CSSA tool, and develop the CSCCRA model into a web application. A current limitation of this study is its lack of practical application, which we plan to address by conducting case studies of three SaaS provider organisations who will use the model to carry out a comprehensive real-world assessment of their cloud service.

Collectively, we anticipate that the implementation of the CSCCRA model will reveal that this inclusive, structured and systematic approach to cloud risk assessment, can deliver objective risk results, saving the CSP time and effort as they mature into the use of the model.

# References

1. Akinrolabu, O., New, S., Martin, A.: Cyber supply chain risks in cloud computing - bridging the risk assessment gap. Open J. Cloud Comput. (OJCC) **5**(1), 1–19 (2018)
2. Badger, L., Patt-Corner, R., Voas, J.: Cloud Computing Synopsis and Recommendations. Recommendations of the National Institute of Standards and Technology. NIST Special Publication 800-146, p. 81 (2012)
3. Boyens, J., Paulsen, C., Moorthy, R., Bartol, N.: Supply Chain Risk Management Practices for Federal Information Systems and Organizations. NIST Special Publication (2015)
4. Dawes, R.M.: The robust beauty of improper linear models in decision making. Am. Psychol. **34**(7), 571–582 (1979)
5. Djemame, K., Armstrong, D.J., Kiran, M.: A risk assessment framework and software toolkit for cloud service ecosystems. In: Computing, pp. 119–126 (2011)
6. Fito, J., Macias, M., Guitart, J.: Toward business-driven risk management for Cloud computing. In: 2010 International Conference Network and Service Management (CNSM), pp. 238–241 (2010)
7. Freund, J., Jones, J.: Measuring and Managing Information Risk: A FAIR Approach. Butterworth-Heinemann (2014)
8. Ghadge, A., Dani, S., Chester, M., Kalawsky, R.: A systems approach for modelling supply chain risks. Supply Chain Manag. Int. J. **18**(5), 523–538 (2013)
9. Gresh, D., Deleris, L.A., Gasparini, L., Evans, D.: Visualizing risk. In: Proceedings of IEEE Information Visualization Conference (2011)
10. Islam, S., Fenz, S., Weippl, E., Mouratidis, H.: A risk management framework for cloud migration decision support. J. Risk Financ. Manag. **10**(2), 10 (2017)
11. Kaliski Jr, B.S., Pauley, W.: Toward risk assessment as a service in cloud environments. In: Proceedings 2nd USENIX Conference Hot Topics in Cloud Computing, pp. 1–7 (2010)
12. Olcott, J.: Input to the Commission on Enhancing National Cybersecurity: The Impact of Security Ratings on National Cybersecurity (2016)
13. Palisade: Monte Carlo Simulation: What is it and How Does it Work? - Palisade (2017)
14. Pearson, S.: Data Protection in the Cloud. Cloud Security Alliance Online, pp. 10–13 (2016)
15. Saripalli, P., Walters, B.: QUIRC: a quantitative impact and risk assessment framework for cloud security. In: 2010 IEEE 3rd International Conference Cloud Computing, pp. 280–288 (2010)
16. Sendi, A.S., Cheriet, M.: Cloud computing: a risk assessment model. In: 2014 IEEE International Conference Cloud Engineering, pp. 147–152 (2014)
17. Sherman, M.: Risks in the software supply chain. In: Software Solution Symposium, pp. 1–36 (2017)
18. Sivasubramanian, Y., Ahmed, S.Z., Mishra, V.P.: Risk assessment for cloud computing Int. Res. J. Electron. Comput. Eng. **3**(2) (2017). ISSN Online 2412-4370
19. Sourcemap: Sub-Supplier Mapping: Tracing Products to the Source with a Supply Chain Social Network, p. 5 (2011)

# Mobile Number Portability Using a Reliable Cloud Database Appliance to Match Predictable Performance

Katelaris Leonidas, Themistocleous Marinos[(✉)],
and Giovanni Roberto

BTO Research, Milan, Italy
{leonidas.katelaris,marinos.themistocleous,
giovanni.roberto}@btoresearch.com

**Abstract.** The great interest for deploying applications in cloud infrastructures is rapidly growing due to its convenience and ease of use. Despite, the large number of different applications migrated to cloud, there are still applications that are not frequently met on cloud infrastructures. Applications defined as time critical or data-intensive are applications of this kind. The need of high resilience alongside with high performance lead these types of applications to run on mainframes, rather than on cloud infrastructures, as cloud is not able to satisfy them under strict Service Level Agreements (SLAs) and without predictable performance. To investigate further this area this paper aims to report on the research issues around time critical and data-intensive applications deployed on cloud and present Mobile Number Portability (MNP) Use Case migration to cloud with predictable performance.

**Keywords:** Predictable performance · Cloud · Data analytics

## 1 Introduction

Cloud service offerings are growing with tremendous speed, under the emergence of even more offerings. Even more companies choose cloud infrastructures to deploy their services, under strict SLAs and guarantees of high availability and performance. Despite the growing and grade improvements on cloud offerings, cloud computing service providers do not serve all types of applications with proficient performance. This happens because, data-intensive or time critical applications could not get ideal performance in cloud without prior predict of performance.

In this paper we demonstrate the MNP Use Case migration to cloud infrastructures using predictable performance suggested by EU project, to meet Key Process Indicators (KPIs) and serve application at ideal performance and high resilience. Mobile Number Portability (MNP), is a major process for mobile network operators, which is in the focus of this paper. The MNP process is taking place when a customer signs a new contract with another operator (the recipient operator). Following, the recipient operator sends the MNP request to the operator (the donator operator) where the customer is currently hosted and asks for the current customer to remove to its network. The MNP process terminates when customer is moved to the new operator.

© Springer Nature Switzerland AG 2019
M. Themistocleous and P. Rupino da Cunha (Eds.): EMCIS 2018, LNBIP 341, pp. 185–190, 2019.
https://doi.org/10.1007/978-3-030-11395-7_17

The lack of a centralized database, alongside with the high complexity of the processes that take place during the MNP process, represent an open issue. The lack of a centralized database in Italy requires strong integration between the different ICT (Information and Communication Technology) systems of the mobile network operators operated in Italy.

## 2 Mobile Number Portability: Requirements and Analysis

As mentioned above the high complexity of the process and the lack of a centralized database for all the domestic phone numbers in Italy arises multiple challenges for mobile number network operators. In an attempt, to give to the reader a better view of the process, the following paragraphs describes the MNP process from the customer point of view as this process is presented in Fig. 1.

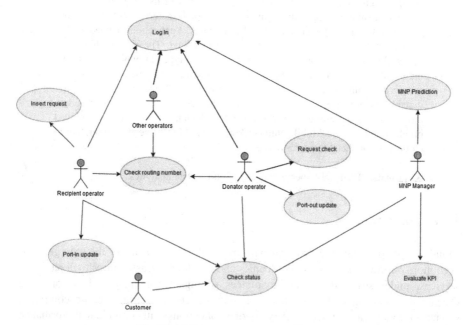

**Fig. 1.** MNP process - use case diagram

1: **Insert MNP Request:** A customer signs a new contract with recipient operator asking for number portability.
2: **Quota Restriction:** At the end of each day (around 19:00 CET) and after all shops (network operator shops) are closed, a system check is performed to check if MNP requests submitted during the day, meet the quota threshold for each operator. Quota for each operator in Italy is set from the Italian Communications authority [1].

3: **Request Check:** During the next three days, multiple checks are made from each of the involved operators such as possibility of blocked number, unpaid bills, ongoing MNP request to third operator etc.

4: **Port-in and Port-out:** After the three days period, early in the morning (e.g., 06:00am–08:00am) the portability of the number is completed with maximum service loss of two hours. The old SIM card is deactivated and it cannot receive service by the donor.

Each of the above steps is subdivided to sub-processes running through each step. Starting from the first step, "Insert MNP Request", the user could visit the shop of a telecommunication provider and ask to move his telephone number to the new provider filling a portability contract form. To be able to get a number portability, a customer gets a Subscriber Identity Module (SIM) card from recipient operator. Most of the times, customers who sign portability contract, they already have a SIM card. The recipient operator activates the new SIM card with a 'new' number, so the customer immediately is able to receive or make calls to the 'new' number. During this time the old SIM card with the customer's number is operated by the donor.

Following, is the second step 'Quota Restriction', where each operator proceeds specific number of requests each day, as a regulatory requirement. All requests over quota are queued in a waiting list, as they are scheduled to be proceeded the next day. This action is taking place every day after 19:30 CET, when all shops (telecommunication provider's shops) close.

Coming after, the step 'Request Check', where donator operator checks if the port out requests are reasonable before proceeding them to the next step. Reasons for decline a port-out request include unpaid bills, blocked number, ongoing number portability to another operator etc. These procedures are taking place during the next three days after the portability number request is submitted.

The final step of the MNP process called 'Port-in Port-out', includes the subprocesses of port-in and port-out. As a result of the successful 'Request Check', all proceeded requests are submitted to the final step. The recipient operator imports all successfully checked numbers to its system. After the completion of port-in, recipient operator informs the donor operator for the completion. Then, the donator removes (port-out), all those numbers from its systems. Actions in this final step are taking place early in the morning (06:00–08:00 CET), with two hours of maximum service lost for the customer.

The above steps compose the MNP process, which is currently running in Italy including high complexity between different systems with the need for strong integration between telecommunication providers. The current status is very time consuming and costly for telecommunication providers, looking ways to reduce cost, time and service failures. To address this issue, a Database as a Service is proposed through EU project called European Cloud Database Appliance (CDBA) [2]. The reliable cloud database appliance deriving from the EU project is proposing a new cloud architecture, which is focused on visualization on service level instead of hardware level. One of the innovations derived from the proposed cloud architecture is that the setup for physical resources that will be consumed by each query-client will be managed during run-time, providing predictable performance for data-intensive applications. To achieve that beyond others, the project behind CDBA will investigate research results from five real-life use cases in three different sectors: Banking, Telco and Retail.

## 3    Mobile Number Portability: Serve Time-Critical Applications in Cloud Infrastructures

As the aim of this paper, is to address the issues around time critical or data-intensive applications and the lack of a suitable solutions in the cloud infrastructures, the authors will present the migration of the Telco's sector Use Case on the cloud platform. Among others, the innovative cloud database appliance deriving from the research project aims to speed up MNP service nationwide providing real-time response and minimizing the risk of the failure.

### 3.1    Cloud Database Appliance Components

The mission of the database appliance is to provide an ultra-scalable operational database with analytical capabilities leveraging an efficient storage engine and be able to scale up on advance hardware platform. Below a brief presentation of cloud database appliance main components is made.

– **Operational Database:** The ultra-scalable operational database is based on a new version of LeanXcale [3] operational database with a new storage engine able to run efficiently in-memory, with full NUMA (Non-uniform Memory Access) awareness.
– **Multicore Hardware Platform:** The hardware where the cloud database appliance will be hosted, will be provided by Atos [4]. The hardware platform will be equipped with 32 CPUs (896 Cores) able to scale up, alongside with 120 TB of main memory in a single computer.
– **Analytical Database:** An in-memory analytical engine will be designed and provided by ActiveViam [5], which will be able to scale up efficiently based on NUMA architecture, integrated with LeanXcale to supply fast analytical queries over operational data.
– **Streaming Analytics Engine:** Data streaming engine is designed able to scale up to several 1000s of cores and well-integrated with LeanXcale supports real-time analytics algorithms over the operational data.
– **Incremental Parallel Analytics Algorithms:** A set of incremental analytic algorithms are designed to run over operational data.

### 3.2    Mobile Number Portability Service in Cloud Database Appliance

The deployment of Mobile Number Portability Service on cloud database appliance embraces risks in time and service failures. Below there is a description of the main risks and requirements for MNP service to run on cloud database appliance.

The current status in Italy for domestic phone numbers is confusing and complicated. Before moving to cloud platform, a major altering has to be made in current processes around domestic phone numbers hosting. According to that, the authors propose a centralized database (Fig. 2), where all domestic phone numbers will be hosted and operated by AGCOM [1], who will be responsible to keep references for all domestic numbers operated by Italian telecommunication providers.

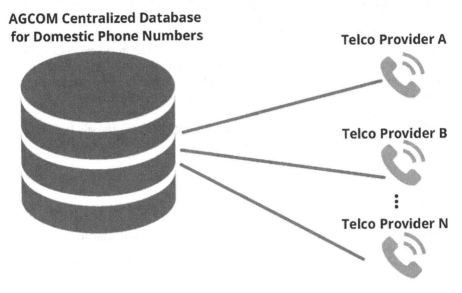

**Fig. 2.** AGCOM centralized database for domestic phone numbers

Below, there is a description of MNP service functionalities and KPIs to be met on cloud database appliance platform. The centralized database where all domestic phone numbers are hosted, will be able to handle about 100 million phone numbers with references for operations by telecommunication providers. Based on that the cloud database appliance should meet the following terms:

- MNP Service process should end in less than 24 h
- Availability of the service must be 99.9%
- Able to manage 100000 MNP requests per day and online check validation (time for response to queries in 2 s)
- Able to Check the status of 1000000 requests per day (response-time in 1 s)
- Able to handle 1 billion requests per hour for check routing number (response time in 0.1 s).

All the above requirements should lead to Reduces TCO (Total Cost of Ownership) and Operations and improve customer experience in MNP service.

## 4 Concluding Remarks

The research that is reported herein is part of a Horizon 2020 European research project called European Cloud-In-Memory Database Appliance with Predictable Performance for Critical Applications (CloudDBAppliance (CDBA)). The project attempts to build a new cloud computing architecture that transfers the concept of mainframe to cloud computing. The proposed architecture will be tested through five use cases from banking, retail and telecom sectors and the use case presented in the previous sections is one of them. Currently the project is half way through and it is expected to be completed in November 2019. In the next months the hardware developments and the software produced for the project will be tested through the 5 use cases.

**Acknowledgement.** This research has been funded by the European Union's Horizon 2020 research and innovation programme under the project CloudDBAppliance (H2020- grant agreement No. 732051).

## References

1. Italian Communications Authority AGCOM: Italian communications authority. https://www.agcom.it
2. Cloud Database Appliance CDBA: Cloud Database Appliance. https://clouddb.eu
3. LeanXcale: LeanXcale. https://www.leanxcale.com
4. Atos: ATOS. https://atos.net
5. In-memory analytical database. https://activeviam.com. ActiveViam. https://atos.net

# Digital Services and Social Media

# Exploratory Research to Identify the Characteristics of Cyber Victims on Social Media in New Zealand

Varun Dhond[1], Shahper Richter[1], and Brad McKenna[2(✉)]

[1] Auckland University of Technology, Auckland, New Zealand
{varun.dhond, shahper.richter}@aut.ac.nz
[2] University of East Anglia, Norwich, UK
b.mckenna@uea.ac.uk

**Abstract.** Cyberbullying is omnipresent among all sections of society who have access to the internet. Vast research has been carried out on this topic around the world however there has not been enough research that is New Zealand based. The objective of this research is to identify the characteristics of cyber victims on social media in New Zealand. We scrutinize the prevalence of cyberbullying in New Zealand among university students based on age, gender and personality. The survey was designed stating the hypotheses developed as a result of the literature review. We gathered the data of sample size n = 158. We conclude that students with openness to experience are more likely to be cyberbullied compared to the other personalities. Whereas, we found no correlation of age and gender with the cyber bullying on a university level. The results from this study can have a positive application in counter cyberbullying programs in New Zealand. This study will a give an impetus for further analytical research in the field of cyber bullying in New Zealand.

**Keywords:** Social media · Cyberbullying · Personality · Cyber victims
New Zealand

## 1 Introduction

The term "cyberbullying" is a combination of the cyber world and the traditional form of bullying. In the last decade, social media has been a major factor for social involvement not only among young adults but also among various other age groups [1]. When compared to the different age groups of the society bullying is more prevalent among the youth population [2]. Social media open a platform of opportunities for everyone, but they have flaws, the consequences of which have been stronger negative feelings and higher rates of depression which may result in the worst possible outcomes like suicide [3].

We define cyberbullying as *the intentional or unintended harm imposed by a person to demean the social value of another through an electronic medium*. In our research, when we say youth we are considering people between the ages of 18 and 30 years who are studying in universities in New Zealand. As indicated in US national data, approximately 15% of youth have been victims of cyberbullying [4]. As relevant

© Springer Nature Switzerland AG 2019
M. Themistocleous and P. Rupino da Cunha (Eds.): EMCIS 2018, LNBIP 341, pp. 193–210, 2019.
https://doi.org/10.1007/978-3-030-11395-7_18

to our research, from previous New Zealand based statistics, 2.6% among 826 participants were bullied in the span of six months in New Zealand where more males were victimized than females on social networking sites (SNS) [5].

Despite much research being carried out in the world, few studies have focused on New Zealand. The reason for that can be because it's a small country, lack of funding, or small-scale implementation of government policies. There has been studies [6, 7], which had targeted Australian adolescents, yet not many researchers has approached New Zealand's social media circuit. Hence, we attempt to identify the likely victims of cyberbullying in New Zealand based on their age, gender and personality. The aim of the research is to design a conceptual model based on factors to get the permutations and combinations of the persons most likely to be cyberbullied. This research can also be considered as a pilot as the data samples collected are *158*. As the nature of this research is exploratory it is important because it's a preliminary stepping stone in New Zealand's social media and bullying co-relation. The following is the research question: *What type of student (age, gender, personality) is most likely to be bullied on social media?*

The next section is a literature review, which will provide us the perspective to design a hypothesis and carry out the research. Following that we present our methodology, findings and results, and finally we discuss and conclude the paper.

## 2   Literature Review

This section begins with assessing the core concepts of cyberbullying and how prevalent it is in society. We will investigate the concepts of cyberbullying, its victims, the causes, and the efforts so far to prevent it.

### 2.1   Cyberbullying

Both bullying and victimization are rampant in the society and have adverse effects on both the victim and the bully [8]. The concept of cyberbullying is defined by Patchin and Hinduja as "wilful and repeated harm imposed through the medium of electronic text" [9]. In the literature, we found nine different types of cyberbullying [10–12] flooding, masquerade, flaming/bashing, trolling, harassment, cyberstalking of cyber threats, denigration, outing, and exclusion. *Flooding* comprises of a monopoly by the bully to avoid the victim posting the contents on social media [11]. *Masquerade* is an act of the bully to log in to social media to use the credentials of the victim to post contents online and chat with other people, causing a threat to others to hamper the reputation of the victim [13]. *Flaming* or *Bashing* involves two users intensely involving in a heated argument and attacks on a personal level in public or in private.

This form of cyberbullying is usually short-lived [13]. *Trolling* implies posting an intentional disagreement with the purpose of provocation to an individual or group of people for engaging in an argument. It is not necessary that the disagreement is an actual opinion of the bully [10]. *Harassment* is the quintessential form of bullying which is a clichéd bully-victim relationship. This form of bullying involves sending offensive messages to the victim which can be prolonged depending on the actions taken over the period of time [13]. *Cyberstalking* and *Cyber threats* may involve sending intimidating, threatening or very abusive messages to the victim with an intention of threat or extortion [13]. *Denigration* is the spreading of untrue or foul rumours about someone in the public domain online. It also involves gossiping about the victims on the public domain and derogating their image online [13]. *Outing* is identical to denigration, requiring the bully to have a personal relationship with the victim. In this form of bullying, the bully posts private, personal and embarrassing information about the victim online [13]. *Exclusion* is ignorance towards the victim in public domains or chat rooms, isolating them leading to psychological distress [14].

From all the types mentioned above, cyberbullying can be caused by ignorance as well as on purpose. While Masquerade, Trolling, Harassment, Cyberstalking, and Outing are intentional forms of cyberbullying, Flaming be an unintentional cyberbullying as someone in a bad state of mind can cause it by unknowingly demeaning someone's social value. Denigration can be both intentional and unintentional as the person starting the hoax can do it intentionally, but the others can pass on the information due to ignorance. Historically, the traditional form of bullying was considered to be an acceptable part of a childhood [15]. Research by [16] theorizes that the repercussions of cyber victimization can be even more hazardous compared to face-to-face bullying. There can be a social ineffectiveness among victims who also face greater interpersonal anxiety [17, 18]. Yet it is difficult to jump to the conclusion that these are the antecedents or consequences of cyberbullying [19, 20]. Compared to traditional bullying, cyberbullying can reach a wider spectrum of victims. For example, the traditional form of bullying can be among a small group of people or a school at maximum and not much evidence is kept circulating around, but the victims of cyberbullying can be the humiliated on a social platform in front of their friends, friends of friends, their family and people can share this act among the people whose numbers are difficult to estimate.

As mentioned in one article [21], the statistics are astounding and are New Zealand based. The Otago-based group named 'Sticks n stones' has surveyed 750 people of which 87% had been victims of cyberbullying. The most frequent victims were teenagers aged 18 and 19, of which 46% have faced cyberbullying. According to NZ attitude and value studies, 27% of those aged 20 to 24 years had been victimized whereas those from age 25 to 29 years have faced cyberbullying in some form or the other.

## 2.2   Cyber Victimization

Peer victimization is not a new concept. Several studies have found multiple peer victimizations such as physical attack, verbal harassment, social exclusion, spreading rumours and cyberbullying [22–24]. Cyberbullying/victimization is the newest of all and is our area of research. A study by [25], found a reciprocal relationship between bullying and victimization. The following study also stated that cyber bullies are also cyber victims at some point in their lives [26]. Different victims are also likely to handle the situation in a different manner: one is likely to take the scenario sportingly by overlooking the whole instance, while some might get offended but will not react to the scenario to maintain their dignity and some could also lose their psychological stability leading to actions like suicide, revenge, threats and self-destructive violence.

In research by [14], we have come across another perspective of children carrying the scars of cyberbullying from their childhood into their adulthood. It urges researchers to gain a better understanding of the antecedents and consequences of the bullying behaviour so that someone can come up with an antidote to the poison named cyberbullying. It was also an interesting finding, because the research was carried out over an online survey and most of the participants were teens and the majority of those were females. The findings clearly state that there is an occurrence of bullying among youth. Multiple occurrences of cyberbullying are prevalent among the youth from the study which includes being disrespectful, social avoidance, threatening etc. Studies have theorized the phenomena of cyberbullying being related to the behaviour of the victims [26–28]. One such study by [29], proposes the aggressive behaviours do not decrease over the course of time but instead, just take the shape of the mould it is currently accessible to. This idea leads us to the conclusion that people with more aggression who were used to traditionally victimising people, when they got access to the internet world are more likely to repeat the actions.

There is a rather interesting study by [30] which labels the characteristics of the person as a dark triad which can lead to them to be a cyber-bullying antagonist. This dark triad comprises Machiavellianism and narcissism. This is an interesting study because of how differently these triads lead to the same destination eventually. People with a Machiavellian triad possess manipulation as their basic characteristic [31]. This leads to cyber-aggression leading to cyber-victimization of one naïve enough to get trapped into the manipulative talks of a person with a Machiavellian personality. The next in the line is narcissism. The person possessing a narcissistic personality has a sense of eminence over others, which makes them a self-proclaimed authority to dominate or victimise others in social and cyber-space [32]. Related work has been carried out with this personality with reference to cyberbullying in the past which comprised anti-social behaviour on Facebook [33], as well as cyberbullying among youth [34].

Hence this research can give us more valuable and interesting insights when factors such as age and gender are taken together with personality to determine likely cyber victims.

## 2.3   Causes of Cyberbullying

Compared to the generation around two decades ago, because of the internet, youth today have an edge to be open to new experiences and satisfy themselves socially without socialising in person. Cyberbullying is the repercussion of this edge. In a research by [5], analysis of different motives like jealousy, bigotry, fear, anger, righteousness and revenge have been mentioned and this is just the tip of the iceberg. There can be so many other reasons for a person to commit cyberbullying. The above-mentioned reasons can lead a person of specific age, gender or personality to become the victim of a cyberbully. Regardless of the vast variety in the frequency of cyberbullying, at reasonable and observational correlation is genuinely reliable [35]. Also, cyber bullies were found to show comparable patterns of psychological similarity as conventional harassers [36]. Hence, what can be the differentiation between traditional bullies and cyber bullies apart from the phone in the hand and internet access? The primary feature recognised is the obscurity that the internet gives, the social idea of the animosity, propelled internet knowledge, high recurrence of web utilisation, and its 24-hour reach [37, 38].

To continue with the argument, bullying others through electronic means furnishes the culprit with the likelihood of remaining unknown, which may build their power differential over the cyber-victim and in addition diminish the view of conceivable countering [39]. The social animosity of cyberbullying is additionally reflected in discoveries demonstrating that it frequently happens through SNS and is more regular among young girls [40].

## 2.4    Past Efforts to Prevent Cyberbullying

A study by [41], has a peculiar algorithm developed by analysing the theories by taking into consideration potential reasons for cyberbullying and a pathway for overcoming those. In their paper, two different theories have been proposed: The Neutralization theory and the Deterrence theory. The aim of the Neutralization theory is to figure out why people are more prone to cyberbullying. The Deterrence theory is an antidote to avoid cyberbullying as stated by the Neutralization theory. According to [41], the 3-dimensionality of the Neutralization theory also signifies how the culprit defends his anamorphic actions. The basis of Deterrence lies in the two building factors, certainty and severity. In this scenario, certainty is termed as the risk of getting caught while in the act of cyberbullying, whereas severity states the sets of penalties to be imposed on committing the specific cyberbullying crime. Their paper has stated that the Neutralization theory has been effective in neutralizing cyberbullying among youth. In a similar context, it has been understood that there is a need to consider other risk variables like the ones at a family level.

In future, if efforts made to monitor the usage of substances, especially alcohol, amongst youth, come up with certain prevention programmes to make people aware of the harmful effects, this might help to show positive results. In the past, the application of data mining concepts and artificial intelligence have been applied to curtail cyberbullying [42]. This has been a recent finding to slow down cyberbullying by enforcing a framework to detect inappropriate content through an SVM linear classifier. Natural Language Processing (NLP) models such as Bag of Words (BoW), Latent Dirichlet Allocation (LDA) and Latent Semantic Analysis (LSA) have proven effective detecting cyberbullying [43]. This has been implemented on Twitter, where the classifier scrutinizes the data to expand the list of predefined words and organize them as per weights and priority to identify the bully features.

In the section above, we have covered the core concepts around cyber victimization. This allows us to gather a perspective and design a hypothesis in the next section.

## 3  Hypothesis Development

Based on the research questions discussed in the introduction, hypotheses were developed for this research.

### 3.1  Age

Age plays an important part in defining the person being cyber victimised. We must draw a hypothesis to propose a theory on which there can be a definite result obtained. "Age is just a number", but is it applicable to cyber victimization? If an individual uses the internet, they may be a victim irrespective of their age [44]. Although age is not a barrier to research for cyberbullying, many researchers have dedicated their time and effort to figure out cyberbullying among youth and its preventive measures. Researchers like [45], have some deep insights about cyber bully victimization among youth. Some studies claim to have disapproved the relatability of age with cyber victimization [46–49], whereas, on the contrary, there are also studies which validate the existence of cyber victimization existing among the youth, especially students [14, 50–53]. We would like to draw a hypothesis stating the vital role age can play for a student to be cyber victimised.

*H1: The age of the student on social media has a direct impact on them being cyber victimised* (Table 1).

**Table 1.** Hypothesis for age

| Hypothesis | Null hypothesis |
|---|---|
| H1a: The younger the student the more is the likelihood of cyber victimization | The age of the student is irrelevant for likelihood to be cyber victimized |
| H1b: The older the student the more is the likelihood of cyber victimization | The age of the student is irrelevant for likelihood to be cyber victimized |

### 3.2  Gender

Gender can also be a valuable variable when it comes to classifying the vulnerability of the population to be studied. A study published by [54] explicitly mentions that gender is an important factor to research for differentiating between cyber and traditional bullying. We can also draw a hypothesis that because females are difficult to be bullied in the public space, their chances of being cyberbullied are higher. By uncovering the literature on traditional bullying methods, it has been discovered that boys are more convoluted in both bullying as well as victimization [55–57]. Other studies have demonstrated females are at a higher risk of cyberbullying because of a lack of receptiveness to traditional bullying compared to the electronic media because females are more affected by bullying psychologically [58].

Based on information from the literature on cyber victimization and the research questions we designed, we can draw the following gender-based hypotheses:

*H2: The gender of the student on social media has a direct impact on their being cyber victimised* (Table 2).

**Table 2.** Hypothesis for gender

| Hypothesis | Null hypothesis |
|---|---|
| H2a: Females are more likely to be cyber victimized | The gender of the student is irrelevant for likelihood to be cyber victimized |
| H2b: Males are more likely to be cyber victimized | The gender of the student is irrelevant for likelihood to be cyber victimized |

### 3.3 Personality

Amongst all the popular theories on personality, the big five factors of [59] are relevant as well as applicable to our research. McCrae and Costa Jr (1997), theorised there are five major personalities of human behaviour: openness, conscientiousness, extraversion, agreeableness and neuroticism.

People with openness to experience generally are open minded people [59]. They welcome new ideas and prefer moving out of their comfort zone and like experiencing new things. These people are also likely to be cyber victims because they tend to be vulnerable when alone while moving out of their comfort zone. People with conscientiousness are workaholics [59]. They possess the virtue of dutifulness and self-discipline. They are generally well-organized and are focused on achieving their goals. People with this personality are less likely to be a cyber-victim or a bully as they are cautious of their environment [59]. People with an extroverted personality are highly social people. They are friendly, attention seeking, enthusiastic and talkative. These kinds of people are most likely to be cyber victimised because of their outgoing nature [59]. The basic equation may suggest that the more the person is in contact with a social group, the more likely they are to be bullied. A study conducted by [60] also says that people with extroversion as their triad have more Facebook friends. The next personality is agreeableness. People with this personality are the compassionate ones. They have a happy-to-help attitude, are courteous, empathetic and unselfish. These people are least prone to cyber-victimisation because of their good behaviour socially. But on the contrary, researchers have also shown that people with openness are more likely to display personal information on social media [61]. The last personality is Neuroticism. The people with this personality are soft targets for cyber bullies because of their vulnerability of being emotionally unstable. They tend to react to very small things which can lead to feuds on social media. They can also be upset easily, and trivial issues can make them angry.

*H3: The personality of the student has a direct impact on their being cyber victimised* (Table 3).

In this section we have designed the hypotheses on which we will base a questionnaire to gather data for analysis. The next section will give us an insight into the step-by-step process of building the questionnaire and executing the online survey.

**Table 3.** Hypothesis for personality

| Hypothesis | Null hypothesis |
| --- | --- |
| H3a: Extroverts are more likely students to be cyber victimized | The personality of a student is irrelevant for likelihood to be cyber victimized |
| H3b: Neurotics are more likely students to be cyber victimized | The personality of a student is irrelevant for likelihood to be cyber victimized |
| H3c: Students with openness to experience are more likely to be cyber victimized | The personality of a student is irrelevant for likelihood to be cyber victimized |
| H3d: Students with agreeable personalities are more likely to be cyber victimised | The personality of a student is irrelevant for likelihood to be cyber victimized |
| H3e: Students with conscientious personalities are more likely to be cyber victimised | The personality of a student is irrelevant for likelihood to be cyber victimized |

# 4 Methodology

Research in the area of cyber victimization is abundant in most technologically advanced countries [62]. Hence, using New Zealand based data, we will carry out our research using exploratory data analysis. The underlying objective of the research is "identifying the characteristics of cyber victims on social media in New Zealand". The three variables we will be discussing for identifying the characteristics of the cyber victims are age, gender and personality.

The main motive behind building this questionnaire is to narrow down the larger context to the most convenient form. The quality of the data obtained heavily relies on the questions in the survey. The two basic rules to designing a questionnaire are relevancy and accuracy [63]. In this context, relevancy means the researchers' understanding of the questions, whereas, accuracy can be defined as the layout of the questionnaire [63]. The questionnaire we will use for the survey is designed with these principles in mind.

For our research and constructing the questionnaire, we are setting the age limit at between 18 and 30 years. Hence to quantify the variable, we will be focusing on asking the age in our questionnaire as a choice between the ranges 18-21 years, 22-25 years, 26-30 years, and 30 years and above. This will give us an idea if the students are getting cyber victimized, the ideal age when the impact of cyber victimization can be maximum. We will also focus on the age-related activities on social media and the actions taken when cyber victimized. In our analysis, we are trying to ascertain whether gender plays a role in cyber victimization. To this end, we will explore whether a gender is more likely to be cyber victimised on social media, and if so, while doing a certain activity on that SNS. By the end of the analysis in this section, we will arrive at a conclusion of cyber victimization with reference to gender on social media and the actions preferred by certain gender when cyber victimized.

Recently efforts have been put into the study to figure out personalities of individuals. This has been an influential factor while determining both the cyber bully and cyber victim [64]. This factor could turn out to be the most interesting part of the study. The research carried out by [59] regarding the five traits from the five-factor model has always been linked to studies of social networking technologies [65]. The five- factor model determines the different personality types of individuals. These personality traits are explained in our hypotheses and will be used now to construct the final segment of our questionnaire. To determine the personalities of the students participating in the survey, we used the big five 15 item scales. These questions were successfully conceptualised and implemented in research done by [65]. The survey was also validated by extensive use of the German Socio-Economic Panel Survey [66]. Each of the five personality traits is assessed by three items. These items are merged to an average score of the respective big five dimensions. Thus, this survey will allow us to get a personality score. We will be using principal component analysis (PCA) in the tool R to derive the personality scores and correlate factors determining cyber victimization.

The survey was distributed by through social media, mobile applications and email. The posts and the email comprised of a hyperlink to the online survey which was created using the survey generating tool *Qualtrics*.

## 5  Findings and Results

In this section, we analyse the data we have collected through the questionnaire and explain cyber victimization in statistics. Initially, we will perform some descriptive statistics on the raw data. Later, we will perform the principal component analysis to determine the personality of each individual respondent. Based on this information, we can later perform the analysis on age and gender to analyse the responses on cyber victimization.

### 5.1  Descriptive Statistics

After completing the online survey, 211 responses were returned. The final number of complete responses used for data analysis was 158. Almost half of respondent's ranges were between 22 and 25 years. The rest of the respondents are almost evenly distributed in the other age groups. The gender variable was also evenly distributed among males and females with 56.96% and 43.04% respectively. A noteworthy fact from the table is that 96.84% of university students use social media which made them ideal candidates to answer the cyberbullying questions.

Facebook is the most preferred social media site among the university students with 69.93% users. The next most popular is YouTube with 41.18% users, followed by Instagram, Snapchat and Twitter. The time spent on social media is somewhat even as the numbers lie close to each other, still, 36.60% students spend around 2 to 4 h a week on social media. Watching others' activity is the most preferred activity for social media users, where 68.63% users prefer doing it. As we discussed in the literature review, to see how the youth in New Zealand prefer using social media, this analysis can be the answer to a certain extent. Chatting with others is also one of the preferred activities on social media, preferred by 44.44%. The other activities (9.15%) include watching videos, browsing through news feeds on social media, researching and browsing for memes.

When asked about being cyberbullied, 73.86% of the students had never been cyberbullied. Only 13.73% of the students were affirmative of being bullied whereas 12.42% were not sure of being cyberbullied. When looking into our findings, most cyberbullying happens on Facebook with 22.82%. The rest of the social media sites are below 10%.

## 5.2   Age

The rate of cyberbullying is low in New Zealand among university students. Students in all age groups were least bullied or they were unsure, but it is apparent that most of them were not bullied based on their age. 113 out of 153 respondents were not bullied, and 83.33% in the age group of 31 years and above were least bullied. Looking at the bullying rate in New Zealand, the most likely to be bullied are from ages 18 to 21 years and 26 to 30 years with 22.22% and 23.08% respectively. One of the noteworthy points is, the number of students saying maybe is like that of the number of students bullied. This gives a vague idea that they either don't want to reveal whether they are bullied, or they might be unclear about the fact of having been bullied on SNS. The (p=) value for this hypothesis 0.32 which is *(p > 0.05)*. Hence, we can accept the null hypothesis for H1 i.e. the age of the students is irrelevant for likelihood to be cyber victimized.

## 5.3   Gender

Total 63 out of 87 (72.41%) of male users and 50 out of 66 (75.76%) of female SNS users have never faced cyberbullying. The *(p=)* value for this analysis is 0.90 which is *(p > 0.05)* greater than the significance level which allows us to accept the null hypothesis for H2. Also, looking at the numbers 14.94% and 12.64% respectively of males and female students having been bullied which are very close to each other. Hence, from the observation and statistical analysis, we can state that gender does not play a substantial role in the cyber victimization of the students as male students are bullied only slightly more compared to female students.

## 5.4   Personality

As mentioned above, we will be using the 15 Likert-Scale questions derived from [59] Each of the 15 questions acts as a sub-variable for each factor from the Five-Factor model.

A principal component analysis (PCA) was conducted on 15 variables with orthogonal rotation (varimax). The procedure was adopted and followed from [67]. The Kaiser-Meyer-Olkin measure verified the sampling adequacy for the analysis, KMO = .69 which is mediocre but well above the acceptable limit of .5 [68]. Two factors, *Ec* and *Ca*, were below the KMO threshold clocking 0.45 and 0.49 respectively. Hence, we had to discard them in the further analysis. Bartlett's test of sphericity, $X^2(78) = 538.63$, $p < .001$, indicated that correlations between items was sufficiently large for PCA. An initial analysis was run to obtain eigenvalues for each component of data.

Assuming the number of samples and Kaiser's criterion, we considered five components for final analysis. The items in the cluster on the same components suggest component 1 represents openness to experience, component 2 is neuroticism and component 3 is extroversion followed by components 4 and 5 that are agreeableness and conscientiousness. From the reliability analysis, the variables openness to experience, neuroticism and agreeableness of the personality data have high reliability ($\alpha$ = 0.89, 0.71, and 0.68). However, the variables extroversion and conscientiousness have low reliability ($\alpha$ = 0.53 and 0.45). As stated by Unwin (2013), still it is not a concern for our data as the threshold for Cronbach's $\alpha$ = 0.3. From the analysis above, we have gathered information that 18.98% respondents possess the personality openness to experience, 20.88% are neurotics, 16.45% are the extroverts, 20.88% possess the personality of agreeableness and 22.81% possess conscientiousness.

The overall percentage of respondents getting cyberbullied is as low as 13.73% whereas, the people who are unsure and responded maybe is 12.42%. The percentage of respondents being bullied is high with the personality openness to experience. With 17.24% of the respondents facing cyberbullying and 20.69% unsure, openness to experience is the personality trait which is slightly more likely to be cyber victimized compared to the other personality traits, whereas, the respondents with the personality trait agreeableness are the least cyberbullied with 82.76%.

## 6 Discussion

We began our research with a framework that included different traits of cyberbullying and its related terminologies. Figure 1 illustrates the conceptual framework around which we designed our research. This framework is a preliminary model that we are proposing to understand the area of this research.

Since the initial phases, we have tried to uncover all the possible areas which concern cyberbullying, and which could have led to the outcome of our research. The area which we specifically tried to uncover in our research are social media users, their characteristics (age, gender, and personality) and how they lead to cyber victimization

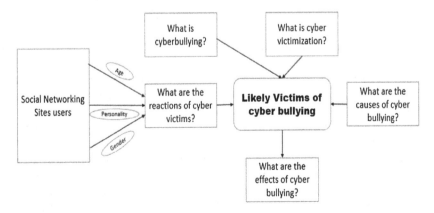

**Fig. 1.** Cyberbullying research framing

of an individual. Based on this conceptual framework, we designed and implemented the methodology explained above. The results we found are, "there is no visible correlation of cyberbullying with respect to age and gender in New Zealand, whereas, the students with the personality trait openness to experience is slightly more prone than people with other personalities".

When we investigated our first factor of the research i.e. the age of the students, there was absolutely no correlation between the age of the university students and cyber victimization. In the literature, we came across a major difference of opinions among different researchers. [44], in his early studies, stated that an individual using the internet is always prone to cyberbullying irrespective of his age. The same view was supported by [62], who state that cyberbullying gradually decreases in adolescence. We have seen studies which proved the relatability of cyber victimization which exists among youth [11, 14, 50–53]. Based on this we designed a hypothesis which said the age of the student on social media has a direct impact on them being cyber victimised. But our results give us a contradictory result validating the null hypothesis. The results are not as strange as they seem because of similar claims made in past studies [46–49]. One of the reasons for these results may be the nature of sample we have collected. The sample population was university students who are older than school children and have bigger problems i.e. career, finance etc. to deal with. Another reason may be reluctance to admit, or ignorance towards the problem.

In previous literature, there has been a major inconsistency while finding a pattern for cyber victimization with respect to gender difference. Still, some literature has led our research to some other perspectives than based on gender disparity. Studies on traditional bullying state that males possess more bullying behaviour than females [18, 69]. Based on the literature we have seen, we presented a hypothesis "the gender of the student on social media has a direct impact on their being cyber victimised." But our research has presented us with contradictory results. Not only have university students of both genders been cyber victimized equally but the students who have never been cyber victimized are also somewhat similar. This means that gender plays no part in the cyber victimization of university students in New Zealand. There should be some rational explanation for this which can be uncovered by qualitative research and interviewing different people with different genders. This will give us a perspective on why gender does not play a part in cyber victimization in New Zealand.

Few studies have been conducted in this domain with the five-factor personality traits by [59], but those few studies have demonstrated how a different personality can play a part in the cyber victimization of an individual [30, 32, 70]. Though the number of students cyberbullied is not substantial, the slight difference between the factors-based result and actual results look significant. The detail regarding the percentage of students belonging to the personality trait of openness to experience is higher than the percentage of total cyberbullied. On the other hand, the percentage of students not cyberbullied with the same personality trait is much lower than the actual number. During hypothesis development, we discussed that the students belonging to the personality trait openness to experience are likely to be cyberbullied, as they could be trying to move out of their comfort zone. Increased novelty seeking that is linked to openness to experience has been associated with internet addiction [71]. The personality trait openness to experience is associated mainly with fantasy, aesthetics, feelings, actions, ideas, and values [72]. It has also been discussed in the research that drug usage by this personality is higher than others [73]. The research conducted by [74], confirms the target youth who are more prone to addictions like smoking, drinking etc. can also be the victims of cyberbullying. This gives us a fair idea how likely the students with the personality trait openness to experience are prone to be cyberbullied. Moreover, the students in a dilemma with the answer 'maybe' for the personality openness to experience also has the higher percentage compared to the total population. Hence, the personality openness to experience is more susceptible to be cyberbullied as compared to its counterparts.

# 7  Conclusion, Limitations and Future Work

The core research topic of this project was to identify the characteristics of the cyber victims on social media in New Zealand. We can demonstrate how age and gender don't play any substantial part in the cyber victimization of students, whereas the personality trait *openness to experience* may lead to cyberbullying by others to a certain extent. This perspective may play an important part in future research in the field of cyber victimization.

As personality plays part in the cyber bullying of an individual, policies, interventions, and monitoring are some of the measures to be taken. Further research can be carried out to determine the earliest age children have access to social media. Based on that number, a small survey can be carried out in a school to determine the personality of every individual child. The children with the personality trait *openness to experience* can be monitored to avoid cyber bullying. Here, some implications of [42] data mining technologies and artificial intelligence methods can be applied for avoiding cyberbullying. In Sect. 5.4 we identified Facebook as the most used social media by the students with personality trait *openness to experience*. This can also help us to monitor the specific social media to evade cyberbullying of these students. Generic internet safety tips and cyberbullying prevention measures can be incorporated at home, in universities, and the social media homepages. In Sect. 2.4 we discussed a recent algorithm proposed by [41]. This algorithm theorises by considering the potential reasons for cyberbullying. It has two factors i.e. Neutralization and Deterrence theories. The neutralization theory aims for the people who are more prone to cyberbullying whereas the deterrence theory acts as its antidote. In such cases, our findings can also contribute as one of the factors. The students possessing the personality trait openness to experience can be aimed in the neutralization theory.

## 7.1  Limitations and Future Work

From the results, we can see the number of students who have never been bullied is high within the age group of 31 years and above. This leads to a counter-argument that, the older the person, the less likely they are to be cyber victimized. Because there has been a gradual drop in the number of people being cyber victimized in later years, we can focus on the younger population. There can be future work in this area of research on school children in New Zealand to see whether young adults i.e. from the age 13 to

19 years having access to the technology are more likely to be cyber victimized. For our research, we analysed 158 responses. Amongst these responses, we had a gender imbalance. Most them are male responses. In future work, we could gather more data with a larger time span. If we got enough data, we could use the random 50% male population and 50% female for analysis purposes. This would give us an accurate ratio of the cyber victim's gender-wise. This could also provide us with the more substantial evidence on whether the victims of either gender are more likely to be cyberbullied.

After conducting the quantitative data analysis and interpreting the results, we have realised there is an immense scope for qualitative research. The qualitative research would give us an interpretive, naturalistic approach to the subject matter [23]. In the research done so far, for example in the quantitative research if we are asking the question "Have you ever been cyberbullied?" in the qualitative research we can first ask the question to a sample population "What does cyberbullying mean to you?" This kind of question in the qualitative research and analysis will give us the implications to the questions to follow in the quantitative research. This could be a good implementation in future work as well. One more important aspect we can monitor is the cultural difference. According to [75], culture is defined as "a collective programming of the mind that distinguishes two different people belonging to two different groups". It is not necessary that two individuals in the same group should be like each other. These can be two completely different individuals who lead their lives in a similar manner [76]. When we look it into the New Zealand perspective, no major study has been found considering this factor. For instance, among the North American communities, Spanish-speaking or Hispanic youth are frequent bullies compared to other ethnicities like African-Americans or Caucasians [69]. Whereas, it is the other way around when it comes to victimization as African-Americans are less bullied compared to the other two ethnicities mentioned above [77, 78]. As per the report published by [79], people in New Zealand can be identified as four major ethnicities: European, Maori, Asian and Pacifica. We tried to implement this factor but unfortunately, the numbers were not on the higher side. Moreover, most of the respondents were either Indians or Europeans. As mentioned above, for the future research if we can gather more numbers, this study can also prove interesting.

In conclusion, the research addresses the gap in the initial phase and has overcome it in later phases. The research gap was in regards with the work done so far in the field cyberbullying in New Zealand. We have implemented the quantitative approach for identifying the characteristics of cyber victims on social media in New Zealand. However, the study also provides us with an insight on how the rate of cyberbullying is low in New Zealand. It has provided a greater clarification surrounding likely leading to the future research outputs.

# Appendix

The survey questions can be requested from the authors.

# References

1. Olweus, D.: Cyber Bullying. Aggression and Violence: A Social Psychological Perspective (2016)
2. Bauman, S., Toomey, R.B., Walker, J.L.: Associations among bullying, cyberbullying, and suicide in high school students. J. Adolesc. 36(2), 341–350 (2013)
3. Cassidy, W., Faucher, C., Jackson, M.: Cyberbullying among youth: a comprehensive review of current international research and its implications and application to policy and practice. Sch. Psychol. Int. 34(6), 575–612 (2013)
4. Holt, M.K., et al.: Multidisciplinary approaches to research on bullying in adolescence. Adolesc. Res. Rev. 2(1), 1–10 (2017)
5. Chandrashekhar, A., Muktha, G., Anjana, D.: Cyberstalking and cyberbullying: effects and prevention measures. Imp. J. Interdiscip. Res. 2(3), 95–102 (2016)
6. Perren, S., et al.: Bullying in school and cyberspace: associations with depressive symptoms in Swiss and Australian adolescents. Child Adolesc. Psychiatry Ment. Health 4(1), 28 (2010)
7. Price, M., Dalgleish, J.: Cyberbullying: experiences, impacts and coping strategies as described by Australian young people. Youth Stud. Aust. 29(2), 51 (2010)
8. Kljakovic, M., Hunt, C., Jose, P.: Incidence of bullying and victimisation among adolescents in New Zealand. N. Z. J. Psychol. 44(2), 57–67 (2015)
9. Hinduja, S. Patchin, J.W.: Cyberbullying statistics (2014). http://www.puresight.com/Cyberbullying/cyber-bullying-statistics.html
10. Bayzick, J., Kontostathis, A., Edwards, L.: Detecting the presence of cyberbullying using computer software (2011)
11. Maher, D.: Cyberbullying: An ethnographic case study of one Australian upper primary school class. Youth Stud. Aust. 27(4), 50 (2008)
12. Willard, N.: Cyberbullying and Cyberthreats. Center for Safe and Responsible Internet Use, Eugene, OR (2006)
13. Willard, N.E.: Cyberbullying and Cyberthreats: Responding to the Challenge of Online Social Aggression, Threats, and Distress. Research Press (2007)
14. Patchin, J.W., Hinduja, S.: Bullies move beyond the schoolyard: a preliminary look at cyberbullying. Youth Violence Juv. Justice 4(2), 148–169 (2006)
15. Limber, S.P., Small, M.A.: State laws and policies to address bullying in schools. Sch. Psychol. Rev. 32(3), 445–456 (2003)
16. Campbell, M.A.: Cyber bullying: an old problem in a new guise? J. Psychol. Couns. Sch. 15(1), 68–76 (2005)
17. Craig, W.M.: The relationship among bullying, victimization, depression, anxiety, and aggression in elementary school children. Pers. Individ. Differ. 24(1), 123–130 (1998)
18. Forero, R., et al.: Bullying behaviour and psychosocial health among school students in New South Wales, Australia: cross sectional survey. BMJ 319(7206), 344–348 (1999)
19. Hodges, E.V., Perry, D.G.: Personal and interpersonal antecedents and consequences of victimization by peers. J. Pers. Soc. Psychol. 76(4), 677 (1999)
20. Roland, E.: Bullying, depressive symptoms and suicidal thoughts. Educ. Res. 44(1), 55–67 (2002)
21. Rates of cyber bullying in New Zealand alarming, in NZ Herald (2016)
22. Awiria, O., Olweus, D., Byrne, B.: Bullying at School-What We Know and What We Can DoCoping with Bullying in Schools (1994)
23. Crick, N.R., Grotpeter, J.K.: Relational aggression, gender, and social-psychological adjustment. Child Dev. 66(3), 710–722 (1995)

24. Williams, K.R., Guerra, N.G.: Prevalence and predictors of internet bullying. J. Adolesc. Health **41**(6), S14–S21 (2007)
25. Jose, P.E., et al.: The joint development of traditional bullying and victimization with cyber bullying and victimization in adolescence. J. Res. Adolesc. **22**(2), 301–309 (2012)
26. Ybarra, M.L., Mitchell, K.J.: Youth engaging in online harassment: associations with caregiver–child relationships, Internet use, and personal characteristics. J. Res. Adolesc. **27** (3), 319–336 (2004)
27. Li, Q.: Cyberbullying in schools: a research of gender differences. Sch. Psychol. Int. **27**(2), 157–170 (2006)
28. Slonje, R., Smith, P.K., FriséN, A.: The nature of cyberbullying, and strategies for prevention. Comput. Hum. Behav. **29**(1), 26–32 (2013)
29. Björkqvist, K.: Sex differences in physical, verbal, and indirect aggression: a review of recent research. Sex Roles **30**(3), 177–188 (1994)
30. Paulhus, D.L., Williams, K.M.: The dark triad of personality: narcissism, machiavellianism, and psychopathy. J. Res. Pers. **36**(6), 556–563 (2002)
31. Geis, F., Levy, M.: Studies in Machiavellianism. Elsevier (1970)
32. Raskin, R.N. Hall, C.S.: A narcissistic personality inventory. Psychological reports (1979)
33. Reidy, D.E., et al.: Effects of narcissistic entitlement and exploitativeness on human physical aggression. Pers. Individ. Differ. **44**(4), 865–875 (2008)
34. Ang, R.P., Tan, K.-A., Talib Mansor, A.: Normative beliefs about aggression as a mediator of narcissistic exploitativeness and cyberbullying. J. Interpers. Violence **26**(13), 2619–2634 (2011)
35. Görzig, A., Ólafsson, K.: What makes a bully a cyberbully? Unravelling the characteristics of cyberbullies across twenty-five European countries. J. Child. Media **7**(1), 9–27 (2013)
36. Görzig, A.: Who bullies and who is bullied online?: A study of 9–16 year old internet users in 25 European countries (2011)
37. Dooley, J., Pyzalski, J., Cross, D.: Cyberbullying and face-to-face bullying: similarities and differences. Zeitschrift für Psychologie/J. Psychol. **217**(4), 182–188 (2009)
38. Heirman, W., Walrave, M.: Assessing concerns and issues about the mediation of technology in cyberbullying. Cyberpsychol.: J. Psychosoc. Res. Cyberspace **2**(2) (2008)
39. Spears, B., et al.: Behind the scenes and screens: insights into the human dimension of covert and cyberbullying. Zeitschrift für Psychologie/J. Psychol. **217**(4), 189–196 (2009)
40. Smith, P.K., et al.: Cyberbullying: its nature and impact in secondary school pupils. J. Child Psychol. Psychiatry **49**(4), 376–385 (2008)
41. Zhang, S., et al.: Friend or foe: cyberbullying in social network sites. ACM SIGMIS Database **47**(1), 51–71 (2016)
42. Zhao, R., Zhou, A., Mao, K.: Automatic detection of cyberbullying on social networks based on bullying features. In: Proceedings of the 17th International Conference on Distributed Computing and Networking. ACM (2016)
43. Xu, J.-M., et al.: Learning from bullying traces in social media. In: Proceedings of the 2012 Conference of the North American Chapter of the Association for Computational Linguistics: Human Language Technologies. Association for Computational Linguistics (2012)
44. Witmer, D.F.: Risky business: why people feel safe in sexually explicit on-line communication. J. Comput.-Mediat. Commun. **2**(4) (1997)
45. Slonje, R., Smith, P.K.: Cyberbullying: another main type of bullying? Scand. J. Psychol. **49** (2), 147–154 (2008)
46. Beran, T., Li, Q.: The relationship between cyberbullying and school bullying. J. Stud. Wellbeing **1**(2), 16–33 (2008)

47. Didden, R., et al.: Cyberbullying among students with intellectual and developmental disability in special education settings. Dev. Neurorehabil. **12**(3), 146–151 (2009)
48. Katzer, C., Fetchenhauer, D., Belschak, F.: Cyberbullying: who are the victims? A comparison of victimization in Internet chatrooms and victimization in school. J. Media Psychol. **21**(1), 25–36 (2009)
49. Varjas, K., Meyers, J., Hunt, M.: Student survey of bullying behavior–revised 2 (SSBB-R2). Georgia State University, Center for Research on School Safety, School Climate and Classroom Management, Atlanta, GA (2006)
50. DeHue, F., Bolman, C., Völlink, T.: Cyberbullying: youngsters' experiences and parental perception. CyberPsychol. Behav. **11**(2), 217–223 (2008)
51. Kowalski, R.M., Limber, S.P.: Electronic bullying among middle school students. J. Adolesc. Health **41**(6), S22–S30 (2007)
52. Ybarra, M.L., Diener-West, M., Leaf, P.J.: Examining the overlap in Internet harassment and school bullying: Implications for school intervention. J. Adolesc. Health **41**(6), S42–S50 (2007)
53. Ybarra, M.L., Mitchell, K.J.: How risky are social networking sites? A comparison of places online where youth sexual solicitation and harassment occurs. Pediatrics **121**(2), e350–e357 (2008)
54. Erdur-Baker, Ö.: Cyberbullying and its correlation to traditional bullying, gender and frequent and risky usage of internet-mediated communication tools. New Media Soc. **12**(1), 109–125 (2010)
55. Boulton, M.J., Underwood, K.: Bully/victim problems among middle school children. Br. J. Educ. Psychol. **62**(1), 73–87 (1992)
56. Lagerspetz, K.M., et al.: Group aggression among school children in three schools. Scand. J. Psychol. **23**(1), 45–52 (1982)
57. O'moore, A. Hillery, B.: Bullying in Dublin schools. Ir. J. Psychol. **10**(3), 426–441 (1989)
58. Stephenson, P., Smith, D.: Bullying in the junior school. In: Bullying in Schools, pp. 45–57 (1989)
59. McCrae, R.R., Costa Jr., P.T.: Personality trait structure as a human universal. Am. Psychol. **52**(5), 509 (1997)
60. Utz, S.: Show me your friends and I will tell you what type of person you are: how one's profile, number of friends, and type of friends influence impression formation on social network sites. J. Comput.-Mediat. Commun. **15**(2), 314–335 (2010)
61. Amichai-Hamburger, Y., Vinitzky, G.: Social network use and personality. Comput. Hum. Behav. **26**(6), 1289–1295 (2010)
62. Vazsonyi, A.T., et al.: Cyberbullying in context: direct and indirect effects by low self-control across 25 European countries. Eur. J. Dev. Psychol. **9**(2), 210–227 (2012)
63. Iarossi, G.: The Power of Survey Design: A User's Guide for Managing Surveys, Interpreting Results, and Influencing Respondents. World Bank Publications (2006)
64. Peluchette, J.V., et al.: Cyberbullying victimization: do victims' personality and risky social network behaviors contribute to the problem? Comput. Hum. Behav. **52**, 424–435 (2015)
65. Vodanovich, S.: Digital Native Well-being and Development in Ubiquitous Spaces (2014). ResearchSpace@Auckland
66. Dehne, M., Schupp, J.: Persönlichkeitsmerkmale im Sozio-oekonomischen Panel (SOEP)-Konzept. Umsetzung und empirische Eigenschaften. Res. Notes **26**, 1–70 (2007)
67. Unwin, A.: Discovering statistics using R by Andy Field, Jeremy Miles, Zoë Field. Int. Stat. Rev. **81**(1), 169–170 (2013)
68. Kaiser, H.F.: An index of factorial simplicity. Psychometrika **39**(1), 31–36 (1974)
69. Haynie, D.L., et al.: Bullies, victims, and bully/victims: distinct groups of at-risk youth. J. Early Adolesc. **21**(1), 29–49 (2001)

70. Christie, R., Geis, F.L.: Studies in Machiavellianism. Academic Press (2013)

71. Ko, C.-H., et al.: The characteristics of decision making, potential to take risks, and personality of college students with Internet addiction. Psychiatry Res. **175**(1), 121–125 (2010)

72. Kuss, D.J., Griffiths, M.D., Binder, J.F.: Internet addiction in students: prevalence and risk factors. Comput. Hum. Behav. **29**(3), 959–966 (2013)

73. Terracciano, A., et al.: Five-factor model personality profiles of drug users. BMC Psychiatry **8**(1), 22 (2008)

74. Chan, S.F., La Greca, A.M.: Cyber victimization and aggression: are they linked with adolescent smoking and drinking? Child Youth Care Forum **45**, 47–63 (2016)

75. Hofstede, G.: Dimensionalizing cultures: the Hofstede model in context. Online Read. Psychol. Cult. **2**(1), 8 (2011)

76. Hofstede, G.: Culture's Consequences: Comparing Values, Behaviors, Institutions, and Organizations Across Cultures. Sage, Thousand Oaks (2001)

77. Nansel, T.R., et al.: Bullying behaviors among US youth: prevalence and association with psychosocial adjustment. JAMA **285**(16), 2094–2100 (2001)

78. Spriggs, A.L., et al.: Adolescent bullying involvement and perceived family, peer and school relations: commonalities and differences across race/ethnicity. J. Adolesc. Health **41**(3), 283–293 (2007)

79. Kenny, K., Fayers, A.: How the ethnic mix in your community is set to change (2015). http://www.stuff.co.nz/national/72557057/How-the-ethnic-mix-in-your-community-is-set-to-change. Accessed 30 Sept 2015

# The Novel Online Comparison Tool for Bank Charges with User-Friendly Approach

Ivan Soukal[(⊠)] [iD]

Faculty of Informatics and Management, Department of Economics,
University of Hradec Kralove,
Rokitanskeho 62, 500 03 Hradec Kralove, Czech Republic
ivan.soukal@uhk.cz

**Abstract.** This paper presents a proposal for the novel comparison tool for bank charges; the online calculator service. The development of this tool was motivated by information asymmetry, which exists on the market of payment accounts to consumer's disadvantage. Our calculator service provides user with the list of the most suitable bank accounts based on his preferences, sorted by monthly fee. It is up to the particular user whether he fills in values of his current usage or future requirements. The results are personalized based solely on user's input. This paper reveals motivation behind our work and presents the current implementation of our proposal including conceptual foundation, workflows, matrix of data for underlying logic and of course user interface. By presenting workflows we stress multidimensional use of our service. Apart for clear benefit for individual user, the data acquired from all users can be used for post-processing, which includes various analyses of user behaviour and resulting user profiling regarding using bank services. The calculator service was already launched for Czech environment on https://uni.uhk.cz/kalkulator/.

**Keywords:** Online services · Digital services · Bank charges
Financial advisor · Online calculators · User experience · User-centered design

## 1 Introduction

Online price comparison agents also known as comparison tool applications (thereinafter as CT or CTs in plural) provide the possibility to compare and contrast products. This comparison is based on a variety of criteria or utilizing at least one criteria filter – price. Price comparison agents belong to a shopbot applications category along with other similar tools such as shopping agents and shopping robots described in research of Zhu et al. [2]. All such applications have one purpose, which is reduction of information asymmetry. Consumer bears a negative impact of information asymmetry concerning the payment accounts market (thereinafter as PA or PAs in plural).

In this paper we would like to present a novel online service for calculating banking fees, which is being developed based on our specification. The application was already launched for Czech environment with URL[1] [1] and presented also here[2]. The proposed

---

[1] https://uni.uhk.cz/kalkulator/.
[2] https://www.bankovnipoplatky.com/kalkulator.html.

© Springer Nature Switzerland AG 2019
M. Themistocleous and P. Rupino da Cunha (Eds.): EMCIS 2018, LNBIP 341, pp. 211–224, 2019.
https://doi.org/10.1007/978-3-030-11395-7_19

service belongs to the category of online comparison agents, however it is unique in its scope, robustness, performance and range of useful data presented to user, based on performed calculation - therefore calculation service. Based on these data consumer can make well-founded decision about the best bank account for him.

Our target market is specific because the information asymmetry regards the very basic feature of any product, which is price. Price information asymmetry is more pronounced in countries with more complex and opaque pricing policy. The Czech Republic belongs to countries with greater information asymmetry. In contrast e.g. Great Britain or Germany have diminished asymmetry. Unlike these two western countries, the Czech banks' tariffs usually include multiple conditional sales and many items representing separate fees. Moreover, fees vary accordingly to the chosen communication channel (e.g. via phone, internet,...) in addition to usual tariff's characteristics, i.e. they are subject of irregular change.

In such situation user can greatly benefit from CT's comparison based on his individual profile, which reflects his requirements and lifestyle. It is a great opportunity for researches at the same time because the consumer willingly provides his unique personal usage record in the process. Moreover, such records are supposed to be precise because users are highly motivated. It is in the user's best interest to provide correct data, otherwise calculation service would not offer helpful results.

In our previous work we based our research on such data in the target market. We performed a retail consumer segmentation by two-step cluster analysis [3], choice optimality study [4] with different influence of geographical preference, desired price modeling [5] based on the current price distribution and recently we started to research consumption variability.

## 2 State of the Art

### 2.1 Impact of Comparison Tools

Information asymmetry is present on the PA market and it negatively influences the optimal choice [4]. The mathematical model of a consumer search for optimal price of PA under the uncertainty [5] shows the main issue concerning the price search – the marginal return on search issue. The traditional approach - when a user performs search and has to calculate the price accordingly a PA tariff - is a time-consuming task. Moreover in the Czech Republic many banks include different types of conditional sales and some tariffs are almost atomized charging each service separately and it also differs according to the communication channel. The search costs can be expressed as a product of an average minute wage and search time, see [5] for full methodology. The search costs are rising with more PAs available. When price distribution is more skewed to the right, the lower is the desired price and of course tariffs are more complex. The search costs are soaring if we take into account that all tariffs are subject of an irregular change. On the other hand, there are savings achieved by finding and opening a cheaper account. The elementary maximization rule then states that a user will continue the search until expected marginal return from search is greater than marginal search costs. The maximization variable differs but one of most usual cases is a maximization of an expected net benefit of searching the set of options (as the difference between the expected maximum utility of searching the brands in the set and the cost of searching these brands) [6]. That is why, from the systematic point of view, shopbots exist – to make a search worthy by minimizing the search costs.

Both academicians, as well as legislative bodies, admit and acknowledge an impact of CTs. From the academic point of view shopbots have a positive impact on both price level as well as price dispersion [e.g. 7, 8]. Another study [9] focused on pricing behaviour by sellers at a price comparison site confirmed strong negative relationship between the number of sellers monitored by comparison site and price. Legislative bodies of the EU rely on CTs in information asymmetry reduction on the retail banking market. The Payment Account Directive (Chap. II/Art. 7) [European Parliament] states the duty to offer consumers of each member country at least one CT through a special website list of the local supervisor authority. CTs are one of main tools to deal with another negative effect of information asymmetry – consumer mobility barrier. Low level of mobility of consumers with respect to retail financial services is to a large extent due to the lack of transparency and comparability as regards the fees and services on offer [10].

## 2.2 Comparators and Calculators

Comparators and calculators are both online digital services for end users, who seek help in deciding which bank account would be the best for their needs. These two services are very different both in their design and implementation. They are different in characteristics of consumers, who use them. Based on the definition of maximizers and satisficers, we can assume that comparators would be used more by satisficers, whereas calculators by maximizers. Satisficers settle for "good enough" option (e.g. bank account), while maximizers strive to make the best possible choice [11, 12]. While there are many comparator services, calculators are very scarce, in some countries even non-existent. However, population consists of both these characteristics [13]. Therefore, we would like to promote use of calculators.

Comparators are in fact only lists of bank accounts from the view of user interface. They are not even web applications from the implementation point of view, only static web pages. Some of them however provide useful sorting options or predefined lists, so consumer can quickly get acquainted with basic characteristics and charges of individual accounts. Usually some basic categorization or filtering is offered, e.g. basic, business, students, suitable for overdraft (i.e. according to the most used service), with high interest etc. Subsequent sorting is done e.g. according to monthly or yearly fee, maximum interest, minimum monthly credit, authorised or unauthorised overdrafts etc. The examples of comparators are summarized in the respective table (Table 1).

Calculators, on the other hand, are actually performing calculation of individual banking fees and as such provide usually more detailed, accurate and personalized information. However, to get personalized information, user has to provide some input data about using his account or choose between several predefined scenarios. The example of calculator is on www.finparada.cz/Bankovni-Ucty-Kalkulacka-Osobnich-Uctu.aspx.

**Table 1.** Examples of comparators of bank accounts

| URL of online service | Categorization/ basic filtering | Sorting | Advanced filtering |
|---|---|---|---|
| www.which.co.uk/money/ banking/bank-accounts | 6 groups | x | x |
| www.knowyourmoney.co. uk/current-accounts | 6 groups | 5 ways | x |
| www.lovemoney.com/ currentaccounts | 2 groups with 5 subgroups | 10 ways | x |
| www.moneysupermarket. com/current-accounts/ | 9 groups | 7 ways | Account benefits, features and types |
| www.uswitch.com/ current-accounts/ | 5 groups | 3 ways | x |
| money.gocompare.com/ currentaccounts/ | 3 groups | 5 ways | x |

## 2.3   User-Friendly Web Interfaces

In development of the proposed calculator service, we have respected web design principles related to user experience (UX for short). UX is commonly recognized in the field of human-computer interaction (HCI). UX approach is focused on how to create outstanding quality experiences rather than merely preventing usability problems [14]. User experience takes a broader view than usability, looking at the individual's entire interaction, feelings and perception [15]. Aesthetics, usability and content are three main design categories, which influence each other and they are all incorporated in overall user experience and preference [16]. There is no established theory, which would specify what exactly on websites is presented by usability, aesthetics and their intersection. There are however many studies, which investigate a connection between usability and aesthetics [e.g. 17].

Lidwell et al. [18] stated that the designs that help people perform optimally are often not the same as the designs that people find most desirable. The question is, which designs should be preferred - those which perform better or those who are liked more by their users. The answer certainly greatly depends on the type of particular website/web service and its purpose. It also depends on user behaviour; particularly we distinguish exploratory and goal-oriented online behaviour [e.g. 19]. Similarly, with web search, there are two commonly recognized types of search tasks - lookup search and exploratory search [20]. In their study, Ellonen et al. confirmed that consumers tend to visit the website in a very goal-oriented manner [21]. This trend would be even more profound in the case of online services with usually quite straightforward process. "Goal-oriented" is in the case of web user interfaces associated with greater impact on usability. Therefore, web service development should reflect web design principles, which are proved to enhance usability.

# 3  Conceptual Foundation

In this study we pursue the goal of developing online web service for specific task. This task is finding the most suitable bank account, which would fit individual's needs and requirements, lifestyle and habits. First we would like to discuss some of the possible strategies, i.e. means of getting information, which could lead the consumer to choosing the best account for him. These strategies are e.g.:

1. getting information from bank assistant
   a. personal visit at bank's office *
   b. via the phone *
2. getting information from other people, who however usually do not have the required knowledge - close related, neighbours, colleagues,...
3. getting information via the internet
   a. on the individual banks' websites *
   b. by online aggregator service, such as comparators of bank accounts or calculator of banking fees
   c. other sources - financial advisor websites, online magazines, news articles, forums, ...

\* repeated for each bank, we are interested in, followed by an analysis and conclusions of gathered information.

The outcome of all these strategies depends greatly on invested time and effort. E.g. regarding case 1, it would be difference if we ask only at one bank´s office or if we explore offer of 10 banks. The more we extend our research, the more time and effort the process consumes, as is typical for all decision-making tasks. Therefore, we suggest that the strategy via the internet by online aggregator service is by far the most efficient of presented strategies.

The importance of comparators and calculators as online services for banking fees is indisputable when consumers are looking for the best account for them. With our online service, we would like to offer the most precise and personalized results to the consumer. Because of that, we chose calculator over comparator in our research. Of course as a result, the suggested calculator may be more suitable for maximizers rather than satisficers.

The following chapters are dedicated to our own proposals of novel calculator service, beginning with information architecture, including data matrix and only quick view on the programmed logic due to space limitations. Finally we will present screenshots of user interface of actual implementation state of our proposal. As was already mentioned earlier, the calculator is being developed at our University and was already launched in Czech language (UI was translated for this study) [1].

# 4  Information Architecture

This chapter is devoted to the conceptual design and information architecture of the proposed new online service for calculating banking fees. The purpose of this service is to provide consumers with breakdown of all bank accounts which fulfil their requirements along with total sum of fees. Our first calculator implementation registers all bank accounts present on the Czech market. The following subchapters describe the process in more detail.

### 4.1    Workflow for One User

First we take a look at this online service from the user's point of view, i.e. his goal in finding the best account. User is presented with a form to fill in the necessary information (for visual design of the form see (Fig. 3)). All fields are optional with applied philosophy that the more information user fills in, the more precise and personalized would be results. Therefore it is in his best interest to provide true and complete information. There are generally three types of information asked from user:

- required services, i.e. which services does he use (or want to use)
- expected frequency of use, i.e. how often does he use (or want to use) these services – applicable only on some of the services, e.g. ATM withdrawals
- additional information – information about user or his behaviour, which could yield benefits or fee discount in some bank accounts (e.g. discounted monthly fee if user is under specified age or if he keeps sufficient credit)

After user fills in all information which he is willing to provide, he sends form data to the server by clicking a relevant button. Calculator service accepts data and performs extensive calculation over them, using in fact a matrix of user data and data about bank

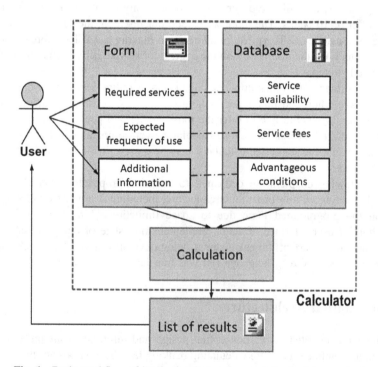

**Fig. 1.** Basic workflow of interaction between user and calculator service

accounts from its database. Types of bank accounts' data correspond with data required from user, as you can see from the following schema (Fig. 1). These are types of data saved for each bank account:

- service availability - reflects if the particular bank account offers the service
- service fee – if the service is available, contains specific sum of money, either fixed or paid periodically monthly or yearly
- advantageous conditions – discounts and benefits based on particular condition or set of conditions (and/or)

After performing the calculation, web service would provide users with list of results (for visual design see (Fig. 4)). In this list there are visually highlighted bank accounts which fulfil the requirements along with the monthly and one-time fee and other additional information. See the whole process as workflow of interactions between user and calculator service in the following figure (Fig. 1).

The process described in the previous figure was related to the individual user. This procedure takes user input, combines it with calculator data and after performing calculation presents results. In other words, for user, calculator service ends with presenting personalized results.

## 4.2    Consolidation and Post-processing of Results

Now we will combine workflows of individual users into the whole workflow of the calculator service. See the following figure (Fig. 2). Data from all users who use this online service are saved, prepared for extensive export of selected views. This export can be then used for post-processing, which includes various analyses of user behaviour and resulting user profiling regarding using bank services. This can be very useful feedback for financial institutions in understanding their clients and hopefully could lead to better designed services and price lists.

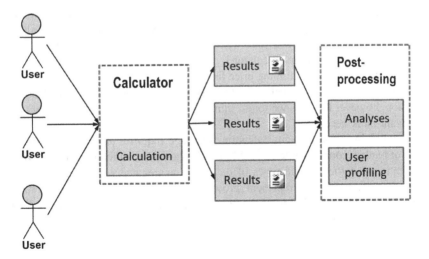

**Fig. 2.** Post-processing of calculation results from all users

The post-processing analyses and user profiling can be of various forms. In our previous research we performed a retail consumer segmentation [3], choice optimality study [4], desired price modeling [5] and recently also consumption variability. Export from the proposed calculator service is designed for easy processing and especially optimized for the syntaxes we prepared in IBM SPSS to automatize routine data refining and supportive analyses. The development on the export module is however not finished yet, so hopefully it will be the subject of our next paper.

### 4.3    Matrix of Data

As was already mentioned, types of bank accounts data correspond with data required from user. However data itself, i.e. individual items about bank accounts, correspond only roughly with individual items of user data, as is shown later in this section (Table 2). We have already established, that user data are extracted from user via the calculator form. Now, where the data about bank accounts come from? All bank institutions have their own website with different environment, i.e. design, navigation, terminology etc. and differently composed price lists. Therefore, the data cannot be downloaded and updated automatically. In the case of our calculator, there is an administrator who checks changes according to bank notices and manages data of individual bank accounts accordingly. This limitation remains to be dealt with.

Now even more important question. What data are required from user and what data are managed for every bank account? The matrix of data was constructed based on extensive analysis of offered bank accounts and user data from our previous research [3, 4]. As for data required from user, they are almost exclusively the data needed for calculation, i.e. personalized results for user. Only brief voluntary survey was added in the end of the questionnaire, which does not benefit user yet we intend to use in our future research on this topic. Types of user data needed for calculation were already discussed in Sect. 4.1 and depicted in relevant figure (Fig. 1), as well as types of data about bank accounts.

Considering bank accounts data, of course it is not possible to include all individual conditions, special offers, profitable packages and unexpected or hidden fees of all bank accounts. We needed to draw a line, whether given condition, offer, package or fee would be implemented in the calculator logic or not. Usually, if there was more than one bank with particular item in the price list, it was included in the matrix of data and consequently in the programmed logic. One bank's specialities were omitted from the calculation, however the ones we found significant were included in the commentary of the relevant bank account.

The following table presents categories of usage inquiries and corresponding categories of bank account data items (Table 2). Categories are different from the types of data mentioned earlier. While types of data were aggregated according to their programmed logic, categories represent groups divided by topic. This categorization reflects also navigational design of the proposed user interface, as you can see later in this paper in presented screenshots.

**Table 2.** Matrix of data - categories/groups of usage inquiries via form

| Categories/groups* | Number of items for user inquiries** | Number of corresponding bank account items*** |
|---|---|---|
| Communication channels and additional services | 7 | 6 |
| Account usage | 6 | 12 |
| Cards | 5 | 17 |
| Cash withdrawals | 6 | 7 |
| Payments – internet banking | 3 | 5 |
| Payments and cash withdrawals at the counter | 5 | 8 |
| Payments – telebanking | 3 | 5 |
| Payments – collection box | 3 | 5 |
| Statements and additional communication services | 4 | 5 |
| Cash withdrawals abroad | 3 | 6 |
| Foreign payments – SEPA payments | 5 | 12 |
| | 50 | 88 |

*corresponds with data about bank accounts in the service's backend.
**we omit the choice of time interval, which is defaulted to "monthly".
***we omit fields, which are used apart from user inquiries ("fixed monthly fee") or which are only informative, not used in calculation (e.g. "bank name", "account type").

You can notice from the previous table, that the numbers are not the same for each group. Where does this disparity come from? Every individual calculation requires different data for its course. Some are similar, such as the calculation for common cash withdrawals, cash withdrawals at the counter and cash withdrawals abroad. However the majority of calculations is specific for each combination of user data and data about bank accounts. Sometimes, it requires more data items on either side. E.g. regarding basic logic about cards, user data includes: the type of first card and optionally the type of second card, i.e. 2 user inputs. However the number of related bank account's data is 11. These data items include fixed fee, monthly fee and number of free cards for every card type in the system (3 types), this makes 9 fields in the database. Another two items are: fixed fee and monthly fee related to the second card, rather than to the specific card type. In this case, price lists of individual bank accounts do not usually use all of the fields, but only some of them depending on selected bank policy. Now see the following table for examples of user inquiries with answers and associated bank account data and field values.

**Table 3.** Examples of user inquiries and bank account data

| Groups of usage inquiries via calculator form | Example of user inquiry and answer | Example of related bank account data and field value |
| --- | --- | --- |
| Communication channels and additional services | Do you use telebanking? (Y/N) | Does the account offer telebanking? (Y/N) What is the fee for using it? (Int/Null) |
| Account usage | What is your minimum balance? (Int/Null) | Does the account offer fee reduction (Y/N, Int) at some level of min. balance? (Int) |
| Cards | What card type do you want as your primary card? (Select: electronic/embossed/premium) | Does the account offer electronic/embossed/premium card? (3x Y/N) With what fee? (3x Int/Null) |
| Cash withdrawals | How often do you withdraw cash from ATM? (Int, Select: monthly, quarterly,...) | What is the fee for using this bank's ATM (Int/Null) and other bank's ATM (Int/Null) |

As you can see from examples in the previous table (Table 3), there is a variety of question answer types, ranging from simple Yes/No to more complex ones. The so far implemented version of our calculator is deterministic, which means it counts with fixed number of service uses per month. Users can choose number of uses for period of time which they choose (per month, per quartal, per half-year, per year), however the application converts them into uses per month in accordance with monthly fees.

## 5   User Interface Overview

In this chapter we present user interface of the proposed calculator (Fig. 3). Fully functional calculator service is running in the Czech environment [1], however its UI was translated for the purposes of this study. After receiving data from user, the calculator service would provide this user with his personalized comparison of bank accounts, based on his inputted values. It depends on the user, whether he fills in values of his current usage or future requirements.

The displayed result is a list of the most suitable bank accounts for this particular user (Fig. 4). This list is based on performed comparison of user data and data about bank accounts such as service availability. Combination of service fees and usage pattern provided by user (i.e. number of expected uses per month) is then calculated into actual numbers. The resulting list of bank accounts is then sorted by final monthly fee for all required services. One-time fees are less frequent, they are used e.g. for issuing new card or activating some service.

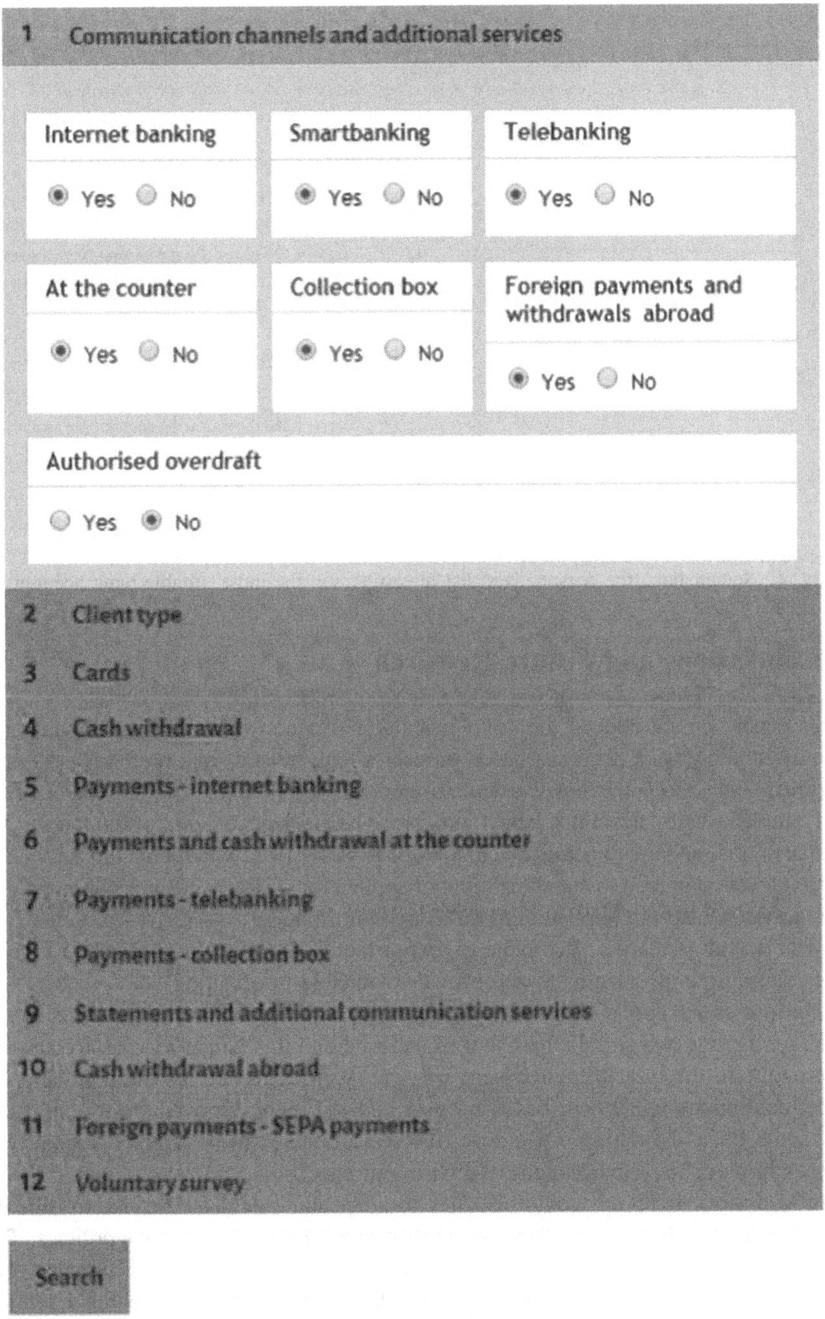

**1  Communication channels and additional services**

| Internet banking | Smartbanking | Telebanking |
|---|---|---|
| ⦿ Yes  ○ No | ⦿ Yes  ○ No | ⦿ Yes  ○ No |

| At the counter | Collection box | Foreign payments and withdrawals abroad |
|---|---|---|
| ⦿ Yes  ○ No | ⦿ Yes  ○ No | ⦿ Yes  ○ No |

**Authorised overdraft**

○ Yes  ⦿ No

**2  Client type**

**3  Cards**

**4  Cash withdrawal**

**5  Payments - internet banking**

**6  Payments and cash withdrawal at the counter**

**7  Payments - telebanking**

**8  Payments - collection box**

**9  Statements and additional communication services**

**10  Cash withdrawal abroad**

**11  Foreign payments - SEPA payments**

**12  Voluntary survey**

Search

**Fig. 3.** Screenshot - user interface of the calculator form

| Bank account | Costs [CZK] | | Comment |
|---|---|---|---|
| | Monthly | One time | |
| Moneta Genius Free & Flexi | 39 | 0 | You have fulfilled the condition (s) for a lower fee for account maintenance. |
| KB My Plus Account | 60 | 0 | There is no lower account maintenance fee for this account. **The calculation did not take into account:** Establishment of standing orders and debit authorization is free of charge for 3 months from the opening of the new account. |
| Oberbank    Žirokonto Plus | 89 | 0 | There is no lower account maintenance fee for this account. **The calculation did not take into account: The** withdrawals from ČSOB ATMs in the Czech Republic with the first Maestro payment card are free of charge. For SEPA with IBAN and type ... more |

**Fig. 4.** Screenshot - the personalized list of results, i.e. the most suitable bank accounts

## 6    Conclusions and Future Research

In this paper was introduced the novel calculator service, which offers comparison of the most suitable bank accounts based on user's requirements and preferences. In this paper was introduced the novel calculator service, which offers a comparison of the most suitable bank accounts based on user's requirements and preferences [22]. Comparison is made with actual calculation of banking fees, which puts this service on the next level compared to standard shopbot applications. However, in accordance with these services, also our service aims to reduce information asymmetry, particularly in payment accounts market. It can be expected that well-designed application considerably saves time of consumers and provides valuable information.

The presented application was under design and development since the end of 2015, i.e. there is two and the half year of work behind this online service. Release for wide public in the Czech environment was the April 2018 [1]. As the next step, we expect continuous refinement based on user and log data, retrieved from application after some time of running. Of course, the service needs to be adapted regularly to changes in particular environment (Czech in our case).

In future research, we would also like to adapt our calculator service to different environment, which requires adapting to other country regarding bank´s policies. This would involve cooperation from the respective country´s researchers in order to offer useful up-to-date service. Finally, we would like to mention our research intention, which we already began to explore, which is the next level from deterministic approach. We intend to deliver even more advanced calculator service, which would be able to reflect stochastic nature of user behaviour. This would be very significant advance from usual deterministic concept used in service design. We also may consider also a different version of the user interface for each gender. There is a significant trend of participation increase e.g. in e-shopping of women in the Czech Republic [23] where our calculator was launched.

**Acknowledgment.** This paper was written with the financial support of specific university research funds allocated to the University of Hradec Králové Faculty of Informatics and Management, the Department of Economics project no. 3/2018, order 2103.

I would like to thank Aneta Bartuskova, Ph.D. for her work on calculator´s development. I would like to thank Lucie Silhabelova and Martin Král for her help with the database and Jan Draessler, Ph.D. for his comments during the design phase.

# References

1. Zhu, H., Siegel, M., Madnick, S.: Enabling global price comparison through semantic integration of web data. Int. J. Electron. Bus. **6**(4), 319–341 (2008)
2. Bartuskova, A., Soukal, I., Draessler, J.: Calculator of banking fees (2018). http://uni.uhk.cz/kalkulator
3. Soukal, I., Draessler, J., Hedvičáková, M.: Cluster analysis of the demand side of the retail core banking services market. E M Ekonomie a Management **14**(4), 102–114 (2011)
4. Soukal, I., Draessler, D.: Price information asymmetry impact on optimal choice – RCBS market case study. In: Kocourek, A. (ed.) 2015 Proceedings of the 12th International Conference on Liberec Economic Forum, Liberec, Czech Republic, pp. 144–153. Technical University of Liberec, Liberec (2015)
5. Soukal, I., Hedvičáková, M., Draessler, J.: Probabilistic model of optimal price search on the retail core banking services market. Int. J. Math. Models Methods Appl. Sci. **6**(2), 386–393 (2012)
6. Pires, T.: Measuring the effects of search costs on equilibrium prices and profits. Int. J. Ind. Organ. (2017, in press). https://doi.org/10.1016/j.ijindorg.2017.10.007. Accessed 22 Nov 2017
7. Tang, Z., Smith, M.D., Montgomery, A.: The impact of shopbot use on prices and price dispersion: evidence from online book retailing. Int. J. Ind. Organ. **28**(6), 579–590 (2010)
8. Iyer, G., Pazgal, A.: Internet shopping agents: virtual co-location and competition. Mark. Sci. **22**(1), 85–106 (2003). https://doi.org/10.1287/mksc.22.1.85.12842
9. Haynes, M., Thompson, S.: Price, price dispersion and number of sellers at a low entry cost shopbot. Int. J. Ind. Organ. **26**(2), 459–472 (2008). https://doi.org/10.1016/j.ijindorg.2007.02.003
10. European Parliament: Directive 2014/92/EU on the comparability of fees related to payment accounts, payment account switching and access to payment accounts with basic features. (L 257/214, Official Journal of the European Union) (2014)
11. Brannon, D.C., Soltwisch, B.W.: If it has lots of bells and whistles, it must be the best: how maximizers and satisficers evaluate feature-rich versus feature-poor products. Mark. Lett. **28**(4), 651–662 (2017). https://doi.org/10.1007/s11002-017-9440-7
12. Schwatz, B.: The Paradox of Choice: Why More Is Less. HarperCollins Publishers, New York (2005)
13. Besharat, A., Ladik, D.M., Carrillat, F.A.: Are maximizers blind to the future? When today's best does not make for a better tomorrow. Mark. Lett. **25**(1), 77–91 (2014)
14. Hassenzahl, M., Tractinsky, N.: User experience - a research agenda. Behav. Inf. Technol. **25**(2), 91–97 (2006)

15. Albert, B., Tullis, T.: Measuring the User Experience: Collecting, Analyzing, and Presenting Usability Metrics, 2nd edn. Morgan Kaufmann, Burlington (2013)
16. Bartuskova, A., Krejcar, O.: Sequential model of user browsing on websites – three activities defined: scanning, interaction and reading. In: Proceedings of the 10th International Conference on Web Information Systems and Technologies, Barcelona, Spain, pp. 143–148 (2014)
17. Lee, S., Koubek, R.J.: Understanding user preferences based on usability and aesthetics before and after actual use. Interact. Comput. **22**(6), 530–543 (2010)
18. Lidwell, W., Holden, K., Butler, J.: Universal Principles of Design Revised and Updated: 125 Ways to Enhance Usability, Influence Perception, Increase Appeal, Make Better Design Decisions, and Teach through Design. Rockport Publishers, Beverly (2010)
19. Moe, W., Fader, P.: Dynamic conversion behavior at e-commerce sites. Manage. Sci. **50**(3), 326–335 (2004)
20. Trattner, C., Lin, Y.L., Parra, D., Yue, Z., Real, W., Brusilovsky, P.: Evaluating tag-based information access in image collections. In: Proceedings of the 23rd ACM Conference on Hypertext and Social Media, pp. 113–122. ACM (2012)
21. Ellonen, H.-K., Wikström, P., Johansson, A.: The role of the website in a magazine business – revisiting old truths. J. Media Bus. Stud. **12**(4), 238–249 (2015)
22. Bartuskova, A., Krejcar, O.: Evaluation framework for user preference research implemented as web application. In: Bădică, C., Nguyen, N.T., Brezovan, M. (eds.) ICCCI 2013. LNCS (LNAI), vol. 8083, pp. 537–548. Springer, Heidelberg (2013). https://doi.org/10.1007/978-3-642-40495-5_54
23. Svobodová, L., Hedvičáková, M.: Actual situation and development in online shopping in the Czech Republic, Visegrad Group and EU-28. In: Sieminski, A., Kozierkiewicz, A., Nunez, M., Ha, Q.T. (eds.) Modern Approaches for Intelligent Information and Database Systems. SCI, vol. 769, pp. 269–279. Springer, Cham (2018). https://doi.org/10.1007/978-3-319-76081-0_23

# An In-Store Mobile App for Customer Engagement: Discovering Hedonic and Utilitarian Motivations in UK Grocery Retail

Joanne Pei-Chung Wang[1(✉)] and Anabel Gutierrez[2]

[1] Digital Marketing and Analytics, Regent's University London, London, UK
S00909316@regents.ac.uk
[2] Digital Marketing and Analytics, University of Kent, Kent, UK
agutierrez@kent.ac.uk

**Abstract.** This paper investigates the hedonic and utilitarian motivations that may influence UK grocery consumers to adopt and use new features proposed for an in-store mobile app. The scope of this research is to develop a conceptual model that reflects the motivations for using an in-store mobile app to engage customers. Two pilots were conducted to explore possible attributes for hedonic and utilitarian motivations found in literature, and factor analysis was used to test their validity. A survey with the final items selected was used to collect data from a large UK grocery retailer resulting in a sample of 633 customers. The results supported that utilitarian motivations for grocery shopping include time convenience, performance expectancy and information availability. For the hedonic motivations, the attributes supported include idea motivation, personalisation, value motivation and experiential shopping. Although previous research conceptualised user control as an important utilitarian motivator, this research found that this attribute correlates similarly to both, hedonic and utilitarian motivations. Possible implications are that regardless of customers' hedonic or utilitarian preferences, it is always essential for customers to have the ability to choose and customise what data and communications they share and receive for successful in-store mobile app engagement.

**Keywords:** Mobile app · Technology adoption · Utilitarian motivation
Hedonic motivation

## 1 Introduction

According to the IGD (Institute of Grocery Distribution), the UK Grocery sector was valued at £179 billion in 2016, of which non-grocery items made up £13 billion and grocery comprised £166 billion [53]. After several years of slumping sales, it has been reported that purchasing levels have been relatively flat, increasing pressure for grocers to compete for market share [39].

There has been substantial growth in online grocery purchasing and in the UK this channel is expected to grow 68% by 2021. The UK is also leading in online grocery

© Springer Nature Switzerland AG 2019
M. Themistocleous and P. Rupino da Cunha (Eds.): EMCIS 2018, LNBIP 341, pp. 225–243, 2019.
https://doi.org/10.1007/978-3-030-11395-7_20

compared to the rest of Europe with 6.9% of UK FMCG (Fast Moving Consumer Goods) sales done online [46]. In April 2016, 48% of Brits were purchasing groceries online via supermarket website and mobile apps for delivery or store collection. Millennials (born between the early 1980s to early 2000s) seem to have a higher propensity for online shopping than other customer segments [11]. Amongst 25–34-year-olds, 23% did all their grocery shopping online, followed closely by 20% of 35–44-year-olds. In contrast, two age segments did not follow this trend. Only 9% of 45–54-year-olds and 5% of shoppers age 55+ did all their grocery shopping online [11].

However, while Mintel forecasts online grocery retailing to reach £16.7 billion in 2021, and UK grocers have invested heavily in developing apps and websites to support delivery and 'click & collect' services, online grocery shopping currently only accounts for an estimated 5% of total grocery sales [10]. About one-quarter of all UK grocery shoppers have purchased groceries online, three-quarters have not, and 24% of Brits had never bought groceries online and had no interest in doing so, rising to 38% of Brits aged 55+ [14]. There are several reasons that customers prefer shopping in-store instead of online, such as the lack of control when choosing fresh products, high delivery charges, limitations in product range or because they find that prices are lower, which might also indicate that they are shopping more at discounters [11].

Nonetheless, it cannot be ignored that smartphones have become a pervasive and integral part of people's lives with an estimated 43.1 million mobile users in the UK [21] Along these lines, if the majority of customers still prefer to purchase groceries in-store, then there are untapped opportunities to create a better shopping experience by adapting grocery mobile apps to serve UK customers where over 90% of retail happens.

## 1.1  Grocery Market Digital Ecosystem

Some retailers, particularly in the US, have designed apps with 'Store Mode', enabling customers to use their mobile in-store to view dynamic store maps, find exact product locations and follow the most efficient routes through a store to fulfil a shopping list. Adding Store Mode features to a retailer's app has been shown to drive five times more shopper engagement while increasing sales and customer loyalty. Research showed not only five times more interactions with the Store Mode app, but also that the average number of shopping list items increased 1.5 times. Those using store mode five or more times in a month are the fastest growing segment of shoppers [45].

Walmart introduced 'Store Mode' in 2012 with functionalities such as a voice-activated shopping list, a 'Scan & Go' feature that provides extensive product information, the ability to access purchase history and conduct e-commerce on the go [35]. If an item on a customer's shopping list is not available in-store, it will let them instantly order it via the app for delivery. By using geofencing technology, the store mode automatically switches on when entering the store and offers localised ads for that particular store, so customers know what is on sale on that day [33].

At the same time, brick-and-mortar supermarkets such as German discounter Aldi are expanding their digital presence, while pure-play online retailers such as Amazon are opening physical stores. Aldi's aggressive brick & mortar expansion across the UK continues apace, but Aldi also launched its first online presence in the UK with a £35 million investment [8], selling wine and non-food items for now. AmazonFresh partnered with Morrisons to offer 1-h delivery to selected postcodes in London in July 2016 [9]. Additionally, Amazon acquired organic foods supermarket Whole Foods, which has nine stores in the UK [39]. Amazon has also made global headlines with its 'just walk out technology' AmazonGo store in Seattle, WA, the beta test was initially open to employees only, and later opened to the public in January 2018 becoming the first brick-and-mortar convenience store with no checkout lines and no cashiers [18, 19].

## 1.2 Customer Loyalty Drivers

Loyalty programmes are a marketing strategy to retain and derive more revenue from customers in the future [37]. Many loyalty programs have shown success by increasing attitudinal as well as behavioural loyalty [15]. However, loyalty is driven by likeability and trust rather than reward schemes and points [11]. This means that for brands the equilibrium between implicit (quality and trust) and explicit (rewards and points) loyalty drivers needs to be achieved in order to 'incentivise the right behaviour and entice people to come back'.

Kantar WorldPanel conducted an interesting study on the drivers of customer loyalty considering the top UK grocery retail brands as perceived by shoppers across five different categories [43]:

- an enjoyable place to shop
- cares about me
- offers good value for money
- convenient
- inertia & proximity

Customer engagement has received considerable attention from researchers due to the strength businesses receive when creating a relationship with the customer [51]. Some arguments give particular importance to the fact that the concept of customer engagement extends to the definition of involvement, attachment and commitment [4]. To date, there is no agreed upon definition of customer engagement. However, Scholer and Higgins [40] define engagement as an active relationship with a brand that is established by the intensity of the customer's psychological state. The authors characterise this psychological state by the emotional connection, sustained attention, brand relevancy and commitment to a brand. Fully engaged customers account for 23% more revenue than average customers, tend to buy more, promote the brand more to others, and demonstrate more loyalty towards the company [12]. However, customer engagement is not a formula that can be applied to all companies, because each customer is different. Brands need to develop strategies to interact with their customers, building relationships with them through personalised messages and discounts, or even inspiring their loyalty and affection [41].

Marketers face a tremendous challenge in raising the public estimation of marketing. Across the UK, 42% of adults distrust brands and as high as 69% distrust online advertising [17]. Furthermore, University of Cambridge Psychometrics Centre reported in Marketing Week [11] that 71% of consumers worldwide feel that marketers use personal marketing data unethically, and 58% have been wary of engaging digitally via apps, email and social media due to concerns about misuse of personal data. Yet, the same study reported that 94% of marketers believe in the importance of using personal data for predictive analytics to engage consumers. This disparity in consumers' versus marketers' perspectives could be problematic and a better understanding of customer engagement drivers is essential.

This research aims to investigate the motivators that influence grocery customer's intention to use an in-store mobile app and to propose a conceptual model that would provide insight into customer intentions to adopt in-store mobile apps. The next section will explain the theory used to explore the different customer's motivations and the initial motivations considered for the conceptual model. Next, the research design and method are presented. The proposed conceptual model is validated in section four followed by the conclusions.

## 2   Research Model

Grocery shopping is perceived as a high-frequency and functionalistic activity [31], and this type of habitual and routine shopping activity is often considered by customers to be a chore [13]. While many factors are known to influence consumers shopping behaviours, utilitarian and hedonic motivators are considered by many researchers to be robust constructs when trying to understand customers' behavioural intentions [2, 3, 44].

Utilitarian shopping motivation reflects the consumer's desire for efficiency, rational and task-oriented efforts [1]. Consumers tend to use technological services, like mobile apps, to simplify a process, in the form of performance expectancy, information availability and time convenience [45]. Additionally, user control can positively affect the outcome and the value of the channel as consumers perceive satisfaction when having more control of the process [27].

In contrast to utilitarian values, hedonic motivators are those factors that tend to trigger consumers' emotions and feelings. While mobile apps are developed with a functional purpose, hedonic values may represent a meaningful way to stimulate the adoption intention of individuals to use mobile apps.

Given the multiple ways grocery retailers are incorporating technologies into their digital ecosystems, this research aims to investigate and test which utilitarian and hedonic motivations influence grocery customer's intention to use an in-store mobile app.

### 2.1   Utilitarian Motivations

**Time Convenience.** Convenience or time savings is defined as the efficiency of shopping found through saving time [1]. Convenience is found to be a strong motivator for consumers to shop online and make use of mobile applications [44] while engaging them in various channels of shopping [1]. Smartphones, and specifically mobile applications, have become personal shopping assistants for customers, primarily due to the convenience aspect of the technology [42].

**Performance Expectancy.** Performance expectancy is a utilitarian value defined by the degree an individual believes that the usage of a technology simplifies the process [46] In the context of mobile apps, the usage of this technology will enable users to accomplish their goal-oriented task [28, 46]. Research has shown that performance expectancy is a strong predictor of the intention of use, meaning that when performance expectancy increases individuals are more likely to continue to use the mobile app [30].

**Information Availability.** Information availability is defined as the availability to acquire information about the product, stores, promotions and other aspects [49]. Mobile applications provide efficient means for consumers to get information with few clicks. For example, mobile apps have the capability of delivering product information on a customer's demand including a product's location, nutritional value, price, offers, reviews, etc. [28].

**User Control.** The last value of utilitarian motivations considered for this research is user control, which is defined as the extent to which users can determine the content and sequence of the transaction [27]. Research has shown that consumers perceive technologies to be of higher value if they are able to have more control of the process and the technology [22] which is extremely important in order to comply with the UK General Data Protection Regulations [24].

## 2.2   Hedonic Motivations

**Idea Motivation.** Hedonic ideas motivation, refers to collecting information about new trends and products, more specifically in the context of shopping it refers to 'keeping up with trends' [2, 26]. Customers enjoy browsing to obtain information about new trends and products, while not making a particular purchase [5]. Also, studies have found that consumers who seek product information more often tend to acquire more personalised and special products, due to their continuous research for latest trends [7]. Mobile applications allow customers to easily access information and promotions about products and services, which has shown to increase the idea shopping motivation [49]. This provides pleasure and positive experience as 'a motive for the ongoing search' [2], which may lead to a final purchase.

**Personalisation.** Personalisation is conceptualised in this research in terms of media richness, the extent to which a channel provides personalised content and emotional messages [16, 29]. Due to information technology and data-mining, many retailers have adopted practices to send personalised messages to individual customers as it can be a cost-effective and practical market tool [36]. Relevant information to individual consumers has shown to improve the effectiveness of mobile commerce strategies [20, 28].

**Value Motivation.** Value motivation focuses on bargain hunting and discount seeking behaviour of customers that explained the excitement of users when looking for discounts and the enjoyment of finding value in a purchase [34, 50]. Research has shown that many consumers that find discounts feel satisfaction and accomplishment [47] Mobile applications have enabled consumers to find inexpensive shopping opportunities and coupons on-the-go while allowing them to share their findings instantaneously with other individuals [3, 50]. Value motivation increases involvement and excitement in the shopping experience, and now mobile devices have enabled individuals to fulfil this need with a few clicks of a button from anywhere [37].

**Experiential Shopping.** Experiential Shopping, also known as 'Adventure Motivation' is a hedonic value that refers to the desire an individual has for an enjoyable, exciting and entertaining shopping experience [3, 48] It has been found that in-store and mobile app usage do not provide the same stimuli, but combining both experiences may have a positive impact on consumers' behaviour [38]. Although different stimulus can be obtained throughout different channels, the usage of a mobile application for in-store shopping can stimulate sensory attributes and create enjoyment through the use of new technologies [22, 38].

### 2.3    Behavioural Intention

Behavioural intention is a well established construct defined by Fishbein and Ajzen as the likeliness of an individual to perform a particular behaviour [22]. Research has found that behavioural intention has been investigated in most studies of m-commerce and mobile applications [52], meaning that the construct is one of the most important to analyse in studies involving mobile technologies and its acceptance when exploring innovative features that may or not attract customers.

This research aims to investigate and test which utilitarian and hedonic motivations influence grocery customer's intention to use an in-store mobile app. Figure 1, illustrates the conceptualisation for utilitarian and hedonic motives to be validated in this research.

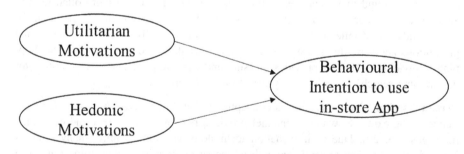

**Fig. 1.** Conceptual model

## 3    Research Design and Method

The collection of data was conducted in a structured manner using a web-questionnaire. This type of survey allows respondents to choose their answers from predetermined options for reliability and validity [32]. Surveys are typically used to test variables simultaneously and the relationship of examined factors [23]. Pilot surveys were created and sent out using Google Forms to a convenience sample in order to test the survey constructs and ensure question clarity (details will be covered later in this report). The actual final customer survey was set up using a different platform. While the pilot survey was sent primarily through social media channels, the final customer survey was sent via email to the customer panel of a large UK grocery retailer.

## 3.1 Survey Design

Two pilot tests were conducted to validate and reduce the 19 items developed from previous research to measure the conceptual model constructs using a 7-point Likert scale. Pre-testing the survey is an important step to generate valuable data [6, 23, 32]. The variations between the surveys are explained below.

**Pilot 1** - Features Focused on using Compatibility, Hedonic & Behavioural Intention *Constructs*

The first pilot test was fielded on 7 Aug 2017, including 19 items sent to a convenience sample. The purpose of the pilot was to identify problems respondents might have with specific questions, improve the quality of the survey for clarity, and narrow down the items that would be more relevant for real customers. The first pilot was sent to a broad age group and various nationalities with a majority based in the UK and US. Respondents were asked to complete the survey and optional open-ended questions were available for feedback or comments in case any difficulties were encountered [32].

An exploratory factor analysis was conducted using SAS Enterprise Guide 7.1 to test the variability and correlation of the constructs. Although the outcome of the first pilot did not support the validity and reliability of the proposed constructs, it revealed valuable insights to improve the questionnaire. The results and the comments provided by the pilot participants informed the re-design of the survey as follows.

Firstly, some items were removed, reworded and/or re-designed to ensure they closely reflected the construct they were measuring. Secondly, a case scenario format (Appendix A) was created describing the use of the proposed in-store mobile app features to ensure participants had the same scenario in mind when evaluating the hedonic and utilitarian dimensions.

Final survey constructs, item attributes and statements are defined in a Table 1 below and were used for the second Pilot.

**Pilot 2** - Scenario-based Survey Using Utilitarian, Hedonic & Behavioural Intention *Constructs*

The second pilot test was fielded on 15 Aug 2017, including ten items sent to a convenience sample. The exploratory factor analysis for this new data showed that all the hedonic questions and most of the utilitarian measures grouped together as anticipated. However, as two of the utilitarian items (UM4 and UM3) were loading high in both factors, both items were reworded to better match utilitarian definitions as conceptualised for the final survey.

**Table 1.** Final survey statements for each item attribute

| Construct | Code | Item attribute | Survey statement |
|---|---|---|---|
| Utilitarian motivations | UM1 | Time convenience | "Using this app while shopping in-store will add convenience and time savings" |
| | UM2 | Performance expectancy | "Using this app will aid and simplify my in-store shopping process" |
| | UM3 | Information availability | "Using this app while shopping in-store will make accessing relevant information available when and where I need it" |
| | UM4 | User control | "The ability to choose what notifications I want to receive, gives me control to use the app in the way that's most useful for me" |
| Hedonic motivations | HM1 | Idea motivation | "I would fancy using the app to discover 'what's new' and get meal ideas" |
| | HM2 | Personalisation | "I like that the app delivers personalised content based on my preferences and favourites…and that I can adjust these preferences" |
| | HM3 | Value motivation | "I would enjoy using the app to find good values and discounts as I navigate through the store" |
| | HM4 | Experiential shopping | "I would enjoy my shopping experience more by using the app" |
| Behavioral intention | BI1 | Behavioral intention | "If the IN-STORE mobile app was developed to assist my grocery shopping, I would prefer this way of shopping over the way I shop today" |
| | BI2 | Behavioral intention | "If these new app features were available, I would regularly use the supermarket's mobile app while shopping in-store" |

## 3.2 Data Collection and Demographics

Respondents were able to access the survey online and answer the questions themselves [23]. Self-completion surveys are known to create less biased answers because there is no social desirability [6]. The final survey was designed with a scenario-based format. Scenarios are used to loosely sketch the user experience in the environment of use, enabling companies to gain valuable user input early in the development stage without having to commit significant resources [25]. Therefore, individuals can indicate their personal opinions without prior knowledge on the topic [23].

The survey presented instructions for participants and was kept as brief as possible to prevent respondent fatigue [6]. The survey was divided into four sections: Scenarios, Participants Intention, Utilitarian and Hedonic Motivations, and sent via email to 2,600 panel members. Demographic questions were not included as this information was captured and available in the panel's member database.

Data quality is an essential measurement in research studies to determine the quality of the survey 'as it influences the validity of the conducted analyses' [23]. Typically, data quality is measured by variables like missing data and time to complete the questionnaire [23], but for the specific study, data quality will mainly focus on the quality of responses.

The study had a 29.34% response rate with a total of 763 respondents, however, when looking at the dataset, it seemed like some respondents did not take the time to differentiate their answers, and therefore we assumed that they did not read the questions and just answered them to enter the panel's prize drawing. Data was cleaned, respondents that answered the questionnaire with same numbers throughout all items were deleted from the dataset. Around 17% of respondents (130) had the same rating for all items. Thus, these were excluded from the study to achieve better data quality and the results. Conceptual validation was conducted with a sample of 633 valid responses.

Table 2 shows that the sample includes 197 male respondents (31%) and 436 females (69%). Regarding age, most respondents were in between the ages of 60 and 69 years old (26%), followed by 50 to 59-year-old (24%). The lowest number of respondents were those aged 20 to 29, which correspond to about 5% of the whole sample.

**Table 2.** Sample characteristics

|  | Frequency | Percent |
| --- | --- | --- |
| Gender | | |
| Female | 436.00 | 68.88 |
| Male | 197.00 | 31.12 |
| Age group | | |
| 20–29 | 30.00 | 4.74 |
| 30–39 | 92.00 | 14.53 |
| 40–49 | 134.00 | 21.17 |
| 50–59 | 149.00 | 23.54 |
| 60–69 | 162.00 | 25.59 |
| 70+ | 66.00 | 10.43 |

# 4   Conceptual Model Validation and Preliminary Results

The raw Cronbach coefficient alpha for hedonic motivations in the final sample is equal to 0.92 and Table 3 illustrates that all items correlation with the total score are acceptable and that none of the items deletion would improve the reliability. However, for the utilitarian motivations, one of the items (UM4) has lower correlation and its removal from the construct would increase the internal reliability to 0.93.

The final validation for the conceptual model using a sample of 633 customers from a large UK grocery retailer is presented in Tables 4 and 5. Despite that user control (UM4) was hypothesised as a utilitarian motivation that increases the value that consumers perceive from technologies when they have more control [23], these research

**Table 3.** Cronbach coefficient alpha with deleted variable

| Construct subscale | Items/deleted variable | Cronbach coefficient alpha | Raw variables correlation with total | Alpha |
|---|---|---|---|---|
| Hedonic motivations | | | | |
| HM1 | Idea motivation | 0.92 | 0.80 | 0.90 |
| HM2 | Personalisation | | 0.79 | 0.90 |
| HM3 | Value motivation | | 0.84 | 0.88 |
| HM4 | Experiential shopping | | 0.82 | 0.89 |
| Utilitarian motivations | | | | |
| UM1 | Time convenience | 0.90 | 0.83 | 0.85 |
| UM2 | Performance expectancy | | 0.84 | 0.85 |
| UM3 | Information availability | | 0.85 | 0.85 |
| UM4 | User control | | 0.61 | **0.93** |

results showed that user control was similarly correlated to both, utilitarian and hedonic motivations. Furthermore, the Cronbach test confirmed that UM4, had low correlation compared to the other items and by removing UM4 the overall reliability could be improved. Validity and reliability for user control as an attribute for utilitarian motivations was not confirmed, we argue that user control might be a fundamental feature for any mobile applications rather than a utilitarian motivation and further research is needed to validate this assumption. Hence, UM4 was removed from the utilitarian construct and factor analysis was conducted to check the validity of the loadings for the final items as illustrated in Table 4.

**Table 4.** Rotated factor pattern loading for the final conceptual model rotated factor pattern

| Items | Factor1 | Factor2 |
|---|---|---|
| Time convenience (UM1) | **0.854** | 0.079 |
| Performance expectancy (UM2) | **0.781** | 0.175 |
| Information availability (UM3) | **0.612** | 0.324 |
| Idea motivation (HM1) | 0.089 | **0.776** |
| Personalisation (HM2) | 0.158 | **0.712** |
| Value motivation (HM3) | 0.251 | **0.692** |
| Experiential shopping (HM4) | 0.291 | **0.631** |

Reliability of the three constructs presented in the proposed model is shown in Table 5, together with the composite mean.

**Table 5.** Final Cronbach's alpha score for each construct of the conceptual model

| Construct subscale | Items | Cronbach's alpha score | Mean |
|---|---|---|---|
| Utilitarian motivators | UM1, UM2, UM3 | 0.93 | 4.66 |
| Hedonic motivators | HM1, HM2, HM3, HM4 | 0.92 | 4.35 |
| Behavioural intention | BI1, BI2 | 0.93 | 3.97 |

While customers rated the utilitarian motivations higher, their final intention to adopt the new app was relatively lower than expected. Although further data analysis is needed to confirm the impact of hedonic and utilitarian motivations have on intention to adopt the new app, preliminary results showed that age has a significant effect on all constructs. For example, comparing participants who are considered Millennials (age 20–39) against those participant that belong to the Gen X or older (age 40–70+) a significant difference is observed in the t-test illustrated in Fig. 2.

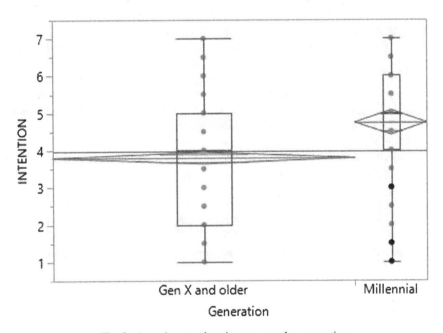

**Fig. 2.** Intention to adopt in-store app by generation

The proposed in-store mobile app features, provide an insight of the hedonic and utilitarian attributes that could make the shopping experience easier and more enjoyable. Consequently, customers may feel more engaged and valued, increasing their loyalty. Further research is needed to provide grocers with greater customer insights and profitability. For example, the millennial generation tend to be more innovative and early adopters of technology, hence the proposed app features may be adequate for targeting this audience. Although only 19% of the participants were Millennials, our results showed that participants who belong to this generation have significantly higher levels of intention to adopt the new app as illustrated in Fig. 2.

## 5 Conclusions

This paper investigates the hedonic and utilitarian motivation that may influence UK grocery consumers to adopt and use new features proposed for an in-store app. Two pilots were conducted to discover valid and reliable attributes to conceptualise the hedonic and utilitarian futures for various new features in a proposed in-store mobile app. Having an engaging and indispensable in-store mobile app can be the key to success, and the validated proposed conceptual model would enable grocers to investigate its impact further.

The final conceptual model using a sample of 633 customers from a large UK grocery retailer provided a valid model that potentially would deliver insight into customer intentions to adopt an in-store mobile app. This research scope is limited to the validation of the conceptual model and further research will be conducted to identify the level of influence that hedonic and utilitarian motivators have in adopting the in-store mobile app proposed. Additionally, different demographics should be tested to determine further relevant segments for which this motivator might vary. As an example, preliminary results indicated that Millennials might be the right target audience for the new app that could enable the grocer to collect data for using a combination of creative approaches and customer analytics.

A random sample from a large UK grocery retailer's customer panel was used for this research, however, some limitations must be noted. For example, the results may be more representative of that specific retailer and cannot be generalised outside the UK context as the data was collected only from participants across the UK. Another limitation is that people on the panel were incentivised with a chance of winning a prize when they participated in the survey which may have influenced their responses, and finally, only 19% of the panel participants belong to the millennial generation.

**Acknowledgements.** We would like to acknowledge the support of SAS UK and the contributions of Patricia Barzotti and Charlotte Nielsen from Regent's University London, MSc Digital Marketing & Analytics.

# A Appendix: Scenario-Based Survey

Introduction:

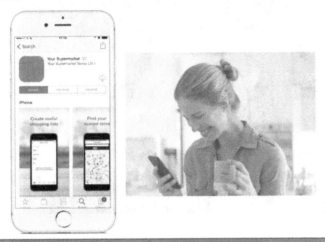

Supermarket mobile apps have many features to facilitate home grocery delivery and store collection, but few offer features for shopping IN-STORE. In this scenario, please IMAGINE you have downloaded your supermarket's app onto your mobile phone. App features have been upgraded to enhance the IN-STORE experience. Suppose you have set your preferences, so the app is displaying the functionalities and notifications you selected. (For these scenarios, we are showing numerous features, but realise that actual customers may not want to use all the options described. Customers would be able to turn preferences on or off, adjust what they want and how often.)

Shopping Lists:

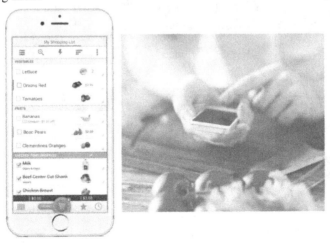

Now imagine you are at home, planning to go to your supermarket for groceries. On your smartphone, you've used your supermarket's mobile app to create a shopping list. You review your list and add a few more items before heading to the store.

Store Map for Your Shopping List:

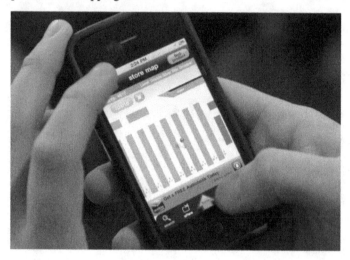

You arrive at your supermarket and receive a message on your mobile asking: "Would you like help locating the items on your shopping list?" You agree, so the app shows you a map of the store with the location of each item on your list, e.g. "Free Range Eggs are on aisle 3."

Meal Ideas with Recipes on the App:

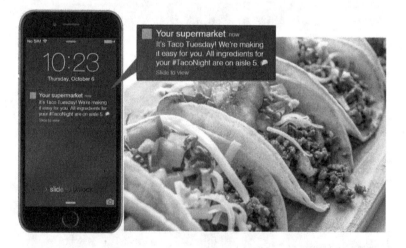

You haven't decided what to make for dinner tonight. Not a problem. You check your app for MEAL DEALS (with recipes & ingredients lists) which are based on your FAVOURITES. Or, you can select in your preferences to automatically receive MEAL IDEAS as a message when you are IN-STORE, e.g. "It's Taco Tuesday! All ingredients for tacos are on aisle 2."

What's Hot:

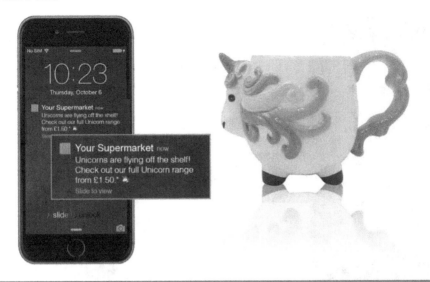

Nearing aisle 11, you receive news about WHAT'S HOT based on your notification preferences, e.g. "Unicorns are flying off the shelf! Check out our full Unicorn range from £1.50."

Your Daily Deal:

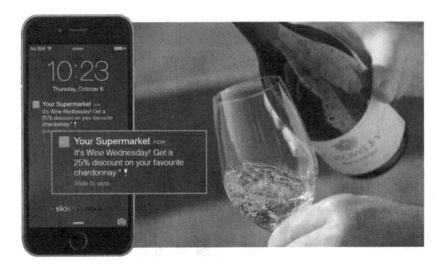

You check for your DAILY DEAL, which is based on our PREFERENCES and PREVIOUS PURCHASES. Or you can choose in your preferences to automatically receive your DAILY DEAL as a message when you are IN-STORE, e.g. "It's Wine Wednesday! Get a 25% discount on your favourite chardonnay."

## In-Store Treats:

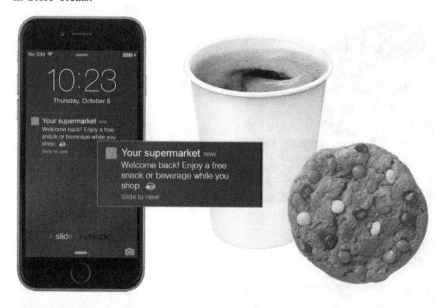

You buy groceries at this supermarket regularly, so every now and then you are rewarded with IN-STORE TREATS. Today your message invites you to the store's café to "come enjoy a free snack or beverage while you shop."

## Contactless Pay with Cashback Rewards:

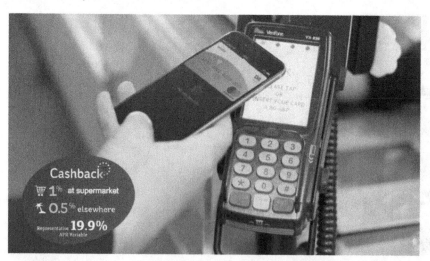

You've finished your shopping and are heading to the till to pay. Imagine you have the supermarket's Cashback Credit Card that offers 1% back on all purchases at this chain, plus 0.5% cashback on purchases from other retailers, and no annual fee. This card is on your mobile app, so you simply pay by tapping your smartphone on the card reader at checkout. It's so safe, quick and easy! The app instantly shows your receipt and how much cash you've earned back.

# References

1. Anderson, E., Simester, D.: Reviews without a purchase: low ratings, loyal customers, and deception. J. Mark. Res. **51**(3), 249–269 (2014)
2. Arnold, M., Reynolds, K.: Hedonic shopping motivations. J. Retail. **79**(2), 77–95 (2003)
3. Babin, B., Darden, W., Griffin, M.: Work and/or fun: measuring hedonic and utilitarian shopping value. J. Consum. Res. **20**(4), 644 (1994)
4. Belaid, S., Behi, A.: The role of attachment in building consumer-brand relationships: an empirical investigation in the utilitarian consumption context. J. Prod. Brand Manag. **20**(1), 37–47 (2011)
5. Bloch, P., Ridgway, N., Sherrell, D.: Extending the concept of shopping: an investigation of browsing activity. J. Acad. Mark. Sci. **17**(1), 13–21 (1989)
6. Bryman, A., Bell, E.: Business Research Methods. Oxford University Press, Cambridge (2011)
7. Burke, R.: Do you see what I see? The future of virtual shopping. J. Acad. Mark. Sci. **25**(4), 352–360 (1997)
8. Butler, S.: Amazon starts UK fresh food delivery. https://www.theguardian.com/technology/2016/jun/09/amazon-starts-uk-fresh-food-delivery
9. Butler, S.: Morrisons expands Amazon deal offering delivery in an hour. https://www.theguardian.com/business/2016/nov/16/morrisons-expands-amazon-deal-offering-delivery-in-an-hour
10. Carroll, N.: Supermarkets - UK - November 2016 - Market Research Report. http://academic.mintel.com/display/748858/
11. Chahal, M.: Are loyalty schemes broken? https://www.marketingweek.com/2016/07/13/are-loyalty-schemes-broken/
12. Clarabridge: Customer Engagement—Why is Customer Engagement important? http://www.clarabridge.com/customer-engagement/
13. Collins, A., Kavanagh, E., Cronin, J., George, R.: Money, mavens, time, and price search: modelling the joint creation of utilitarian and hedonic value in grocery shopping. J. Mark. Manag. **30**, 719–746 (2014). http://www.tandfonline.com/doi/abs/10.1080/0267257X.2013.839572
14. Criteo: UK FMCG Trend Report: Taking Stock of the Future of Grocery. http://www.criteo.com/insights/uk-fmcg-trend-report-taking-stock-of-the-future-of-grocery/
15. Daams, P., Gelderman, K., Schijns, J.: The impact of loyalty programmes in a B-to-B context: results of an experimental design. J. Target. Meas. Anal. Mark. **16**(4), 274–284 (2008)
16. Daft, R., Lengel, R.: Organizational information requirements, media richness and structural design. Manag. Sci. **32**(5), 554–571 (1986)
17. Davies, J.: The global state of consumer trust in advertising in 5 charts. https://digiday.com/marketing/global-state-consumer-trust-advertising-5-charts/
18. Del Rey, J.: Amazon's store of the future is delayed. Insert 'Told ya so' from sceptical retail execs. https://www.recode.net/2017/3/27/15072084/amazons-go-future-store-delayed-opening
19. Del Rey, J.: Amazon Go, a high-tech version of a 7-Eleven, will finally open on Monday - with no checkout lines and no cashiers. https://www.recode.net/2018/1/21/16914188/amazon-go-grocery-convenience-store-opening-seattle-dilip-kumar
20. Durlacher Research: Internet Portals. Durlacher Research, London (2000)
21. eMarketer.com: Mobile Trends That Will Reshape the UK in 2017 https://www.emarketer.com/Article/Mobile-Trends-That-Will-Reshape-UK-2017/1014901

22. Fishbein, M., Ajzen, I.: Beliefs, Attitude, Intention and Behavior: An introduction to Theory and Research. Addison-Wesley, Reading (1975)
23. Fröhlke, M., Pettersson, L.: What factors influence a consumer's intention to use a mobile device in the grocery shopping process? A quantitative study of Swedish grocery shoppers. Lund University Publications. http://lup.lub.lu.se/luur/download?func=downloadFile&rec ordOId=7439512&fileOId=7439516
24. ICO: Guide to the General Data Protection Regulation (GDPR). https://ico.org.uk/for-organisations/guide-to-the-general-data-protection-regulation-gdpr
25. Jordan, M., Geiselhart, E.: Scenario boards can be used to improve validation of early product and service concepts. http://94westbound.com/. Available from: http://94westbound.com/wp-content/uploads/2013/01/Scenario-Boards-article.pdf
26. Kim, H.W., Chan, H.C., Gupta, S.: Value-based adoption of mobile internet: an empirical investigation. Decis. Support Syst. **43**(1), 111–126 (2007)
27. Kleijnen, M., Lee, N., Wetzels, M.: An exploration of consumer resistance to innovation and its antecedents. J. Econ. Psychol. **30**(3), 344–357 (2009)
28. Lee, S., Kim, K.J., Sundar, S.S.: Customization in location-based advertising: effects of tailoring source, locational congruity, and product involvement on ad attitudes. Comput. Hum. Behav. **51**(Part A), 336–343 (2015). https://doi.org/10.1016/j.chb.2015.04.049
29. Li, M., Dong, Z., Chen, X.: Factors influencing consumption experience of mobile commerce. Internet Res. **22**(2), 120–141 (2012)
30. Kang, J.-Y.M., Johnson, K.K.P., Wu, J.: Consumer style inventory and intent to social shop online for apparel using social networking sites. J. Fashion Mark. Manag.: Int. J. **18**(3), 301–320 (2014)
31. Maher, J., Marks, L., Grimm, P.: Overload, pressure, and convenience: testing a conceptual model of factors influencing women's attitudes toward, and use of, shopping channels. https://www.acrwebsite.org/search/view-conference-proceedings.aspx?Id=8091
32. Malhotra, N.K.: Marketing Research: An Applied Orientation, 6th edn. Pearson Education, Upper Saddle River (2010)
33. Marvin, R.: 5 Ways @WalmartLabs is Revolutionizing Mobile Retail. http://uk.pcmag.com/feature/72345/5-ways-walmartlabs-is-revolutionizing-mobile-retail
34. McGuire, W.: Psychological motives and communication gratification. In: Blumler, J.F., Katz, J. (eds.) The Uses of Mass Communications: Current Perspectives on Gratification Research, pp. 167–196. Sage, Beverly Hills (1974)
35. McNamee, B.: The Resolute Digital Retail Mobile Readiness Report. https://doc-14-2g-apps-viewer.googleusercontent.com/viewer/secure/pdf/dno3b0og2iq9kv91ojahvq2499k7b 8tc/2a4gb52epu5ihp4d4k7brepecrc6ectj/1504872525000/gmail/06221871698039594192/ ACFrOgC2PgmcICc5UEEhvREJu_FBQQShPg3xoL0RCIHTl_O9Ym2vM0khM6g419_cU wRfQQrKQw0dJUVJNubn–6bpiMlvzE6bkFLQ5Uzfh4GzoxryhaUJAdlbkpqzFo=?print=tr ue&nonce=lgla3r59c7e3e&user=06221871698039594192&hash=mivulqcqlhhm5gmkd3els ok2aasg5915
36. Morey, T., Forbath, T., Schoop, A.: Customer data: designing for transparency and trust. Harvard Bus. Rev. **93**, 96–105 (2015). https://hbr.org/2015/05/customer-data-designing-for-transparency-and-trust
37. Noone, B., Mount, D.: The effect of price on return intentions: do satisfaction and reward programme membership matter? J. Revenue Pricing Manag. **7**(4), 357–369 (2008)
38. Ono, A., Nakamura, A., Okuno, A., Sumikawa, M.: Consumer motivations in browsing online stores with mobile devices. Int. J. Electron. Commer. **16**(4), 153–178 (2012)
39. Rigby, C.: Amazon gains UK stores with the acquisition of Whole Foods Market – Internet Retailing. http://internetretailing.net/2017/06/amazon-gains-uk-stores-acquisition-whole-foods-market/

40. Scholer, A.A., Higgins, E.T.: Exploring the complexities of value creation: the role of engagement strength. J. Consum. Psychol. **19**(2), 137–143 (2009)
41. Selligent: ASDA Case Study: location targeting and personalisation in retail. http://www.selligent.com/customers/retail/asda
42. Siwicki, B.: Future success in stores depends on nimble use of mobile tech. http://www.thedrum.com/opinion/2015/05/27/future-success-stores-depends-nimble-use-mobile-tech
43. TCC.: UK Shopper Loyalty Study. https://www.tccglobal.com/blog/article/uk-shopper-loyalty-study/
44. To, P., Liao, C., Lin, T.: Shopping motivations on internet: a study based on utilitarian and hedonic value. Technovation **27**(12), 774–787 (2007)
45. Tode, C.: Store mode significantly increases retail app engagement levels: report—Retail Dive. http://www.retaildive.com/ex/mobilecommercedaily/store-mode-significantly-increases-retail-app-engagement-levels-report
46. Venkatesh, V., Thong, J., Xu, X.: Consumer acceptance and use of information technology: extending the unified theory of acceptance and use of technology. MIS Q. **36**(1), 157–178 (2012)
47. Wagner, T.: Shopping motivation revised: a means-end chain analytical perspective. Int. J. Retail Distrib. Manag. **35**(7), 569–582 (2007)
48. Webster, J., Trevino, L., Ryan, L.: The dimensionality and correlates of flow in human computer interactions. Comput. Hum. Behav. **9**(4), 411–426 (1993)
49. Wolfinbarger, M., Gilly, M.: Shopping online for freedom, control, and fun. Calif. Manag. Rev. **43**(2), 34–55 (2001)
50. Yang, K.: Consumer technology traits in determining mobile shopping adoption: an application of the extended theory of planned behaviour. J. Retail. Consum. Serv. **19**, 484–491 (2012)
51. Zainol, Z., Yasin, N.M., Omar, N.A., Hashim, N.M., Osman, J.: The effect of customer-brand relationship investments on customer engagement: an imperative for sustained competitiveness. J. Pengur. **44**, 117–127 (2015)
52. Zhang, L., Zhu, J., Liu, Q.: A meta-analysis of mobile commerce adoption and the moderating effect of culture. Comput. Hum. Behav. **28**, 1902–1911 (2012). http://ejournals.ukm.my/pengurusan/article/viewFile/11145/3700

# Information Quality of Web Services: Payment Account Online Comparison Tools Survey in the Czech Republic and Slovakia

Ivan Soukal[(⊠)]

Department of Economics, Faculty of Informatics and Management,
University of Hradec Kralove,
Rokitanskeho 62, 500 03 Hradec Kralove, Czech Republic
ivan.soukal@uhk.cz

**Abstract.** The paper is focused on the comparison and calculation of retail payment accounts. The latest development of digital services within the frame of a FinTech leaves out the product comparison so far and therefore a consumer has to rely on these online tools. Six comparison tools were found and analyzed in two selected countries. The information quality test was performed based on the EU methodology regarding accuracy and full price, relevance, language and concision, detail, uniformity, comparability, and verifiability. The user test profile is a retail mainstream client with e-banking preference. All comparison tools but one failed in the information quality test. Some of them provided a correct result for only 33% of compared offers. Most of the misguiding and incorrect results came from a miscalculation of specific conditional sales issues and ATM withdrawal from other bank's network service. Only one comparison tool passed with the share of correct and plausible results above 90%. Unsatisfactory results can be explained by the incompleteness of CTs, not being up-to-date issues and by a specific pricing policy different from e.g. United Kingdom or Germany. The last part suggests possible ways how to improve current unsatisfactory situation by creating a test framework that would complement the Directive 2014/92/EU.

**Keywords:** Shopbot · Online comparison tool · Information quality
Payment account · Price calculation · Relevance · Language · Detail
Uniformity · Comparability · Verifiability

## 1 Introduction

Digitalization and digital services are paid great attention concerning a banking industry. The latest trend of FinTech [5–7] brought new third parties, new challenges and new services that were 10 years ago unimaginable such as multiple account direct access home budget management. Nevertheless, only very little attention is paid to the services for a product selection phase that consists of a market overview and decision making, i.e. the choice of the service provider itself. There are web services that are supposed to help a future user to pick the right one for him or her (instead of a "shopping tour" or the need to contact an advisor). The question of this paper is whether such application are providing helpful information or not.

© Springer Nature Switzerland AG 2019
M. Themistocleous and P. Rupino da Cunha (Eds.): EMCIS 2018, LNBIP 341, pp. 244–257, 2019.
https://doi.org/10.1007/978-3-030-11395-7_21

This paper is focused on online price comparison tools (thereinafter as CT or CTs in plural). Such applications provide a consumer the ability to compare and contrast products based on a variety of criteria or utilizing at least one criteria filter – price. One of the most frequent areas for CTs usage is a sector of financial services. The scope of this paper is CTs for retail core banking services (thereinafter as RCBS). RCBS term relates to basic day-to-day needs that are common to all payment accounts (thereinafter as PA) in the EU. PAs prices in the Czech Republic and Slovakia can consist of many small fees for individual services and many small conditional sales. The latest EU-wide study [2] finds that banking fees are one of the main reasons for consumer complaints, particularly in terms of a lack of transparency that impedes consumers from making well-informed choices, the comparability of fees and pricing. Therefore, any user can greatly benefit from CT deployment because investing his/her time in individual price search and calculation would be highly time-consuming and tedious process. Within the scope of this paper are online and free of charge RCBS CTs focused on the banks' PAs offer in two countries - the Czech Republic and Slovakia.

Both academicians, as well as legislative bodies, admit and acknowledge an impact of comparison tool applications. From the academic point of view shopbots have a positive impact on both price level as well as price dispersion, see e.g. [9, 17]. Another study [8] focused on pricing behavior by sellers at a price comparison site confirmed a strong negative relationship between the number of sellers monitored by comparison site and price. EU performed a survey (11 countries involved) that confirmed the influence of CTs. 78% of consumer groups have a normal or good perception concerning the CTs and 35% of comparison tool users answered that the use of a comparison tool usually resulted in a purchase [4].

Such influence creates high demands on information quality. Its strong impact creates a situation when incorrect or misguiding comparison may easily influence user's behavior in an undesirable manner. Therefore, price accuracy of offers and a guarantee of impartiality were considered to be the areas in most need of concern by all stakeholders [3]. Also, any precise comparison can be misunderstood if a comparison result or GUI of an input form is not organized in a user-friendly manner. This includes also incorporating features enabling consumers to extract the information that is most relevant to their individual needs. It may seem inferior compared to the quality of information issue. However, as Kim and Ha [10] show that users have difficulty in browsing such sites because of the amount of information gathered and the uncertainty surrounding web environments.

## 2 Methodology

The main goal is to assess a quality of information and basic elements enhancing the consumer experience regarding RCBS CTs available in the Czech Republic and Slovakia. Surveyed CTs are narrow provided service in the sense that they only allow price comparing of a single product type of which consumers are already aware of. For such applications was suitable methodology presented on the European Consumer Summit [4]. It is based on the previous survey in 11 EU countries and recommendations of consumer protection intuitions, regulators, business representatives, and EU representatives, see more in [3]. The main focus is on core principles which are consisted of quality of information, transparency and impartiality of comparison, compliance, and redress criterion. Additionally, it defines experience enhancers as user-friendliness and comprehensiveness. This survey is focused on the first core principle – the quality of information. Quality of information was assessed through:

1. relevance and clarity:
   a. relevance: information provided by CT should be relevant for comparing offers from a consumer perspective.
   b. language and concision: CT input/output form should be written in simple language, avoiding complex legal and technical terms. CT should not go beyond the level of detail necessary to enable consumers to make a meaningful comparison.
   c. detail: CT give the possibility to consumers to access more detailed information if they so wish, by applying where appropriate a layered information structure.
2. comparability:
   a. uniformity: CT should provide the same set of information, in uniform manner.
   b. comparability: CT should separate or distinguishing services which are not identical or mentioning the differences.
3. verifiability: CTs should enable consumers to easily verify the information, by indicating the contact information of the seller.
4. accuracy and full price: CT provide comparison exactly to the offer as it is made available by the seller and with the final product price.

All above quality criteria were assessed dichotomically with one exception – accuracy and full price. Price calculation is rather more complex concerning RCBS offer than e.g. flat TV or perfume offer. Regular input form consists of much more parameter, see e.g. [16] and the rules in a calculation are much more complex as well. Therefore, it was chosen to use a scale. Price calculation assessment scale:

1. correct: final price is exactly accordingly a bank's tariff, i.e. it matches verification calculation result,
2. plausible: it is very likely that final price would be as CT calculated. This result corresponds to the situation of conditional sale that is not included in the CT's calculation but it is easy to achieve. Therefore, it is very likely that consumer would manage to meet it.
3. misguiding: it may be possible that final price would be as CT calculated. This result corresponds to the situation of conditional sale that is not included in the CT's calculation and it is hard to achieve.
4. incorrect: final price calculation does not correspond a bank's tariff or it is impossible to clearly state what conditional sale(s) caused a price deviation.

The scale allows assessing the result in a much better resolution which is necessary because the final price in the Czech Republic and also in Slovakia usually depends on a larger variety of conditional sales. CTs are not able to reflect all possible conditional sales and those which are reflected may not be taken into account correctly. There-fore, such conditions had to be individually assessed and divided into two groups – easy to achieve and hard to achieve. Example of the first one is already mentioned – a low amount of payment or balance below the monthly average wage (886 € in Slovakia, 1068 € in the Czech Republic), turnover below 50% of the average wage and ATM withdrawal over 10% of the average wage. Some banks in Slovakia regards the payment card usage. Regarding this feature, there were left default settings of usage frequencies as it is in a CT. This caused that for the same PA different CTS displayed different price. The next issue is that some tariffs are almost atomized charging each service separately and moreover it differs accordingly the communication channel. The price verification was performed by own calculation based on the banks' tariffs including described assessment of the conditional sales.

The test profile was based on typical consumer patterns of RCBS usage [14] and updated accordingly RCBS offer change in recent years. The test profiles resulted in exclusive electronic banking user as a mainstream profile, see Table 1 below. All features and services usage are frequencies per month.

**Table 1.** Test user profile – retail mainstream client with e-banking preference (per month features)

| Demanded services and main features | |
| --- | --- |
| Minimal turnover | 608 € |
| Minimal balance | 458 € |
| Incoming payment | 3 |
| Direct payment; internet or smart baking | 5 |
| Standing order; internet or smart baking | 3 |
| Direct debit; internet or smart baking | 1 |
| Domestic ATM withdrawal; own bank's network | 3 |
| Domestic ATM withdrawal; another bank's network | 1 |
| Statements | Electronic |

The comparison tools behavioral experiment [4] showed that likelihood of being chosen is practically zero if an offer is listed on the fifteenth place or further. Therefore, CTs calculation was verified only for the first fifteen PAs listed on.

## 3   Results

The survey was performed in the first quartile of 2018. Our research identified three RCBS CTs in each country that met the criteria of (Table 2):

1. Czech Republic:
   a. Měšec Osobní účty – srovnání; thereinafter as Mesec; URL: https://www.mesec. cz/produkty/osobni-ucty/,
   b. Finparáda kalkulačka osobních účtů, thereinafter as Finparada; URL: http:// www.finparada.cz/Bankovni-Ucty-Kalkulacka-Osobnich-Uctu.aspx,
   c. Kalkulátor bankovních poplatků*; thereinafter as KBP; URL: https://www. bankovnipoplatky.com/kalkulator.html,

2. Slovakia:
   a. Finančná Hitparáda Běžné účty; thereinafter as Finhit; URL: https://www.
      financnahitparada.sk/bezne-ucty,
   b. Finančný kompas Účet – porovnanie; thereinafter as Finkomp; URL: https://
      www.financnykompas.sk/ucet,
   c. Plať menej – běžné účty, thereinafter as Menej; URL: http://www.menej.sk/
      bezne-ucty/.


*this CT was 2 months after the survey replaced by a different application. The
results do not concern this new CT.

## 3.1    Non-price Criteria Assessment

At first, there are presented results of non-calculation criteria. The most complex
criterion results (price calculation) are presented in the Tables 3, 4 and 5.

**Table 2.** CTs assessment of non-price criteria assessment

|                          | Mesec | Finpar | KPB | Finhit | Finkom | Menej |
|--------------------------|-------|--------|-----|--------|--------|-------|
| Relevance                | No    | Yes    | No  | Yes    | Yes    | Yes   |
| Language and concision   | No    | Yes    | Yes | Yes    | Yes    | Yes   |
| Detail                   | Yes   | Yes    | No  | Yes    | Yes    | Yes   |
| Uniformity               | Yes   | Yes    | Yes | Yes    | Yes    | Yes   |
| Comparability            | No    | Yes    | Yes | No     | No     | No    |
| Verifiability            | Yes   | Yes    | No  | No     | No     | Yes   |

The relevance criterion (offer available to the retail mainstream user) was not met
by two CTs. Mesec included offers of institutions that are not present in all regions of
the country. Moreover, some of them are in the capital only and/or are focused on
affluent clients only (J&T bank, PPF bank). These offers are not relevant for the
mainstream retail client. KPB displayed additional information next to some PAs
brand. This information was usually: "turnover condition met" or "balance condition
met". The reason why the relevance criterion was not met is that these accounts (2 in
total) were displayed in spite of the fact that required balance or turnover was not met
by the test profile set in the input form. The rest of the CTs showed the adequate scope
and relevant offers to the retail mainstream user.

The language-concision criterion was not me by just one CT. CT should not to go
beyond the level of detail necessary to enable meaningful comparison but also it should
not go below that level. Mesec CT uses a different approach to comparison which offers
maintenance fee as a default comparison and then two additional criteria. Although it
may be beneficial for specified search query or satisficer [12] user, who wants just some
criterion to be met and does not want to go through complete comparison and optimize

the search. However, it is not concise for a general comparison because a user has to add at least three results up in order to obtain complete information.

The detail criterion was not met by BKN CT. BKN offers detail button next to some accounts but the information is too brief and detailed overview of the pricelist was not present at all. All other CTs provides "detail" button next to each account that opens a page with tariff details including conditional sales. Finhit, Finkom and Mesec provide an icon which displays on hover conditional sales details reducing interaction costs. Three mentioned CTs also provide a detailed ad-hoc comparison by services.

The uniformity criterion was met by all surveyed CTs. All offers were displayed in the same manner without any text highlighting or extra icons. The only factor that partially disrupts the uniformity of the result page is present at the Finhit result page. The first two items under the comparison table's heading are not PAs but consumer credit ads displayed in very similar graphics that is used for PAs comparison.

The comparability criterion showed the first larger issue in comparison. Only two CTs separate or distinguishing services which are not identical or mentioning the differences. This ability was additionally confirmed by the test of at the branch over a counter service. Four CTs displayed PAs that does not offer an option of over a counter service without any sort of separation. It is true that Mesec shows a disclaimer that some services are not provided by all PAs which may distort a result. Nevertheless, this disclaimer is not visible until a user scrolls down the bottom of the page which leaves great space for overlooking it. Finpar does not display products that do not meet all the demanded services at all. KNB displays a secondary comparison results with a notice that accounts are compared by price only and so with no regard to the range of demanded services distinguishing it from the valid offers.

The verifiability criterion was met by Mesec, Finpar and Menej CTs. All of them offered a direct link to the product page or at least the page of offering bank. Although KBP offers this as well, it was not functional for all offers. Links to four offers' providers were not valid anymore (404 error page). The rest of the CTs display only the logo and the title of a provider and users have to search the product page themselves.

## 3.2   Price Criteria Assessment

The next tables present the results concerning the accuracy and price calculation. Each table contains the result for two CTs. The first column with figures, labeled as "CT", is consisted of final prices in € which were calculated by a CT for each PA. The second column with figures, labeled as "Dev", is consisted of the difference between the price calculated accordingly the bank's tariff and the price calculated by a CT. Therefore, an accurate and full price has the "Dev" value zero. There is one rare case.

There are mostly positive deviations but Finpar showed one deviation below zero. This means that the CT calculated a higher price that user would pay in reality.

Mesec comparison includes only 11 banks' PAs because the range of the CT is wider than of other surveyed CTs and listed among results credit unions as well. The rest of CTs got 15 bank PAs in the comparison. The accuracy share was 33% (3 PAs were correct results). There were four incorrect and three misguiding results. 2 cases of ATM withdrawal from other bank's network charge omission (Air Bank, Komerční banka).

**Table 3.** Price calculation assessment for Mesec and Finpar CTs (amounts in €)

| Mesec | | | | Finpar | | | |
|-------|-----------|-----|------|-------|-----------|-----|------|
| Bank | Offered PA | CT | Dev | Bank | Offered PA | CT | Dev |
| mBank | mKonto | 0 | 0 | Equa bank | Běžný účet | 0 | 0 |
| Equa bank | Běžný účet | 0 | 0 | mBank | mKonto | 0 | 0 |
| Air Bank | Malý tarif | 0 | 1.0 | Raiffeisenbank | eKonto Smart | 0 | 0 |
| Komerční banka | Můj účet | 0 | 3.6 | Unicredit bank | U konto | 0 | 0 |
| J&T banka | Běžný účet | 0 | 1.2 | Creditas | běžný účet | 0 | 0 |
| Česká spořitelna | Premier konto | 0 | 40.8 | Air Bank | Malý tarif | 0.7 | 03 |
| Expobank | VIP konto | 0 | 21.6 | Moneta | Tom účet | 0.8 | 0 |
| Creditas | Běžný účet | 0 | 0 | Fio banka | Osobní účet | 1.2 | −1.2 |
| J&T banka | Běžný účet premium | 0 | 40.4 | Sberbank | Fér Aktiv | 1.5 | 0 |
| PPF banka | Běžný účet | 0 | 3.0 | Komerční banka | Můj účet Plus | 1.5 | 0 |
| Moneta | Free & Flexi | 0 | 0 | ČSOB | Plus Konto | 1.6 | 0 |
| Wüstenrot bank | Běžný účet "A" | 0 | 0 | Era banka | Poštovní účet | 1.6 | 0 |
| Československé úvěrní družstvo | | Non-bank | | Moneta | Free & Flexi | 1.9 | 0 |
| Moravský peněžní ústav | | Non-bank | | Komerční banka | Můj účet | 3.5 | 0 |
| Artesa | | Non-bank | | Česká spořitelna | Účet s MZF | 3.5 | 0 |

Moneta calculation omitted to include a card maintenance fee and the PPF Bank calculation did not take into account that the bank distinguishes and charges outgoing payments to other banks. The rest of the non-accurate results were misguiding ones. The deviation was caused by assumption that user meets criteria usually connected with very high account balance or amounts of investments in the bank (offers of J&T banka, Česká spořitelna, Expobank). These features were not a part of the input form. 3 cases were account offered by non-bank institution (credit unions) which are beyond the scope of the paper.

Finpar was accurate in 87% of cases (13 PAs). 1 result was incorrect and 1 was plausible. The first case contained a mistake in fee for ATM withdrawal from other bank's network (Air Bank). The plausible result (Fio banka) regards the ATM withdrawal from another bank's network. There is a specific conditional sale available: cardholder gets a free ATM withdrawal from other bank's network per every 160 € spent via payment card at terminals or payment gateways during one calendar month. The result is plausible because a general possibility of obtaining one conditional sale is high.

KBP CT was accurate in 27% cases (4 PAs). Five results were incorrect and six were misguiding. Incorrect results are mostly connected to an ATM withdrawal from other bank's network issue (ČSOB, Era Bank, Moneta, Air Bank). It was not included in the calculation or it was incorrectly considered as own bank's ATM withdrawal. The last incorrect calculation relates to an omission of outgoing payments charges (Expobank). 6 misguiding results are connected to the same issue that was mentioned in the relevance assessment. There was a notice that the price is calculated with an

**Table 4.** Price calculation assessment for KBP and Finhit CTs (amounts in €)

| KBP | | | | Finhit | | | |
|---|---|---|---|---|---|---|---|
| Bank | Offered PA | CT | Dev | Bank | Offered PA | CT | Dev |
| Equa bank | Běžný účet | 0 | 0 | Unicredit bank | U konto | 0 | 0 |
| Expobank | Global | 0 | 11.7 | Unicredit bank | U konto Tandem | 0 | 0 |
| mBank | mKonto | 0 | 1.1 | Fio banka | Osobný účet | 0 | 3.6 |
| Moneta | Genius Gold | 0 | 18.4 | mBank | mKonto | 0 | 0 |
| Sberbank | Fér Mini | 0 | 5.4 | Oberbank | Účet Klasik | 2.0 | 3.7 |
| Sberbank | Fér Optimal | 0 | 7.8 | BKS bank | Premium konto | 3.5 | 0 |
| Unicredit bank | U konto | 0 | 11.7 | Prima Banka | Osobný účet | 3.9 | 2.0 |
| Expobank | Active | 0.1 | 5.7 | Raiffeisenbank | Účet | 4.5 | 7.0 |
| Fio banka | Osobní účet | 0 | 0 | Oberbank | Účet Výhoda | 5.0 | 0.7 |
| Raiffeisenbank | eKonto Smart | 0.2 | 6.3 | Poštová banka | Užitočný účet | 5.0 | 0 |
| Air Bank | Malý tarif | 0.7 | 0.2 | Slov. sporiteľňa | Osobný účet | 5.9 | 4.9 |
| ČSOB | Plus Konto | 1.3 | 0.3 | VÚB | Učet so základnými funkciami | 6.0 | 0 |
| ČSOB | Premium | 1.3 | 34.0 | OTP Bank | Aktívny účet | 6.0 | 3.1 |
| Era banka | Poštovní účet | 1.3 | 0.3 | ČSOB | ČSOB Pohoda | 6.0 | -2.9 |
| Moneta | Free & Flexi | 1.5 | 0.4 | Tatra banka | Tatra Personal | 7.0 | 0 |

assumption of meeting turnover or balance condition next to six PAs. However, the test profile, as it was set in the CT's input form, did not meet any of them. The calculation itself was not incorrect but it is not relevant to display the results for a different comparison setting.

Finhit CT had a share of correct results 53% (8 PAs). Four results were incorrect, two were misguiding and one was plausible. The incorrect result (Oberbank Klasik) was caused by the omission of outgoing payments charges. The bank allows only the first outgoing payment to be for free in two groups (automatic and electronic trans-actions), then every outgoing payment is charged each. Unlike the Czech banks, some of the Slovakian banks charge outgoing payments and this was the reason of incorrect result for Slovenská sporiteľňa. Incorrect results for Fio and Raiffeisenbank was caused by the ATM withdrawal from other bank's network issue when only the first with-drawal in the month is for free. The same service was a cause of plausible result for Oberbank Výhoda. Oberbank distinguishes ATMs of ČSOB (contracted partner) and other banks' ATMs. The calculation treated all ATM withdrawals as if they were done from ČSOB's network only which might be possible but not sure. A misguiding result of OTP Bank was caused by an assumption that user meets the balance condition which

**Table 5.** Price calculation assessment for Finkomp and Menej CTs (amounts in €)

| Finkomp | | | | Menej | | | |
|---|---|---|---|---|---|---|---|
| Bank | Offered PA | CT | Dev | Bank | Offered PA | CT | Dev |
| mBank | mKonto | 0 | 0 | mBank | mKonto | 0 | 0 |
| Unicredit bank | U konto | 0 | 0 | Slov. sporiteľňa | Osobný účet exclusive | 0 | 13.8 |
| ČSOB | ČSOB Pohoda | 0 | 3.1 | Unicredit bank | U konto | 0 | 0 |
| Privat Banka | Konto Plus | 2.0 | 0 | Privat Banka | Konto Plus | 0 | 2.0 |
| Oberbank | Účet Klasik | 2.0 | 3.7 | Privat Banka | Standard konto | 0 | 5.0 |
| Unicredit bank | Štandardný účet | 3.0 | 0 | Poštová banka | Základný bankový produkt | 0 | 11.0 |
| ČSOB | Účet Extra Pohoda | 3.0 | 11.9 | Slov. sporiteľňa | Osobný účet | 0 | 5.0 |
| Fio banka | Osobný účet | 3.6 | 0 | Prima Banka | Osobný účet (min. card payment 780 € p.m.) | 0 | 0 |
| Fio banka | Platobný účet so základnými finkciami | 4.2 | 0 | Prima Banka | Osobný účet (min. card payment 480 € p.m.) | 1.0 | 2.5 |
| Prima Banka | Osobný účet | 5.0 | 0.9 | OTP Bank | Štandardný účet | 3.0 | 9.0 |
| Tatra banka | Štandardný legislatívny účet | 5.0 | 0 | OTP Bank | Aktívny účet | 3.0 | 6.1 |
| Privat Banka | Standard konto | 5.0 | 0 | ČSOB | ČSOB Pohoda | 3.0 | 0.1 |
| VÚB | VÚB účet | 5.0 | 0 | Tatra banka | Tatra personal | 3.5 | 10.1 |
| OTP Bank | Aktívny účet | 5.0 | 7.0 | BKS bank | Premium konto | 3.5 | 0 |
| Slov. sporiteľňa | Osobný účet | 5.5 | 5.3 | Prima Banka | Osobný účet | 3.9 | 2.0 |

was over the Slovakian average wage. A misguiding result concerning ČSOB was caused by conditions of 50% account maintenance fee sale that is likely to be met (card usage condition).

Finkomp CT had a share of correct results 60% (9 PAs). Three results were incorrect and three results were misguiding. The incorrect result (Oberbank Klasik) was caused by the omission of outgoing payments charges. The bank allows only the first outgoing payment to be for free in two groups (automatic and electronic transactions), then every outgoing payment is charged each. Prima Banka result was incorrect because the calculation did not include a bonus of 0.5% of total amount spent by card per month which is a conditional sale from a maintenance fee. Incorrectly were taken into account fees for outgoing payments for Slovenská sporiteľňa. A misguiding result of OTP Bank was caused by an assumption that user meets the balance condition which was over the Slovakian average wage. The rest of misguiding result were two accounts of ČSOB where there was included conditional sale on maintenance fee. The conditions are beyond the amounts set is methodology.

Menej CT was accurate in 33% cases (5 PAs). There were six seven incorrect results and four misguiding ones. An incorrect result of Prima banka Osobný účet came from the omission of ATM withdrawal from another bank's network fee. It was not possible to find why the result of Osobný účet (min. card payment 480 € p.m.) is wrong because the deviation does not correspond to either conditional sale for card payments and neither to ATM withdrawal from another bank's network fee. Poštová banka incorrect result came from not including a card maintenance fee and ATM withdrawal from another bank's network fee which are not a part of a free package. The latter charge was also a cause of incorrect result for OTP Bank Štandardný účet (ATM withdrawal from another bank's network is not a part of the package) and the same mistake concerns Privat banka PAs. A misguiding result of both Slov. sporiteľňa PAs prices were caused by an assumption that user meets criteria connected with high account balance, amounts of investments in the bank or turnover. A misguiding result of OTP Bank Aktívny účet was caused by an assumption that user meets the balance condition which was over the Slovakian average wage. A misguiding result concerns Tatra Bank because CT presumed that user achieves 50% conditional sale on maintenance fee (condition of wife account and husband account in Tatra or usage of at least 2 "bank innovations" like spending report, voice biometry, smart banking etc.).

## 4   Discussion

There is one fact that has to be taken into consideration before the results interpretation. Both Czech and Slovak retail banks' offers differ from the western European countries ones, e.g. in Great Britain or Germany. Unlike these two western countries the Czech and Slovak banks' RCBS tariffs are much more complex with multiple conditional sales and many items representing separate fees. Banks in Great Britain usually charge overdrafts instead of RCBS services and Germany applies much fewer fee types concerning RCBS. Therefore, generally unsatisfactory results cannot be seen only as CTs failure because the problem at some point rises from pricing policy. Moreover, tariffs are a subject of irregular change. This problem is in accordance with findings of [1] regarding the main weakness of all shopbots. Other studies [11, 18] also identified various factors such as the product category, number of sellers, and market imperfections that diminish a positive influence of CTs and shopbots in general. This may lead to a situation described by Smith [13]: "*In spite of the wealth of information provided by shopbots, shopbot customers remain asymmetrically informed about critical product attributes*". Therefore, accordingly [13] consumers are then using a brand and prior positive experience as proxies.

The general result interpretation is clear – all CTs but one showed unsatisfactory performance and do not provide adequate quality of information. Most of the problems were caused by the omission of the ATM withdrawal from other bank's network issue or specific rules related to it. Such rules relate to an amount of withdrawn money, user activity (mostly card usage) or having another bank as a contracted partner that acts then as own ATM network. The next most frequent problem is related to the conditional sales of the maintenance fee. These sales were achieved by different ways but mostly it includes user's turnover, PA balance or a total amount of money at the bank and user's activity (card usage, outgoing payments). However, there are also very specific conditions to be met in order to obtain a sale. Therefore, as mentioned in the previous paragraph, the level of inaccurate results (e.g. misguiding) comes from the overall complexness. Similar issues were discovered in test of the comparison tool in Poland "Porównywarka kont bankowych" at kontomierz.pl portal, see [15]. The table below summarizes the results (Table 6).

**Table 6.** A concise overview of calculation accuracy

| Result/CT | Czech Republic | | | Slovakia | | |
|---|---|---|---|---|---|---|
| | Mesec | Finpar | KBP | Finhit | Finkom | Menej |
| Correct | 4 | 13 | 4 | 8 | 9 | 5 |
| Plausible | 0 | 1 | 0 | 1 | 0 | 0 |
| Misguiding | 3 | 0 | 6 | 2 | 3 | 4 |
| Incorrect | 5 | 1 | 5 | 4 | 3 | 6 |
| Share of correct | 33% | 87% | 27% | 53% | 60% | 33% |
| Share of correct + plausible | 33% | 93% | 27% | 60% | 60% | 33% |

Only the Finpar CT can be considered as reliable and recommendable, i.e. offering very good information quality. It offers very accurate price calculation and it met all other criteria concerning other information quality features such as relevance, detail, uniformity, comparability and verifiability. The rest of the CTs performed unsatisfactorily or very poorly in price calculation.

The results of Menej and KBP have to be commented in a greater detail since their performance was the worst one. Menej CT high incorrect results occurrence comes from the fact that this CT does not distinguish between own bank's ATM network and another bank's ATM network. It is a major flaw because this condition is present in a large share of tariffs. Another possible issue of Menej CT and KBP as well might be an update frequency. Some incorrect results might be caused rather than a wrong calculation by an update lag. It is likely because two months after our survey, the KBP was replaced by a completely different CT. It is just a speculation but since the site owners knew that KBP is going to be replaced, they completely neglected an update process.

Although the results of the verifiability criterion results seem as a serious problem, it is not. Although the CTs did not provide a direct link, there was a bank brand and the precise product title. Therefore, it is just a matter of a simple and short search to find the PA provider's website. Although, due to different websites and different locations of tariffs lists it significantly increases user's interaction costs.

Unlike verifiability, the comparability issue is more serious. I find it highly misguiding to include accounts that do not offer all the demanded services in the comparison. Only two CTs were able to separate accounts efficiently. An additional test for such feature is e.g. over a counter service at the low-cost banks. The mBank does not offer payments or cash operations to be done at the branch over a counter. Yet it was present in a comparison list of four CTs when the option of payment over a counter was chosen. It seems that some CTs do not even have a rule that checks this type of a condition which is unsatisfactory.

Other criteria such as language, detail and uniformity showed no or only rare problems which were not of a serious matter. Therefore, those criteria were met and mustn't be a part of a future research because they do not separate good and bad performing CTs, unlike comparability and price accuracy criteria.

Unsatisfactory results of comparability and price accuracy criteria should be studied further. The paper [14] presents also a specific user profile which is consisted also of services used abroad. These services are typically connected to business trips or vacations. What would be the results like in case of e.g. ATM withdrawals abroad? A similar problem is a user with mixed preference regarding a communication channel. The smallest cluster in [14] utilizes most of the PA instrument through the Internet or smart banking. However, some services such as the creation of a standing order or a direct debit are done at the branch over a counter. The range of services is then grater and so a change for possible error is greater as well.

Possible way how to provide a consumer tools with adequate information quality relies on the idea of accreditation. The Directive 2014/92/EU states an obligatory duty for an EU member country to provide RCBS CT and that such CT has to provide accurate and up-to-date information. The means how to assure accurate and up-to-date information were not specified and were supposed to be included in the EU national law transposition. Nevertheless, the act no. 452/2016 coll. (transposition of the Directive 2014/92/EU) did not specified this requirement any further in the Czech Republic. However, it stated that Czech National Bank and Czech Trade Inspection Authority are supposed to publish a list of CTs that meet the requirements. In other words, give them an approval or accreditation concerning quality. Neither of them published any CT yet. Therefore, Czech National Bank and Czech Trade Inspection Authority should prepare a test framework to verify accuracy and recentness of the information provided by the CT. Creation of an application that would test possible combination of the consumer choices would be the most robust but also the least possible way due. The most feasible approach seems to identify typical consumer profiles or specific combination of test profiles that would contain the full range of services available for a comparison. Accreditation or being published on the list of approved CTs would regularly depend on passing this test. The downside of this problem is that without a cooperation from the side of the banks the accreditation institution would have do all the confirmation calculation by themselves. The calculation would be done in a similar way as it was in this paper which is time consuming and rather tedious task. However, then any consumer could easily choose the reliable CT by picking only those with an accreditation.

# 5  Conclusion

The goal of the paper was to assess the information quality level of the RCBS CTs in the Czech Republic and Slovakia. The information quality was assessed in seven dimensions (accuracy and full price, relevance, language and concision, detail, uniformity, comparability, and verifiability). Six CTs were found and analyzed in the survey. Although the literature generally acknowledges and appreciates an impact of shopbots [4, 9, 17, 19], the survey found some serious issues concerning the data quality. The results were in all cases but one unsatisfactory. Except the "Finparáda kalkulačka osobních účtů" all other CTs failed in delivering of adequately precise comparison mainly regarding the price accuracy.

The major issues problem rises not just from the incompleteness of CTs' databases but also from the pricing policy itself. Some tariffs are almost atomized charging each service separately and moreover, it differs accordingly the communication channel. The next issue with the same effect was a variety of conditional sales. Therefore, the costs of monitoring, updating and redesigning the CT are soaring. This is a problem since all the surveyed CTs are for free and just one displays advertisement.

A consumer should not rely on RCBS CTs completely with just one exception of "Finparáda" CT. Most of the CTs failed in information quality test and there are no means available now to distinguish high information quality CT from the rest. Therefore, it is suggested to start providing an accreditation or the list of approved CTs by the national regulatory bodies: national bank and trade inspection authority. The EU legal environment as well as national one allows it and even suggests it since the end of the year 2016 and yet there is no result available. The most feasible approach seems to identify typical consumer profiles or specific combination of test profiles that would contain the full range of services available for a comparison. Then the CT's results would be compared to regulator's one and assessed. The list of approved CTs or an option to show that the CT was accredited would be the signal of quality for a consumer. The principle of the invisible hand of the market would then separate reliable CTs from the rest to the benefit of all users.

**Acknowledgment.** This paper was written with the financial support of Specific Research Project "Investments within the Industry 4.0 concept" 2018 at Faculty of Informatics and Management of the University of Hradec Králové to the Department of Economics. I would like to thank Aneta Bartuskova, Ph.D. for her valuable comments. I would like to thank Lucie Silhabelova for her help with the calculator's database.

# References

1. Baye, M.R., Morgan, J.: Temporal price dispersion: evidence from an online consumer electronics market. J. Interact. Mark. **18**(4), 101–115 (2004). https://doi.org/10.1002/dir. 20016
2. European Banking Authority. Consumer trends report 2016. http://www.eba.europa.eu/ documents/10180/1360107/Consumer+Trends+Report+2016.pdf. Accessed 12 Mar 2018

3. European Commission: Comparison Tools: Report from the Multi-Stakeholder Dialogue (2013). http://edz.bib.uni-mannheim.de/daten/edz-a/gdgv/13/comparison-tools-report-ecs-2013_en.pdf. Accessed 12 Mar 2018
4. European Commission: Study on the coverage functioning and consumer use of comparison tools and third party verification schemes for such tools (2013). https://ec.europa.eu/info/sites/info/files/final_report_study_on_comparison_tools_2013_en.pdf. Accessed 16 Mar 2018
5. Gai, K.K., Qiu, M.K., Sun, X.T.: A survey on FinTech. J. Netw. Comput. Appl. **103**, 262–273 (2018). https://doi.org/10.1016/j.jnca.2017.10.011
6. Gomber, P., Kauffman, R.J., Parker, C., Weber, B.W.: On the fintech revolution: interpreting the forces of innovation, disruption, and transformation in financial services. J. Manag. Inf. Syst. **35**(1), 220–265 (2018). https://doi.org/10.1080/07421222.2018.1440766
7. Gozman, D., Liebenau, J., Mangan, J.: The innovation mechanisms of fintech start-ups: insights from SWIFT's innotribe competition. J. Manag. Inf. Syst. **35**(1), 145–179 (2018). https://doi.org/10.1080/07421222.2018.1440768
8. Haynes, M., Thompson, S.: Price, price dispersion and number of sellers at a low entry cost shopbot. Int. J. Ind. Organ. **26**(2), 459–472 (2008). https://doi.org/10.1016/j.ijindorg.2007.02.003
9. Iyer, G., Pazgal, A.: Internet shopping agents: virtual co-location and competition. Mark. Sci. **22**(1), 85–106 (2003)
10. Kim, J.W., Ha, S.H.: Price comparisons on the internet based on computational intelligence. PLoS ONE **9**(9), e106946 (2014). https://doi.org/10.1371/journal.pone.0106946
11. Ma, Z., Liao, K., Lee, J.J.-Y.: Examining comparative shopping agents from two types of search results. Inf. Syst. Manag. **27**(1), 3–9 (2010). https://doi.org/10.1080/10580530903455072
12. Schwartz, B.: The Paradox of Choice: Why More Is Less. HarperCollins Publishers, New York (2005)
13. Smith, M.D.: The impact of shopbots on electronic markets. J. Acad. Mark. Sci. **30**(4), 446–454 (2002). https://doi.org/10.1177/009207002236916
14. Soukal, I., Draessler, J., Hedvičáková, M.: Cluster analysis of the demand side of the retail core banking services market. E & M Ekonomie a Manag. **14**(4), 102–114 (2011)
15. Soukal, I., Draessler, J.: Retail core banking services comparison tools and the quality of information. In: Novak, P., Jurigova, Z., Kozubikova, L., Zlamalova, J. (eds.) Finance and Performance of Firms in Science, Education and Practice, pp. 994–1009. Tomas Bata University, Zlin (2017)
16. Soukal, I., Hedvičáková, M.: Retail core banking services costs optimization. Procedia Technol. **1**(1), 177–182 (2012)
17. Tang, Z., Smith, M.D., Montgomery, A.: The impact of shopbot use on prices and price dispersion: evidence from online book retailing. Int. J. Ind. Organ. **28**(6), 579–590 (2010). https://doi.org/10.1016/j.ijindorg.2010.03.014
18. Yuan, S.T.: A personalized and integrative comparison-shopping engine and its applications. Decis. Support Syst. **34**(2), 139–156 (2003). https://doi.org/10.1016/S0167-9236(02)00077-5

# An Organizational Scheme for Privacy Impact Assessments

Konstantina Vemou[(⊠)] and Maria Karyda

Department of Information and Communication Systems Engineering,
University of the Aegean, 83200 Samos, Greece
{kvemou,mka}@aegean.gr

**Abstract.** The importance of Privacy Impact Assessment (PIA) has been emphasized by privacy researchers and its conduction is provisioned in legal frameworks, such as the European Union's General Data Protection Regulation. However, it is still a complicated and bewildering task for organizations processing personal data, as available methods and guidelines fail to provide adequate guidance confusing organisations and PIA practitioners. This paper analyzes the interplay among PIA stakeholders and proposes an organizational scheme for successful PIA projects.

**Keywords:** Privacy impact assessment · Privacy management
Privacy governance · GDPR

## 1 Introduction

With the advent of information technology, information privacy, the concept of controlling how one's personal information will be processed and shared has become an emerging study field [1]. Several conceptual models, legal frameworks and self-regulation frameworks have been proposed, aiming at protecting one's privacy while allowing organizations to operate and provide personalized services [2–4]. However, several personal data breach incidents, such as the recent Facebook–Cambridge Analytica scandal [5], show that privacy practices so far have only partially succeeded in privacy protection. At the same time, concerns over privacy are rising [1, 6–9], especially among Web 2.0 users, who share vast amounts of personal data over the internet. Moreover, the European Union recently adopted a new legal framework, the General Data Protection Regulation (Regulation (EU) 2016/679, also known as EU GDPR), enforcing privacy rights of data subjects and introducing new obligations for organizations to apply privacy practices.

In this context, a shift towards applying privacy-by-design principles [10] and privacy risk management on information systems processing personal data has emerged. Privacy Impact Assessment (PIA) aims at identifying and mitigating privacy risks imminent in new systems [11]. The importance of PIA is underlined by two facts: (a) several legal frameworks, such as Canada's Privacy Act and the EU GDPR, mandate its conduction and (b) Data Protection Authorities (DPAs) worldwide have

© Springer Nature Switzerland AG 2019
M. Themistocleous and P. Rupino da Cunha (Eds.): EMCIS 2018, LNBIP 341, pp. 258–271, 2019.
https://doi.org/10.1007/978-3-030-11395-7_22

published generic guidelines on conducting them (e.g. [12, 13]), while the International Organization for Standardization recently published a PIA guidelines standard (ISO/IEC 29134) [14].

However, PIA conduction remains a complicated task for organizations processing personal data. Although several methods and guidelines on PIA conduction have been published by Data Protection Authorities, they follow different approaches and provide limited assistance on how to organize a PIA project, especially with regard to the management and organizational approach needed, e.g. on how to assign the roles involved in a PIA project, how to identify related responsibilities for privacy protection and how to manage stakeholders involved. Some approaches require the project manager of a new process or system to take responsibility of the PIA conduction (e.g. [15]), while others assign this task to the Data Protection Officer of the Organization (DPO) (e.g. [12]). In both cases the person organizing a PIA needs to collaborate with other stakeholders (e.g. the project manager needs to consult the DPO). Furthermore, existing approaches make no reference to the role of senior management, despite the fact that their commitment is a mandate [16].

To fill this gap, this paper proposes an organizational scheme for PIA conduction, identifying and describing involved roles. To illustrate the applicability of the scheme, we provide two examples that further explain the issue of responsibility assignment and stakeholder communication in the case of two projects processing personal data. Our research contributes both theoretically, by complementing existing frameworks lacking organizational aspects of PIA projects (identifying roles and responsibilities) and practically, by providing support to organizations conducting PIAs (stakeholder analysis and example of interactions, directions for responsibilities assignment).

In the next section, organizational guidelines as identified in existing PIA methods are presented. In Sect. 3, our organization scheme with roles and responsibilities involved in PIAs is analysed, followed by its application in two example cases in Sect. 4. Conclusions and areas for further research are presented in Sect. 5.

## 2 Existing Guidelines for PIA Organization

During the past years several PIA methods have been proposed, either in academic papers (e.g. [17, 18]) or in policy-oriented papers, published from Data Protection Authorities around the world (e.g. [12, 19, 20]). Moreover, a PIA guidelines standard (ISO/IEC 29134) was published recently from the International Organization for Standardization [14]. Apart from following different approaches, existing methods provide little or no guidance with regard to the organisational aspects of a PIA project, especially with regard to the responsibilities that need to be assigned to different roles, as well as with regard to interactions and communication between them Table 1 summarizes different organizational roles as identified in current PIA methods. Methods have been identified through exhaustive literature research and selected based on their references in academic papers.

In most guidelines for PIA projects accountability for PIA conduction is not mentioned, while in other approaches the whole organization is considered accountable (e.g. the Controller in [19], the RFID Application Operator in [21]). In [17], certain roles that need to be aware of privacy risks are identified, such as the organization's corporate risk management, marketing staff and upper management; however, none of these is explicitly assigned accountability to conduct PIA. However, [13–15] and [22] point at the top management of the organization to hold accountability of PIA conduction.

At the same time, there are different approaches with regard to the person responsible for organizing and implementing a PIA project. Some guidelines expect the project manager to conduct the PIA (e.g. [15, 18, 20]), while others assign the responsibility to the stakeholder that will benefit by the project, in other words the project owner (e.g. [13, 19]). Others, such as [12] and [14] assign the role to the person responsible for Personally Identifiable Information (PII) protection (e.g. a risk manager or the organization's Data Protection Officer).

Sign-off of the PIA report (the PIA's outcome) demonstrates organization's commitment to protect privacy during the new PII processing activity and therefore is an important step of PIA methods. Some methods explicitly assign this responsibility to a specific role within the organization, while others implicitly mention it by designating a space for name and signature in provided PIA report templates. Proposed officials to sign-off the PIA report include senior managers and executives (e.g. [13, 22]) as well as the project manager (e.g. [12]).

After the PIA report is signed off, a role responsible to revisit it any time it is necessary and be the contact point for future questions concerning privacy protection needs to be defined. Most guidelines propose the person responsible for PII protection to own the report after its completion (e.g. [17, 21, 23]), while others propose the responsibility to be assigned to senior management (e.g. [13, 15]).

Also, although it is not part of the PIA process, responsibilities for implementation of PIA recommendations and residual risks ownership after the PIA sign-off are indicated in most of proposed PIA report templates. However, such roles are vaguely defined ([12, 14, 23]), with the exception of CNIL guidelines [19] mentioning the project owner as the person responsible to implement recommendations. In addition, residual risks' owner is not defined, although risk owners, senior managers within the organization and the project owner are mentioned in some of the guidelines.

Conclusively, available guidelines on PIA projects adopt different approaches in roles and responsibilities assignment, whenever these roles are identified. Also, little or no guidance on how these roles interact is provided. As a result, PIA practitioners are provided with limited assistance on how to organize a PIA project. There is need for a comprehensive assignment of roles within a PIA conduction project and explanation of how the project will be affected by the outcome of their work.

## 3   An Organizational Scheme for PIA Projects

In this section, we propose an organizational scheme for PIA conduction: we explain terms for responsibilities, followed by PIA stakeholder analysis and propose assignment of roles in PIA projects. The latter also includes an example of a PIA workflow that shows how each role interacts with the other stakeholders. The proposed organizational scheme is based on existing PIA guidelines, ISO 29134 as well as ISO 27005

**Table 1.** Identified PIA roles and responsibilities in PIA methods

| Role description | Systematic PIA methodology | DPIA process under EU GDPR | UK PIA code of practice | New Zealand PIA toolkit | Australian ICO PIA guide | CNIL PIA method | Canada directive on PIA | PIAF methodology | ISO 29134 | RFID PIA | HIQA PIA in health and social care |
|---|---|---|---|---|---|---|---|---|---|---|---|
| Accountable for PIA conduction | X | X | X | X | X | Controller | Head of government institution | Chief executive officer | Top management | RFID app operator | Senior management |
| Responsible for PIA project | X | Project manager | DPO/risk manager | X | Project manager | Project owner | Senior executive responsible for project | Project manager | Responsible for PII protection/ project manager | X | Project team |
| Responsible for PIA report sign-off | X | X | Senior management (large projects/ high risks) project leader (small projects) | X | X | X | Senior officials/ executives/ legal services unit | X | Risk owner (management by signing acceptance statement) | X | Senior management |
| Owner of residual risks | X | X | X | X | Project manager and the organization | X | Approval from respective minister | Project manager and the organization | Risk owner | X | X |
| Responsible for recommendations implementation | X | X | X | X | X | Project owner | X | X | Risk owner | X | X |
| Ownership of the PIA report after sign-off | Privacy responsible | X | X | X | X | X | Senior official | Chief executive officer | X | Data privacy/ security official | X |

for information security risk management. To propose this organizational scheme, we analyzed existing PIA guidelines and identified stakeholders and needs for responsibilities assignment. Then we compared proposals for responsibilities assignment in current PIA methods, and consulted respective roles and responsibilities from ISO 29134 and ISO 27005 for information security risk management. Finally, we identified necessary interactions among stakeholders throughout the PIA steps described in ISO 29134.

### 3.1 Terms for Responsibilities

Our analysis concluded in three levels of responsibility. First of all, there is need to define a person having legal responsibility to carry out an action and will be imposed with penalties by legal authorities in case of incompliance (**Liable**). Also, internal to the organization, there is need to define a person authorized to approve an action and ensure it will be accomplished (**Accountable**) and a person authorized to actually carry out the action (**Responsible**).

### 3.2 Stakeholders Involved

After analyzing relevant literature and framework, we have identified stakeholders involved in a PIA project, focusing on internal entities of the organization affecting or being affected by the PIA. External stakeholders, such as consumers and privacy advocates' associations were considered out of scope for this PIA organizational scheme, as they do not share the organizations' responsibilities to protect privacy. However, they may be consulted during certain PIA phases. An exception is the reference to DPAs which may have legal authority to review and approve PIA reports.

**Senior Management.** The entity legally representing the organization (management board).

**Project Owner.** The business unit of the organization succeeding its goals by processing personal data. The business unit that requested the project implementation.

**Project Manager (PM).** The person responsible to organize and carry out the project, according to requirements set out by the project owner and other business units, e.g. the legal department posing requirements for legal compliance. The project manager could reside in the business unit of the project owner, in the IT department of the organization or even an external company in cases the project implementation is outsourced.

**PIA Project Manager (PIA PM).** The person assigned the responsibility to organize and carry out the assessment, producing the PIA report. The PIA PM skills should include risk management, project organization and privacy protection and could originate from an abundance of business units, such as internal audit, legal compliance, data protection officers' supporting team, even the Project Owner department. The PIA PM needs to be accompanied by a team of members with skill in risk management and privacy protection and knowledge of the business processes involved in the project, as well as the project itself.

**Data Protection Officer (DPO).** The person assigned the role to organize legal compliance for PII protection and report whether the privacy protection strategy of the organization is applied. The Data Protection Officer also provides advice during privacy impact assessments, taking into account the nature, scope, context and purposes of the processing.

Other roles:

**Chief Information Security Officer (CISO).** The person responsible to apply the security strategy of the organization, by developing a security management program, assign security related roles and propose security controls to protect important information assets of the organization that may also include PII.

**Data Protection Authority (DPA).** The external authority that may audit the report (if applicable by law) or review and provide recommendations. It could be an Information Commisioners' Office, a Data Protection Authority, or a Supervisory Authority as outlined in EU GDPR.

### 3.3   Identifying Roles and Interactions

Overall, as any organization processing personal data is considered as a PII controller, liability for privacy protection is assigned to its senior management (management board). This is the top management establishing the organization's strategies and directing all business operations. Also, establishing a risk management process for privacy lies within the organizations' senior management responsibilities. Extending this, senior management should be liable for PIA conduction and implementation of recommendations, in cases it is provisioned in the organization's legal context.

On the other hand, accountability, to ensure a PII process is developed following privacy preserving practices and ensure privacy risk assessment is performed during the project development lies within the business unit that has asked for it (Project Owner). This is the business unit that assigns the project to a specific project manager (within the unit, or in another unit of the organization such as IT department if it involves IT systems development, or even to a contractor external to the organization). The project owner should inform the DPO of the organization, seek its consultation for the project, as well as ensure DPO assigns responsibility to perform a PIA. The person who will actually organize and perform the assessment is the PIA Project Manager and should be provided with necessary resources (DPO and the Project Owner shall ensure these are provided). The PIA PM will identify the needs and skills for PIA team members and will also establish a consultation plan with any external stakeholders, in case this is considered necessary.

During PIA conduction, PIA PM and the PIA team should consult DPO about both privacy threats and their impact on data subjects. The organization's CISO should also be consulted, as some of the threat sources are actually security threats and security-related controls may be necessary in order to mitigate privacy risks. PIA PM should also be in direct communication with the Project Manager to ensure recommended changes and controls are not only viable to implement, but also the most appropriate in the context of the project.

The outcome of the PIA is a report including a description of the PII processes, main stakeholders and assets involved in the project, privacy risks evolving from the project (threats and their likelihood, as well as impact they could have on the data subjects' privacy), recommendations for changes in the processes implemented within the project, recommendations for implementation of organizational and technical controls, reasoning for the selection of such controls and residual risks (after the implementation of the recommendations). While its creation is included in the responsibilities of the PIA PM, the sign-off of such a report should lie within the responsibility of the Project Owner who will ensure the project and related PII processing will be amended according to recommendations. For this, the DPO of the organization may be consulted. In addition, the DPO shall ensure the project will not continue unless PIA report is signed-off. In some legal contexts, such as EU GDPR (for high-risk PII processing operations)[1] and Victoria Privacy and Data Protection Act of 2014, an external review and sign-off of the PIA report is required. However, such a sign-off does not refute the need for the Project Owner to take internal responsibility for signing-off the PIA report and by this officially warrant for the project continuation according to recommendations.

This leads to the next responsibility, the implementation of recommended changes and controls. While the Project Owner is accountable for the amendment of the project and application of recommended controls, the project manager will actually be responsible for their implementation (by assignment to the development team). In any case, residual risks ownership remains the Project Owner's responsibility. Although controls' implementation and acceptance of residual risks are typically not part of the PIA process, related responsibilities are presented in this section as they form the result and fulfill the goal of such a process.

After the PIA process is completed and besides other actions to implement recommended changes, the project owner should deliver the report to the person responsible for privacy protection within the organization (DPO). From this moment on, the Data Protection Officer will be the owner of the report, will maintain applicable documents and ensure its review. Review can be performed at regular intervals, or any time it is mandated, due to significant changes in the PII processing or the legal environment of the organization. The Data Protection Officer shall investigate whether significant changes affect the project outcome and ask for a new PIA cycle if necessary. Respectively, the DPO shall act as a contact point for external audits, e.g. from the Data Protection Authorities.

In the following we present an organizational scheme (Table 2), while high-level communications among PIA stakeholders are demonstrated within an example of project process in Figs. 1 and 2.

---

[1] Article 36 of EU GDPR does not mention sign-off but requires prior consultation with the supervisory authority prior to processing "where a data protection impact assessment under Article 35 indicates that the processing would result in a high risk in the absence of measures taken by the controller to mitigate the risk". The report is one of the elements to be provided to the supervisory authority during the consultation.

**Table 2.** Organizational scheme for PIA projects

| Role description | Liability | Accountability | Responsibility |
|---|---|---|---|
| PIA conduction | Senior management | Project owner | PIA project manager |
| PIA report sign-off | Senior management | Data protection officer | Project owner |
| Implementation of controls | Senior management | Project owner | Project manager |
| Ownership of residual risks | Senior management | Project owner | Project owner |
| Ownership of PIA report/updates | Senior management | Data protection officer | Data protection officer |
| External audit contact point | Senior management | Senior management | Data protection officer |

# 4  Applying the Organizational Scheme

In this section, we illustrate how the proposed organization scheme is applied for supporting PIA projects in two example cases: a university alumni records system and a hospital medical records system. The first case was selected because universities involve special organizational structures and the role of a special team (from the School of IT studies) resembles the role of contractors in cases of outsourced IT projects, while the second case was selected because of the sensitivity of involved personal data.

## 4.1  Case 1: Alumni Records System

**Project Description.** University "A" decided to create an alumni relations office. This will be implemented as a new administration office and will support students with job offers and trend news on their study field. At the same time, graduates will be able to provide their feedback and proposals about the educational programs of the university, based on their work experience, as well as start conversations and mentor other students. The alumni relations office will be supported by a customer relations management system (alumni records system) which will be implemented by a dedicated team of students in the School of IT studies of the university and a website in which all communications will take place (alumni records system). Account information for logging on the website, contact details (email, telephone, and address), detailed biographical information and posts or messages exchanged are some examples of personal information that will be stored and processed by the alumni relations office.

**Stakeholders' Analysis and Their Role in the PIA Project.** The rector acts as the senior management of the university and will be considered as the PII controller. The project owner of the system will be the new administrative unit that will be set (alumni relations office), which will set a project manager. In this case the project manager will be a professor from the School of IT studies, managing a team of students implementing the system. The new administrative team's head will also inform the Data

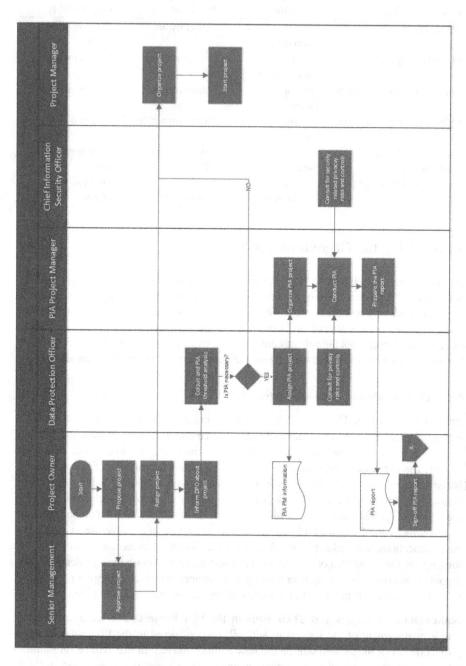

**Fig. 1.** Interactions between PIA stakeholders (Figure 1/2)

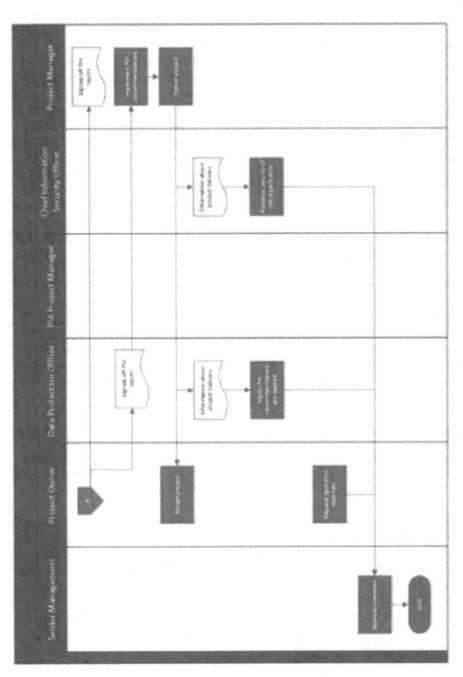

**Fig. 2.** Interactions between PIA stakeholders (Figure 2/2)

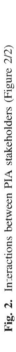

protection officer assigned by the rector for ensuring privacy protection in the context of personal data processing activities.

When the DPO is informed about the project and the new office's function, will assess whether a PIA is necessary. In this case as personal data are involved in the project, the decision will be affirmative and the DPO will assign a PIA PM.

The role will be assigned to a professor from the School of Law studies, specializing in data protection. His team will include post graduate students studying risk management, IT and public relations, as well as a member from the team that designed the proposal of the new administrative unit. With the initial analysis of the new office business processes and the involved information system (alumni system), the PIA team will start the assessment, which will also be updated in later stages of the IT project. The DPO will be consulted for privacy risks originating from the system under development and their impacts on alumni students and will also involve the CISO of the university (from the IT department of the university), as well as the Project manager of the project, in order to select the appropriate organizational and technical measures to recommend. Then the PIA team will create the PIA report which will also document the rationale of each decision for measures recommendations as well as residual risks stemming from the project.

The head of the alumni relations office will sign-off the PIA report and inform the PM of any changes that need to be implemented in the process covered by the IT system or any measures necessary. The PM will revise the requirements of the system according to the recommendations in the PIA report and then will proceed with the implementation. During delivery, the DPO will verify privacy recommendations were applied to the project, and CISO will be asked to assess the security of the system. Then the alumni relations office head will inform the rector about the project implementation and will request the start of operations for the system. The rector will take into account the DPO and CISO's opinions and will grant authorization to operate.

## 4.2 Case 2: Patient Records System

**Project Description.** Hospital "B" decided to create a patient records system which will be used by caregivers (doctors and nurses) in the context of offering medical services. The new system will provide information on the patient's medical history and support doctors towards accurate diagnosis and treatment selection. Also, as in emergency cases there is little time to ask for full patient history, this system will also benefit emergency medical services' (e.g. ambulances) caregivers, providing first line medical support. The hospital business unit that will be assigned the role of maintaining this record is the Department of Hospital Organization, an existing administration office, dealing with managing records and organizing cooperation between different hospital departments.

Information processed by the system concerns medical records, such as patients' medical history and care by specific doctors (e.g. physical examinations, test results, x-rays, administration of drugs and therapies, orders for the administration of drugs and therapies), vaccination history, known hereditary illnesses of family members, allergies, habits affecting health (e.g. smoking, alcohol intake, exercise) and other sensitive personal information.

**Stakeholders' Analysis and Their Role in the Project.** The Hospital Manager administering the hospital along with the management board will be considered as the senior management of the hospital. The project owner of the system will be the Department of Hospital Organization, which will set a project manager. In this case the project manager will be a member of the IT department as the main scope of the project will be achieved via a new information system. The Department of Hospital Organization's head will also inform the Data protection officer assigned by the Hospital Manager for ensuring privacy protection in the context of personal data processing activities.

As the project involves processing of sensitive personal data, the DPO will decide a PIA is necessary and will assign a PIA PM. The role will be assigned to a member from his team, specializing in data protection and internal audit. PIA team will include a set of doctors of different disciplines, a member of the legal department of the hospital, as well as a member from the team that designed the proposal of the new system. The DPO will be consulted for privacy risks originating from the system under development and their impacts on patients and will also involve the CISO of the organization, as well as the Project manager, in order to select the appropriate organizational and technical measures to recommend. Then the PIA team will create the PIA report which will also document the rationale of each decision for recommendations as well as residual risks stemming from the project.

The head of Department of Hospital Organization will sign-off the PIA report and inform the PM of any changes or measures that need to be implemented in the IT system. The PM will revise the requirements of the system according to the recommendations in the PIA report and then will proceed with the implementation. During delivery, the DPO will verify privacy recommendations were applied to the project, and CISO will be asked to assess the security of the system. Before asking authorization to operate, the DPO of the organization will inform the DPA about the new system and provide the PIA report for consultation. As soon as the DPA approves the PIA report, the DPO will inform the head of Department of Hospital Organization in order to proceed with the request for the start of operation. The hospital manager will take into account the DPO and CISO's opinions, as well as the outcome of the consultation with the DPA to grant authorization to operate the system.

# 5  Conclusions and Further Research

In this paper, we propose an organizational scheme for PIA projects conduction. Reconciling vague and contradicting recommendations from existing PIA guidelines, the proposed scheme describes roles and responsibilities assignment among PIA stakeholders and demonstrates high level interactions of these roles, thus contributes to existing PIA frameworks lacking organizational aspects and providing guidance to organizations undertaking such projects.

Although the proposed organizational scheme was created with EU GDPR in mind, it can be applied in different legal contexts as focus is on internal organization of the PIA project. Also, the involvement of external reviewers (DPAs), whenever mandated by law, is provisioned. This scheme is also independent of the decision to outsource development of an IT system, as a distinct role for the project manager is defined and interactions with other stakeholders are described.

The aim of this research was to define an organization scheme to support the implementation of PIA projects that currently lack adequate support and related guidelines, by defining roles and responsibilities and describing high-level communication and interaction among stakeholders during all stages and phases of a PIA process. We have also shown the application of the scheme on two diverse, relative scenarios. Furthermore, the essential role of senior management, that is to establish a risk management framework and provide adequate support (mandate, resources, etc.) is explicitly exhibited and highlighted to raise awareness.

Open issues for further research include the expansion of the organizational scheme for cases when an external company (e.g. legal/advisory) is assigned the responsibility of PIA conduction in favor of the organization. Also, this organizational scheme can be extended to include more directions for interaction among stakeholders (e.g. which roles should be consulted in each step, which roles should be informed after each PIA step) and embedded in an optimized PIA method to support PIA practitioners. Last but not least, the organizational scheme's applicability to real case studies should be studied.

# References

1. Pavlou, P.: State of the information privacy literature: where are we now and where should we go. MIS Q. **35**(4), 977–988 (2011)
2. Schwaig, K.S., Kane, G.C., Storey, V.C.: Compliance to the fair information practices: how are the Fortune 500 handling online privacy disclosures? Inf. Manag. **43**(7), 805–820 (2006)
3. Spiekermann, S., Novotny, A.: A vision for global privacy bridges: technical and legal measures for international data markets. Comput. Law Secur. Rev. **31**(2), 181–200 (2015)
4. Moores, T., Dhillon, G.: Do privacy seals in e-commerce really work? Commun. ACM - Mob. Comput. Oppor. Chall. **46**(12), 265–271 (2003)
5. BBC: Facebook scandal 'hit 87 million users', 04 April 2018. http://www.bbc.com/news/technology-43649018. Accessed 20 May 2018
6. European Commission: Flash Eurobarometer: data protection in the European Union: citizens perceptions. Analytical report (2008)
7. European Commission: Special Eurobarometer 431: data protection. Report (2015)
8. European Commission: Special Eurobarometer 443: e-privacy. Report (2016)
9. Gigya: The 2017 State of Consumer Privacy and Trust report. https://www.gigya.com/resource/report/2017-state-of-consumer-privacy-trust/. Accessed 20 May 2018
10. Cavoukian, A.: Privacy by design: the definitive workshop. A foreword by Ann Cavoukian, Ph.D. Identity Inf. Soc. **3**(2), 247–251 (2010)
11. Clarke, R.: Privacy impact assessment: its origins and development. Comput. Law Secur. Rev. **25**(2), 123–135 (2009)
12. UK Information Commissioner's Office (ICO): Conducting Privacy Impact Assessments: Code of Practice (2014). https://ico.org.uk/media/for-organisations/documents/1595/pia-code-of-practice.pdf. Accessed 02 Mar 2018
13. Treasury Board of Canada Secretariat (Canada TBS): Directive of Privacy Impact Assessments (2010). https://www.tbs-sct.gc.ca/pol/doc-eng.aspx?id=18308. Accessed 02 Mar 2018

14. International Organization for Standardization (ISO): ISO/IEC 29134 Information Technology – Security Techniques—Privacy Impact Assessment – Guidelines (2017)
15. Wright, D.: Making privacy impact assessment more effective. Inf. Soc. **29**(5), 307–315 (2013)
16. Wright, D., Finn, R., Rodrigues, R.: A comparative analysis of privacy impact assessment in six countries. J. Contemp. Eur. Res. **9**(1), 160–180 (2013)
17. Oetzel, M.C., Spiekermann, S.: A systematic methodology for privacy impact assessments: a design science approach. Eur. J. Inf. Syst. **23**(2), 126–150 (2014)
18. Bieker, F., Friedewald, M., Hansen, M., Obersteller, H., Rost, M.: A process for data protection impact assessment under the European general data protection regulation. In: Schiffner, S., Serna, J., Ikonomou, D., Rannenberg, K. (eds.) APF 2016. LNCS, vol. 9857, pp. 21–37. Springer, Cham (2016). https://doi.org/10.1007/978-3-319-44760-5_2
19. Commission Nationale de l'Informatique et des Libertes (CNIL): Privacy Impact Assessment (PIA) Methodology (2018). https://www.cnil.fr/en/PIA-privacy-impact-assessment-en. Accessed 22 Apr 2018
20. Office of the Australian Information Commissioner (OAIC): Guide to undertaking privacy impact assessments (2014). https://www.oaic.gov.au/agencies-and-organisations/guides/guide-to-undertaking-privacy-impact-assessments. Accessed 02 Mar 2018
21. Spiekermann, S.: The RFID PIA–developed by industry, endorsed by regulators. In: Wright, D., De Hert, P. (eds.) Privacy Impact Assessment. LGTS, vol. 6, pp. 323–346. Springer, Dordrecht (2012). https://doi.org/10.1007/978-94-007-2543-0_15
22. Health Information and Quality Authority of Ireland (HIQA): Guidance on Privacy Impact Assessment (PIA) in Health and Social Care (2017). https://www.hiqa.ie/reports-and-publications/health-information/guidance-privacy-impact-assessment-pia-health-and. Accessed 20 May 2018
23. Office of the Privacy Commissioner (OPC) New Zealand: Privacy Impact Assessment Toolkit (2015). https://www.privacy.org.nz/news-and-publications/guidance-resources/privacy-impact-assessment/. Accessed 02 Mar 2018

# How Social Media Can Afford Engagement Processes

Xiaoxiao Zeng[1], Brad McKenna[1(✉)], Shahper Richter[2],
and Wenjie Cai[3]

[1] University of East Anglia, Norwich, UK
{xiaoxiao.zeng,b.mckenna}@uea.ac.uk
[2] Auckland University of Technology, Auckland, New Zealand
shahper.richter@aut.ac.nz
[3] University of Greenwich, London, UK
w.cai@greenwich.ac.uk

**Abstract.** The increasing popularity of social media has led many organizations to find new ways of customer engagement. This paper presents an initial pilot study to explore the affordance of social media in engagement processes. By applying the affordance theory and Porter's process for engagement model, we used a case study approach to examine the case company's Facebook and Twitter content to identify the engagement possibilities of social media. Our preliminary results show that social media opens a new channel for organisations to engage with their customers. We present a preliminary theoretical model to understand the how the functional affordances of social media are socialised in engagement processes, which ultimately gives rise to socialised affordances.

**Keywords:** Social media · Engagement · Functional affordances
Socialised affordances

## 1 Introduction

The utilization of social media has generated a considerable body of research in the last decades. For example, social media and engagement [1, 2], social media and electronic word of mouth [3], social media and branding [4]. Social media represents a significant innovation for customer engagement, it allows information changes among customers and influences potential customer decisions [5]. Social media has changed the way companies communicate with customers, hence, allowing companies to organize a variety of customer engagement strategies [6]. Social media is important for customer engagement, yet our understanding remains limited. Although there exists a wide range of research in social media and customer engagement [7–9], none of this research explores how the features of social media afford engagement processes. Therefore, there is need for researchers to investigate how social media can afford the customer engagement. This study aims address the gap by using "Affordances" theory [10]. To explore the possibilities of social media in the engagement process, we drew up the following question: *How do affordances of social media tools facilitate the customer engagement process?*

M. Themistocleous and P. Rupino da Cunha (Eds.): EMCIS 2018, LNBIP 341, pp. 272–279, 2019.
https://doi.org/10.1007/978-3-030-11395-7_23

## 2 Social Media and Customer Engagement

Many scholars have examined brands and customer relationships on social media [11–14]. Gensler and Völckner [4] say that social media enable dynamic and real-time interaction between company and customer, while this new change also lets brand managers lose control of their brand. Hence, social media is a double-edged sword, it is important for brand managers to understand customer needs and cope with customer issues in this new environment.

It is necessary for firms to know how they are using social media applications, specifically, for what content they should post to serve their business objectives [15]. Naaman and Boase [16] examine the characteristics of social activity and pattern of communications on Twitter, called "social awareness streams". Based on their work, Lovejoy and Saxton [17] proposed an "Information-Community-Action" microblog message classification in organizational level. Harder and Howard [18] used this classification to build their analysis of "One Book Nova Scotia" activity. They split the tweets into three separate categories: Information, which represents information functions, like offer news, highlights; Conversation, which provides direct interaction with the community, for example, @participants or direct conversations; Action-orientation, which engages followers to participate in something, such as events.

## 3 Theoretical Framework

Affordances represent the concept of "action possibilities" as perceived by the environment [10]. The existence of affordances is when opportunity for action is available and affordances are properties of the relationship between an object and a social entity [19]. Therefore, when applying affordance to technology, the interaction of animal & environment would be replaced by human & artefact [20]. Affordance theory has been applied by some scholars to understand the relationship between technological artefacts and organizations, and how technology creates possible interactions that affect organizations [21–23]. Leonardi [22] argues that technology affordances are usually the same or similar across different organizational environments because the material characteristics or features of the technology limit people's use of it. Majchrzak and Lynne Markus [24] interpret technology affordances use in information systems as "an action potential, that is, to what an individual or organization with a particular purpose can do with a technology or information system" (p. 832).

Treem and Leonardi [23] explore social media use in organizations, they identified the affordances of *Visibility, Editability, Persistence,* and *Association.* The affordance of persistence allows for growing content, sustaining knowledge and communication over time. The editability of social media affords more purposeful communication, this means the asynchronous text-based conversation gives users the time to improve information quality, targeting content and regulating personal expressions. The affordance of association allows individuals to connect with others or content, it supports social connections and enables relevant or emergent connection.

# 4    Methodology

## 4.1    Case Study – The Dairy

Our case study is a dairy farm (hereafter referred to as The Dairy) in the south west region of the United Kingdom, which produces milk, cream, butter and yoghurt. The Dairy aims to build brand awareness and engage more with its customers. The Dairy has three core customer groups: national retailers (49%), local independent businesses (30%) and local dairy ingredients to food manufacturers (21%).

## 4.2    Data Collection

Data was collected through Facebook and Twitter. For triangulation purposes of social media data [25], we also used additional data collected from the case company's website. We used Netlytic to collect primary data from public tweets by using the search criteria of relevant hashtags (not named here due to anonymity), and The Dairy's Twitter handle posts between 26 June 2017 and 26 July 2017. We also downloaded posts from The Dairy's Facebook page. Posts were collected using R by using the same search criteria we used for Twitter. We gathered 1712 posts consisting of 4 events, 62 videos, 111 text status updates, 334 links, and 1215 photos.

## 4.3    Data Analysis

We used text analysis to investigate how The Dairy promotes participation through social media activities. Text analysis results are analysed through coding form in Excel. We also analysed data from the company's website. This helped us to understand The Dairy's brand-expression and how they successfully transform customers from their website to social media platforms.

# 5    Preliminary Findings and Discussion

## 5.1    Understanding Customer Needs and Motivations

It is important for firms to know what their customers expect from them [26]. Porter and Donthu [27] argue that satisfying social and psychological needs motivate customers to participate in various social media platforms. Therefore, the engagement processes model is rooted in the notion that customer engagement is based on the value created when companies or brands help them meet their needs [28]. Social media provide a good way for firms to understand their customers through the Internet. Two socialising affordances in understanding customer needs were derived from the data: embedded social media analysis features and two-way communication.

**Embedded Social Media Analysis Features.** The Dairy applied the embedded features from their social media platforms to help them monitor customers; this validates Treem and Leonardi [23] arguments that social media afford companies visibility to visualize the customer preference and behaviours. The Dairy uses Twitter analytics to help them understand their follower's interests and what types of posts they expect to see. In the past, usually firms analysed customer preferences by sending questionnaires or collect from face-to-face interviews, all of which are inconvenient and time-consuming [29]. These embedded analysis tools make it more convenient for firms to understand customer motivations and preferences.

**Two-Way Communication.** The Dairy posts many messages, while at the same time they also receive a lot comments and feedback from customers. It illustrates the functional affordances of persistence and editability [23]. This finding also verifies the change of social media marketing [30, 31]. Indeed, social media affords multi-way communication for firms, which not only enable them talk to customers but also allow customers talk to companies and customers communicate with each other. Firstly, companies can initially ask their audience about their preferences or post questions on social media platforms, which is the traditional way of communication. The Dairy uses Facebook and Twitter to collect large numbers of customer opinions. We found that the company posts a lot messages for gathering opinions about their products and brands.

> *We've always believed that in life you get out what you put in - and this ethos is no different in our dairy. If you can tell us what you think makes our milk taste so uniquely different and delicious, then you could win a lovely prize! Get guessing...* (Facebook, 2013-05-11).

Secondly, customers also can express their experience and opinions freely and users have more control over the content [32]. The Dairy withdrew several products in August 2014 because there has been an unfortunate error at one of their farms. This incident received lots of negative comments from customers. Some customers expressed their worries or complained about The Dairy. The negative comments damaged The Dairy's image in the public (see below).

> *Please let us know what the common substance is – it's bad enough that our household has already drank 4 pints and are already a way into a second 4 pint (both dated 25th Aug). I'm not looking to throw a fit or blame coincidental symptoms of a bug but my toddlers have drunk the milk straight – the environment agency's word is useless without us knowing if we've been drinking bleach, chlorine and more* (Facebook, 2014-08-18).

This example demonstrates that social media platforms provide two-way communication for customers and organisations, it not only enables marketing managers to communicate with customers and seek responses in social media network's comments sections, but also allows for customers to communicate freely about the products in public.

## 5.2 Promote Participation

Social media enable firms to engage audiences and generate useful business insights [33]. The Dairy created different types of content and launched different activities on social media. There are three socialising affordances in engagement processes derived from our data: *brand-expression*, *encouraging content creation*, and *creating enjoyable experiences*.

**Brand Expression.** Social media can be a powerful tool to spread brand-expression and enhance brand awareness [34]. The Dairy's brand-expression is "delicious things" which was developed based on customers' comments. It illustrates the social media affordances of visibility and editability [23]. The Dairy explains that "*Delicious things says everything we want to say about the natural goodness, the care, the attention and the expertise you can taste every time you try one of our delicious products*". We conclude that customers hold positive views about the products and the brand. People talked a lot about the clotted cream and butter. There are also plenty of descriptive words like "good", "yummy", "fantastic" and "amazing". The Dairy strategically uses customer-generated content to build their brand-expression and show what customers say about their products to the public.

**Encourage Content Creation.** As highlighted by Treem and Leonardi [23], social media afford editability which enables more purposeful content creation, the association allows individuals to connect with others through social media functions (e.g., likes/shares), and the affordance of persistency enables the company to grow content. The Dairy encourages content creation through two aspects: firstly, by posting different types of content to involve participants; secondly, encouraging their fans to like or share the content they produce.

**Create Enjoyable Experience.** Research shows that people would have favourable attitudes towards a firm, which provides them with enjoyable experiences [27]. The Dairy uses social media to provide a variety of enjoyable experiences to engage its existing customers and potential customers, like competitions and recipes. This finding validates Treem and Leonardi [23]'s statement that social media affords individual editability to craft and compose messages, which can aid to target content and improving content quality. The company launched lots of competitions to increase this involvement.

> *Competition time! Following on from last years 'How many balloons in a Smart Car' is this years 'How many balloons in a Mini'. Let us know your answers by 4 pm today and you could be in with a chance to win some The Dairy goodies! (Facebook, 2016-02-24).*

### 5.3    Motivate Cooperation

Social media affords users the visibility to identify the network connections and the ability of association to support and build social connections [23]. Therefore, identifying influencers and cooperating with them can greatly contribute to higher customer engagement. Harder and Howard [18] suggest managers should engage different types of participants to facilitate the engagement processes. Gruzd and Haythornthwaite [35] add that it is necessary to involve community members into social media activities. Hence, two socialising affordances of social media in motivating cooperation were derived from datasets: finding influencers and constructing networks.

**Find Influencers.** It is necessary for organizations to find the influential actors quickly in the network [36]. Li and Lin [8] suggest companies should build interactions and cooperation with influencers. The Dairy builds interactions with some potential influencers to spread brand awareness.

**Construct Networks.** We found that The Dairy has direct connections with wide range of users. We grouped the participants into 3 groups. The first group is *dairy* *related organizations*: a local market, a herb farm, a bakery, and a baker. The second group we named *other organizations* (organizations that do not directly relate to dairy), which contains travel agencies, financial companies, and hotels. The third group are *individual users* who generally are fans of The Dairy.

## 6 Affordance of Social Media in the Engagement Processes

Our preliminary theoretical model (Fig. 1) was developed based on the discussion above. The first column is based on Treem and Leonardi [23], and the second on Porter and Donthu [27]. The functional affordances of social media are "socialized" through engagement processes. Social media affords visibility, editability and persistence, which makes it possible for The Dairy to understand customer needs and motivations and promote more participation. The functional affordances of social media should be socialized by human actions. By this, we mean, The Dairy managers need to use Twitter or Facebook and related technologies to carry out a series of activities such as "mentions" find influencers, and establish Facebook groups to support engagement processes.

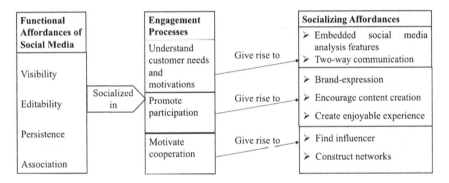

**Fig. 1.** Preliminary research model.

## 7 Conclusion

In this paper, we have presented the findings of our pilot study to explore the affordances of social media in engagement processes of an organisation and how those socialising affordances help organisations to increase engagement. We introduced social media and engagement related literature and adopted an affordances theoretical lens to guide the research. This study contributes to the understanding of social media and social media use in engagement processes [37, 38]. By basing our theoretical development on empirical data from this pilot study, we provide a more rigorous model for the next stages of our research. We attempted to answer how socialising affordances helps organisations increase engagement. The next stage of the research is for further investigation to validate our research model. Bryman and Bell [39] suggest in-depth interviews can help generate deep insights into the complex business environment. Therefore, our future stages involve in-depth interviews to validate our theoretical model.

## References

1. Noguti, V.: Post language and user engagement in online content communities. Eur. J. Mark. **50**(5/6), 695–723 (2016)
2. Ibrahim, N.F., Wang, X., Bourne, H.: Exploring the effect of user engagement in online brand communities: evidence from Twitter. Comput. Hum. Behav. **72**, 321–338 (2017)
3. Brown, J., Broderick, A.J., Lee, N.: Word of mouth communication within online communities: conceptualizing the online social network. J. Interact. Mark. **21**(3), 2–20 (2007)
4. Gensler, S., et al.: Managing brands in the social media environment. J. Interact. Mark. **27** (4), 242–256 (2013)
5. Gallaugher, J., Ransbotham, S.: Social media and customer dialog management at Starbucks. MIS Q. Exec. **9**(4), 197–212 (2010)
6. Hennig-Thurau, T., Wiertz, C., Feldhaus, F.: Does Twitter matter? The impact of microblogging word of mouth on consumers' adoption of new movies. J. Acad. Mark. Sci. **43**(3), 375–394 (2015)
7. Mollen, A., Wilson, H.: Engagement, telepresence and interactivity in online consumer experience: reconciling scholastic and managerial perspectives. J. Bus. Res. **63**(9–10), 919–925 (2010)
8. Li, Y.-M., Lin, C.-H., Lai, C.-Y.: Identifying influential reviewers for word-of-mouth marketing. Electron. Commer. Res. Appl. **9**(4), 294–304 (2010)
9. Hamilton, K., Alexander, M.: Organic community tourism: a cocreated approach. Ann. Tour. Res. **42**, 169–190 (2013)
10. Gibson, J.J.: The theory of affordances. In: Shaw, R.E., Bransford, J. (eds.) Perceiving, Acting and Knowing, pp. 67–82. Lawrence Erlbaum Associates, Hillsdale (1977)
11. Habibi, M.R., Laroche, M., Richard, M.-O.: The roles of brand community and community engagement in building brand trust on social media. Comput. Hum. Behav. **37**, 152–161 (2014)
12. Popp, B., Woratschek, H.: Introducing branded communities in sport for building strong brand relations in social media. Sport Manag. Rev. **19**(2), 183–197 (2016)
13. Brownstein, M.: Overreliance on social media will damage your brand. Adage (2010). http://adage.com/article/small-agency-diary/overreliance-social-media-damage-brand/143779/. Accessed 17 July 2017
14. Hudson, S., et al.: The influence of social media interactions on consumer–brand relationships: a three-country study of brand perceptions and marketing behaviors. Int. J. Res. Mark. **33**(1), 27–41 (2016)
15. Van Looy, A.: Social Media Management. STBE. Springer, Cham (2016). https://doi.org/10.1007/978-3-319-21990-5
16. Naaman, M., Boase, J., Lai, C.-H.: Is it really about me? Message content in social awareness streams. In: Proceedings of the 2010 ACM Conference on Computer Supported Cooperative Work. ACM, New York (2010)
17. Lovejoy, K., Saxton, G.D.: Information, community, and action: how nonprofit organizations use social media. J. Comput.-Mediat. Commun. **17**(3), 337–353 (2012)

18. Harder, A., Howard, V., Sedo, D.R.: Creating cohesive community through shared reading: a case study of One Book Nova Scotia. Can. J. Libr. Inf. Pract. Res. **10**(1), 1–21 (2015)
19. Hutchby, I.: Technologies, texts and affordances. Sociology **35**(2), 441–456 (2001)
20. Zheng, Y., Yu, A.: Affordances of social media in collective action: the case of Free Lunch for Children in China. Inf. Syst. J. **26**(3), 289–313 (2016)
21. Markus, M.L., Silver, M.S.: A foundation for the study of IT effects: a new look at DeSanctis and Poole's concepts of structural features and spirit. J. Assoc. Inf. Syst. **9**(10/11), 609–632 (2008)
22. Leonardi, P.M.: When flexible routines meet flexible technologies: affordance, constraint, and the imbrication of human and material agencies. MIS Q. **35**(1), 147–167 (2011)
23. Treem, J.W., Leonardi, P.M.: Social media use in organizations: exploring the affordances of visibility, editability, persistence, and association. Ann. Int. Commun. Assoc. **36**(1), 143–189 (2012)
24. Majchrzak, A., Lynne Markus, M.: Encyclopedia of Management Theory: Technology Affordances and Constraints Theory (of MIS), pp. 832–836. SAGE, Thousand Oaks (2013)
25. McKenna, B., Myers, M.D., Newman, M.: Social media in qualitative research: challenges and recommendations. Inf. Organ. **27**(2), 87–99 (2017)
26. Agostini, J.-M.: The case for direct questions on reading habits. J. Advert. Res. **2**, 28–33 (1964)
27. Porter, C.E., et al.: How to foster and sustain engagement in virtual communities. Calif. Manag. Rev. **53**(4), 80–110 (2011)
28. van Weezel, A., Benavides, C.: How to engage the audience? A study on using Twitter to engage newspaper readers. In: Friedrichsen, M., Mühl-Benninghaus, W. (eds.) Handbook of Social Media Management. MEDIA, pp. 703–713. Springer, Berlin (2013). https://doi.org/10.1007/978-3-642-28897-5_41
29. Lin, J., Ryaboy, D.: Scaling big data mining infrastructure: the Twitter experience. ACM SIGKDD Explor. Newslett. **14**(2), 6–19 (2013)
30. Tuten, T.L.: Advertising 2.0: Social Media Marketing in a Web 2.0 World. Praeger, London (2008)
31. Mangold, W.G., Faulds, D.J.: Social media: the new hybrid element of the promotion mix. Bus. Horiz. **52**(4), 357–365 (2009)
32. Vollmer, C., Precourt, G.: Always on: Advertising, Marketing, and Media in an Era of Consumer Control (Strategy + Business). McGraw-Hill, New York (2008)
33. Culnan, M.J., McHugh, P.J., Zubillaga, J.I.: How large US companies can use Twitter and other social media to gain business value. MIS Q. Exec. **9**(4), 243–259 (2010)
34. Ashley, C., Tuten, T.: Creative strategies in social media marketing: an exploratory study of branded social content and consumer engagement. Psychol. Mark. **32**(1), 15–27 (2015)
35. Gruzd, A., Haythornthwaite, C.: Enabling community through social media. J. Med. Internet Res. **15**(10), 248 (2013)
36. Gruzd, A., Mai, P., Kampen, A.: A how-to for using Netlytic to collect and analyze social media data: a case study of the use of Twitter during the 2014 Euromaidan Revolution in Ukraine. In: Sloan, L., Quan-Haase, A. (eds.) The SAGE Handbook of Social Media Research Methods, pp. 513–529. SAGE, Los Angeles (2017)
37. Wei, W., Miao, L., Huang, Z.J.: Customer engagement behaviors and hotel responses. Int. J. Hosp. Manag. **33**, 316–330 (2013)
38. Cabiddu, F., de Carlo, M., Piccoli, G.: Social media affordances: enabling customer engagement. Ann. Tour. Res. **48**, 175–192 (2014)
39. Bryman, A., Bell, E.: Business Research Methods. Oxford University Press, Oxford (2015)

# e-Government

# GE-government: A Geographic Information Based E-government Citizens' Adoption Framework

Hassan K. Dennaoui and Angelika I. Kokkinaki[✉]

46 Makedonitissas Avenue, Engomi, P.O. Box 24005, 1700 Nicosia, Cyprus
hassan.dennaoui@gmail.com, kokkinaki.a@unic.ac.cy

**Abstract.** The research aim is to investigate the Geographic Information (GI) influence on e-government adoption by citizens and introduce the GI based E-government citizens' adoption framework (GE-government). A thorough literature review was executed examining how GI is relevant to E-government services and identify the GI aspects that may affect e-government adoption by citizens. The literature review showed no evidence of any published e-government model considering GI as an independent factor having impact on e-government citizens' adoption. Moreover, it identified the most common E-government adoption influential factors. We studied the GI impact through the GE-government adoption model by assessing its significant influence. The research findings offered an additional value supporting the E-government's implementers in enhancing the E-government citizens' adoption. This paper proposes a factor that could affect E-government adoption modelling and has not been identified in the literature, so far. The paper concludes with a proposed framework and outlines future research.

**Keywords:** Geographic information · Geographic information system
Digital government · E-government · E-services · Adoption

## 1 Introduction

The aim of this research is to investigate the relevant importance of geographic information (GI) as an influential factor enriching the government e-services adoption models by citizens. More specifically, this research examined how GI affects e-government adoption and proposed a new GI-based e-government (GE-government) citizens' adoption framework. According to the literature review, there is no evidence of any published e-government citizens' adoption models considering GI as an independent factor having an impact (direct or indirect) on e-government citizens' adoption. The proposed GE-government citizens' adoption framework will offer the government the necessary guidance in order to increase the inhabitants' adoption of its e-services.

E-government, as per The World Bank Group [71], encompasses the use of E-government services that transform relations with citizens, businesses, and other arms of government. The e-government services can serve a variety of different ends: better delivery of government services to citizens, improved interactions with business and industry, citizen empowerment through access to information, or more efficient

© Springer Nature Switzerland AG 2019
M. Themistocleous and P. Rupino da Cunha (Eds.): EMCIS 2018, LNBIP 341, pp. 283–301, 2019.
https://doi.org/10.1007/978-3-030-11395-7_24

government management. E-government employment may lead to less corruption, increased transparency, greater convenience, revenue growth, and/or cost reductions. Studies on the subject have been conducted in different contexts including developed countries [18, 25, 51, 59, 60] as well as in developing countries [32, 44].

A reoccurring theme in many studies is the development and examination of adoption models for E-government initiatives, which are based on adoption theories [19, 55, 67]. As substantiated by the extensive literature review we have conducted, proposed e-government adoption models that study the impact over the users' adoption for the government E-services, have not taken under consideration the influence of Geographic Information.

Geographic Information (GI), as defined by Goodchild [27], refers to the location or information linked to a place or property on or near Earth and the knowledge about the location of something and its description at a specific time or time interval. GI was represented historically as the information available or stored on paper maps or in analogue format.

Recently, GI has been used widely in advanced Information Systems and E-services like E-land Administration System, E-tourism System, Disaster Management System, and many others, to provide the potential users with advanced usability, flexibility, usefulness, information accuracy while at the same time maintain less complexity. Therefore, GI coupled with relevant tools and applications are expected to influence interactions among different stakeholders in various societal settings over the time [28].

In this paper, together with the main influential factors as identified in the literature, we also examine whether there is evidence to suggest that the GI factor exercises influence over the E-government adoption and if so what aspects of it could be proposed for a new GI based E-government citizens' adoption framework. The remaining of this paper is structured as follows. Section two introduces a brief literature review section about the E-government, the GI related components that are relevant as well as GI aspects that relate to E-government services adoption. Section three introduces a conceptual model for the GI based E-government adoption framework with a brief on the identified influential factors. Section four outlines the main research findings and in section five the paper concludes with future research direction.

## 2  Literature Review: E-government, Geographic Information and Their Interrelation

The E-government dimensions, as described by Bonham [11], Fang [24], Yildiz [73], Reddick [54], Ramaswamy and Selian [53], Turban [63], ITU [40], Chavan and Rathod [16], Ashaye and Irani [10], are the following:

- Government to Government – G2G
- Government to Businesses – G2B
- Government to Citizens – G2C
- Government-to-Nonprofit (G2 N)
- Government-to-Employee (G2E)

- Government-to-Civil Societal Organizations (G2CS)
- Citizen-to-Citizen (C2C)

The World Bank Group [71] definition covers multiple perspectives including Information Technology, Reforming Public Sector, Relationship with partners, Benefits, Dimensions, Political Reasons and Citizens Focus. This definition is totally aligned with the research objective of studying the E-government Citizens' adoption models and the importance of using the Geospatial Technology to enhance the Citizens adoption of the E-government services and fortify the G2C (Government to Citizen) dimension relation.

According to Rogers [55] definition, Adoption is the decision of "full use of an innovation as the best course of action available". A detailed literature review on technology adoption theories has been conducted derived from the need for a thorough understanding of the adoption theories origins and an overview of some key adoption theories used in the technology, business, and many other sectors to assess the success of any concept implementation. Many technology adoption theories were adopted and validated over the last four decades to understand the user's technology acceptance [37, 67] where user can be an individual, household, organization or community. The three main technology adoption theories and models: include Technology Acceptance Model – TAM [19], Diffusion of Innovation theory – DOI [55] and Unified Theory of Acceptance and Use of Technology – UTAUT [67].

Factors influencing the citizens and overall society to adopt E-government technology have been studied by Carter and Bélanger [15] and Warkentin et al. [69] including the "intention" by Gilbert [26] and the "willingness" of the citizens to use E-government and many adoption models have been proposed and tested between 2005 (Web 2.0 official launching [51]) and 2016 in developing and developed countries (countries categorization according to the World Bank). We have identified that most of the identified models used TAM described by Venkatesh and Davis [65] as the most "well-established, well-tested, powerful, robust and parsimonious model for predicting user acceptance of technology". As the TAM is testing the adoption of technology at the individual level [17], and since we are assessing the citizens' technology adoption, the upcoming conceptual G-government Citizen's Adoption model will be based on the TAM [19], considered as one of top mature Technology Adoption Models, widely used and tested over the last two decades in various information systems including E-services.

Social factors, including Word of Mouth – WOM [7], Favoritism – FA [6, 7], Digital Divide – DD [5, 7], Website Design – WD [6, 7], Internet & Computer Skills Confidence – ICSC [6, 7], Fear of Job Loss Belief – FJLB [7], Religious Belief – RB [7], Attitude – AT [7, 71], Resistance to Change – RC [57], Trust in Internet – TI [7, 32] and Trust in Government – TG [14, 32] were also considered as potential influential factors on the E-government citizens' adoption and tested in almost all the E-government citizens' adoption models. Accordingly, the "Social", representing the grouping of the social factors, will be inserted in the conceptual GE-government Citizen's Adoption model and tested in order to extract the significant influential social factors over the E-government citizens' adoption.

Moreover, some demographic factors, including Gender – GE [5, 68, 71], Age – AG [5, 7, 68, 71], Level of Income – LI [1, 7] and Level of Education – LE [5, 7, 62, 68] were considered also as potential influential factors on the E-government citizens' adoption and tested in various E-government citizens' adoption models. Accordingly, the "Demographics", representing the grouping of the demographic factors, will be inserted in the conceptual G-government Citizen's Adoption model and tested in order to extract the significant influential demographic factors over the E-government citizens' adoption.

The interrelation between E-government adoption and Geographical Information has not been formally studied, yet in our literature review, we have identified E-services that incorporate GI technologies and are used widely by citizens. A few indicative examples follow.

There is a wide range of Disaster Management Systems (DMS) that are geo-enabled Crowd-sourced Emergency Services, currently used to improve the response of the government to an incident, critical event or disaster. Through such systems, citizens collaborate dynamically, employ geospatial E-government services, and ultimately support the governmental disaster/emergency agencies through a variety of means. It is worth noting that situational awareness is improved by the assimilation of accurate real-time geo-information via the DMS's interactive map that extends incidents' location with all relevant and supportive spatial and non-spatial information so to enhance the on-event decision making, improve the future analysis of the government's response to disasters & Incidents and support the proper development of a preventive disaster management plans [12, 30]. Another interesting GI-based E-service is the Complaints Management System that increased the response efficiency of the local government. A case study that demonstrates such potentials is the adoption of a Complaints Management System in Amsterdam in 2007; citizens' complaints were addressed within two working days for 80% of the reported incidents. The improved throughout was attributed to the accurate pinpointing of the relevant location in the incident or complaint that significantly affected the operational response process [33, 35, 61]. The E-participation application is another Web GI based E-government application is usually launched by local governments and municipalities to offer their citizens expected capabilities; for example, citizens have the ability to visualize the urban planning of any new development, submit their feedback and reactions to what is proposed, chat and communicate with local government decision makers and thus improving the citizens' participation in all governments' future policy making and service delivery [38, 47, 49, 61].

A variety of GI-based E-tourism Applications exist and some are included in e-governmental platforms dedicated to tourism. These services include advanced querying capabilities like the nearest facilities, search by address, identification of the shortest route between two points of interest, and develop a Tour plan with multiple scenarios (html5). Very recently, those applications support 3D displaying of the touristic sites in order to offer more attractions to tourists as well as increase their familiarity with the sites to be visited. As part of the experience sharing, those applications support the insertion of blogs or reviews on each visited site as a kind of sharing the travelers' experience [46, 52, 58, 73]. Lately, many countries started the adoption of the GI-based E-elections Management Application, a geospatial based E-government application that offers services for the pre-election period, as well as after the electoral process is finished. Some indicative pre-election services include the online registration of voters, retrieval of information about the election process or procedure such as the Voters' (Citizens') location, the polling station, the shortest path to the polling station with directions, location of the voters' assemblies, location of the buses, taxis or any available transportation system with schedules and routes, etc. Situation Analysis is also supported and the results may be visualised in maps, plots and reports in real time. Such visual representation enhances the citizens' capability of sharing their observations and opinion about the overall election procedure and execution directly on the application or through the integration with the social media apps [9, 23, 31, 39].

Through the cases mentioned above, it is evident that the impact of the GI enabled E-services on citizens' adoption of such services should be examined in more detail. Accordingly, There is a need to test the impact of the GI based E-services and applications over the adoption of E-government services among citizens and therefore it is interesting to develop a framework for examining such adoption influences more thoroughly.

## 3 GE-Government: E-government Citizens' Adoption Framework Encompassing Geographic Information

The factors having influence over citizens' adoption, as identified in the literature, include the TAM adoption theory factors, Perceived Ease of Use and Perceived Usefulness, Social factors as well as demographics. We considered GI factor as an independent potential direct and moderate influential factor over the independent TAM factors, the Website Design social factor and direct influential factor over the E-government citizens' adoption dependent factor. Figure 1 illustrates the different elements of the GE-government Citizens' Adoption conceptual framework. In this research, we have tested the proposed framework with regards to the significance of the GI factor's role in enhancing the E government adoption and the research findings are summarized in the next section.

Table 1 summarizes the proposed hypotheses as well as the relevant independent and dependent factors.

Since there is a need to assess the impact of various factors on the E-government citizens' adoption and study those factors' impact on a large sample, a survey has been conducted based on 446 questionnaire collected out of 500 distributed where the convenient sampling method has been applied since the survey's participants were selected from public and private organizations and agencies that we have access to. The developed questionnaire was partially based on previous research as identified in the literature, with close ended questions following the Five-point Likert scale for all non-demographic questions. Content validity has been employed to examine the validity of the research instrument through face-to-face interviews with 3 experts in the relevant fields. Following that, a pilot test with 10 respondents was conducted. A cover letter was attached with the questionnaire to clarify the purpose of conducting this research survey.

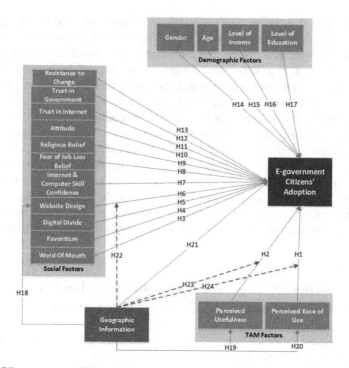

**Fig. 1.** GE-government (GI based E-government) citizens' adoption conceptual framework

**Table 1.** Summary of proposed hypotheses

| HN | Research hypothesis | Ind. factor | Dep. factor |
|---|---|---|---|
| H1 | High level of perceived ease of use has positive influence on the E-government citizens' adoption | PEOU | EGovAdop |
| H2 | High level of perceived usefulness has positive influence on the E-government citizens' adoption | PU | EGovAdop |
| H3 | High level of positive word of mouth has positive influence on the E-government citizens' adoption | WOM | EGovAdop |
| H4 | Low level of favouritism has positive influence on the E-government citizens' adoption | FA | EGovAdop |
| H5 | Digital divide has influence on the E-government citizens' adoption | DD | EGovAdop |
| H6 | High level of website design has positive influence on the E-government citizens' adoption | WD | EGovAdop |
| H7 | High level of internet & computer skills Confidence has positive influence on the E-government citizens' adoption | ICSC | EGovAdop |

(continued)

**Table 1.** (*continued*)

| HN | Research hypothesis | Ind. factor | Dep. factor |
|---|---|---|---|
| H8 | Low level of fear of job loss belief has positive influence on the E-government citizens' adoption | FJLB | EGovAdop |
| H9 | Low level of religious belief has positive influence on the E-government citizens' adoption | RB | EGovAdop |
| H10 | High level of positive attitude has positive influence on the E-government citizens' adoption | AT | EGovAdop |
| H11 | High level of trust in Internet has positive influence on the E-government citizens' adoption | TI | EGovAdop |
| H12 | High level of trust in government has positive influence on the E-government citizens' adoption | TG | EGovAdop |
| H13 | Low level of resistance to change has positive influence on the E-government citizens' adoption | RTC | EGovAdop |
| H14 | Male is more E-government adopter than Female gender | GE | EGovAdop |
| H15 | Younger and middle age are more E-government adopters than older age groups | AG | EGovAdop |
| H16 | Higher level of income are more E-government adopters than lower Level of Income groups | LI | EGovAdop |
| H17 | Higher level of education are more E-government adopters than lower Level of Education groups | LE | EGovAdop |
| H18 | The GI has influence over the website design of the E-government applications | GI | WD |
| H19 | The GI has influence over the perceived usefulness of the E-government applications | GI | PU |
| H20 | The GI has influence over the perceived ease of use of the E-government applications | GI | PEOU |
| H21 | GI has positive influence on the E-government citizens' adoption | GI | EGovAdop |
| H22 | The GI increase the level of positive influence of the website design on the E-government citizens' adoption | GI & WD | EGovAdop |
| H23 | The GI increase the level of positive influence of the perceived usefulness on the E-government Citizens' Adoption | GI & PU | EGovAdop |
| H24 | The GI increase the level of positive influence of the perceived ease of use on the E-government citizens' adoption | GI & PEOU | EGovAdop |

A multivariate statistical approach, that is Exploratory Factor Analysis (EFA), was used because it offers the advanced statistical tools that help the researcher in measuring (a) the independent variables' influence (Social except digital divide, TAM and GI factors) over the corresponding measured dependent variable (E-government Adoption), (b) the strength & correlation between the independent variables and the corresponding measured dependent variable, and (c) the depth, breadth & validity of the measurement scales [71, 75]. This statistical technique is widely where many E-government researchers have used it including but not limited to: Alomari [7], Harfouche [75], Al-Shafi and Weerakkody [8].

A Binary Logistic Regression Modelling Analysis (BLRMA), also employed in Harfouche [75], Al-Shafi and Weerakkody [8] for analysing the relationship between one dependent variable (binary variable) and multiple independent variables (Malhotra [74]), has been followed in order to analyse the relation between the E-government citizens' adoption dependent variable (binary variable) and the independent variables (Social except digital divide, TAM and GI) identified in the conceptual framework. The data analysis process continued by using the Pearson Chi-square statistical tool that tests the relationship between two categorical variables whether they are binary (two categories) or more than two categories [75]. Accordingly, the Pearson Chi-square was first used to analyse the relation between the GI independent variables and the other 3 independent variables (Website Design, Perceived Usefulness and Perceived Ease of Use) within the conceptual framework. The study of those relationships helps in getting clear response to the proposed research questions. Then, the Pearson Chi-square was used to explore the impact of the Demographic and Digital Divide variables (independent categorical variables) on the E-government Adoption (binary variable).

During the data analysis process, a third validity technique, the construct validity, was used to measure and rate, from the responses of the participants, (i) the degree of influence of each factor in the proposed framework over the E-government citizens' adoption, (ii) the degree of influence of the geographic information factor in the proposed framework over the E-government citizens' adoption, (iii) the degree of influence or moderation of the GI over other factors.

Finally, the data representation process followed by developing charts, graphs, tables and statistics in order to give figures and number for further interpretation.

Therefore, the GE-government citizens' adoption conceptual framework has been developed based on TAM model and the Literature Review has identified the influential E-government citizens' adoption factors and a list of hypothesis has been proposed for testing and interpretation. Hence, we have (i) selected a large and representative sample of the targeted population for latter generalization purposes, (ii) collected their response on the formal close ended addressed questions already deducted in majority from previous researchers' questions, (iii) analysed the collected feedback and (iv) interpreted the final results that should highlight the accepted and rejected proposed hypothesis. Therefore, this study (a) relied on a large collected data that is heavily expressed in numerical forms and (b) required complex statistical analysis to study, in the proposed conceptual framework, each measurable variable or factor influence over the citizens including the GI factor as well as the correlation between those factors.

# 4   Research Findings

Five hundred survey questionnaires were distributed, while 446 were collected with fully filled questions, during the period of October – November 2016 which represents a successful questionnaire collection rate of 89.2%. From the collected questionnaires, only 409 were actually used for the analysis representing 91.7% of the total collected questionnaires since the remaining (8.3%) belongs to participants who responded to be oblivious to any E-government services (2.5%) or be unaware of any Geographic Information or mapping services (2.5%) or both (3.3%).

From the (409) accepted participants who are aware of the E-government and Geographic Information, a percentage of (83.4%) used the E-government services previously whereas the rest (16.6%) did not. Furthermore, (88%) of our survey participants had used Geographic Information services before and (12%) did not.

The participants were (55.3%) male and (44.7%) female with a majority of respondents between 20 and 50 years old (91.6%). The majority of the respondents have a level of income between 500 and 2,500 USD (79.7%). In addition, the majority of the respondents are well educated with a minimum College degree (90.9%), where (57.1%) participants are holders of Higher Education degree. The religion of the participants was (66.7%) Muslims, (26.5%) Christians and (6.8%) decided not to disclose their religion. (55.5%) of the respondents are working in the private sector and around (15.9%) selected the "Other" response option corresponding to an "Employee in Public or Private Sector" participant's owner of a small business. (69.9%) of the respondents live in Cities or urban areas and (30.1%) live in villages or rural areas. Almost all the respondents have internet access in their region of residence (98.8%). The survey shows that (44.4%) of the respondents prefer the use of internet at home, (16.4%) at work and the (39.6%) have not expressed any preference. In addition, (55.6%) of the respondents prefer to execute their E-government transactions at home, (20%) at work and (24.4%) did not have any preference. Finally, we can realize that the majority of respondents prefer to use the tools that offer mobility such as mobile, tablet and laptop (76.8%), (11.5%) prefer to use the desktop and (11.7%) has no preference.

## 4.1   Framework Testing

The research questionnaire reliability was tested using the Reliability Analysis test in SPSS which calculate the Cronbach's coefficient alpha values for the overall questionnaire and the research framework's factors. According to Field [76] and Hinton et al. [77], the Cronbach's coefficient alpha measures the reliability and examines the inter-consistency of the data collected. Moreover, Hinton et al. [77] proposed four reliability categories based on a value range: Excellent Reliability (above 0.9), High Reliability (0.7–0.9), High Moderate Reliability (0.5–0.7) and Low Reliability (below 0.50). The overall questionnaire Cronbach's coefficient alpha value, based on 20 standardized items/questions, is 0.846 considered as High Reliability value.

To identify the factors' potential grouping according to their correlation, the Exploratory Factor Analysis (EFA) was executed using the Principal Component Analysis (PCA) extraction method with the Varimax – Kaiser Normalization Rotation Method. The EFA will help in identifying the factors that can be grouped together in common components, having relationships between each other, in order to be analyzed separately using the Binary Logistic Regression Analysis. The EFA performed on the 16 independent variables or 5 – Likert Scale items, proposed as the potential influential factors over the dependent variable EGovAdop in the Literature Review, shows a KMO (Kaiser-Meyer-Olkin) of (0.812) considered as high and acceptable, since it exceeds the (0.5) minimum value required to accept the PCA Factor Analysis results, and a Bartlett's Test of Sphericity with high significance (0.000). The EFA results discovered the existence of 16 components where only 4 components have eigenvalues exceeding 1, considered as important components for analysis according to Hair et al. (1998). The Table 2 shows the initial eigenvalues and the total variance of the 4 components extracted.

**Table 2.** Initial eigenvalues & total variance with 16 items

| Comp. | Initial eigenvalues | | | Extraction sums of sq. loadings | | | Rotation sums of sq. loadings | | |
|---|---|---|---|---|---|---|---|---|---|
| | Total | % of Var. | Cum. % | Total | % of Var. | Cum. % | Total | % of Var. | Cum. % |
| 1 | 4.687 | 29.296 | 29.296 | 4.687 | 29.296 | 29.296 | 2.536 | 15.853 | 15.853 |
| 2 | 1.545 | 9.658 | 38.954 | 1.545 | 9.658 | 38.954 | 2.358 | 14.736 | 30.589 |
| 3 | 1.387 | 8.669 | 47.623 | 1.387 | 8.669 | 47.623 | 2.298 | 14.361 | 44.950 |
| 4 | 1.072 | 6.697 | 54.320 | 1.072 | 6.697 | 54.320 | 1.499 | 9.370 | 54.320 |

The Table 3 shows the distribution of the 16 factors across the four extracted components having a factor loading of above (0.4), defined as the minimum preferable in the IS research (Carter et al. [78], Dwivedi et al. [79], Straub et al. [80]) except for the ICSC factor (0.388), and with no cross-loading of the variables where none exceeds the (0.4) in the other components.

**Table 3.** EFA factors loading with 16 items

| Factors | PEOU | PU | WOM | FA | WD | ICSC | FJLB | RB | AT | TI | TG | RC | GI&WD | GI&PU | GI&PEOU | GI |
|---|---|---|---|---|---|---|---|---|---|---|---|---|---|---|---|---|
| 1 | 0.723 | 0.769 | 0.609 | 0.595 | 0.490 | | | | | | | | | | | |
| 2 | | | | | | | | | | | | | 0.515 | 0.716 | 0.836 | 0.761 |
| 3 | | | | | | 0.388 | | 0.692 | 0.548 | 0.666 | 0.677 | | | | | |
| 4 | | | | | | 0.839 | 0.794 | | | | | | | | | |

The Internet & Computer Skills Confidence (ICSC) independent variable, having a factor loading less than (0.4) has been removed and thus the relevant hypothesis (H7) was automatically rejected. Accordingly, the above analysis indicates the following:

- The Component 1 groups the Technology Adoption Model (TAM) factors PEOU & PU with WOM, FA and WD social factors.
- The Component 2 groups the GI based factors, GIWDEGov, GIPUEGov, GIPEOUEGov and GIEGovAdop, related directly to the dependent EGovAdop.
- The Component 3 groups the Trustworthiness social factors TI & TG with AT and RTC social factors, and the ICSC will be removed from the Component 3 factors as having a factor loading less than (0.4).
- The Component 4 groups only the Belief social FJLB and RB factors together.
- All the components except the Component2 are totally or partially of social factors.
- All the factors, with factor loading exceeding 0.4 and no cross-load across the other components, are valid and thus the data collected and the results can be considered as reliable and valid.

Based on the EFA results, we started the test of the E-government Citizens' Adoption Framework through various testing method on the framework's influential factors:

- The four components extracted from the EFA – PCA were tested using the Binary Logistic Regression.
- The Pearson Chi-square was performed to check the correlation between the GI independent factor and the other three independent factors (WD, PU and PEOU).
- The Pearson Chi-square was applied in order to examine the relation between the Demographics' factors and the EGovAdop dependent factor.
- All the tested factors were analysed according to their relevant proposed hypotheses in Chapter 4 – Conceptual Framework.

The overall GE-government Citizens' Adoption Framework was tested with a df (number of factors tested) equal to 15 representing the independent factors defined as potential influential factors over the E-government Citizens' Adoption (EGovAdop) dependent factor. The model significance (Sig.) was equal to (0.000) which confirms the excellent model fit, the model $-2$ Log likelihood was equal to (174.008) which indicates that model fits well and the Cox-Snell R2 was equal to (0.243). The Sig. value, calculated for the overall model based on Hosmer-Lemeshow goodness-of-fit test and for the components based on the Omnibus tests of model Coefficient, represents the P value that should be less than (0.05) to consider the factor, component or model significant. The $-2$ Log likelihood, that should be a small value close to 0, reflects how much the model or the component fits. The Cox-Snell R2, ranging from 0 to 1, measures how well the prediction of the dependent factor based on the independent factors and should be bigger enough from 0. The results of the Binary Logistic Regression are summarized in the Table 4:

**Table 4.** Binary logistic regression extracts

| HN | Factors | Coef. (B) | df | Sig. (P) | Odd Ratio (Exp. B) | Confidence (95%) Interval | |
|----|---------|-----------|----|----------|--------------------|---------------------------|--|
| | | | | | | Lower | Upper |
| H1 | PEOU | - 0.095 | 1 | 0.688 | 0.909 | 0.570 | 1.449 |
| H2 | PU | 0.553 | 1 | 0.033 | 1.738 | 1.045 | 2.888 |
| H3 | WOM | 0.631 | 1 | 0.002 | 1.879 | 1.265 | 2.791 |
| H4 | FA | 0.301 | 1 | 0.074 | 1.352 | 0.972 | 1.880 |
| H6 | WD | 0.281 | 1 | 0.202 | 1.324 | 0.860 | 2.040 |
| H21 | GI | 1.202 | 1 | 0.000 | 3.328 | 1.941 | 5.704 |
| H22 | GI & WD | 0.673 | 1 | 0.002 | 1.960 | 1.277 | 3.010 |
| H23 | GI & PU | - 0.185 | 1 | 0.491 | 0.831 | 0.490 | 1.407 |
| H24 | GI & PEOU | - 0.063 | 1 | 0.816 | 0.939 | 0.553 | 1.595 |
| H10 | AT | 0.525 | 1 | 0.011 | 1.690 | 1.127 | 2.535 |
| H11 | TI | - 0.332 | 1 | 0.172 | 0.718 | 0.446 | 1.156 |
| H12 | TG | 0.882 | 1 | 0.000 | 2.415 | 1.490 | 3.914 |
| H13 | RTC | 0.556 | 1 | 0.010 | 1.744 | 1.141 | 2.666 |
| H8 | FJLB | - 0.475 | 1 | 0.003 | 0.622 | 0.452 | 0.855 |
| H9 | RB | - 0.320 | 1 | 0.032 | 0.726 | 0.542 | 0.972 |

The results of the Pearson Chi-Square results are summarized in the Table 5:

In this study, we have tested and identified, through various analysis tools such as Exploratory Factor Analysis – PCA, Binary Logistic Regression and Pearson Chi-Square, the factors that have significant influence over the E-government Adoption. The Table 6 shows the proposed hypotheses along with the test result which classify every hypothesis as accepted or rejected hypothesis.

Based on the Table 6 findings, the GI based E-government (GE-government) Citizens' Adoption conceptual framework was adjusted and the final GI based E-government (GE-government) Citizens' Adoption framework is illustrated in the Fig. 2.

**Table 5.**  Pearson chi-square extracts

| Factor1 | Factor2 | Asymp. Sig. 2 sided (P) | Pearson Chi-Square Value | Contingency Coefficient | |
|---|---|---|---|---|---|
| | | | | Approx. Sig. | Value |
| GI | PEOU | 0.000 | 125.254 | 0.000 | 0.484 |
| GI | PU | 0.007 | 33.089 | 0.007 | 0.274 |
| GI | WD | 0.000 | 205.506 | 0.000 | 0.578 |
| EGov Adop | Gender | 0.079 | 3.087 | - | - |

| Factor1 | Factor2 | Asymp. Sig. 2 sided (P) | Pearson Chi-Square Value | Contingency Coefficient | |
|---|---|---|---|---|---|
| | | | | Approx. Sig. | Value |
| EGov Adop | Age | 0.000 | 31.947 | 0.000 | 0.482 |
| EGov Adop | LI | 0.536 | 3.135 | - | - |
| EGov Adop | LE | 0.000 | 47.325 | 0.000 | 0.322 |

**Table 6.**  Summary of tested hypotheses

| HN | Hypothesis Accepted | HN | Hypothesis Accepted |
|---|---|---|---|
| H1 | NO | H13 | YES |
| H2 | YES | H14 | NO |
| H3 | YES | H15 | YES |
| H4 | NO | H16 | NO |
| H5 | YES | H17 | YES |
| H6 | NO | H18 | YES |
| H7 | NO | H19 | YES |
| H8 | YES | H20 | YES |
| H9 | YES | H21 | YES |
| H10 | YES | H22 | YES |
| H11 | NO | H23 | NO |
| H12 | YES | H24 | NO |

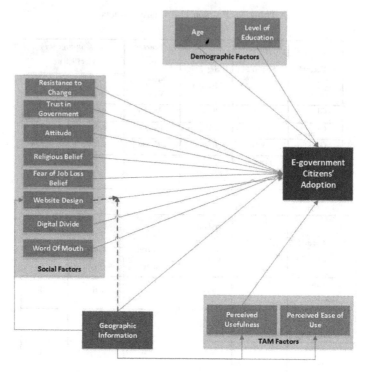

**Fig. 2.** Final GE-government citizens' adoption framework

## 5   Conclusion

The essential aim of this research was to assess the role of the Geographic Information (GI) in E-government Citizens' Adoption. Previously, most of the researcher looked at the Geographic Information, based on its GIS component, as part of the IT factor and assessed its impact on the E-government implementation, where in this research we highlighted on the existence of the Geographic Information as a concept and focused on its impact on the E-government adoption. We have set various objectives that cover all the research aspects including the introduction of a new e-government adoption framework and identification of all the e-government adoption influential significant factors. Between the conceptual and the final e-government citizens' adoption research framework, many hypotheses were rejected, some proposed factors were removed and the remaining factors were retained and identified as significant influential factors according to the study executed in Lebanon. The research findings confirm the relation between the Geographic Information and the E-government citizens' adoption by identifying a new factor, Geographic Information, as influential over the citizens' adoption of the government E-services. Also, it proposes the GE-government Adoption framework to be considered as a new framework in the E-government adoption. This needs to be examined further in the future. We could identify various direct and moderate influential role of the GI factor over the E-government adoption. The GI factor shows a strong direct influence over the E-government adoption, strong direct influence over the Website design, Perceived Ease of Use and less over the Perceived Usefulness, and finally a strong moderate indirect role over the Website Design which has been considered as non-influential as a standalone factor but turned into influential factor when associated to GI. Therefore, the GI should be considered in any future studies and included, as potential influential factor, in any new E-government proposed conceptual frameworks to assess and examine its influential role over the E-government adoption in both developed and developing countries as it showed strong significant, direct and moderate, role over various factors in the current research setting. This research has contributed in theory and practice to the e-government through many perspectives.

In theory, we have introduced a new E-government (GE-Government) citizens' adoption framework, we confirmed the geographic information influential role over the e-government adoption, we identified a significant relation between website design and perceived ease of use as well as a significant relation between fear of job loss and religious belief, and finally a significant relation between attitude, trust in government and resistance to change. Such theoretical findings need to be examined in deep in any future research.

In practice, the research contributes in three main perspectives. The first practical perspective is about the availability of a new GE-government framework ready to be tested in developed and developing countries to evaluate the impact of various factors mainly the GI in order to build an e-government implementation plan, before any new e-services' implementations or upgrades that guarantee citizens' adoption. The second practical contribution lies mainly in the role of the geographic information in improving the e-government adoption and enhancing the e-government websites design, simplicity and usefulness. The research shows a strong citizens' intention to use the e-government websites if empowered by the GI components, mainly mapping component, since it gives a more appealing design to the users. The final practical contribution lies in the identification of the group of people that the government should target when promoting its services or preparing its e-government's awareness marketing roadmap and campaigns, showing a concentration within the young to middle aged citizens' groups having at least a college degree or higher.

# References

1. Abu Nadi, I.K. Sanzogni, L. Sandhu, K., Woods, P.: Success factors contributing to E-government adoption in Saudi Arabia. SIIC J. (2008)
2. Akkaya, C., Wolf, P., Krcmar, H.: A comprehensive analysis of E-government adoption in the german household. In: 11th International Conference on Wirtschafts informatik, 27th February – 01st March 2013, Leipzig, Germany (2013)
3. Al Awadhi, S., Morris, A.: Factors influencing the adoption of E-government services. J. Softw. **4**, 584–590 (2009)
4. Al Hujran, O., Aloudat, A., Altarawneh, I.: Factors influencing citizen adoption of E-government in developing countries: the case of jordan. Int. J. Technol. Hum. Interact. **9**(2), 1–19 (2013)

5. Alateyah, S.A., Crowder, R.M., Wills, G.B.: Identified factors affecting the citizen's intention to adopt E-government in Saudi Arabia. World Acad. Sci. Eng. Technol. Int. J. Soc. Bus. Psychol. Hum. Sci. Eng. **7**(8), 244–252 (2013)

6. Alghamdi, S., Beloff, N.: Innovative framework for E-government adoption in Saudi Arabia: a study from the business sector perspective. Int. J. Adv. Comput. Sci. Appl. **7**(1), 655–664 (2016)

7. Alomari, M.K.: Discovering citizens reaction toward EGOVERNMENT: factors in E-government adoption. JISTEM – J. Inf. Syst. Technol. Manag. **11**(1), 05–20 (2014)

8. Al-Shafi, S., Weerakkody, V.: E-government Adoption in Qatar: investigating the citizens' perspective. J. Comput. Inf. Syst. (2009)

9. Aphane, J.: Delimitation, voter registration and election results – a modern day GIS perspective. In: Geospatial Africa 2015, South Africa (2015)

10. Ashaye, O.R., Irani, Z.: E-government implementation factors: a conceptual framework. J. Mod. Account. Audit. **10**(2), 241–247 (2014)

11. Bonham, G., Seifert, J., Thorson, S.: The transformational potential of E-government: the role of political leadership. In: The 4th Pan European International Relations Conference of the European Consortium for Political Research, University of Kent, Canterbury, UK (2001)

12. Bott, M., Young, G.: Croudsourcing for better governance: the role of crowdsourcing for better governance in international development. Fletcher J. Hum. Secur. **27**, 47–70 (2012)

13. Brynard, P.A., Hanekom, S.X.: Introduction to Research in Public Administration. Van Schaik (1997)

14. Bwalya, K.J.: Determining factors influencing e-government development in the developing world: a case study of Zambia. J. e-Gov. Stud. Best Pract. (2017)

15. Carter, L., Bélanger, F.: The utilization of e-government services: citizen trust, innovation and acceptance factors. Inf. Syst. J. **15**, 5–26 (2005)

16. Chavan, G.R., Rathod, M.L.: E-governance and its implementation. SRELS J. Inf. Manag. **46**(1), 17–24 (2009)

17. Chong, A.Y.L., Ooi, K.B., Lin, B.S., Raman, M.: Factors affecting the adoption level of c-commerce: an empirical study. J. Comput. Inf. Syst. **50**(2), 13–22 (2009)

18. Davidrajuh, R.: Realizing a new e-commerce tool for formation of a virtual enterprise. Ind. Manag. Data Syst. **103**, 434–445 (2003)

19. Davis, F.D.: Perceived usefulness, perceived ease of use, and user acceptance of information technology. MIS Q. **13**, 319–340 (1989)

20. Davis, F.D.: Perceived usefulness, perceived ease of use, and user acceptance of information technology. MIS Q. **13**(3), 319–340 (1989)

21. Dimitrova, D.V., Beilock, R.: Where freedom matters: Internet adoption among the formerly socialist countries. Gaz.: Int. J. Commun. Stud. **67**(2), 173–187 (2005)

22. Evans, D., Yen, D.C.: E-government: an analysis for implementation: framework for understanding cultural and social impact. Gov. Inf. Q. **22**(3), 354–373 (2005)

23. Everton, N., Waithaka, H., Watene, G.: A distributed geospatial information system for managing elections: a case study of Kenya. Int. J. Sci. Res. (IJSR) **2**(9), 158–161 (2013)

24. Fang, Z.: E-government in digital era: concept, practice, and development. Int. J. Comput. Internet Manag. **10**(2), 1–22 (2002)

25. Frank, L.: Architecture for integration of distributed ERP systems and e-commerce systems. Ind. Manag. Data Syst. **104**, 418–429 (2004)

26. Gilbert, D., Balestrini, P.: Barriers and benefits in the adoption of E-government. Int. J. Public Sect. Manag. **17**(4), 286–301 (2004)

27. Goodchild, M.: Twenty years of progress: GIScience in 2010. J. Spat. Inf. Sci. **1**, 3–20 (2010)

28. Goodchild, M., Palladino, J.R.: Geographic information system as a tool in science and technology education. Specul. Sci. Technol. **18**, 278–286 (1995)
29. Goodchild, M.F.: Geographic information systems. In: Hanson, S. (ed.) Ten Geographic Ideas that Changed the World, pp. 60–86. Rutgers University Press, New Brunswick (1997)
30. Grant, A., Razdan, R., Shang, T.: Coordinates for change: how GIS technology and geospatial analytics can improve city services. Government Designed for New Times, 32–43 (2012)
31. Gupta, A.K.C., Kumar, P., Kumar, N.V.: Development of geospatial map based election portal. In: The 2014 ISPRS Technical Commission VIII Symposium International Archives of the Photogrammetry, Remote Sensing and Spatial Information Sciences, vol. 10, Hyderabad, India, pp. 1149–1152 (2014)
32. Gupta, K.P., Singh, S., Bhaskar, P.: Citizen adoption of E-government: a literature review and conceptual framework. Electron. Gov. Int. J. **12**(2), 160–185 (2016)
33. Hassan, A.A.: E-grievance System in Local Government: Case Study, Amsterdam, The Netherlands, International Institute for Geo-information Science and Earth Observation, University of Twente (2010)
34. Heeks, R.: Information systems and developing countries: Failure, success, and local improvisations. Inf. Soc. **18**, 101–112 (2002)
35. Hickel, C., Blankenbach, J.: From Local SDI to E-government, case study in municipalities in the south of Hesse, FIG Working week (2012)
36. Hofheinz, A.: The internet in the Arab World: playground for political liberalization. IPG J. (2005)
37. Hu, P.J., Chau, P.Y.K., Sheng, O.R.L., Tam, K.Y.: Examining the technology acceptance model using physician acceptance of telemedicine technology. J. Manag. Inf. Syst. **16**, 91–112 (1999)
38. Ijeh, A.: Geofencing as a Tool for Urban Planning, UN-HBITAT E-Governance and Urban Policy Design in Developing Countries Report, 84–102 (2014)
39. International IDEA: An Overview of the Electoral Risk Management Tool (ERM Tool), Stockholm, Sweden (2013)
40. ITU E-government Implementation Toolkit: A Framework for e-Government Readiness and Action Priorities 1 (2009)
41. Kamal, M.M., Themistocleous, M.: A conceptual model for EAI Adoption in an E-government Environment. In: Paper presented at the European and Mediterranean Conference on Information Systems (EMCIS), Costa Blanca, Spain (2006)
42. Kim, K., Prabhakar, B.: Initial trust and the adoption of B2C E-commerce: the case of internet banking. ACM Sigmis Database **35**, 50–64 (2004)
43. Kumar, R., Best, M.L.: Impact and sustainability of E-government services in developing countries: lessons learned from Tamil Nadu, India. Inf. Soc. **22**(1), 1–12 (2006)
44. Kurunananda, A., Weerakkody, V.: E-government Implementation in Sri Lanka: lessons from the UK. In: Proceedings of the 8th International Information Technology Conference, Colombo, Sri Lanka (2006)
45. Maguire, D.J.: GIS: A tool or science. Birmingham City University UK (2010)
46. Marson, T., Badaruddin, M., Azizan, M.: GIS base tourism decision support system for Langkawi Island, Kedah, Malaysia. Theor. Empir. Res. Urban Manag. **10**(2), 21–35 (2015)
47. Moody, Rebeccca: Assessing the role of GIS in E-government: a tale of E-participation in two cities. In: Wimmer, Maria A., Scholl, Jochen, Grönlund, Åke (eds.) EGOV 2007. LNCS, vol. 4656, pp. 354–365. Springer, Heidelberg (2007). https://doi.org/10.1007/978-3-540-74444-3_30
48. Mossenburg, K., Tolbert, C., Stansbury, M.: Virtual Inequality: Beyond the Digital Divide. George Washington University Press, Washington DC (2003)

49. OECD: Citizens as Partners – Information, Consultation, and Public Participation in Policy-Making. OECD e-Book (2001)
50. OECD: The E-Government Imperative, OECDE-Government Studies: OECD, Paris (2003)
51. O'reilly, T.: What Is Web 2.0: Design Patterns and Business Models for the Next Generation of Software, Published on O'Reilly (2005). (http://www.oreilly.com/)
52. Pandagale, P.U., Mundhe, M.R., Pathan, A.: Geospatial information system for tourism management in Aurangabad city- a review. Int. J. Res. Eng. Technol. 3(5), 720–724 (2014)
53. Ramaswamy, M., Selian, A.N.: On the dimensions of e-government interactions. Issues Inf. Syst. 8(2) (2007)
54. Reddick, C.G.: A two stage model of e-government growth: theories and empirical evidence for U.S. cities. Gov. Inf. Q. 21(1), 51–64 (2004)
55. Rogers, E.M.: Diffusion of Innovations, 4th edn. Free Press, New York (1995)
56. Saunders, M., Lewis, P., Thornhill, A.: i(3rd edition). Prentice Hall, Harlow (2003)
57. Schwester, R.W.: Examining the barriers to E-government adoption. Electron. J. E-Gov. 7 (1), 113–122 (2009)
58. Shah, S.A., Wani, M.A.: Application of geospatial technology for the promotion of tourist industry in Srinagar city. Int. J. U-E-Serv. Sci. Technol. 8(1), 37–50 (2015)
59. Siau, K., Long, Y.: Synthesizing e-government stage models- a meta-synthesis based on meta-ethnography approach. Ind. Manag. Data Syst. 105, 443–458 (2005)
60. Siau, K., Tian, Y.: Supply chains integration: architecture and enabling technologies. J. Comput. Inf. Syst. 44, 67–72 (2004)
61. Stachowicz, S.: Geographical data sharing – advantages of web based technology to local government. In: 10th EC GI & GIS Workshop, ESDI State of the Art, Warsaw, Poland (2004)
62. Susanto, T.D.: Individual acceptance of e-government: a literature review. Soc. Digit. Inf. Wirel. Commun. J. (2013). ISBN: 978-0-9891305-2-3
63. Turban, K., Lee, W.: Electronic Commerce, A Managerial Perspective. Prentice Hall, Upper Saddle River (2008)
64. Vassilakis, C., Lepouras, G., Fraser, J., Haston, S., Georgiadis, P.: Barriers to electronic service development. e-Service Journal 4(1), 41–63 (2005)
65. Venkatesh, V., Davis, F.D.: A theoretical extension of the technology acceptance model: four longitudinal field studies. Manag. Sci. 46(2), 186–204 (2000)
66. Venkatesh, V., Morris, M., Davis, G., Davis, F.: User acceptance of information technology: toward a unified view. MIS Q. 27, 425–478 (2003)
67. Voutinioti, A.: Determinants of User Adoption of e-Government Services in Greece and the role of Citizen Service Centres. In: 6th International Conference on Information and Communication Technologies in Agriculture, Food and Environment, https://doi.org/10.1016/j.protcy.2013.11.033 (2013)
68. Wangpipatwong, S., Chutimaskul, W., Papasratorn, B.: Understanding citizen's continuance intention to use e-government website: A composite view of technology acceptance model and computer self-efficacy. Electronic Journal of E-Government 6(1), 55–64 (2008)
69. Warkentin, M., Gefen, D., Pavlou, P., Rose, G.: Encouraging citizen adoption of e-government by building trust. Electron. Mark. 12, 157–162 (2002)
70. Williams, M.D., Rana N.P., Roderick S., Clement M.: Gender, age and frequency of internet use as moderators of citizens' adoption of electronic government. In: Proceedings in Twenty Second Americas Conference on Information Systems, San Diego (2016)
71. World Bank: Building Blocks of e-Governments: Lessons from Developing Countries, Development Economics Vice Presidency and Poverty Reduction and Economic Management Network (PREM Notes for Public Sector), No. 91 (2004)

72. Yan, X., Wang, Y.: Development of Zaozhuang tourism information system based on WebGIS. Int. J. Comput. Sci. Issues **9**(6), 249–252 (2012)
73. Yildiz, M.: A general evaluation of the theory and practice of e-government (In Turkish). In: Acar, M., Ozgur, H. (eds.) Cagdas Kamu Yonetimi-1, pp. 305–328. Nobel Publications, Istanbul (2003)
74. Malhotra, N.K., Baalbaki, I.B., Bechwati, N.N.: Marketing Research: An Applied Orientation. Published by Pearson Education, Inc., Arab World edition (2013)
75. Harfouche, A.: Big brother is watching you: inhibitors and enablers of public E-services in Lebanon. In: tGov workshop 2010 (tGOV 2010). Brunel University, West London, March 2010
76. Field, A.: Discovering Statistics Using SPSS, 2nd edn. Sagem Publications, London (2005)
77. Hinton, P.R., Brownlow, C., McMurvay, I., Cozens, B.: SPSS Explained, East Sussex. Routledge Inc., England (2004)
78. Carter, L., Schaupp, L., Evans, A.: Antecedents to E-file adoption: the US perspective. In: Proceedings of the 41st Annual Hawaii International Conference on System Sciences, p. 216 (2008)
79. Dwivedi, Y.K., Choudrie, J., Brinkman, W.P.: Development of a survey instrument to examine consumer adoption of broadband. Ind. Manag. Data Syst. **106**, 700–718 (2006)
80. Straub, D., Boudreau, M.C., Gefen, D.: Validation guidelines for IS positivist research. Commun. Assoc. Inf. Syst. **13**, 380–427 (2004)

# Factors Affecting Intention to Use E-government Services: The Case of Non-adopters

Stellios Rallis[1], Dimitrios Chatzoudes[1], Symeon Symeonidis[2(✉)], Vasillis Aggelidis[1], and Prodromos Chatzoglou[1]

[1] Department of Production and Management Engineering, Democritus University of Thrace, Vasillisis Sofias 12, 67100 Xanthi, Greece
strallis@gmail.com, dchatzoudes@yahoo.gr, {vangelid,pchatzog}@pme.duth.gr
[2] Department of Electrical and Computer Engineering, Democritus University of Thrace, University Campus, Kimmeria, 67100 Xanthi, Greece
ssymeoni@ee.duth.gr

**Abstract.** 'E-government' is an extremely interesting research field, with numerous academic and practical implications. Its empirical investigation gives rise for significant observations, since the existing international literature offers several research gaps. The aim of the present study is twofold: (a) to develop an original conceptual framework (research model) examining the factors that have an impact on the intention to use of e-government services, (b) to empirically test that framework, using primary data collected from non-adopters of e-government located in Greece. The proposed framework is tested using data collected with a newly-developed structured questionnaire in a sample of Greek internet users. The ten independent factors incorporated into the proposed research framework are measured with a series of questions (items) which have been adopted from various other studies found in the international literature. The empirical data are analyzed using the 'Structural Equation Modeling' technique. The main findings suggest that Perceived Usefulness, Peer Influence, Computer Self-efficacy, and Perceived Risk are the main factors affecting the intention of non-users to use e-Government services.

**Keywords:** e-Government · Intention to use · Non-adopters · Perceived usefulness · Peer influence · Structural equation modelling

## 1 Introduction

Information and communication technologies (ICT) are the main factors having an impact on the success of e-government services that are offered to citizens [34, 39]. During the last two decades, many studies and frameworks (research models) have examined the adoption, the experience, and the interaction of e-government information systems with society and organizations [3, 28, 33, 51].

© Springer Nature Switzerland AG 2019
M. Themistocleous and P. Rupino da Cunha (Eds.): EMCIS 2018, LNBIP 341, pp. 302–315, 2019.
https://doi.org/10.1007/978-3-030-11395-7_25

Numerous definitions have been given, during the last decade, for e-Government. According to [24], e-Government provides government data and administration via online services, while [4] defines e-Government as a tool that is used in order to offer public administration services.

This study examines the intention of non-users to use e-government services. This examination is conducted through the development and the empirical testing of a conceptual framework that includes factors that were adopted from other international research attempts after an extensive literature review. One dependent factor (intention to use) and ten independent factors, which have never been studied collectively in the past, were incorporated into the proposed research model.

Despite the plethora of studies on e-government during the recent years, [41] argue that there is a research gap on the investigation of the factors that have an impact on the intention of non-users to adopt e-government services. This paper contributes to the study of a critical area, examining the behavioral attitude of non-users, thus highlighting the factors affecting their intention to use e-government services. Such an approach still lacks in the relevant literature.

In the following section, a brief theoretical and literature review is being conducted, focusing: (a) on models that have been extensively used in the literature and (b) on the empirical results of previous studies. Section 2.3 presents the proposed hypotheses, while Sect. 3 includes a brief analysis of the research methodology. Section 4 analyzes the empirical results (hypothesis testing). Finally, the main conclusions of the study are presented in Sect. 5.

# 2 Literature Review and Hypotheses Development

Many previous studies defined e-Government using different approaches. [49] defined e-Government as a digital connection between citizens and businesses, on the one hand, and government agencies, on the other. This interaction is being conducted without the physical presence of both parties. According to [51], e-government is a pathway that provides public assistance to citizens, through ICT technologies.

## 2.1 Theoretical Background

Some of the most well known theories of human behavior concerning the use of ICT system are the following:

*Diffusion of Innovation (DOI):* The diffusion of innovations among individual citizens and various groups of citizens, is defined by the corresponding theory [38]. [19] showed that e-government concepts are not easily accepted from other domains.

*Theory of Reasoned Action (TRA):* This theory of human behavior examines the intention and behavior of technology users, based on behavioral beliefs, subjective norms, and attitudes [21, 31].

*Theory of Planned Behavior (TPB):* As an extension of TRA, TPB makes the addition of 'perceived behavioral control', which refers to the 'selfish' behavior that depends on people's perceptions [1]. [42] indicated that the feeling of a technology user concerning the ability to successfully use an online system is measured through his attitude and intention.

*Technology Acceptance Model (TAM) and TAM2:* This model, which is based on perceived usefulness and perceived ease of use, was developed for computer acceptance behaviors. Perceived usefulness measures the value a user receives by using an Information System, while perceived ease of use measures how easily users can learn to operate the same system [17].

*Motivational Model:* It describes the intrinsic motivation of a person, arguing that a person wishes to feel responsible for its social environment [18].

*Model of PC Utilization:* According to [45], the factors that influence the use of a computer are the social interests of the user and the complexity of the system.

*Social Cognitive Theory:* A well-known theory for human behavior, which is based on the argument that every person is being influenced by its environment [6].

*Unified Theory of Acceptance and Use of Technology (UTAUT):* The unified theory of acceptance and use of technology (UTAUT) is based on previous models of technology acceptance and describes the intention and actual usage of a system [46].

## 2.2  Previous Studies

A plethora of previous studies have dealt with factors of adoption, quality and other relevant factors of e-Government services. [41] investigated the attitude of 337 non-users and users of e-government services in the Netherlands, from one rural and one urban municipality. Results showed that rural residents switch their behavioral attitudes between periods of pre-adoption and post-adoption more often, in comparison with urban residents. [19] examined 377 respondents from seven cities of India, in order to validate a comprehensive adoption model, named UMEGA. Empirical findings revealed that this model can be used for e-Government adoption, since it satisfactorily predicts the phenomenon under examination. In order to measure the adoption of e-government services in Turkey, [31] used the UTAUT model, significantly expanding the factor of 'trust', on a survey of 529 citizens. Empirical results revealed that the factors Performance expectancy, Social influence, Facilitating conditions and Trust of Internet have a significant impact on the intention to use e-government services, while the effect of Effort expectancy and Trust in government were found to be trivial (non-significant). The study of [30] examined the Experience and Trust of citizens towards e-Government services in India. The findings reported an obvious shift of users to electronic services and technological innovations. The quality of local e-Government online services was examined by [39], who recognized the different types of services offered by e-government platforms. Another study which investigated the effect of quality of e-Government services was conducted by [27]. The authors developed a research model that classifies e-services according to their service features. Finally, [43] constructed a conceptual framework and examined the success of e-government systems in Serbia. Results revealed that System Quality, Information Quality and Service Quality have a positive effect on the intention to use.

The proposed model of the present study is based on the previous empirical work of [29, 37, 41], who examine the different perceptions between users and non-users of e-government services. The present study examines only the case of non-users, an approach rarely adopted in the relevant literature.

### 2.3  Conceptual Framework

The present paper developed its conceptual framework based on the findings and suggestions of recent international empirical studies. The proposed framework includes one dependent factor (intention to use e-Government services) and ten independent factors. The corresponding research hypotheses are analytically presented below (Table 1).

**Table 1.** Summary of hypotheses

| | |
|---|---|
| H1: | Perceived risk has a negative effect on the intention to use e-Government services |
| H2: | Trust in e-Government has a positive effect on the intention to use e-Government services |
| H3: | Perceived usefulness has a positive effect on the intention to use e-Government services |
| H4: | Perceived ease of use has a positive effect on the intention to use e-Government services |
| H5: | Perceived Quality has a positive effect on the intention to use e-Government services |
| H6: | Perceived Quality of Internet (Communication) has a positive effect on the intention to use e-Government services |
| H7: | Internet experience has a positive effect on the intention to use e-Government services |
| H8: | Computer self-efficacy has a positive effect on the intention to use e-Government services |
| H9: | Self-image has a positive effect on the intention to use e-Government services |
| H10: | Peer Influence has a positive effect on the intention to use e-Government services |

## 3  Research Methodology

The present study is empirical (based on primary data), explanatory (examines cause and effect relationships), deductive (tests research hypotheses) and quantitative (analyses quantitative data that are collected with the use of a structured questionnaire). In that direction, a newly-developed structured questionnaire was developed and tested on 513 randomly selected non-users, residing in Greece.

The questionnaire was based on previous relevant studies, which provided useful insights considering the appropriate factors and measures (items). All items measuring the various research factors were measured using a five-point Likert scale, ranging from one (totally disagree) to five (totally agree). Table 2 presents the factors of the study and the sources of their measurement.

**Table 2.** Factor measurement

| Factor | Definitions | Reference |
|---|---|---|
| B. Internet Experience | The level of experience in using the Internet | [11, 15, 47] |
| C. Perceived Quality of Internet (Communication) | The existence of a decent Internet connection and its quality | [2, 35] |
| D. Computer Self-Efficacy | An individuals perceptions of his ability to use computers for the accomplishment of a certain task | [48] |
| E. Trust in e-Government | The level of trust in government, as well as trust in the reliability of the enabling technology (trust of the Internet) | [7, 8, 16] |
| F. Perceived Usefulness | The degree to which a person believes that using a particular system would enhance his job performance | [9, 17, 44] |
| G. Perceived Ease of Use | The degree to which a person believes that using a particular system would be free of effort | [9, 17, 22] |
| H. Perceived Quality | Consumer judgment about e-government services, including overall excellence or superiority | [12] |
| I. Perceived Risk | An individuals subjective feelings of possible losses from using e-government | [32, 36] |
| J. Self-Image | The degree to which an individual perceives that use of e-government will enhance his status in the social system | [8, 40] |
| K. Peer Influence | The degree to which peers influence the use of the system | [25] |
| L. Intention to Use | An individuals will to use e-government in the near future | [9, 10] |

The research instrument (questionnaire) was tested for both its content and construct validity.

As far as the test for the content validity is concerned, it was performed using a pilot study approach, where twenty (20) citizens were asked to fill in the final draft of the questionnaire and make comments concerning their level of understanding. Their comments were then used in order to make the final adjustments to the questionnaire that was sent out to the participants.

After collecting the appropriate empirical data, each of the eleven research factors was evaluated for its unidimensionality and reliability, using Exploratory Factor Analysis (EFA) (construct validity test). The results are presented in Table 3. For determining the appropriateness of the factor analysis, the following measures were examined: (a) the statistical test of Kaiser-Mayer-Olkin (KMO) (values over 0,7 are satisfactory, while values over 0,5 are acceptable); (b) the Bartletts test of Sphericity (it should be statistically significant, at the 0,05 level); (c) the correlations of the entry table (correlations should be statistically significant, at the 0,05 level). For determining the percent of the total variance that is explained by the proposed factor(s), Total Variance Explained (TVE) was used. TVE should be more than 50%. For testing the significance of the items, their factor loadings were examined. For a sample size of more than 150 observations a loading over 0,40 is considered significant [14, 23, 26]. The results of the factor analysis indicate that the factors included in the proposed model are both valid and reliable. More specifically, KMO is higher than .700 (except for the second order factor Trust), TVE is higher than 60.000, factor loadings are higher than the .700 and Cronbach a is also higher than .700 threshold for all factors.

**Table 3.** Unidimensionality & reliability

| Factor | Items | KMO | TVE | Factor loadings | Cronbach a | Mean | St. dev. |
|---|---|---|---|---|---|---|---|
| B. Internet Experience | 1–3 | .725 | 75.120 | .864–.872 | .830 | 3.38 | 1.07 |
| C. Perceived Quality of Internet (Communication) | 1–4 | .801 | 70.590 | .817–.854 | .861 | 3.64 | 0.84 |
| D. Computer Self-Efficacy | 1–3 | .700 | 73.442 | .820–.888 | .818 | 2.85 | 1.02 |
| E1. Trust (Internet) | 1–3 | .699 | 70.918 | .811–.867 | .795 | 2.86 | 0.78 |
| E2. Trust (Government/ Public Services) | 1–4 | .855 | 82.147 | .880–.934 | .927 | 2.09 | 0.96 |
| E3. Trust (e-Government) | 1–4 | .836 | 75.990 | .828–.909 | .894 | 2.73 | 0.89 |
| E. Trust | E1, E2, E3 | .635 | 62.641 | .705–.848 | .700 | 2.56 | 0.69 |
| F. Perceived Usefulness | 1–4 | .828 | 80.093 | .859–.921 | .917 | 3.70 | 0.85 |
| G. Perceived Ease of Use | 1–4 | .839 | 80.385 | .864–.928 | .918 | 3.41 | 0.95 |
| H. Perceived Quality | 1–4 | .795 | 67.636 | .724–.880 | .838 | 3.25 | 0.73 |
| I. Perceived Risk (Security) | 1–3 | .721 | 76.763 | .849–.893 | .848 | 3.64 | 0.95 |
| J. Self-Image | 1–3 | .731 | 84.997 | .890–.945 | .911 | 2.28 | 1.04 |
| K. Peer Influence | 1–3 | .702 | 73.175 | .829–.887 | .816 | 3.04 | 0.94 |
| L. Intention to Use | 1–3 | .703 | 72.567 | .825–.880 | .811 | 3.11 | 0.92 |

# 4 Results

The results of the descriptive analysis show that, the participants consider that their Internet Experience is average (B = 3.38), while their Self-Efficacy is below average (D = 2.85). They also perceive that the Usefulness and the Ease of Use of e-Government services is moderately high (F = 3.70 and G = 3.41 respectively), while the Quality of the same services is acceptable (H = 3.25). Despite that, they consider that the Risk of using these services is rather high (I = 3.64) and this is probably why they do not Trust them (E = 2.56). As a result, they are rather reluctant to use e-Government applications (L = 3.11). However, considering that the sample consists only of people who currently do not use e-government applications, it is rather promising that they are slightly positive in using them sometime in the future.

The results of the correlation analysis are presented in Tables 4 and 5. Firstly, it seems that from the four demographic variables that are examined in this study, Gender and Family Income are significantly related only to a limited number of the factors incorporated in the proposed model (Table 4). On the other hand, Age and Education are related to most of the factors, especially with Internet Experience and Computer Self Efficacy. It should also be underlined that none of the four demographic variables are related to the dependent factor of this study (Intention to use e-Government). Secondly, the results presented in Table 5 reveal that there is a statistically significant relationship between almost all factors, something that supports their adoption in the proposed research model. Additionally, it should be stressed out that, none of the correlation scores is higher than .600 (actually, most of them are lower than .300).

**Table 4.** Correlation analysis A

|  | Gender | Age | Education | Family income (monthly) |
|---|---|---|---|---|
| B. Internet Experience | −.158** | −.393** | .309** | |
| C. Perceived Quality of Internet (Communication) | | −.156** | .175** | |
| D. Computer Self-Efficacy | −.141** | −.281** | .170** | |
| E. Trust | | | | |
| F. Perceived Usefulness | | | | |
| G. Perceived Ease of Use | | −.147** | .150** | |
| H. Perceived Quality | | .093* | | |
| I. Perceived Risk (Security) | | .123** | | |
| J. Self-Image | | .106* | | |
| K. Peer Influence | | .154** | .094* | .107* |
| L. Intention to Use | | | | |

**Table 5.** Correlation analysis B

|  | B | C | D | E | F | G | H | I | J | K |
|---|---|---|---|---|---|---|---|---|---|---|
| B. Internet Experience | 1.000 | | | | | | | | | |
| C. Perceived Quality of Internet (Communication) | .385** | 1.000 | | | | | | | | |
| D. Computer Self-Efficacy | .591** | .432** | 1.000 | | | | | | | |
| E. Trust | .100* | .291** | .264** | 1.000 | | | | | | |
| F. Perceived Usefulness | .119** | .266** | .186** | .208** | 1.000 | | | | | |
| G. Perceived Ease of Use | .444** | .354** | .468** | .190** | .433** | 1.000 | | | | |
| H. Perceived Quality | | .181** | .186** | .392** | .360** | .313** | 1.000 | | | |
| I. Perceived Risk (Security) | −.151** | | −.147** | −.174** | | −.128** | −.135** | 1.000 | | |
| J. Self-Image | −.115** | | | .151** | .103* | | .196** | | 1.000 | |
| K. Peer Influence | | .106* | | | .166** | .276** | | .204** | | .326** | 1.000 |
| L. Intention to Use | .114** | .197** | .245** | .224** | .507** | .320** | .291** | −.170** | .265** | .432** |

**. Correlation is significant at the 0.01 level (2-tailed).
*. Correlation is significant at the 0.05 level (2-tailed).

The validity of the proposed research model as well as the subsequent hypotheses are tested using the structural equation modelling technique.

To evaluate the fit of the (modified) overall model, the chi-square ($X^2$) value and the p-value were estimated. These values indicate a satisfactory fit of the data to the (modified) overall model. However, the sensitivity of the $X^2$ statistic to the sample size enforces to control other supplementary measures of evaluating the overall model, such as the Normed-$X^2$ index (2.97), the RSMEA (Root Mean Square Error of Approximation) index (.061), the RMR (Root Mean Square Residual) (.043), the CFI (Comparative Fit Index) (.960) and the GFI (Goodness of Fit Index) (.972), that all indicate a very good fit. Furthermore, for testing the measurement model, the significance of the factor loadings, the Construct Reliability (C.R.) and the Variance Extracted (V.E.) were estimated and the results indicated that all loadings are significant at the $p < 0.05$ level. Additionally, C.R. and V.E. for all factors (constructs) were satisfactory (Table 6).

**Table 6.** Goodness of fit estimation

| CMIN/DF | CFI | GFI | TLI | RMR | RMSEA |
|---|---|---|---|---|---|
| <5 | >.900 | >.900 | >.900 | <.050 | <.100 |
| 2.927 | .960 | .972 | .925 | .043 | .061 |

The predictive power of the model is satisfactory since it can explain 43% of the variation of the dependent factor (Intention to Use e-Government), but also the variation of some of the most important of the other factors, such as Perceived Usefulness, Perceived Ease of Use, Perceived Quality (32%, 30% and 26% respectively).

Analyzing the results of Fig. 1 and Table 7, it becomes obvious that Perceived Usefulness, Peer Influence, Computer Self Efficacy and Perceived Risk have the highest direct impact on Intention to Use (.382, .355, .177 and −.139 respectively). Further, Perceived Ease of Use has the highest indirect effect on Intention to Use (.175). Overall, while some of the initial hypotheses have been rejected, many more new ones have been emerged and were incorporated into the final modified model presented in Fig. 1.

The following observations can be made after reviewing the empirical results of the study (see Table 7 and Fig. 1):

- Perceived usefulness directly affects intention. This is also confirmed by the Technology Acceptance Model (TAM) of [17]. Moreover, this impact is not only statistical significant, but it is also quite strong (r = 0.38).
- Perceived risk has a negative effect on intention. This conclusion is in line with the studies of [32] and [20]. For example, a loss of communication between user and server may have a negative impact on users' trust and, therefore, in their intention to further use the online services.

– Peer influence positively affects intention. The same conclusion was reached by
  [25]. A possible reward from the immediate social environment predisposes the user
  towards using e-Government services.
– Moreover, computer self-efficacy has a direct positive effect on intention. [48] argue
  that people with increased computer self-efficacy easily understand the functions of
  online services, thus increasing their confidence and their general intention to use
  such systems (Table 8).

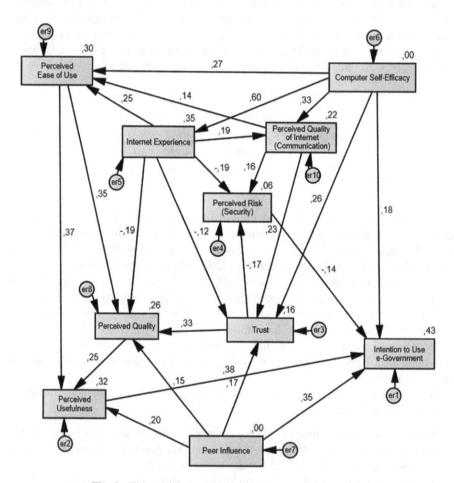

**Fig. 1.** The modified conceptual framework of the study.

**Table 7.** Standardized direct, indirect and total effects

|  |  | D | B | C | G | H | E | F | K | I |
|---|---|---|---|---|---|---|---|---|---|---|
| B. Internet Experience | D | .596 |  |  |  |  |  |  |  |  |
|  | I | .000 |  |  |  |  |  |  |  |  |
|  | T | .596 |  |  |  |  |  |  |  |  |
| C. Perceived Quality of Internet (Communication) | D | .325 | .193 |  |  |  |  |  |  |  |
|  | I | .115 | .000 |  |  |  |  |  |  |  |
|  | T | .440 | .193 |  |  |  |  |  |  |  |
| G. Perceived Ease of Use | D | .270 | .254 | .143 |  |  |  |  |  |  |
|  | I | .214 | .028 | .000 |  |  |  |  |  |  |
|  | T | .484 | .282 | .143 |  |  |  |  |  |  |
| H. Perceived Quality | D | .000 | −.191 | .000 | .345 |  | .333 | .000 | .151 |  |
|  | I | .149 | .073 | .126 | .000 |  | .000 | .060 | .055 |  |
|  | T | .149 | −.118 | .126 | .345 |  | .333 | .060 | .206 |  |
| E. Trust | D | .257 | −.116 | .230 | .000 | .000 |  | .000 | .165 |  |
|  | I | .032 | .045 | .000 | .000 | .000 |  | .084 | .000 |  |
|  | T | .289 | −.071 | .230 | .000 | .000 |  | .084 | .165 |  |
| F. Perceived Usefulness | D | .000 | .000 | .000 | .371 | .252 | .000 |  | .204 |  |
|  | I | .217 | .075 | .085 | .087 | .000 | .084 |  | .052 |  |
|  | T | .217 | .075 | .085 | .458 | .252 | .084 |  | .256 |  |
| I. Perceived Risk (Security) | D | .000 | −.189 | .165 | .000 | .000 | −.170 | .000 | .000 |  |
|  | I | −.089 | .044 | −.039 | −.017 | .000 | .000 | −.035 | −.028 |  |
|  | T | −.089 | −.145 | .126 | −.017 | .000 | −.170 | −.035 | −.028 |  |
| L. Intention to Use | D | .177 | .000 | .000 | .000 | .000 | .000 | .382 | .355 | −.139 |
|  | I | .095 | .049 | .015 | .175 | .096 | .056 | .000 | .101 | .000 |
|  | T | .272 | .049 | .015 | .175 | .096 | .056 | .382 | .456 | −.139 |

D. Computer Self-Efficacy, K. Peer Influence

**Table 8.** Accepted hypotheses

| Causal paths (hypotheses) |  | Estimate | p | Result |
|---|---|---|---|---|
| H1 | Perceived risk Intention to use | −0.14 | 0.000 | Accepted |
| H3 | Perceived usefulness Intention to use | 0.38 | 0.000 | Accepted |
| H8 | Computer self-efficacy Intention to use | 0.18 | 0.000 | Accepted |
| H10 | Peer influence Intention to use | 0.35 | 0.000 | Accepted |

## 5 Conclusions

The present study proposed a new conceptual framework in an attempt to identify the main factors affecting the intention of non-users to use e-Government services. According to [41], there is a significant research gap in the examination of the behavior of non-users of e-Government services. More specifically, little is still known about the factors that have the most significant impact on their behaviour. The proposed conceptual framework of this study has been developed after an extensive literature review and has been empirically tested on a sample of 513 internet users.

The main conclusion drawn from the empirical results is that both researchers and practitioners should examine and manage a bundle of factors (dimensions), which seem to be highly interrelated, when considering the use of e-Government applications from non-users. Thus, they should not only pay attention to enhancing a rather limited number of factors, since the emergence of various indirect effects underlined the need for a more integrated approach.

As far as the impact of each individual factor on the intention of non-users to use e-Government is concerned, it is concluded that although Perceived Usefulness is found to have the highest direct impact, Peer Influence seems to have the highest total (direct and indirect) impact. [25] also found that external resources, such as television/news, significantly influence not only early-adopters, but also non-adopters of e-Government. By providing proper information to citizens (through the internet or in the form of leaflets), the state can bend the bias that exists towards online services [5, 50].

Of course, special focus should be given in enhancing the level of perceived usefulness [46]. Citizens are more interested in usefulness, as the effect of perceived ease of use (which sometimes is mainly indirect, as in this case) is often reduced after a short period of time. In that direction, e-Government services should add value to citizens, offering access to useful information. There is no meaning in developing services that offer very little information and utility, while, at the same time, discourage citizens from future use. A useful application will attract the attention of the public and create more users in the near future.

In line with [13] and [48] findings, who suggest that State officials should fight computer illiteracy, since only self-efficient citizens will adopt e-Government, the results of the current research have shown that computer self-efficacy is positively related with the intention of non-users to use e-Government services.

Finally, the State should implement all the necessary mechanisms in order to enhance the level of trust citizens exhibit on the use of similar applications, effectively protect their privacy and transactions in an impersonal medium such as the internet, and, thus, convince citizens that the level of their exposure to various risks associated with the use of these applications is as low as possible. The above suggestions are in line with the ones also proposed by [16].

# References

1. Ajzen, I.: The theory of planned behavior. Organ. Behav. Hum. Decis. Process. **50**(2), 179–211 (1991). https://doi.org/10.1016/0749-5978(91)90020-T
2. Al-Somali, S.A., Gholami, R., Clegg, B.: An investigation into the acceptance of online banking in Saudi Arabia. Technovation **29**(2), 130–141 (2009). https://doi.org/10.1016/J.TECHNOVATION.2008.07.004
3. Alateyah, S.A., Crowder, R.M., Wills, G.B.: Identified factors affecting the citizen's intention to adopt e-government in Saudi Arabia. Int. J. Soc., Hum. Sci. Eng. **7**(8), 601–606 (2013). https://doi.org/10.7763/IJIMT.2014.V5.527

4. Alghamdi, I.A., Goodwin, R., Rampersad, G.: E-government readiness assessment for government organizations in developing countries. Comput. Inf. Sci. **4**(3), 3 (2011)
5. Alghamdi, S., Beloff, N.: Towards a comprehensive model for e-government adoption and utilisation analysis: the case of Saudi Arabia. In: 2014 Federated Conference on Computer Science and Information Systems, pp. 1217–1225, September 2014. https://doi.org/10. 15439/2014F146
6. Bandura, A.: The explanatory and predictive scope of self-efficacy theory. J. Soc. Clin. Psychol. **4**(3), 359–373 (1986). https://doi.org/10.1521/jscp.1986.4.3.359
7. Bélanger, F., Carter, L.: Trust and risk in e-government adoption. J. Strateg. Inf. Syst. **17**(2), 165–176 (2008). https://doi.org/10.1016/J.JSIS.2007.12.002
8. Carter, L., Bélanger, F.: The utilization of e-government services: citizen trust, innovation and acceptance factors. Inf. Syst. J. **15**(1), 5–25 (2005). https://doi.org/10.1111/j.1365-2575. 2005.00183.x
9. Cheng, T.E., Lam, D.Y., Yeung, A.C.: Adoption of internet banking: an empirical study in Hong Kong. Decis. Support Syst. **42**(3), 1558–1572 (2006). https://doi.org/10.1016/J.DSS. 2006.01.002
10. Cheong, J.H., Park, M.: Mobile internet acceptance in Korea. Internet Res. **15**(2), 125–140 (2005). https://doi.org/10.1108/10662240510590324
11. Cho, J.: Likelihood to abort an online transaction: influences from cognitive evaluations, attitudes, and behavioral variables. Inf. Manag. **41**(7), 827–838 (2004). https://doi.org/10. 1016/J.IM.2003.08.013
12. Colesca, S.E.: Increasing e-trust: a solution to minimize risk in egovernment adoption. J. Appl. Quant. Methods **4**, 31–44 (2009)
13. Compeau, D.R., Higgins, C.A.: Computer self-efficacy: development of a measure and initial test. MIS Q. **19**, 189–211 (1995)
14. Conway, J.M., Huffcutt, A.I.: A review and evaluation of exploratory factor analysis practices in organizational research. Organ. Res. Methods **6**(2), 147–168 (2003)
15. Corbitt, B.J., Thanasankit, T., Yi, H.: Trust and e-commerce: a study of consumer perceptions. Electron. Commer. Res. Appl. **2**(3), 203–215 (2003). https://doi.org/10.1016/ S1567-4223(03)00024-3
16. Dashti, A., Benbasat, I., Burton-Jones, A.: Developing trust reciprocity in electronic-government: the role of felt trust. In: Proceedings of the European and Mediterranean Conference on Information Systems, Izmir, Turkey, pp. 1–13. Citeseer (2009)
17. Davis, F.D.: Perceived usefulness, perceived ease of use, and user acceptance of information technology. MIS Q. **13**(3), 319 (1989). https://doi.org/10.2307/249008
18. Deci, E.L., Ryan, R.M.: Intrinsic motivation. In: The Corsini Encyclopedia of Psychology, pp. 1–2. Wiley, Hoboken, January 2010. https://doi.org/10.1002/9780470479216. corpsy0467
19. Dwivedi, Y.K., Rana, N.P., Janssen, M., Lal, B., Williams, M.D., Clement, M.: An empirical validation of a unified model of electronic government adoption (UMEGA). Gov. Inf. Q. **34** (2), 211–230 (2017). https://doi.org/10.1016/j.giq.2017.03.001
20. Featherman, M.S., Pavlou, P.A.: Predicting e-services adoption: a perceived risk facets perspective. Int. J. Hum Comput Stud. **59**(4), 451–474 (2003). https://doi.org/10.1016/ S1071-5819(03)00111-3
21. Fishbein, M., Ajzen, I.: Belief, Attitude, Intention, and Behavior: An Introduction to Theory and Research. Addison-Wesley Publishing Company, Reading (1975)
22. Gefen, D., Straub, D., Mack, J., Distinguished, R.: The relative importance of perceived ease of use in IS adoption: a study of e-commerce adoption. J. Assoc. Inf. Syst. **1**(8) (2000)
23. Hayton, J.C., Allen, D.G., Scarpello, V.: Factor retention decisions in exploratory factor analysis: a tutorial on parallel analysis. Organ. Res. Methods **7**(2), 191–205 (2004)

24. Huai, J.: Quality evaluation of e-government public service. In: 2011 International Conference on Management and Service Science (MASS), pp. 1–4. IEEE (2011)
25. Hung, S.Y., Chang, C.M., Yu, T.J.: Determinants of user acceptance of the e-Government services: the case of online tax filing and payment system. Gov. Inf. Q. **23**(1), 97–122 (2006). https://doi.org/10.1016/J.GIQ.2005.11.005
26. Hurley, A.E., et al.: Exploratory and confirmatory factor analysis: guidelines, issues, and alternatives. J. Organ. Behav.: Int. J. Ind. Occup. Organ. Psychol. Behav. **18**(6), 667–683 (1997)
27. Jansen, A., Ølnes, S.: The nature of public e-services and their quality dimensions. Gov. Inf. Q. **33**(4), 647–657 (2016). https://doi.org/10.1016/j.giq.2016.08.005
28. Kaliannan, M., Awang, H., Raman, M.: Technology adoption in the public sector: an exploratory study of e-government in Malaysia. In: Proceedings of the 1st International Conference on Theory and Practice of Electronic Governance, pp. 221–224 (2007). https://doi.org/10.1145/1328057.1328103
29. Karahanna, E., Straub, D.W., Chervany, N.L.: Information technology adoption across time: a cross-sectional comparison of pre-adoption and post-adoption beliefs. MIS Q. **23**, 183–213 (1999)
30. Kumar, R., Sachan, A., Mukherjee, A.: Qualitative approach to determine user experience of e-government services. Comput. Hum. Behav. **71**, 299–306 (2017). https://doi.org/10.1016/j.chb.2017.02.023
31. Kurfal, M., Arifolu, A., Tokdemir, G., Paçin, Y.: Adoption of e-government services in Turkey. Comput. Hum. Behav. **66**, 168–178 (2017). https://doi.org/10.1016/j.chb.2016.09.041
32. Lee, M.C.: Factors influencing the adoption of internet banking: an integration of TAM and TPB with perceived risk and perceived benefit. Electron. Commer. Res. Appl. **8**(3), 130–141 (2009). https://doi.org/10.1016/J.ELERAP.2008.11.006
33. Nam, T.: Determining the type of e-government use. Gov. Inf. Q. **31**(2), 211–220 (2014). https://doi.org/10.1016/j.giq.2013.09.006
34. Osman, I.H., et al.: COBRA framework to evaluate e-government services: a citizen-centric perspective. Gov. Inf. Q. **31**(2), 243–256 (2014). https://doi.org/10.1016/j.giq.2013.10.009
35. Pikkarainen, T., Pikkarainen, K., Karjaluoto, H., Pahnila, S.: Consumer acceptance of online banking: an extension of the technology acceptance model. Internet Res. **14**(3), 224–235 (2004). https://doi.org/10.1108/10662240410542652
36. Pires, G., Stanton, J., Eckford, A.: Influences on the perceived risk of purchasing online. J. Consum. Behav. **4**(2), 118–131 (2004). https://doi.org/10.1002/cb.163
37. Ramayah, T., Maruf, J.J., Jantan, M., Osman, M.: Technology acceptance model: is it applicable to users and non users of internet banking. In: The Proceedings of the International Seminar, Indonesia-Malaysia, the Role of Harmonization of Economics and Business Discipline in Global Competitiveness, Banda Aceh, Indonesia, pp. 14–15 (2002)
38. Rogers, E.M.: Diffusion of Innovations. Free Press, New York (1995)
39. Sá, F., Rocha, Á., Pérez Cota, M.: From the quality of traditional services to the quality of local e-Government online services: a literature review. Gov. Inf. Q. **33**(1), 149–160 (2016). https://doi.org/10.1016/j.giq.2015.07.004
40. Sang, S., Lee, J., Lee, J.: E-government adoption in ASEAN: the case of Cambodia. Internet Res. **19**(5), 517–534 (2009). https://doi.org/10.1108/10662240910998869
41. Seo, D.B., Bernsen, M.: Comparing attitudes toward e-government of non-users versus users in a rural and urban municipality. Gov. Inf. Q. **33**(2), 270–282 (2016). https://doi.org/10.1016/j.giq.2016.02.002

42. Shareef, M.A., Kumar, V., Kumar, U., Dwivedi, Y.K.: e-Government adoption model (GAM): differing service maturity levels. Gov. Inf. Q. **28**(1), 17–35 (2011). https://doi.org/10.1016/j.giq.2010.05.006
43. Stefanovic, D., Marjanovic, U., Delić, M., Culibrk, D., Lalic, B.: Assessing the success of e-government systems: an employee perspective. Inf. Manag. **53**(6), 717–726 (2016). https://doi.org/10.1016/j.im.2016.02.007
44. Suh, B., Han, I.: Effect of trust on customer acceptance of internet banking. Electron. Commer. Res. Appl. **1**(3–4), 247–263 (2002). https://doi.org/10.1016/S1567-4223(02)00017-0
45. Thompson, R.L., Higgins, C.A., Howell, J.M.: Personal computing: toward a conceptual model of utilization. MIS Q. **15**(1), 125 (1991). https://doi.org/10.2307/249443
46. Venkatesh, V., Morris, M.G., Davis, G.B., Davis, F.D.: User acceptance of information technology: toward a unified view. MIS Q. **27**(3), 425 (2003). https://doi.org/10.2307/30036540
47. Wang, Y., Wang, Y., Lin, H., Tang, T.: Determinants of user acceptance of internet banking: an empirical study. Int. J. Serv. Ind. Manag. **14**(5), 501–519 (2003). https://doi.org/10.1108/09564230310500192
48. Wangpipatwong, S., Chutimaskul, W., Papasratorn, B.: Understanding citizen's continuance intention to use e-government website: a composite view of technology acceptance model and computer self-efficacy. Electron. J. e-Gov. **6**(1), 55–64 (2008)
49. Ebrahim, Z., Irani, Z., Al Shawi, S.: A strategic framework for E-government adoption in public sector organisations. In: AMCIS 2004 Proceedings, pp. 1116–1125 (2004)
50. Ziemba, E., Papaj, T., Descours, D.: Assessing the quality of e-government portals-the polish experience. In: 2014 Federated Conference on Computer Science and Information Systems (FedCSIS), pp. 1259–1267. IEEE (2014)
51. Ziemba, E., Papaj, T., Żelazny, R.: A model of success factors for e-Government adoption - the case of Poland. Issues Inf. Syst. **14**(2), 87–100 (2013)

# Agile Development in Bureaucratic Environments: A Literature Review

Gerald Onwujekwe[✉] and Heinz Weistroffer

Department of Information Systems, Virginia Commonwealth University,
Richmond, VA, USA
{onwujekwegn, hrweistr}@vcu.edu

**Abstract.** For the past decade, agile development approaches have achieved a good level of success. It does appear however that not all development environments have the same level of agile readiness, hence an organization's prevalent culture may be a mismatch with the agile development approach adopted. In this paper, we report on a structured literature review of information systems development projects that were conducted in a public sector or government organization. We posit that public sector and government organizations are commonly found to be bureaucratic in nature and we investigate how this impacts the project implementation using agile methodology. We document the challenges encountered in implementing these projects and some approaches to resolving these challenges.

**Keywords:** Agile development · Government · Bureaucracy · Public sector Projects · Literature review

## 1 Introduction

It is common knowledge that the traditional waterfall approach to product and software development is not always adequate for the increasingly dynamic and rapid business environment of modern society. This is because such approaches rely on detailed and upfront specification of project requirements before development can commence and real-world projects do not always follow the sequential process that the waterfall approach prescribes. Furthermore, in the waterfall approach, a working version of a product does not appear until towards the end of the project. At this point, it is difficult, perhaps impossible to accommodate changing customer requirements. Due to these challenges with the waterfall approach, organizations are increasingly migrating to the agile method of development. Agile approaches focus on rapid life cycle development of a product through short and quick iterations that feature frequent customer participation and user involvement to get immediate feedback and requirements updates to be used in the next iteration. Agile approaches fast track the realization of the development product, and through iterative and incremental design, ensure that value is delivered on an ongoing basis throughout the development cycle. Thus, the project teams are able to continuously bring the product under development in alignment with the client's business needs throughout the process, adapting to the changing requirements. In its basic form, it offers a plain framework that could help development and project teams, given a constantly evolving functional,

M. Themistocleous and P. Rupino da Cunha (Eds.): EMCIS 2018, LNBIP 341, pp. 316–330, 2019.
https://doi.org/10.1007/978-3-030-11395-7_26

non-functional and methodical landscape, maintain a focus on the speedy delivery of business value. Consequently, the merits of agile software development are that organizations are able to reduce in a measurable way the overall risk associated with software development. Agile advocates that the only way to truly know whether information technology (IT) initiatives are consistently meeting business requirements is to actively involve the business area (the "customer") in the regular review and refinement of fully functional, fully tested system capabilities and agile works on the premise that detailed user requirements specification documents and prototype screens are no substitute for getting direct feedback from the customer's hands-on review of working capabilities in their solutions [1]. Making user experts available as part of the team gives developers rapid feedback on the implications to the user of their design choices. The user experts, seeing the evolving software in its earliest stages, learn both what the developers misunderstood and also which of their requests do not work as well in practice as they had thought [2]. No amount of detailed planning – even by the most experienced IT resources – can accurately predict the changes that will occur during the course of a project, and as a result, agile approaches replace upfront planning with incremental planning based on the collaborative work between the project team and the customer. Working jointly with the customer provides staff with an ongoing opportunity to more easily adapt solutions (and supporting documentation) to reflect the changes that occur within the organization – and external to the organization – as the project progresses [1].

The research questions we ask in this study are:

R1. Does the bureaucratic nature of public sector and government organizations impact the use of agile methodologies for information systems development?

R2. Are there steps that can be taken or ways to adapt agile methodologies to suit bureaucratic organizational cultures?

R3. Are there projects that have been implemented with agile methodologies in a bureaucratic setting whose results show that the bureaucratic nature of public sector organization negatively impacts the use of agile methodologies?

## 2   Government and Public Sector Organizational Culture

Organizational culture is described as the sum total of beliefs, meanings and values, the accepted behaviors and the political environment of a company [17, 18]. In essence it can be defined as the pattern of basic assumptions, and shared norms that are accepted and used by the organization. Implicit is the 'routinized' character of peoples' day-to-day activities that become internalized such that they may be autonomous. Such behavioral routines create repeated patterns of behavior [3]. Agile method authors clearly state that the organizational culture in which the agile method is embedded could have an impact on its use and they also make it clear that certain types of culture would make the successful use of an agile method difficult [4]. Beck [21] remarked that extreme programming (XP) is ineffective in organizations whose actual values are at odds with the XP values. We refer to "actual values" because many organizations have professed values differing from or contradicting the values revealed by their actions. In XP, you have a set of practices intended to express and reinforce a certain set of values. If an organization's actual values are secrecy, isolation, complexity, timidity, and disrespect, expressing the opposite values through a new set of practices will cause trouble rather than create improvement.

Bureaucracy is a form of organization based on strict rules and responsibilities attached to positions, not persons [5]. Within a bureaucratic context the emerging culture will be influenced by its endemic structure and culture—this is 'the way we do things around here' [3]. A structured rationality is endemic within bureaucratic environments; hence, they are common to government public sector departments [5]. It must be said here that not all government and public sector organizations are bureaucratic in nature. There are some government organization that may be less bureaucratic than some private sector organizations. Bureaucracy is not usually popular with those who undergo its effects, as it is thought of as a huge machinery, grinding slowly, with no feelings and no regard for the concerns of individuals [5]. Cynicism about the federal bureaucracy is widespread and the general public often views federal employees as aloof, uncaring bureaucrats who are unresponsive to their requests [6]. Bureaucrats make decisions by processing information with reference to predetermined rules, and accordingly, management emphasis is on order, uniformity, and consistency where organizational hierarchies provide channels for decision-making [19]. Predetermined rules that are inherent in bureaucratic environments do not seem to be consistent with the nature of agile methodology. Agile practitioners are known to make quick decisions on the fly based on the prevailing circumstances. Unlike in power-oriented government organizations, where decision-making is based on hierarchy, the best ideas resulting in the best decisions do not have to come from the top hierarchy in an agile team.

# 3 Review and Assessment Methodology

## 3.1 Literature Search Process

The methodology of evaluating, synthesizing and classifying academic literature is necessary for the advancement of knowledge, facilitating the development of new theories [16], identifying gaps in the collective published knowledge bank [15], and discovering opportunities for future research endeavors [20].

In order to identify the articles that were relevant for our study, we conducted a literature search of previously published works. We queried electronic library databases including Science Direct, ISI Web of Science, ACM Digital Library, Scopus, Emerald, Springer, Taylor & Francis, EBSCO, and JSTOR, with related keywords (see Table 1). The reference sections of identified articles were also used to find more articles. Because we did not find many journal articles relevant to the subject area, we also included conference papers. Literature in interrelated areas and subjects, such as agile adoption and agile manufacturing were excluded from the present study.

The literature search was conducted in April and May 2018. Following the procedure outlined in Fig. 1, we identified fifty-one (51) papers at the end of stage one (Identification). At the end of the second stage (screening), we had thirteen (13) papers remaining. After concluding the third stage (eligibility), we were left with eight (8) papers for this review.

**Table 1.** Database of sources and search term used

| S/N | Electronic database | Search terms |
|---|---|---|
| 1 | Google Scholar | Agile government, Agile Public Sector, |
| 2 | ACM Digital Library | Agile Bureaucracy, SCRUM Government, |
| 3 | IEEE Xplore | SCRUM Public Sector, |
| 4 | Web of Science | Extreme Programming government, |
| 5 | Science Direct - Elsevier | Extreme Programming Public Sector |
| 6 | Springer | |
| 7 | Wiley | |
| 8 | ProQuest | |
| 9 | Ebscohost | |
| 10 | JSTOR | |
| 11 | DTIC | |

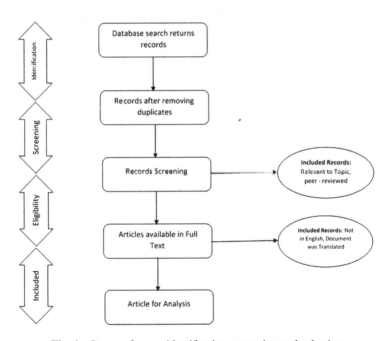

**Fig. 1.** Stages of paper identification, screening and selection

Table 2 shows the distribution of the articles by journal/conference of publication and year of publication. Four of the articles included in the review are conference articles and the other four are journal articles.

**Table 2.** Papers by journal/conference and year

| No. | Journal/conference | 2007 | 2008 | 2011 | 2012 | 2016 | Total |
|---|---|---|---|---|---|---|---|
| 1 | International Journal of Information Management | 1 | | | | | 1 |
| 2 | Journal of Management and Projects | | | | | 1 | 1 |
| 3 | IEEE IT Professional | | | 1 | | | 1 |
| 4 | HICCS Conference | | 1 | | | | 1 |
| 5 | IEEE | | | 1 | | | 1 |
| 6 | Agile 2008 Conference | | 1 | | | | 1 |
| 7 | Public Contract Law Journal | | | 1 | | | 1 |
| 8 | CrossTalk: Journal of Defense Software Engr. | | 1 | | 1 | | 1 |
| | Total | 1 | 2 | 3 | 1 | 1 | 8 |

## 3.2  Analytical Framework

The framework for our literature review and analysis is shown in Fig. 2. This framework was adapted from Roztocki and Weistroffer, 2015. The literature review focused on the elements that comprised the 'perspective'. The perspective includes research focus such as the type of project, the country of research, agile methodology used in the project, the challenges encountered in the process and the step taken to resolve the challenges. The research approach includes the sources of the data and the unit of analysis. The outcomes will feature the themes and trends in the papers we surveyed, identifying areas of consensus or contradiction, and specific actionable results.

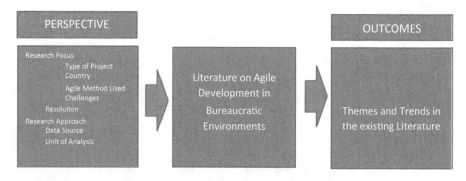

**Fig. 2.** Framework for literature review and analysis

Figure 3 shows the chart for the country of research based on the surveyed paper. 50% of the research papers analyzed were conducted in the United States while Brazil, Canada, UAE and UK have one paper each. The US dominance is in part due to the fact that various government organizations in the US are pushing for the use of agile methodologies in systems development including the FBI and the Department of Defense (DoD).

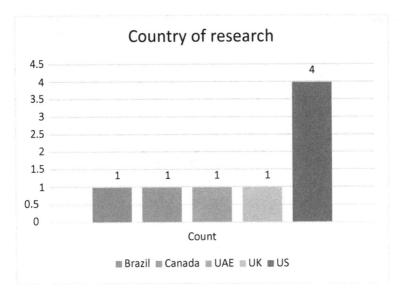

**Fig. 3.** Papers by country of research

Figure 4 below shows the papers surveyed by type of project. Software Development is the most common project encountered in the literature review, taking up 50% of the count for the type of project in the papers reviewed. This could be an indication that software development is the most common IS development that government and public sector organizations engage in. The other types of project include Knowledge Management System, IT Procurement and Business Process Re-engineering (BPR).

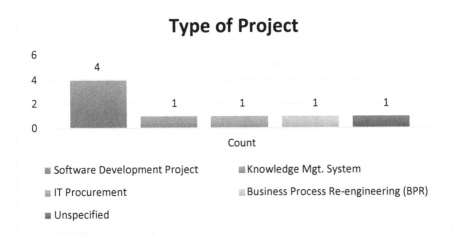

**Fig. 4.** Papers by type of project

The unit of analysis of the paper surveyed in the review is shown in Fig. 5. Seven of the eight papers focused on the organization. Bearing in mind that these papers all represent an attempt to use agile methodology in a government or public sector setting, it is not surprising that most projects were done within the level of the organization. However, one of the papers has a national focus in its approach and it was a call for all government organizations to adopt agile in their information systems development.

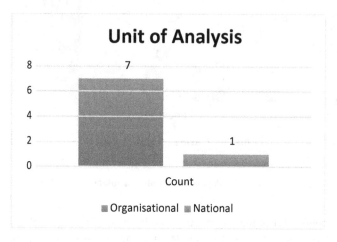

**Fig. 5.** Papers by unit of analysis

SCRUM turns out to be the most commonly used agile methodology. This is shown in Fig. 6. Other agile methodologies used in the reviewed papers are Iterative Application Development (IAD), Test Driven Development (TDD) and Extreme Programming (XP). Two papers did not focus on any specific agile methodology.

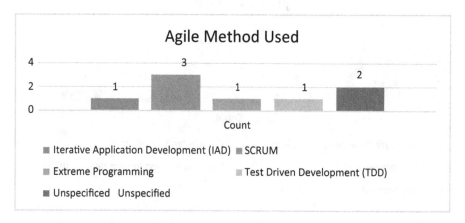

**Fig. 6.** Papers by agile method used

# 4   Observations and Implications

Our analysis of the papers reviewed in this study revealed several interesting findings. We found that each of the papers have highlighted several challenges that were deemed to impact or negatively impacted the adoption of agile methodology in the organization. Some of the papers discussed the resolution of some of the challenges while others did not. We discuss these challenges and their resolution.

## 4.1   Paper 1 – Agile Development in a Bureaucratic Arena – A Case Study Experience: Berger [3]

**Challenges**

a. The iterative nature of agile process requires speedy decision-making. Business managers, accustomed to high degree of culpability were not able to make these decisions as quickly as necessary because they were still driven by their need to satisfy higher authorities and external legislation and regulations.
b. For this bureaucratic setting the generation of trust, which was necessary to foster collaboration and co-operation, was problematic. Evidence illustrates that there was a lack of trust not only between the Developers and the organizational stakeholders, but also amongst the Business Managers themselves that impacted upon the ability to foster an integrated development environment.
c. Linked to this is the issue of team fusion. Evidence posits that collaborative working practices required for Agile development proved difficult. Getting consensus from Business Managers to move development forward was particularly problematic.
d. The bureaucratic working patterns of 'one person, one job' engendered a sense of 'ownership' of key business processes which bound key stakeholders to discrete working cultures that undermined the team fusion that was necessary for consensus and fast iterative development.
e. The Joint Application Development (JAD) workshops utilized for requirements gathering where agreeing to core development activities were crucial became complicated. Business Managers had difficulty in coming to a consensus due to their individual agendas, as each believed their own priorities to be paramount.

## 4.2   Paper 2 – Agile Method Application in a Public Sector Education Foundation: Date et al. [10]

**Challenges**

a. Challenges related to resistance to change by management in relation to allowing self-managing and self-organizing teams.
b. Communication problems between managers and staff. Stakeholders were not available to validate the product of a completed cycle. Without this the next cycle cannot start and continuing the project without validation means running the risk of creating rework and to delay the delivery of the final product.

c. It was observed that the managers used excessive control over activities and processes, for example, there was stiffness to control spending, the lack of openness to dialogue between employees from different sectors and departments.

## 4.3   Paper 3 – The FBI Gets Agile: Fulgham et al. [8]

**Challenges**

a. The project started with waterfall method but couldn't proceed further with the methodology. With the project design and requirements decided up front, the development team couldn't adapt to make improvements or desired changes.
b. The project included a large software development and management team of almost 300 people, which led to communication challenges, particularly among the software developers.
c. The FBI's large size and the project's political nature presented challenges as to how best to provide for external oversight without overburdening the Sentinel team.
d. Government contracting practices pose a significant problem for the adoption of agile methodologies in the federal government. Government agencies often prefer firm-fixed-price contracts, because they're simpler to administer and don't require the government to incur as much risk. However, such contracts are largely incompatible with the premises of agile development. They involve little flexibility and are based on the premises of stable requirements and upfront planning.
e. Federal regulations mandate implementing an earned value management (EVM) system for all government development projects. EVM is heavily dependent on the quality and completeness of a project's baseline plan, while agile projects are founded on the premise that you can't determine the complete scope and requirements upfront.

**Resolution**

a. Adhering to the agile tenant of small teams, the FBI selected a group of FBI employees and government contractors from the original large team to create a development team of approximately 15 members and a business team of approximately 30 members. The manageable team size let the FBI be more selective in its staffing and led to a more collaborative environment.
b. The development team is organized to share responsibility. No developer owns an area of work, although some take responsibility in their areas of expertise. This lack of a hierarchy results in more collaborative design decisions, where the group can override one person's ideas.
c. Also, the Sentinel team forged a strong relationship with upper management. Fulgham serves as the team's representative to other FBI executives and outside entities, and CTO.
   Jeff Johnson serves as co-executive sponsor for the program. Johnson relocated his office to the development team's area for daily contact with the team. He's the final arbiter for project decisions and helps remove any project-level barriers. Having access to high-level executives significantly reduces the time for major decisions and provides beneficial support to the Sentinel team.

d. The FBI's agile approach to Sentinel includes a combination of "cost plus" and "time and materials" contracting structures. These contracting vehicles, while more difficult to administer than firm fixed-price contracts, more naturally allow for iterative changes in requirements and plans. The FBI meets EVM requirements by using a bracketed project-tracking approach that combines the value metrics of traditional EVM with the burn down charts and velocity metrics commonly used in agile project management.

### 4.4  Paper 4 – A Case Study: Introducing Extreme Programming in a US Government System Development Project: Fruhling et al. [12]

**Challenges**

a. Traditional plan-driven methods are the mainstay in the military, partly because they are considered by some to have less risk and they support Capability Maturity Model Integration (CMMI) level-5 certification. (Most Department of Defense (DoD) projects are required by law to be CMMI level-3 compliant). Also, plan-driven methods are more consistent with the hierarchical structured military culture.
b. In the US Strategic Command contracting environment, it is not uncommon for development teams to be actively participating in multiple projects simultaneously and even for team members to be assigned to multiple projects with different teams. This was the case with the team participating in the Phase 1. Occasionally, there were competing priorities that interrupted work-flow.
c. Another issue that caused problems was scope creep. About the third week of Phase 1 it was determined that the user interface would need considerable changes and it would be helpful to have Human Factor Engineer (HFE) involvement. The HFE was not available to assist in the timely manner that the XP team needed. Further, this person seemed to be reluctant to participate in the XP process. Perhaps, partly due to the perception that the XP process was infringing on the HFE's current job responsibility as the chief designer of all the user interface modifications. Also the HFE was not included in the initial task selection discussion and was not integrated into the XP Pilot team originally.
d. The most frequent point made by interviewees was the importance of timely, complete, and accurate communication among the development project team. Meetings were scheduled and not everyone was available to attend and therefore, decisions were made, but not always completely and accurately communicated to everyone.

### 4.5  Paper 5 – Agile Adoption Experience: A Case Study in the U.A.E: Hajjdiab and Taleb [11]

**Challenges**

a. Agile master or agile coach is an essential role during agile adopting process in any organization. Agile coach is considered a consultant for the team in every step of a project using any agile method, such as Scrum, where is responsible for providing guidance and help to succeed in adopting agile. Entity S management recognized the need to hire a contractor as an agile master. However, the position was not filled due to financial constraints.

b. Another challenge is the absence of a pilot project in the transition from the previous traditional method to the scrum method. Conducting a pilot project was a recommended step in the adoption of agile development for the first time and was advised by the "Introduction to Agile Development" training course the project team attended. However, Entity S management thought that was a waste of time and resources and did not implement that.

c. The highly bureaucratic environment of Entity S meant that the agile team has to secure approvals and sign offs before moving forward with every step of the implementation. The time consumed by this process was affecting further development of the project.

d. The management of Entity S who were still influence by the heavy documentation of traditional methods required the team to create more documentations which created extra activities, took more time and took the focus away from actual implementation.

**Resolution**

a. Agile Master has a critical role to play to ensure successful outcomes. Obviously entity S needs to hire an Agile Master for at least six months to increases the chance of succeeding in the agile adopting process.

b. A pilot project must be selected when first adopting agile. The pilot project should be carefully selected as follows:
The project duration should be near the middle of what is the average for an organization. It should be small enough to be done by one team.
It should not be critical to the organization.

c. Agile development offers a new way of comprehensive documentation that takes less time and effort. This is another issue that needs to be supported by the upper management and agreed upon from the beginning of the project.

## 4.6    Paper 6 – Toward a More Agile Government: The Case for Rebooting Federal IT Procurement: Balter [7]

**Challenges**

a. Both conceptually and practically, Waterfall assumes that contracting agencies can accurately forecast a Project's requirements in advance, yet due to the often-unique nature of government systems, software contractors typically face challenges to which they have never been exposed, rendering predicting future needs an inherently futile task.

b. The traditional procurement model, which leans heavily on waterfall's central tenets, demands specificity in planning, funding, and acquisition, and requires the contractors and COs to attain a certain level of "predictive precision" simply not found in the ever-changing world of technology. As such, by requiring that all specifications be outlined up front, the current procurement model encourages agencies to attempt an inevitably unsuccessful endeavor and thereby increases project risk.

c. Because it is impossible for COs to resolve all unknowns at the onset of procurement, they often err on the side of caution and compound errors by over-documenting requirements and making erroneous assumptions. This risk is further exacerbated as a result of waterfall's insistence on delaying testing until late in the development cycle, meaning mistakes often do not become apparent until corrections are cost-prohibitive, especially given the size of typical government procurements.

d. Government contracts are not written for agile, as a matter of public policy, government contracting typically requires agencies to prefer competition at the cost of project deliverables. Secondly, government programs generally involve significant lead times—forcing funding to be mapped out well in advance—rendering a "develop as you go" method counterintuitive.

**Resolution**

a. Before federal IT procurement can embrace agile methodology, best practices education is required on two levels. First, Contracting Officers (COs) must learn best practices for agile contracting. Second, technical officers within the agency must learn best practices for agile project management in the government sector.

b. Many COs may not know what agile development is, let alone that it is a potential contracting vehicle and how best to implement it. The White House Office of Science and Technology Policy (OSTP) should oversee the joint efforts of the General Services Administration (GSA), the White House OMB, and the Office of Federal Procurement Policy (OFPP) to educate COs as to agile contracting best practices.

**4.7   Paper 7 – DoD Agile Adoption: Necessary Considerations, Concerns, and Changes: Lapham [13]**

**Challenges**

a. One particular stumbling block for the adoption of Agile tends to be capstone technical review events such as preliminary design review and critical design review. Agile methods typically do not produce the types of documentation expected at these milestones. Instead, they provide working prototypes and, in some cases, a subset of requirements implemented as usable software. Therefore, expectations and criteria for acceptance need to be established at the beginning of the contract that meet both the contractual needs and allow for the use of agile methods.

b. Each agile team usually conducts regular reflection and adaption called retrospectives.
The government team needs to understand and support this way of doing business. Otherwise, using Agile will have less than optimal results.

c. Customer collaboration is usually accomplished by having continuous contact with the end user. In many instances, the end user is an integral member of the iteration team. This is not always practical in the department of defense (DoD) environment, especially with joint programs and the myriad of stakeholders DoD software-reliant systems serve. In addition, the real end user is an operational person who may not have any experience in the acquisition career field while the acquirer may or may not have operational experience.

d. The team composition for agile developers is different than on traditional teams. Thus, the government should consider that their team would also have a different composition. Two important positions that are new to most government teams are agile advocate and end-user representative. An agile advocate provides real-time answers to immediate agile issues for the government team.

**Resolution**

a. The contractor and government usually solve this end user problem by agreeing on a proxy for the end users' day-to-day interaction and inviting end users to all demos.
b. Many of the agile concepts are not new, but the subtleties and nuances of each agile method can be new to the uninformed. To overcome this, all DoD PMO staff should be trained in the contractor's method of choice.

### 4.8   Paper 8 – Executing Agile in a Structured Organization: Government: Scott et al. [14]

**Challenges**

a. Client engagement varies. Their participation may be challenging to get and to keep past requirements sign off.
b. Communication and collaboration are hampered when conforming to the hierarchical structure.
c. Decision making is slow due to the top down single direction flow of information.
d. Delays in approvals often result in unauthorized work.
e. Authority to make work-related decisions by the team is limited due to the hierarchical structure.
f. The complexity of our process can obscure the end goals and diminish motivation of the team's effort.
g. Many Project Managers have 3 or more projects at varying stages of development, so they are continually switching context from one project to another.

## 5   Conclusion

As par our research questions, we asked if the bureaucratic nature of public sector and government organizations impacts the use of agile methodologies for information systems development. Based on the projects that were conducted in the reviewed papers, it is evident that using agile methodology for information systems development in a government or public sector organization does present challenges that appear to be directly linked to the bureaucratic environment of these organizations. We further asked if there are steps that can be taken to mitigate these challenges and adapt agile methodologies to bureaucratic cultures, and our literature review identifies the steps that were taken in these projects to resolve some of the challenges encountered. Some of the projects encountered in this study were deemed to be successful while others were not. Based on the reviewed papers, the authors believe that those projects that failed are due to a lack of advance knowledge on the challenges of using agile methodology for system development in a bureaucratic environment. Further research in this area is necessary to confirm this.

We feel that our research contributes to practice and scholarship in the following ways:

- Our findings may serve as guide for government and public sector organizations to be aware of the practices inherent in their bureaucratic culture that could hamper the adoption or use of agile methodology in systems development.
- Based on the nature of the challenges encountered in the projects investigated in this paper, government and public sector organizations may anticipate the problem areas that occur frequently and take preparative steps.
- Government and public sector organizations intending to use agile in their projects may learn from the measures taken in the projects investigated in this research to resolve some of the challenges encountered during the implementation of the project.
- Our findings may serve academic researchers to develop a more comprehensive framework that can guide bureaucratic organizations in the use of agile approaches in systems development.

# References

1. Cooke, J.L.: Everything You Want to Know about Agile How to Get Agile Results in a Less-than-agile Organization. IT Governance Publishing, Ely, Cambridgeshire (2012)
2. Cockburn, A., Highsmith, J.: Agile software development, the people factor. Computer **34**, 131–133 (2001)
3. Berger, H.: Agile development in a bureaucratic arena—a case study experience. Int. J. Inf. Manag. **27**, 386–396 (2007)
4. Strode, D.E., Huff, S.L., Tretiakov, A.: The impact of organizational culture on agile method use. In: 2009 42nd Hawaii International Conference on System Sciences, pp. 1–9 (2009)
5. Hofstede, G., Hofstede, G.J., Minkov, M.: Cultures and Organizations: Software of the Mind; Intercultural Cooperation and Its Importance for Survival. McGraw-Hill, New York (2010)
6. Johnson, R.N., Libecap, G.D.: The Federal Civil Service System and the Problem of Bureaucracy: The Economics and Politics of Institutional Change. University of Chicago Press, Chicago (1994)
7. Balter, B.J.: Toward a more agile government: the case for rebooting federal it procurement. Public Contract Law J. **41**, 149–171 (2011)
8. Fulgham, C., Johnson, J., Crandall, M., Jackson, L., Burrows, N.: The FBI gets agile. IT Prof. **13**, 57–59 (2011)
9. Alter, R., Lau, E., Saya, S.: Towards a more agile public governance. OECD Observer 24–25 (2014)

10. Date, R.N., Pinochet, L.H.C., Pereira Bueno, R.L., Nemoto, M.C.M.O.: Agile method application in a public sector educational foundation. Revista de Gestão e Projetos 7, 75–94 (2016)
11. Hajjdiab, H., Taleb, A.S.: Agile adoption experience: a case study in the U.A.E. In: 2011 IEEE 2nd International Conference on Software Engineering and Service Science, pp. 31–34 (2011)
12. Fruhling, A., McDonald, P., Dunbar, C.: A case study: introducing eXtreme programming in a US government system development project. In: Proceedings of the 41st Annual Hawaii International Conference on System Sciences (HICSS 2008), p. 464 (2008)
13. Lapham, M.A.: DoD Agile Adoption: Necessary Considerations, Concerns, and Changes. Carnegie-Mellon Univ Pittsburgh PA Software Engineering Inst (2012)
14. Scott, J., Johnson, R., McCullough, M.: Executing agile in a structured organization: government. In: Agile 2008 Conference, pp. 166–170 (2008)
15. Roztocki, N., Weistroffer, H.R.: Information and communication technology in transition economies: an assessment of research trends. Inf. Technol. Dev. 21, 330–364 (2015)
16. Webster, J., Watson, R.T.: Analyzing the past to prepare for the future: writing a literature review. MIS Q. Minneap. 26, R13 (2002)
17. Bliss, W.G.: Why is Corporate Culture Important? Workforce. How Organizational Culture Influences Outcome Information Utilization (1999)
18. Hodges, S.P., Hernandez, M.: How organizational culture influences outcome information utilization. Eval. Program Plan. 22, 183–197 (1999)
19. Carnall, C.A.: Managing Change in Organisations. Prentice Hall International, Upper Saddle River (1990)
20. Urbach, N., Smolnik, S., Riempp, G.: An empirical investigation of employee portal success. J. Strateg. Inf. Syst. 19, 184–206 (2010)
21. Beck, K., Andres, C.: Extreme Programming Explained: Embrace Change, 2nd edn. Addison-Wesley, Boston (2015)

# Transparency Driven Public Sector Innovation: Smart Waterways and Maritime Traffic in Finland

Vaida Meskauskiene[✉], Anssi Öörni, and Anna Sell

Information Systems, Åbo Akademi University, Turku, Finland
{vaida.meskauskiene,anssi.oorni,anna.sell}@abo.fi

**Abstract.** Finland is set to take the lead in developing maritime digitalization and autonomous shipping. This transformation rests on transparency efforts by Finnish government, characterized by participatory democracy and co-creation of services in public sector, the end of innovation deficit in public services through introduction of dedicated innovation budgets and open data movement for re-usability purposes. The research employs action research methodology and aims to analyse two forms of transparency driven innovation that took place during 2016–2018 as part of waterway digitalisation initiative by Finnish Transport Agency: 'Open Data Innovation' as opening up government processes and data and 'Open Door Innovation' approach as transforming service delivery. Both approaches initially resulted in number of innovative services, unintended consequences occurred in later stages of digitalization phase due to the lack of interest from businesses and greater public. We conclude with lessons learned and share recommendations for government to succeed in digitalizing one of the most conservative industries.

**Keywords:** Transparency · Public sector innovation · Smart government
Open data · Digitalisation · Maritime industry

## 1 Introduction

Finland is a maritime nation with several hundreds of seafaring and shipbuilding tradition and home to one of the most conservative industries in the world – maritime. The country's location on the northern fringes of Europe, long distances to Europe's main markets and challenging winter conditions all place Finland in a special position in relation to many other EU countries. Finland is very dependent on shipping and international trade for its national prosperity and wellbeing and about 90% of its exports and 80% of its imports are carried by Baltic sea [1]. Maritime industry is one of the key industries of Finland and includes very diverse actors in all global market segments, such as marine industry, shipping, ports and port operations, classification, financing and insurance, public sector (Finnish Transport Agency (FTA), Finnish Safety Agency (Traffi), Navy, research institutes and universities). In 2016, the total turnover of all activities associated with the maritime sector was approximately EUR 13 billion (the survey included 1,750 Finnish limited companies operating in the

© Springer Nature Switzerland AG 2019
M. Themistocleous and P. Rupino da Cunha (Eds.): EMCIS 2018, LNBIP 341, pp. 331–350, 2019.
https://doi.org/10.1007/978-3-030-11395-7_27

maritime cluster) [2]. Finnish companies alone employed 48,800 people in activities directly associated with the maritime sector. The value created by the cluster was estimated at around EUR 4 billion and created significant amount of exports.

Maritime industry has long been regarded in Finland as a traditional industry, where major innovations are born inside large corporations [1]. Understanding that maritime industry is conventional, closed, and not as flexible as desired, in recent years Finnish Government acted as partner and mediator for big corporations and startups and funded numerous national (2014–2017, €100 mln) and co-funded international EU development programmers (2015–2018, €100 mln) of the Finnish maritime cluster [3]. Keeping up with the pace of technological development requires maintaining the sufficient financial and scientific resources for innovation activities especially in the times of crisis. Because of the 2008 economic downturn shipbuilding orders broadly halted from 2009 to 2010 and shipping volumes decreased. To counter the unemployment and loss of know-how during the downturn, the Finnish government and regional administrations have established support functions to preserve the industry, including training programs, developing R&D networking between the firms in- and outside of the marine industry and, also universities and innovation grants paid for developing more environmentally friendly ships. These innovations proven crucial today, due to new Environmental legislation entered into effected since Jan 2018. Thus, innovations created by the public sector also affect the overall functioning of the Finnish shipbuilding and marine industry and maritime cluster [4].

Maritime is also one of the last industries affected by digitalization due to primary reason: connectivity at sea has been limited until very recently. With improving satellite data transmission, Arctic area coverage, deployed 5G connectivity, decreasing costs of sensors, enables full scale deployment of internet of things (IoT), enabling dramatic development how data, sensoring and Artificial Intelligence (AI) solutions can be utilised to support decision making, optimize processes, reduce resources and environmental impact. Intelligence built on top of big data collected by sensors installed on ships open up new possibilities for environmental monitoring, ensure transparency, enable public scrutiny and make shipping more environment-friendly. The increasing importance of the IT sector is a cross-cutting trend in the maritime cluster that brings together global industry forerunners, agile start-ups as well public sector to transform maritime sector thought automation and develop the world's first autonomous shipping solution. Ministry of Economic Affairs and Employment together with Finnish Marine Industries updated strategic research agenda for the time period 2017–2025, with the vision to become the world's leading country of digital maritime excellence [3]. Along with the vision, the world's leading digital ecosystem for marine industry - One Sea was established in Finland with the aim to create an environment suitable for autonomous ships by 2025. Trade dependency on sea transportation, freezing ports as well as shallow and difficult to navigate archipelago have been a catalyst for Finnish government in the past to develop innovative Arctic technology and know-how, the Baltic Sea having served as a test bed for prototyping. It's not a surprise that a globally unique feature of the ecosystem is its approximately 127 km$^2$ test area located off the west coast of Finland, open to all organizations wishing to test autonomous maritime traffic, vessels or technology [5].

Governmental agencies, such as FTA and legislation bodies have practiced an early adaptor mentality, paving the way to digitalization, automation and ultimately towards remote navigation. The high proportion of foreign trade transported by sea makes it essential that sea routes are well-functioning, reliable, safe and environmentally friendly. Good maritime connections are vital for the competitiveness of Finland's businesses and economy and for the Finnish society in general. In 2016, intelligent waterways initiatives and open data movement in Marine Traffic started to materialize in Finland, along with the announced dedicated government support for autonomous ship to become reality by 2025, and produced number of innovative experimental projects as a part of digitalisation initiative by Finnish Transport Agency (FTA) during 2016–2018. It is a unique opportunity to witness Finnish maritime transformation where government is set to play a major role. As new drivers for innovation emerge to fulfill ambitious goals of becoming a global pioneer in maritime digitalization, at the same time tensions arise from within the industry characterized by conservative culture deeply rooted in its traditions, while government gives a sense of stability having had a track record in adopting innovative solutions to address complex challenges it has faced through history. From information systems point of view, this makes research setting particularly interesting, relevant to practice and unique. Moreover, the innovation literature most often concerns ICT or other rapidly developing technology industries whereas the maritime related research may be viewed as a traditional industrial branch thus dominated in maritime industry and engineering subjects.

The remainder of the research paper is structured as follows: in literature review, we highlight the importance of public sector as a great source of open innovation, as well as place emphasis on transparency of information - the key starting point in smart government innovation projects. Our work employs action research methodology and reveals two forms of transparency driven innovation that crystalized in public sector during 2016–2018 smart waterway digitalisation initiatives: 'Open Data Innovation' as opening up government processes and data and 'Open Door Innovation' approach as transforming service delivery. Both approaches initially resulted in number of innovative services, unintended consequences occurred due to the lack of interest from businesses and greater public in later stages digitalization initiative. We conclude with lessons learned, share recommendations for government to succeed in digitalizing one of the most conservative industries.

## 2   Literature Review

### 2.1   Smart Government and Innovation in Public Sector

Smart government is used to characterize activities that creatively invest in emergent technologies coupled with innovative strategies to achieve more agile and resilient government structures and governance infrastructures to cope with complex and uncertain environments. Scholl and Scholl [6] outline a set of smart government elements: openness and decision making, open information sharing and use, stakeholder participation and collaboration, and improving government operations and services, all through the use of intelligent technologies as they act as a facilitator of innovation, sustainability, competitiveness, and livability. Gil-Garcia [7] emphasizes greater interorganizational collaboration, information sharing and integration as a core aspect of a smart state, which is not an end state or smart government dealing with complex social problems. Key and We [8] move further down the spectrum by more narrowly viewing smarter government as enabling smart information technology government operations such as establishing a government-wide, fee-based IT expert center/clearing house, organizing cross-agency birds of a feather working groups for every IT field; providing an infrastructure for educational training and easy online access to technical papers; and instituting procurement strategies. Smart government is build upon smart governance, which is defined as the creation, execution, and implementation of activities backed by the shared goals of citizens and organizations, who may or may not have formal authority or policing power" [9]. While there is an emerging consensus regarding its definition, the concept smart government has yet to be rigorously developed in research. A few studies have described some elements and characteristics of smart government and it varies with some governments are focusing on public sector innovation that has very little to do with emergent technologies and are characterized by large varieties of data sources including open and big data and others are focusing more on emergent technologies [10]. Gil-Garcia provide perspectives on the nature of smart governments and summarises its smart initiatives into two categories: on how smart governments are opening up public sector processes and data, and transforming service delivery to become smarter [10]. In summary, smart government challenges continually push public sector, at all levels, to explore innovative strategies that change internal processes and structures, for improved service delivery and new transparency requirements for communications with their users [11, 12], therefore more clear definition on information transparency requirements is needed as a starting prerequisite for smart government innovation activities.

## 2.2 Role of Transparency in Public Sector Innovation

Transparency of the public sector data and processes is one of the most important enablers of expansive use of digital services aimed at supporting value creation for society. Transparency has been defined as "the perceived quality of intentionally shared information from a sender" [13]. It implies openness, communication, and accountability. A transparent organization provides information in such a way that the stakeholders involved can obtain a proper insight into the issues that are relevant for them [14]. To put it succinctly, highly transparent processes can be characterized as the contact points between customers and organizations, at which the customers are allowed to interact with the process. Transparency is morally important, as it enhances an attitude of honesty openness and a commitment to truth; may enhance dynamic efficiency and innovation and is necessary condition for corporate social responsibility [15]. Without transparency, organizations performing well cannot distinguish themselves from ones that perform badly. This will limit the incentive to product and process innovation and necessity to increase value creation in the social and ecological dimensions [14, 16]. Recent research suggests there are three primary aspects of transparency relevant to management practice: *information disclosure, clarity, and accuracy* [13]. To increase transparency, organizations should actively infuse greater disclosure, clarity, and accuracy into their communications with stakeholders. This is also in organizations' self-interest for organizational transparency that is known to drive organizational performance [17]. Meijer analysed the history of concept and practice of government transparency over the past 250 years, using The Netherlands as a case study, and identified two major phases in this process: in the 1$^{st}$ one, transparency and openness are associated with the possibility of monitoring representatives of citizens in a representative democracy; in the 2$^{nd}$ – with participatory democracy of citizens, provided with the necessary information to "engage on an equal basis with government agencies and officials" [18]. Government transparency is nowadays associated with internet-driven information and communication technology (ICT), the open data movement [19] that aims to "deliver value to the public by creating additional, often unanticipated public-facing applications from that data" [20] and with open government portals [21]. Widespread availability of Internet and digital services were drivers for e-government participation, online service provision and reinforced benefits of openness: citizen sourcing in public decision-making and policies; co-production and collaborative service delivery for social and economic value [20]. But, as transparency within open government is closely associated with the open data movement, this risk is reinforced by the possibility of even the simple "open (government) data" expression losing its accountability-related meaning, focusing on the technical aspects of data release rather than on the goal of its release (accountability), blurring "the distinction between the technologies of open data and the politics of open government" [22]. We focus on the value of transparency within public sector innovation, and we follow Linders and Wilson's [20] two subgoals of transparency: releasing information for public accountability purposes and the intent to make data publicly available for re-usability purposes.

## 3  Methodology

Our study aims to fill the gap by investigating smart government innovation practices through transparency initiatives in Finnish Maritime Traffic Agency based on ethnographic observations and 59 in-depths interviews conducted in 2017–2018. It involves municipal and local officials, business representatives from large and small companies, leaders and public figures from different associations and One sea ecosystem, lecturers, researchers, students and start-up developers in Maritime industry Cluster. Additionally, the following archival data has been used in the research: Project Documentation, Posts in discussion forums, communication material on company websites, Press Releases, Critical Incidents/technical failure reports, Measures/KPIs of Success, Annual reports, Strategy documents, policy briefings. In specific, we aim to answer these questions: (1) what are the key issues in building innovation in smart waterways and maritime traffic? (2) how different transparency initiatives by government help or hinder to deliver innovations in waterways? As our research subject is relatively new one, the research intended here has attempts to generate new theory on the basics of existing constructs. Therefore a case study research is chosen, which is generally recommended as a suitable research design for theory building [23, 24]. Employing action research design will allow to intimately connect with the empirical reality of maritime industry and employ hands-on approach [25], which is often problematic for outside researchers. In the case of transformative nature of maritime industry, the issues involved are often of political control, the content matter tends to be complicated characterized by its complexity of domain specific knowledge, the stakeholders are large network of ecosystem players involved that are many in number and often time pressed and not easily accessible due to presence required at sea. The researcher has been actively involved in the digitalization of sea infrastructure project as consultant for the period of about 1.5 years. Besides the possibility to closely observe an organization, an action research approach has other well-noted methodological advantages: it enables researcher to revisit the organization after they are no longer involved directly in the project, and ensure the research results will be of guaranteed practical relevance, as fairway unit management is closely involved in research effort in progress [26].

## 4 Analysis of Smart Waterways and Maritime Traffic in Finland

Following the strategic implementation guidelines for the Finnish smart maritime technology solutions by 2025 [3], it was essential for the Ministry of Transportation and Communications (LVM) to start initiatives aiming to not only transform maritime sector to the digital age but direct all its activities to place Finnish maritime cluster in the leading role of digital maritime technology. In 2016 government, kick started maritime digitalization programs in two ways: by increasing operational efficiency of FTA services or by creation of new software applications, digital service offerings and added value for customers by opening data from public authorities. In Finland LVM deals with matters concerning the safety of waterborne traffic, aids to maritime navigation (ATNs), legal issues concerning shipping and maritime environmental legislation. Navigational instruments are preventive in nature to avoid groundings or collisions, and they include, for example, speed limits, sea-lanes, routeing of ships, ship reporting systems and Vessel Traffic Services (VTS). Internationally, navigational standards are embodied in the Convention on the International Regulations for the Prevention of Collisions at Sea (COLREG), SOLAS, IALA (International Association of Marine Aids to Navigation and Lighthouse Authorities) recommendation on waterway marking and related IMO guidelines [27]. In total, Finland has approximately 20,000 km of public, mapped fairways recorded on maps. Approximately 8,300 km of coastal fairways and 8,000 km of inland waterways are maintained by FTA. These fairways are marked with more than 34,000 maritime aids to navigation (including lighthouses, buoys signs and leading beacons) [28]. Despite the many dangerous spots, serious accidents occur infrequently due to safety-minded organisations and knowledge accumulated over one hundred years by FTA and preventive services.

FTA for maritime affairs consists of two major functions: VTS and waterway infrastructure service (cartography, ATNs, waterway markings and maintenance). The condition of waterways is very crucial from the point of view of shipping safety; the depth and breadth of a waterway and its safety devices – channel alignment and buoyage – all are important aspects. VTS aim to improve the safety and effectiveness of ship traffic. The VTS centers inform ships of the traffic situation, the conditions of waterways and safety devices, severe weather and ice conditions and other issues concerning the safety of navigation and follow situation in the area in real time based on information transmitted by AIS, radars, cameras and VHF radios. Finnish government decided VTS will be transferred to the new company on 1st January 2019. The aim of the new company is to promote the utilization of traffic control data in support of the development of new digital services, promote new business, improve the digital business environment for traffic and boost the growth of the Finnish maritime transport market [29]. This initiative means that the remaining FTA organization will be smaller; more constrained with resources and competence shortage, and will need to find new ways of partnering and co-creating digitalization of services.

## 4.1 Open Door Innovation Approach as Transforming Service Delivery

In 2016 FTA released new vision document "Smart routes and intelligent traffic - for you" aiming at reaching the target state described in the 2025 strategic research document [3]. There are several strategic goals that, when met through innovation projects, point FTA operations and decisions towards the target state of smart government:

- Renewed ecosystem for mobility and transport;
- Reliable digital services and greater operational efficiency;
- Services based on a well-functioning and safe infrastructure;
- Skilled professionals and an innovative organisational culture.

Anne Berner, Minister of Transport & Communications of Finland highlighted that "Finland is a forerunner of digital vessel services. Intelligent automation in fairways is the key to enhancing maritime safety, reducing emissions and improving productivity". When analyzing FTA strategic goals for maritime affairs, it became clear that any innovation must contribute to three key criteria:

1. Maritime Safety;
2. Transport and Service Efficiency;
3. Environmentally sustainable development and reduction in traffic emissions. Traditional innovation acquisition process in public sector is highly inflexible and follows strict rules and regulations, while OI processes are by design open and have few rules. European government agencies are either working with a group of pre-approved vendors and contractors who are responding to requests for proposals, which are then internally vetted before a solution proposed by a vendor is implemented; or, innovations are driven by policy mandates as a source of innovation in the public sector [30]. These forms of internal innovation creation following the standards of the bureaucratic governance process is called 'closed innovation' [31]. FTA agency was able to create so called 'Open Door' innovation acquisition approach by stepping outside of the formalized innovation acquisition process with contractual relationships by literally opening up the innovation process to amateur problem solvers, i.e. anybody who had a novel technological solution or unique way to address problems in maritime service provisioning, was able to approach the agency and present it to the team, which often followed by joined experiments arranged in testing areas in the field as well as provided technical support. In case testing results yielded desired outcomes, innovation when was acquired through digital dynamic procurement process or was indirectly acquired by FTA's maintenance contractors. In 2016 The Finnish Transport

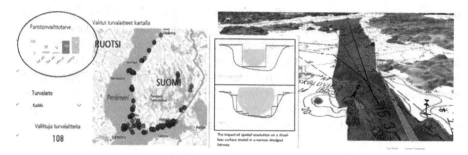

**Fig. 1.** Open door innovation streamlined service provision by digitizing physical aids to navigation into predictive maintenance platform, but failed to deliver instruments for bathymetric model in fairways (FTA)

Agency is made a digital leap in procurement by introducing online portal for government competitive tenders– all the way from publishing the call for tenders to announcing the final decision. Using the portal reduced physical paper pushing, and its automation and checks boosted the efficiency and reduce costs of both drawing up calls and submitting tenders. Agency was able to receive easily comparable, higher-quality tenders which was also open to the foreign supplier market. For FTA, this will mean receiving the most competitive and innovative tenders. Cost-effective competitive bids were made using the piloted version of the dynamic procurement system (KASSU) during 2016 with agile tools that accelerated the procurement process and generate savings in both costs and resources. It was possible to divide work into appropriate packages with regard to adequate market competition. The faster, fully digital procurement process also saved resources on both the client's and contractor's side, led to shorter times to procurements. Funding decisions were given quickly, often work needed to be launched as quickly as possible.

Open door approach worked well and did deliver successful project results in terms of digitalizing aids to navigation and streamlining service provision for more proactive/predictive fairway maintenance. However, more complex calls for innovation, such as Bathymetric model implementation of a sea bed data required deep Sw knowledge well as combination of GIS, machine learning capabilities and data visualization capabilities, received '0' proposals (see Fig. 1). Old network of supplier companies were running over capacity with their sw resources, while new comers form ICT sector were not actively participating in FTA calls for innovation traditionally dominant by companies with deep maritime experience and special hardware skills. As digitalization was more expanding into maritime, deep sw skills were more and more appreciated, and cannot be supplied by usual suspects. When it became obvious that open door approach is not open, but in fact – *semi open*.

Our data suggests that whereas FTA used versatile communication channels in Open door initiatives, they were used to target a historically established community of users directly, timely and explicitly. While rest of the public was informed with press releases, info decks and information about the past events published only several days after it actually happened. In other words, there was no possible way of informing large community of sw developers to attend open events, meet officials and learn about operational problem statements on time. Traditional innovation acquisition instruments limited FTA to involve larger community of problem solvers who were not a part of the formal acquisition process. The standard and only current practice to communicate to public the need for novel maritime solutions is directly tied to RFP. The existing RFP process, using language that is maritime industry standard and terms only known to professionals with background in maritime affairs or education as master mariners. High level of uncertainty about the capabilities of the new solvers, such s as start-ups form ICT field, most often prompted public officials to opt for less risky options: to work with preferred suppliers whom they trust based on a long history of successful collaboration, or as a last resort, let new comer companies though lengthy field trials and travail in order to prove their trustworthiness.

### 4.2 Open Data Innovation Approach as Opening-Up Government Processes, Data

Finnish public administrations have extensive data resources at its disposal (from field information to environmental, weather, climate, maritime, transport, economic, legislative, statistical and cultural material) which could generate significant financial and social benefits if used The Finnish Open Data Programme 2013–2015, set up by the Ministry of Finance, defined the goals which have made opening up data a part of daily work in FTA. Open data was officially declared an important factor in all development, planning and purchases that FTA does and Open API's were a key factor when renewing old and designing new information systems. FTA aim was is to share the Digitraffic service data - Real time traffic information it collects for operative purposes. Openly to everyone according to open data principles:

– without usage restrictions, with open licensing
– without cost
– through self-service electronic API's or by file downloads.

Since 2016, Digitraffic has become fully open data and expanded to cover information not only form road and rail but also marine traffic. FTA has chosen Creative Commons 4.0 as it's open data license. Currently open data API provides following information:

1. Marine warnings
2. Harbor schedules (gathered from the Portnet-system)
3. Vessel location AIS (Automatic Identification System)
4. Vessel and harbor metadata
5. Ice breakers.

As part of European Maritime Day 18th May 2016 in Turku City of Helsinki, Finnish Meteorological institute and Strategic Research Council of the Academy of Finland organized a workshop discussing maritime digital revolution and open data. The basic understanding behind the workshop was that digitalization means taking advantage of the big maritime data. The workshop focused on sources of open ocean data, opportunities and challenges of maritime digitalization and sharing how the open data have been utilized in maritime service sector and industry. It was widely agreed that open data policy is generating new business opportunities, but some data collected by the authorities should be freely available for a classified users only. In general, research institutes and other public agencies were considered to have a pivotal role in boosting new business opportunities by providing access to their data holdings as well as requesting companies to share their data too. The workshop discussed also on development of downstream applications. It was noted that for a large community of users and service providers would create a competitive markets where best and most user friendly applications are naturally developed. Following the event, in June 2016 a new Google group was created by FTA - meri.digitraffic.fi to facilitate open discussion among developers on terabytes of unstudied maritime data. It's customer support team is comprised of internal FTA experts, who provide regulatory guidelines and confirms that there are no legal obstacles for data publication and external International Sw consulting company experts, who have customer centered attitude and are very agile in daily operations. This mode proved to work well and FTA avoided early pitfalls of open data initiatives, where poor data management and overstretched public sector employees were cause of civic app failure in government initiative. Possibility to discuss in both English and Finnish attracted international participants and open release application was developed as cross collaboration effort between British and Finnish developers. Open data initiatives resulted in 3 published application. One of them was a novel offering, designed to spot abnormal behavior of vessels, however haven't got much public expose as it was names a test application and shortly deleted. The 1$^{st}$ public app 'Aluskartta.com' which also got a little advertisement across governmental pages, was developed by one of the open internet forum- country defense forum members who shared interest in military and navy technology. Few months later the second application 'Boat watch' was released by navigational sw company Pocket Mariner as a test app, but shortly it has been developed into more sophisticated commercial version (Fig. 2).

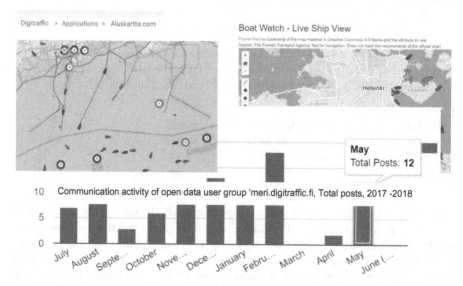

**Fig. 2.** Open data resulted in similar applications and lack of activity in open data user group (FTA)

The group activity was focused on primarily reporting the bugs or requesting more data to be opened. Out of 41 members, only 6 developers were relatively active with posts, couple of these were students driven by possibility to learn coding practices with GIS data, while the rest represented successfully growing SME companies in maritime navigational sw. and equipment. What united all of these users was deep interest in maritime affairs, proceeded by experience at sea as enthusiast or captains and formal master mariner's education. Companies valued open data, and greeted with enthusiasm to open access to ice breakers, in couple of instances developers asked to provide data also from other Nordic countries to get better scalability for their apps and to save costs, as similar data was very costly to obtain in other Nordic countries. However, compared to road and railway Open data groups, Maritime's activity was sporadic and initial enthusiasm slowed towards the beginning of 2018. Developers wanted to have release of bathymetric sea bed data sooner, but were asked about the possible data formats in 2018 when it was way too late for most companies, who have purchase the data sets from commercial data providers. This was not surprising to have '0' replies for desirable formats of new data sets. Also the initial open data sets were somewhat limiting, the data has been to some extend already available in one form or the other. Developers, with similar maritime experience or interest, were guided by limited data set availability which resulted in applications similar in functionality, limited impact for FTA and limited civic benefit. Developers struggled to envision solutions that would greatly complement provision of FTA services, such as needed redevelopment of public feedback channels, or solve operational challenges. The FTA maritime unit did little to attract large numbers of open data users with ICT background, which was becoming a crucial trend to incorporate advanced sw knowledge in maritime field that was shifting form hardware to sw platform approach. In terms of information transparency dimensions, open data was opaque in terms of both clarity – was very hard to comprehend for non-mariners, while mariners could not easily envision solutions to solve operational challenges in servicing fairway infrastructure. Disclosure of data was slower than developers expected and maritime officials were not keen to release new data sets that would potentially produce radical innovations or generate great developer interest to open even more data. It could be argued that also accuracy of open data was heart by FTA regulatory requirement to include following statement when publishing developer apps: 'Not for navigation. Does not meet the requirements of the official chart', as FTA was not able to check the accuracy or timeliness of the data of ECS systems, ie plotter and navigation software.

Our findings also support the preliminary assessment prepared by Ministry of Finance, in September 2015 [32] which suggests that research into the impacts of open data is just beginning and more systematic follow-up and improved methodologies will be needed in the future. We conclude open data initiatives should be part of a more comprehensive digitalisation policy, including the principles of digitalization of fairway services. Moreover, managing Open data release at FTA and operational service provision work was usually done in separate sub-units, who had little interaction and did not share common targets. This disconnect between open door for service provision and open data initiatives greatly hampered joined innovation activities towards 2025 and its potential success. Second disconnect was observed in user communities, where prevailing knowledge was maritime and hardware related, while experienced ICT developers did not flock in high numbers. Along our findings, the government report [32] proposed further steps for moving from the opening of data resources to data utilization and data competence enhancement. The third disconnect was between cultures: the digitalization culture that brought a sense of urgency to experiment clashed with and old-fashioned maritime culture not willing to change established ways of doing things for the sake of safety.

## 5  Lessons Learned

National-level policies for the for implementing OI in maritime affairs have been designed relatively recently (with official action procedures released in 2016) and FTA is still in rather early stages of innovation implementation process [33], despite it's efforts to practice of early technology adaptor mentality, deployment of number of successful experimental innovation in the field, and publishing a crowed sourced application to track sea traffic in real time. Number of open innovation projects and publicly released open data sets in maritime unit have been mediocre in comparison to other units of transportation, such as roads and railways there amount of budget allocated, number dedicated test sites and resulted innovative apps have doubled or tripled in size in comparison to waterways. FTA's maritime unit, characterized without prior experience of opening up the formal innovation creation process, with multidimensional practices that include range of technological, legal, organizational and outcome related aspects of innovations has been one of the last to activate open data initiatives. Therefore important to understand not only how government organization perceive the challenges of open innovation, but the factors that hinder or may foster the implementation. Main issues identified in our research study include the lack of interest and slowness to react to calls for innovation from developers in both open door and open data initiatives; quality of radical innovations provided by companies (due to widespread availability of IoT solutions and prevailing hardware competence amongst companies involved in marine ecosystem); low quality of user ideas (excessive use of similar datasets leading to numerous similar apps), officials' skeptical attitudes towards user ideas and new comer companies in innovation space, and the lack of transparency in supportive processes/structure/resources in public service organizations. We further discuss how these main organizational transparency issues can be resolved (see Table 1) by accessing its three key dimensions underpinning transparency suggested by Schnackenberg and Tomlison: disclosure, clarity, accuracy [13]. To address varying and, in certain aspects, low degree of information transparency, we identify key organizational capabilities and related actions that FTA maritime organization should take: **competence, communications, commitment and culture.**

**Table 1.** How to improve transparency of government information and foster innovation.

| What was learned? | Transparency dimensions |
|---|---|
| Problem statements, strategic priorities and guidelines published by officials to direct developers innovation effort toward operational challenges | Clarity |
| Start-ups and developers from ICT domain invited to 'shadow' ongoing work in FTA organizations to better understand particularities of maritime services operations and accelerate reciprocal trustworthy relationships | Clarity, disclosure |
| Common communication practices towards members form both communities, joined shared events and discussion forums | Clarity, disclosure |
| Target setting in place and in line with strategic research programs to force public officials to publish data in a timely manner | Disclosure |
| Coordination of data standardization, structured data models, open APIs, decentralised data management, provision of real time and raw data whenever possible by legislation or deregulation | Accuracy |
| Common repositories for crowdsourced data and applications, open source coding practices to foster community engagement | Disclosure |
| Stronger coordination by government officials towards direct interaction between two communities for competence exchange | Clarity, disclosure |
| Culture shift form 'fair of un-know' to leadership in experimenting with new technology/crowdsourcing concepts and risk-taking attitude | Accuracy, disclosure |

**Competence.** Greater *clarity* of information can be achieved by increasing competence of organizational stakeholders exchanging the information. Organizations can more clearly communicate with stakeholders through messages that accommodate the knowledge and information requirements of the stakeholder [34]. Conveying information with *clarity* involves understanding the perspective of the stakeholder audience who may also not be as familiar with internal organizational processes, routines, and jargon [13]. Unlike FTA organizational insiders, ICT developers and open user community often have unique interests, needs, and concerns that are built upon software development knowledge processes, yet be unfamiliar with particularities of maritime technology and terminology. Thus often FTA agency is more likely to abandon the idea to invite external non-professional problem solvers into their innovation process as there is an obvious knowledge gap that takes time to even explain the problem area. The maritime technology oriented R&D teams hired and partially outsourced to ICT companies to develop answers in-house and might feel that it is their core job to know it all, the result is oftentimes that solutions from non-professional problem solvers are not accepted [35]. We believe that broad participation of users, rather than strictly with maritime background, is likely to increase the probability of generating services that contribute not only to the private businesses as open data community showed, but also to public value. We argue, OI and end-user generated practices help make conflicts of different user and value perspectives explicit and more transparent, thus stimulate the generation of entirely new services or new ways of streamlining provision of existing services – versatility in competence and attitudes, that has been missing in both the open door and open data communities. We have also learned that competences of users in open data and FRP calls directly affected how they participate in innovation activities, which support previous research [36]. Developing transparent procedures and relevant online resources to help citizens develop their knowledge and skills in innovation, tapping into outlets and events to facilitate users' learning process is vital for fostering open innovation in the public sector, that has been suggested as an effective strategy by Ministry of Employment and the Economy in Finland [3].

**Communications.** Open innovation strategy requires a rich, intense, and open dialogue, where different communication channels enable organisations to create the transparency of service development process. Having a firm understanding on the information requirements of stakeholders is important to successfully increase organizational *disclosure* through open information systems [13]. To accomplish this, Google user group for Open data in maritime traffic was created. Although relatively small in terms of number of users, it provided opportunities for small developer companies and maritime enthusiast with sw knowledge to collaborate (in some cases across the countries) and report bugs, suggest ideas, request additional data from FTA, in other words moved knowledge from one context to another [37]. However, other means of communication were not so successful. Versatility of communication channels can reach different innovator audiences, facilitate the participation of users in their innovation process, enable the transferring of certain development tasks and knowledge to users, and help users develop their knowledge and skills during the process [38, 39]. Our data suggests that whereas FTA used versatile communication channels in Open door initiatives, they were used to target a historically established community of users directly, timely and explicitly. While rest of the public was informed with press releases, info decks and information about the past events published only several days after it actually happened. In other words, there was no possible way of informing large community of sw developers to attend open events, meet officials and learn about operational problem statements on time. Traditional innovation acquisition instruments limited FTA to involve larger community of problem solvers who were not a part of the formal acquisition process. The standard and only current practice to communicate to public the need for novel maritime solutions is directly tied to RFP. The existing RFP process, using language that is maritime industry standard and terms only known to professionals with background in maritime affairs or education as master mariners. Salge et al. showed that too much openness does not support the innovation process unless a guided approach is used [40]. Organization scan influence *clarity* though use of framing that render information content more understandable [13]. Therefore problem statements in the OI process need to be written in plain language to make them understandable to amateur problem solvers, such as sw developer enthusiasts, but open ended enough to allow for suggested innovations from ICT start-up community the FTA has not thought about itself. As addressed by the majority of sw developers, to foster open innovation, FTA need to set up multiple communication channels, including both e-communication tools and direct contact approaches, and at different levels, e.g. use common sense to reach out to state-of-the-art knowledge outlets, such as start-up community open spaces, to meet the heterogeneous demands of citizens. By doing so, public sector can facilitate open access to information, encourage larger participation, raise awareness and support their own capacity-building. Unlike successful experiments through open door innovation processes that typically followed with press releases, FTA marine unit did little to openly advertise new public apps and not surprisingly, citizens didn't check governmental websites to discover them.

**Commitment.** In public sector, strategic objectives of FTA are set up on the basis of government policies, which in turn determine resource allocation. If organizations often face resource constraints and competitive dynamics that render efforts toward *disclosure* – completeness of information transparency difficult to achieve [41]. In our research setting FTA unit managers appear to have a variety of leadership, resource allocation, and third-party alternatives to influence *accuracy*. Researchers suggested that to build a capacity for candid interactions and disclose reliable information with stakeholders organizations must promote honesty and hire authentic leaders [42, 43]. While for other FTA (road and railway) agencies open data mandate allowed to innovate in an open format through release of various data sets, the mandate was a burden to maritime as they have been avoiding to release bathymetric and environmental data early on in 2016 to enforce more versatile release of apps and sustainable implementation of OI. Developer companies could not afford to wait and instead purchased the needed data from other commercial providers, which resulted reluctance to provide feedback on desirable formats of forthcoming release of bathymetric data. Research suggest the dominance of private interests encourages narrowly instrumental motivation for participation and lose focus on public interests [44]. Without clear leadership, developers in open community tended to focus on self-interest or their company interests and ignore commitment of users as citizens, sharing public innovations during their engagement in innovation process. It could have been argued that the commitment was needed across all levels, not only at politicians, ministry, but also most senior leadership level at FTA maritime and public officials, who have impact on strategic direction and tactical implementation. FTA organization structure eventually followed strategy 2025 and as example, have institutionalized several roles of Innovation Management, filled by internal people who were most knowledgeable at a time to lead the way and promoted experiments, internal innovation and open data the most, as well as encouraged other to follow the path. It turned out that problem was on most senior maritime unit management level: open data release was steady since launch of the program in 2016 as performance targets were tight to financial rewards. As soon as these were dropped, senior management lost its interest in open data release. However the latest restructuring resulted in transferring of all innovation managers to public company VTS, thus it remains unclear and worrying who can lead public innovation openly at FTA maritime unit. In line with research findings on the first generation failures of civic apps, releasing open data was a chore with no tangible, unpredictable benefits but also subjected FTA department to unwanted public scrutiny [45]. Commitment should be set up at different levels including target setting and key performance indicators concerning relevant OI activities. Taken together, these factors suggest that managing transparency is a complicated endeavor requiring organizations to balance internally defined objectives against the interests of divergent stakeholder groups [13].

**Culture.** Organizational culture influences level of information *disclosure* to its stakeholders [42]. According to our research investigation, both participants in open doors and open data communities in general considered public service organization easy to approach and cooperative, but slow to react and lacking enthusiasm toward external participation. Being innovative and doing innovative things implies certain amount of risk taking, and by definition public officials are risk adverse. All public sector managers in FTA were trained to define very clearly deliverables for any contract or RFP call, while open innovation relies to solve problems that doe not have predefined solutions. This was counter intuitive to the way their structure operates. High level of uncertainty about the innovation outcomes and about the capabilities of the solver communities most often prompted public officials to opt for less risky options: to work with preferred suppliers whom they trust based on a long history of successful collaboration, or as a last resort, let new comer companies though lengthy field trials and travail in order to prove their trustworthiness. *Accuracy* is related to correctness of information provided by organization, which is a challenge for FTA operating in complex, highly nationally and internationally regulated environment. Organizations ability to successfully navigate complex data and master the technical aspects of compiling needed data to develop reliable information perceived as ability to convey accurate information [13]. Regulatory bodies request FTA information that is highly technical and subject to compliance with national and IMO regulations and standards, however the new digiticed ECS data would require constant effort of testing terabytes of new data to reach acceptable level of quality assurance. Traditionally testing of paper charts has been an internal, time-consuming activity carried out by FTA professionals and master mariners, resulting in trelase of data accuracy of 100% every two weeks. FTA was not able to test the accuracy or timeliness of the data of ECS systems, ie plotter and navigation software in order to meet performance standards of the IMO Official Electronic Navigation System (ECDIS). To counter that, FTA released public statement that advised users should have printed charts when navigating and requested developers to include the following statement when publishing their apps with FTA's digital data: 'Not for navigation. Does not meet the requirements of the official chart'. Declaring innovations as inaccurate is counterproductive. Instead, we believe government should focus on finding new ways or organizing data performance test as digitalization only going to increase in the future. The maritime safety policy is very detailed, for example with regard to ship construction and equipment, and there is less there is room for experimentation and innovations, however standards are still lagging behind any other industry. More attention has been paid to make policies more encouraging for continuous improvement [46]. By nature, maritime safety is a very complex issue and it is as much related to culture than anything else. Besides policy instruments, such complex issues as language, authority and communication are all determined by individual and institutional relationships. Several studies have pointed out to the safety culture of the maritime industry, which is in many ways, old-fashioned: there is a high tolerance for accepting incidents and near misses in the maritime community; mariners are not proactive on safety issues; Pilots and VTS centers cannot command ships, only give advice; it is still the basis of maritime law that the ship master is in absolute charge of his vessel [46, 47]. The law was guiding this practice in the past when there were no ways to follow a ship after it left a port and no effective means to swiftly communicate between the cargo owner and a ship master. Digitalization and connectivity has change the maritime operating context, but regulation and culture remains backward looking. When compared to other industries, e.g. aviation, this practice seems quite odd especially when thinking about safety culture on the organizational or industry-wide levels, which are probably a greater cause of accidents than the actions of a single officer on board [27]. Successful policy changes are needed to change old-fashioned safety culture of the maritime industry and reflect the complexity of inter-relationships and the multiplicity of centers of authority rather than a single person.

Organizational culture is slowly changing at FTA maritime unit from closed innovation paradigm to open, where experimentation is a part of trial and error process and new learning is encouraged form mistakes. In the past existing culture did not allow to take innovation related risks: failing was not acceptable in public institution of welfare state and things simply could not go wrong because maritime always place safety first above all. With strategic vision 2025 and designated innovation budgets, encouraging small scale experiments with new technology and new data was gradual but probably the safest way to innovate in maritime.

New practices for developing competences, building commitment and improving communication together foster establishment of experimental, innovation embracing culture where different contributor roles are valued. As our research shows, both open door and open data approaches to public sector innovation have its strengths and weaknesses (missing accountability for the impact of the open data; open door ecosystem was semi-open) resulting in different transparency deficits. Combining the two would be the best approach in terms of resource utilization and innovation results.

# 6 Conclusions

The case demonstrates the benefits of making maritime information transparent through government efforts to open data and open its doors in terms of both engaging maritime enthusiasts and harnessing the potential for service innovations from the private sector.

What we have learned during open data initiatives in maritime sector is not special to the world of smart government but comparable to other domains of collective, decentralized creativity common in software development platforms. Closer examination of open door policy revealed how service delivery in infrastructure provisioning and maintenance can be transformed through innovations from community-based private organizations that are effective at instrumenting new technologies based on the transparency and guidance provided by government into potential fixes, which is not fundamentally different from how successful public-private partnerships work.

What we uncovered as unique in our study was the management of required competence. It proved more complex than in any other traditional markets as digitalisation challenged prevailing skillset in rather homogeneous maritime ecosystem. Innovating through open data required at least basic skillset of maritime specific knowledge and familiarity with definitions, something that was traditionally present among software developers who happen to be maritime enthusiasts or with relevant master marine education. The existing skill set gap in open data community isolated larger proportion of Finnish developers, who would have been invaluable in delivering wide range of applications for wider community and citizens. Another type of skills, such as advanced software knowledge in geographical information systems, machine learning and computer vision became obvious shortage in open door innovation community, historically excelling at hardware competence, and became a showstopper in the most radical innovation projects. This could been easily avoided with on-line training, educational seminars, and communicating guidance on policy briefings as well as sharing insights on key operational challenges facing infrastructure services. And more importantly, the two transparency driven initiatives should have been blended in form the very beginning of government innovation programs.

Smart government initiatives in maritime are complex and cuts across functions and sectors. Only senior leaders can orchestrate such a complex system and, as quoted by Kotter would dare "to make the status quo seem more dangerous than launching into the unknown" [48]. Government officials have identified potential drawbacks of both approaches to transparency as potential threat to navigational safety. This reasoning is deeply rooted in traditional maritime culture where historically any introduction of incremental innovation in maritime (such as new navigational instruments, processes or vessels) placed safety first into the equation of potential benefits. The safety has been and is a challenge in a marine environment, where unpredictable force of nature is always present and cannot be controlled 100%. Therefore conservative culture still strongly prevails amongst most experienced, leading officials in the public sector of waterway and marine traffic unit: *an introduction of new is a risk to safety for society at large*. The issue of talent gap contributes to the case of visionary committed leadership. After all, it's far easier to introduce bottom-up innovation and implement change if you have people with the right competences around, who also have a pulse on technology and positive believe it can benefit the society at large.

# References

1. Liuhtio, K.: The maritime cluster in the Baltic Sea region and beyond. Centrum Balticum Foundation, 18 May 2016
2. Karvonen, T., et al.: The Finnish maritime cluster: towards the 2020s. In: Ministry of Economic Affairs and Employment. University of Turku (2016)
3. Finnish Marine Industries: A Strategic Research Agenda For The Finnish Maritime Cluster 2017–2025
4. Makkonen, T., Inkinen, T., Saarni, J.: Innovation types in the Finnish maritime cluster. WMU J. Marit Aff. **12**, 1–15 (2013)
5. Business Finland, 16 May 2018. https://www.businessfinland.fi/en/whats-new/news/2018/finland-takes-the-lead-in-developing-maritime-digitalization-and-autonomous-shipping/
6. Scholl, H.J., Scholl, M.C.: Smart governance: a roadmap for research and practice. In: iConference 2014, pp. 163–176 (2014). http://dx.doi.org/10.9776/14060
7. Gil-Garcia, J.R.: Towards a smart state? Inter-agency collaboration, information integration and beyond. Inf. Polity **17**, 269–280 (2012). https://doi.org/10.3233/IP-2012-000287
8. T., W. C. Key: Smart IT. In: IEEE IT Proceedings, pp. 20–23, February 2009

9. Bingham, L.B., Nabatchi, T., O'Leary, R.: The new governance: practices and processes for stakeholder and citizen participation in the work of government. Public Adm. Rev. **65**(5), 547–558 (2005)
10. Gil-Garcia, J.L., Helbig, N., Ojo, A.: Being smart: emerging technologies and innovation in the public sector. Gov. Inf. Q. **31**, I1–I8 (2014)
11. Bertot, J.C., Jaeger, P.T., Grimes, J.M.: Using ICTs to create a culture of transparency: e-Government and social media as openness and anti-corruption tools for societies. Gov. Inf. Q. **27**(3), 264–271 (2010)
12. Reddick, C.G., Turner, M.: Channel choice and public service delivery in Canada: comparing e-government to traditional service delivery. Gov. Inf. Q. **29**(1), 1–11 (2012)
13. Schnackenberg, A.K., Tomlison, E.C.: Organizational transparency: a new perspective on managing trust in organization-stakeholder relationships. J. Manag. **42**(7), 1784–1810 (2014). https://doi.org/10.1177/0149206314525202
14. Kaptein, M.: Developing and testing a measure for the ethical culture of organizations: the corporate ethical virtues model. J. Organ. Behav. **29**, 923–947 (2008)
15. Dubbnik, W., et al.: CSR, transparency and the role of intermediate organisations. J. Bus. Ethics **82**, 391–406 (2008)
16. Graafland, J.J., Eijffinger, S.: Corporate social responsibility of Dutch companies: benchmarking, transparency and robustness. De Economist **152**, 1–24 (2004)
17. Berggren, E., Bernshteyn, R.: Organizational transparency drives company performance. J. Manag. Dev. **26**, 411–417 (2007)
18. Meijer, A.: Government transparency in historical perspective: from the ancient regime to open data in the Netherlands. Int. J. Public Adm. **38**(3), 189–199 (2015). https://doi.org/10.1080/01900692.2014.934837
19. Davies, T.: Open data barometer: 2013 global report (2013). www.opendataresearch.org/
20. Linders, D., Wilson, S.C.: What is open government? One year after the directive. In: 12th Annual International Conference on Digital Government Research (Dg.o 2011), pp. 262–271. ACM, College Park (2011)
21. Lourenço, R.: An analysis of open government portals: a perspective of transparency for accountability. Gov. Inf. Q. **32**(3), 323–332 (2015). https://doi.org/10.1016/j.giq.2015.05.006
22. Yu, H., Robinson, D.G.: The new ambiguity of 'open government'. UCLA Law Rev. Discl. **59**, 178–208 (2012). https://doi.org/10.2139/ssrn.2012489
23. Eisenhardt, K.: Building theories from case study research. Acad. Manag. Rev. **14**(4), 532–550 (1989)
24. Yin, R.: Case Study Research: Design and Methods (1989)
25. Reason, P., Bradbury, H. (eds.): Handbook of Action Research: Participative Inquiry and Practice. Sage, London (2000)
26. Gill, J.: Research as action: an experiment in utilising the social sciences. In: Heller, F. (ed.) The Use and Abuse of Social Science. Sage, London (1983)
27. Kuronen, J., Tapaninen, U.: Maritime safety in the Gulf of Finland. Center for Maritime Studies, University of Turku (2009)
28. https://www.liikennevirasto.fi/web/en/waterways#.WxAgi0iFM2w
29. https://www.liikennevirasto.fi/web/en/-/traffic-control-functions-of-the-transport-agency-into-a-special-assignment-company#.Ww65HkiFM2z
30. Arundel, A., Casali, L., Hollanders, H.: How European public sector agencies innovate: the use of bottom-up, policy-dependent and knowledge-scanning innovation methods. Res. Policy **44**(7), 1271–1282 (2015). https://doi.org/10.1016/j.respol.2015.04.007
31. Felina, T., Zenger, T.R.: Closed or open innovation? Problem solving and the governance choice. Res. Policy **43**(5), 914–925 (2014). https://doi.org/10.1016/j.respol.2013.09.006

32. Kauhanen-Simanainen, A., Suurhasko, M.: From open data to innovative knowledge exploitation: open data program 2013–2015 final report. Ministry of Finance Publications, 31 September 2015. http://vm.fi/julkaisu?pubid=6902

33. Lee, S.M., Hwang, T., Choi, D.: Open innovation in the public sector of leading countries. Manag. Decis. **50**(1), 147–162 (2012). https://doi.org/10.1108/00251741211194921

34. Wolfe, R.A., Putler, D.S.: How tight are the ties that bind stakeholder groups? Organ. Sci. **13**, 64–80 (2002)

35. Katz, R., Allen, T.J.: Investigating the Not Invented Here (NIH) syndrome: a Look at the performance, tenure, and communication patterns of 50 R&D project groups. R&D Manag. **12**(1), 7–20 (1982). https://doi.org/10.1111/radm.1982.12.issue-1

36. Spital, F.: An analysis of the role of users in the total R&D portfolios of scientific instrument firms. Res. Policy **8**(3), 284–296 (1979)

37. Gray, P.H., Parise, S., Iyer, B.: Innovation impacts of using social bookmarking systems. MIS Q. **35**, 629–643 (2011)

38. Bogers, M., Afuah, A., Bastian, B.: Users as innovators: a review, critique, and future research directions. J. Manag. **36**, 857–875 (2010)

39. von Hippel, E.: Democratizing Innovation. The MIT Press, Cambridge (2005)

40. Salge, T.O., Farchi, T., Barrett, M.I., Dopson, S.: When does search openness really matter? A contingency study of health-care innovation projects. J. Prod. Innov. Manag. **30**(4), 659–676 (2013). https://doi.org/10.1111/jpim.12015

41. Chen, M., Miller, D.: Competitive dynamics: themes, trends, and a prospective research platform. Acad. Manag. Ann. **6**, 135–210 (2012)

42. O'Toole, J., Bennis, W.: What's needed next: a culture of candor. Harvard Bus. Rev. **87**(6), 54–61 (2009)

43. Walumbwa, F.O., Luthans, F., Avey, J.B., Oke, A.: Authentically leading groups: the mediating role of collective psychological capital and trust. J. Organ. Behav. **32**, 4–24 (2011)

44. Langergaard, L.L.: Understanding of 'users' and 'innovation' in a public sector context. In: Sundbo, J., Toivonen, M. (eds.) User-Based Innovation in Services, pp. 203–226. Edward Elgar, Cheltenham (2011)

45. Lee, M.J., Almirall Mezquita, E., Wareham, J.: Open data & civic apps: 1st generation failures - 2nd generation improvements. Commun. ACM **59**(1), 82–89 (2016)

46. Lappalainen, J.: Transforming maritime safety culture – evaluation of the impacts of the ISM Code on maritime safety culture in Finland. Publications from the Centre for Maritime Studies University of Turku A46 2008 (2008). http://www.merikotka.fi/metku/Lappalainen_2008_transforming_maritime_safety_cultu

47. Hänninen, H.: Negotiated risks - the Estonia accident and the stream of bow visor failures in the Baltic ferry traffic. Doctoral Thesis, Helsinki School of Economics, A-300 (2007)

48. Kotter, J.P.: Leading change: why transformation efforts fail. Harvard Bus. Rev. (1995)

# Healthcare Information Systems

# Analysis of the Readiness for Healthcare Personnel Adopting Telerehabilitation: An Interpretive Structural Modelling (ISM) Approach

Mahadi Bahari[1]([⊠]), Tiara Izrinda Jafni[2], Waidah Ismail[3]([⊠]),
Haslina Hashim[2], and Hafez Hussain[4]

[1] Information Service Systems and Innovation Research Group,
Azman Hashim International Business School (Information Systems),
Universiti Teknologi Malaysia, Johor Bahru, Malaysia
mahadi@utm.my

[2] School of Computing, Faculty of Engineering, Universiti Teknologi Malaysia,
Johor Bahru, Malaysia

[3] Faculty of Science and Technology, Universiti Sains Islam Malaysia,
Nilai, Malaysia
waidah@usim.edu.my

[4] PERKESO Rehabilitation Centre, Malacca, Malaysia

**Abstract.** Telerehabilitation (TeleRehab) is the modern innovation used for rehabilitation service. Evidence in favor of readiness among healthcare personnel in adopting TeleRehab is limited. Since "readiness" is a crucial prerequisite to the successful implementation of an innovation, studying the healthcare personnel readiness for TeleRehab is mandatory to gain a better understanding of the relationships among the factors. The main aim of this paper is to determine the relationship among the readiness factors of healthcare personnel and to identify the most influential factors from the recommended readiness list with the help of ISM approach. The study has been conducted in three different phases: the identification of readiness factors from reviewing the literature, interviews with personnel healthcare, and determining the relationship among the readiness factors and its most influential factor. Twelve (12) relevant readiness factors have been identified from reviewing the literature and interviews with experts. Through the use of ISM, five (5) factors have been identified as driver factors; another five (5) factors have been identified as the linkage factors and two (2) factors have been identified as the dependence factors. No factor has been identified as autonomous factor. Out of which, one (1) factor has been identified as top-level factor and one (1) bottom level factor. Clear understanding of these readiness factors will help healthcare institutions to better prioritize and manage their human resource, healthcare personnel in an efficient and effective way to adopt TeleRehab. The proposed structured model developed will help to understand relationship of the readiness factors.

**Keywords:** Telerehabilitation · Readiness factor · Healthcare personnel
Interpretive Structural Modelling (ISM)

© Springer Nature Switzerland AG 2019
M. Themistocleous and P. Rupino da Cunha (Eds.): EMCIS 2018, LNBIP 341, pp. 353–368, 2019.
https://doi.org/10.1007/978-3-030-11395-7_28

# 1 Introduction

The implementation of telerehabilitation (TeleRehab) has been well implemented in developed countries such as Canada [1], Italy [2], and the United States [3]. There has also been an increase in implementation of TeleRehab in developing countries such as Pakistan [4], and South Africa [5]. The acceptance and implementation of TeleRehab in these countries are attributed to the attitude and willingness of patients, healthcare personnel, and healthcare organizations who are receptive to new technologies.

In addition, the demand for better rehabilitation recovery encourages patients with chronic pain who receive physical therapy to accept TeleRehab as an alternative rehabilitation method. The advantages of TeleRehab such as cost-effectiveness [6] and barriers reducer (e.g., time, distance) [7, 8] has been well documented and has shown that it can improve healthcare. Considering these factors, TeleRehab service is one of the innovations to be adopted in Malaysia to improve its healthcare specifically in rehabilitation of patients.

Some studies have highlighted the importance of healthcare personnel's role as a trigger for the acceptance of innovation [9], The readiness of healthcare personnel is crucial as they are main users and gatekeeper in the healthcare institution and this affects their acceptance for this new innovation. However, the influence of the readiness of healthcare personnel for TeleRehab has not been well investigated [10].

In this study, we seek to determine the readiness factor that influence healthcare personnel for TeleRehab adoption as it is important to ensure the project's effectiveness and success. This study will also focus on the interaction or relationship between determined factors from the literature review and interview sessions by formulating a model of readiness factors that influence healthcare personnel for TeleRehab. The aim of the study is to focus on formulating a model of readiness factors that influence healthcare personnel for TeleRehab.

To explore this domain, we applied the Interpretive Structural Modelling (ISM) approach to determine the most readiness factors impact or influence healthcare personnel for TeleRehab adoption. The paper is organized as follows: Sect. 2 presents a brief literature review, Sect. 3 outlines the research methodology used and Sect. 4 details the finding of the study. Finally Sect. 5 concludes and discusses the contribution of the study.

# 2 Literature Review

To achieve the main objective, a comprehensive literature review is performed to develop a list of readiness factors. This requires a qualitative approach by means reviewing the relevant literature from various electronic databases, including ScienceDirect, Scopus, PubMed, Web of Science, SAGE, IEEE Xplore and ACM Digital Library. All articles were then filtered according to inclusions (i.e., paper related to TeleRehab readiness) and exclusions (i.e., paper that applied TeleRehab in others component such as TeleRehab adoption and TeleRehab implementation). Any duplicating factors (i.e., based on their characteristics) was then merged and treated as similar. As a result, 12 variables were identified as the readiness factor that influences healthcare personnel for TeleRehab. These readiness factors are discussed below.

(1) *Awareness:* The awareness towards TeleRehab is referring to the individual who is concerned or is aware for the needs of existing and new innovation in healthcare [8, 9] and towards the potential advantage and disadvantage of TeleRehab [12]. It is important for the healthcare personnel to keep up-to-date or is aware of the new TeleRehab innovations to ensure they are always ready to apply something new for the benefit of patients and healthcare field.

(2) *Comfort:* It refers to the openness of the individual or healthcare personnel to accept technology and use it [8, 11, 12]. The positive perception of the technology affects the condition of the healthcare personnel in adopting the new technology [15]. If they perceive that the new innovation of TeleRehab can benefit both the patients and themselves (i.e., ease the rehabilitation service delivery), they will be more comfortable using it.

(3) *Satisfaction and willingness:* Satisfaction indicates whether the healthcare personnel is satisfied with the current method of delivery of services to the patients which can influence the acceptance of use for TeleRehab [8, 11, 12]. While, willingness refers to the healthcare personnel who is willing to implement the new innovation to improve and replace the current system [9, 13, 14]. These variables are related to each other since satisfaction of healthcare personnel leads to the willingness to accept, learn, and adopt TeleRehab.

(4) *Connectivity:* Connectivity refers to the speed and quality of internet connection for data exchange between the healthcare institution and patient's house [8, 14]. Secure and stable internet connection allows the improvement of the behavior change of using communication in the health information technology [17].

(5) *Skills:* Other than medical skills, computer skills are essential and important for TeleRehab. Lack of exposure to computer skills of the healthcare personnel is one of the major issues, which need to be solved before the adoption of new innovation [16]. The healthcare personnel needs time to learn and master computer skills, thus allowing them to use it [18]. Good qualification, adequate training, and experience enables the healthcare personnel to use and implement TeleRehab effectively [9, 16].

(6) *Hardware and software:* Generally, hardware are tools, machinery equipment used in the physical aspect of telecommunications network infrastructure, while software is the common term used to describe any operating system or programs used by the computer [16, 19]. The hardware required for healthcare service are a laptop, desktop, monitor, TV-based conferencing, and PC-based conferencing [18]. Both patient and healthcare institutions need necessary of hardware and software for adopting TeleRehab [4].

(7) *Concern:* Concern as a readiness factor in this study is seen from the view point of the healthcare personnel. There are three aspects that need to be examined. First is the concern and awareness of the healthcare personnel of whether their medical expertise is adequate to implement and use new innovation (TeleRehab) [14]. In cases whereby, their medical expertise does not fulfill the requirement for the new innovation, additional training is needed. Second, the concern of

handling the daily quota of patients for rehabilitation by the healthcare personnel [18]. The number of daily quotas for each healthcare personnel will affect the time and quality of the healthcare they provide to patients. This is due to the extra time and effort needed as the patients are from both healthcare organizations and in their own homes. Third is the concern of healthcare personnel of the return on investment of using TeleRehab. To implement TeleRehab requires a big investment at the start however it does not immediately provide high return to the patients [17–19]. Due to this, the healthcare personnel will start to compare using TeleRehab against the usual rehabilitation practice and their concern on this matter will affect their receptiveness on using new innovation in their healthcare delivery.

(8) *Planning:* Planning new innovation starts with the idea followed by the involvement of responsible individual or group with good implementation plan [8, 12, 20]. The contribution of the effective champion as the individual who issues ideas of innovation, push for approval of the innovation and resolve the innovations barriers [21] is very important in the adoption of TeleRehab. In this regard, top management may provide a medium for healthcare personnel to issue ideas for improvement. Through the ideas, the innovation planning to enhance the rehabilitation service delivery can be carried out.

(9) *E-Healthcare knowledge:* This refers to the knowledge about what accurately e-Healthcare is about and its contribution to the healthcare [10]. The healthcare personnel with advanced and up-to-date knowledge could potentially become innovators or champions by producing great ideas for TeleRehab service. TeleRehab service offers many advantages to advance the limitation of current service delivered at a healthcare institution. It also affects the readiness level of healthcare personnel in accepting new innovation [14]. In addition, it is important to understand the readiness concept before implementing this innovation to avoid loss of money, time, and effort [10].

(10) *Learnability:* The learnability is the ability of the individual to learn the new knowledge such as being able to learn the new system and the belief that it is more productive to use the system [14, 22]. The exposure to new innovation of TeleRehab allows healthcare personnel to understand and quickly learn about it. Subsequently, the resistance to change can be reduced since the exposure to the advantages of TeleRehab in providing good rehabilitation service.

(11) *Resistance to change:* The resistance to change is one the negative impacts to the need of the healthcare institution to adopt TeleRehab [14]. The resistance to change occurs when healthcare personnel perceive this new innovation as less innovative than any existing technology already used in the healthcare institution. In addition, the healthcare personnel also tend to resist change if their patients will not be able to gain access and utilize it for recovery [12].

(12) *Financial benefits:* A good innovation if new technology can provide financial benefits to the patients and also healthcare institution [23]. The start-up cost, ongoing cost, cost related to a loss returns, and potential savings to put against these costs are the variables in financial benefits factor [23]. Some studies mention that TeleRehab service will benefit the patients due to the cost reduction to get rehabilitation service in the long term [6, 24]. TeleRehab service offers to

overcome the cost, distance, and time barrier for the rural patients to get rehabilitation services [18]. However, the new roles and responsibilities created
through the introduction of TeleRehab also allow the healthcare personnel to
receive the financial benefits [23]. The healthcare personnel needs more time and
effort to tackle TeleRehab at the beginning of the adoption. Therefore, the
healthcare institution tends to deliver incentives which benefits the healthcare
personnel [23].

In order to comprehensively assess TeleRehab readiness among healthcare personnel, the relevant readiness factors must be recognized. The consideration of these
readiness factors thus improves the quality of planning of TeleRehab programs in
healthcare institution.

## 3   Research Methodology

To analyze the readiness factors of healthcare personnel for TeleRehab adoption, all
twelve (12) factors identified while reviewing the literature (as listed in Table 1) were
considered. For developing a structural relationship among these factors and to find the
prominent factors that influence healthcare personnel for TeleRehab, the ISM is used.

**Table 1.** Factors influencing readiness of healthcare personnel for TeleRehab

| Serial no. | Factor | Reference |
|---|---|---|
| 1 | Awareness | [9, 11, 14] |
| 2 | Comfort | [9, 13–15] |
| 3 | Satisfaction and willingness | [9, 13, 14] |
| 4 | Connectivity | [9, 16–18] |
| 5 | Skills | [9, 16, 18] |
| 6 | Hardware and software | [4, 9, 16, 18, 19] |
| 7 | Concern | [18, 19, 25, 26] |
| 8 | Planning | [9, 14, 20, 21] |
| 9 | e-Healthcare knowledge | [12, 14] |
| 10 | Learnability | [14, 22] |
| 11 | Resistance to change | [12, 14] |
| 12 | Financial benefits | [6, 23, 24] |

The basic idea of ISM is to use the knowledge and experience of healthcare
personnel to construct a multilevel of the structural model [25]. The flowchart for the
ISM approach [27] is shown in Fig. 1.

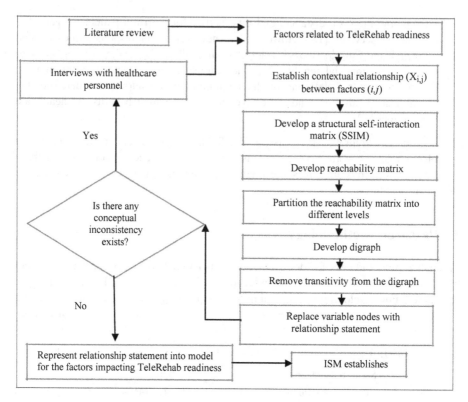

**Fig. 1.** Flowchart diagram for preparing the ISM for factors of TeleRehab readiness

The eight steps involved in the ISM methodology are as follow [26, 27]:

- **Step 1: Generation an ISM implementation group** - Identify a group of healthcare personnel with related knowledge, skills, experience, and work background related to study area.
- **Step 2: Recognition and selection the key elements** - Prepare a list of key elements (factors).
- **Step 3: Formation of the structural self-interaction matrix (SSIM)** - Identify pairs of elements and format the pair-wise relationship between elements.
- **Step 4: Development the reachability matrix** - Develop the reachability matrix to verified for transitivity of the relation. Transitivity is when factor "A" is related to factor "B" and factor "B" is related to factor "C", the factor "A" is necessarily related to factor "C".
- **Step 5: Division the reachability matrix into different levels** - Divide reachability matrix to generate the digraph. The transitivity links are removed.
- **Step 6: Development of ISM** - Convert the digraph into an ISM by replacing element nodes with the statement.

- **Step 7: Check for consistency** - Review the developed ISM model for conceptual inconsistency.
- **Step 8: Conduct the MICMAC analysis** - Classify key elements using MICMAC analysis.

## 3.1   Data Gathering

The first step in the development of ISM is the identification of healthcare personnel's opinion. We conducted one case study at one rehabilitation center in Malaysia. We interviewed eight (8) physicians, twenty-five (25) therapists and fifteen (15) nurses in a semi-structured way. The purpose of conducting these interviews was to explore intensively the opinions of selected healthcare personnel on their readiness for Tele-Rehab. The interviewees were carefully selected based on their experience and involvement with rehabilitation services. At the end of this step, we are able to identify and develop the contextual relationship among the twelve (12) identified factors.

## 3.2   Structural Self-Interaction Matrix (SSIM)

The contextual relation is selected to evaluate the connection between the variety of factors that affect TeleRehab readiness. The relationship between two factors, $i$ and $j$ and the linked direction of this relationship was classified into four alphabets. The alphabets used to as the direction of the relationship between any two factors ($i$ and $j$) are V, A, X, and O, as follows:

- V: factor $i$ will influence on factor $j$;
- A: factor $j$ will influence on factor $i$;
- X: factors $i$ and $j$ will influence each other;
- O: factors $i$ and $j$ have no correlation with each other.

**Table 2.**  Structural self-interaction matrix (SSIM)

| Factor no. | 12 | 11 | 10 | 9 | 8 | 7 | 6 | 5 | 4 | 3 | 2 | 1 |
|---|---|---|---|---|---|---|---|---|---|---|---|---|
| 1 | V | V | V | A | V | X | O | O | A | A | A | – |
| 2 | X | V | X | A | X | X | X | A | A | A | – | |
| 3 | A | V | V | A | V | X | A | A | A | – | | |
| 4 | V | V | V | O | V | V | X | V | – | | | |
| 5 | O | V | X | A | A | V | X | – | | | | |
| 6 | O | V | V | O | X | O | – | | | | | |
| 7 | A | X | V | O | V | – | | | | | | |
| 8 | X | X | V | A | – | | | | | | | |
| 9 | O | X | V | – | | | | | | | | |
| 10 | A | O | – | | | | | | | | | |
| 11 | A | – | | | | | | | | | | |
| 12 | – | | | | | | | | | | | |

The SSIM for the factors is summarized in Table 2. The following cases provide support as examples:

- Factor 1 helps achieve factor 10, implying that as "awareness" increases the "learnability" increases as well. Thus, the relationship between factors 1 and 10 is denoted by "V" in the SSIM.
- Factor 5, "skills" can be achieved by factor 3, "satisfaction and willingness". Computer skills would promote the satisfaction and willingness of healthcare personnel to adopt TeleRehab. Thus, the relationship between these two factors is denoted by "A" in the SSIM.
- Factors 8 and 6 help achieve each other. Factor 8, "planning", and factor 6, "hardware and software" help achieve each other. Thus, the relationship between these factors is denoted by "X" in the SSIM.
- No relationship exists between "e-Healthcare knowledge" (i.e., factor 9) and "concern" (i.e., factor 7), and hence, the relationship between these factors is denoted by "O" in the SSIM.

### 3.3   Initial Reachability Matrix

In this step, the SSIM is converted into a binary matrix, which known as initial reachability matrix. Here, the SSIM alphabets of V, A, X, and O is substituted by 1's and 0's as per the case [28]. The reachability matrix follows simple rules as follows:

- If $(i, j)$ value in the SSIM is V, $(i, j)$ value in the reachability matrix will be 1 and $(j, i)$ will be 0
- If $(i, j)$ value in the SSIM is A, $(i, j)$ value in the reachability matrix will be 0 and $(j, i)$ will be 1
- If $(i, j)$ value in the SSIM is X, $(i,j)$ value in the reachability matrix will be 1 and $(j, i)$ will be 1
- If $(i, j)$ value in the SSIM is O, $(i, j)$ value in the reachability matrix will be 0 and $(j, i)$ will be 0.

Following these rules, the initial reachability matrix for factors is developed as depicted in Table 3.

**Table 3.** Initial reachability matrix

| Factor no. | 1 | 2 | 3 | 4 | 5 | 6 | 7 | 8 | 9 | 10 | 11 | 12 |
|---|---|---|---|---|---|---|---|---|---|---|---|---|
| 1 | 1 | 0 | 0 | 0 | 0 | 0 | 1 | 1 | 0 | 1 | 1 | 1 |
| 2 | 1 | 1 | 0 | 0 | 0 | 1 | 1 | 1 | 0 | 1 | 1 | 1 |
| 3 | 1 | 1 | 1 | 0 | 0 | 0 | 1 | 1 | 0 | 1 | 1 | 0 |
| 4 | 1 | 1 | 1 | 1 | 1 | 1 | 1 | 1 | 0 | 1 | 1 | 1 |

(continued)

**Table 3.** (*continued*)

| Factor no. | 1 | 2 | 3 | 4 | 5 | 6 | 7 | 8 | 9 | 10 | 11 | 12 |
|---|---|---|---|---|---|---|---|---|---|---|---|---|
| 5 | 0 | 1 | 1 | 0 | 1 | 1 | 1 | 0 | 0 | 1 | 1 | 0 |
| 6 | 0 | 1 | 1 | 1 | 1 | 1 | 0 | 1 | 0 | 1 | 1 | 0 |
| 7 | 1 | 1 | 1 | 0 | 0 | 0 | 1 | 1 | 0 | 1 | 1 | 0 |
| 8 | 0 | 1 | 0 | 0 | 1 | 1 | 0 | 1 | 0 | 1 | 1 | 1 |
| 9 | 1 | 1 | 1 | 0 | 1 | 0 | 0 | 1 | 1 | 1 | 1 | 0 |
| 10 | 0 | 1 | 0 | 0 | 1 | 0 | 0 | 0 | 0 | 1 | 0 | 0 |
| 11 | 0 | 0 | 0 | 0 | 0 | 0 | 1 | 1 | 1 | 0 | 1 | 0 |
| 12 | 0 | 1 | 1 | 0 | 0 | 0 | 1 | 1 | 0 | 1 | 1 | 1 |

## 3.4   Final Reachability Matrix (FRM)

The final reachability matrix is obtained by incorporating the transitivity as enumerated in Step 4 earlier. The final reachability matrix is presented in Table 4. This table shows the contextual relation in which if factor "A" is related to factor "B" and factor "B" is related to factor "C", the factor "A" is necessarily related to factor "C". In this table, the driving power and dependence power of each factor are also shown along with their level. The driving power of a particular factor is the sum of factors which it may help achieve while the dependence is the sum of factors which may help achieve it.

**Table 4.** Final reachability matrix (FRM)

| Factor no. | 1 | 2 | 3 | 4 | 5 | 6 | 7 | 8 | 9 | 10 | 11 | 12 | Driving power | Level |
|---|---|---|---|---|---|---|---|---|---|---|---|---|---|---|
| 1 | 1 | 1* | 0 | 0 | 1* | 0 | 1 | 1 | 0 | 1 | 1 | 1 | 8 | IV |
| 2 | 1 | 1 | 1* | 0 | 0 | 1 | 1 | 1 | 0 | 1 | 1 | 1 | 9 | III |
| 3 | 1 | 1 | 1 | 1* | 1* | 0 | 1 | 1 | 0 | 1 | 1 | 0 | 9 | III |
| 4 | 1 | 1 | 1 | 1 | 1 | 1 | 1 | 1 | 0 | 1 | 1 | 1 | 11 | I |
| 5 | 0 | 1 | 1 | 1* | 1 | 1 | 1 | 1* | 0 | 1 | 1 | 0 | 9 | III |
| 6 | 0 | 1 | 1 | 1 | 1 | 1 | 1* | 1 | 0 | 1 | 1 | 0 | 9 | III |
| 7 | 1 | 1 | 1 | 1* | 0 | 1* | 1 | 1 | 0 | 1 | 1 | 0 | 9 | III |
| 8 | 0 | 1 | 0 | 1* | 1 | 1 | 1* | 1 | 1* | 1 | 1 | 1 | 10 | II |
| 9 | 1 | 1 | 1 | 0 | 1 | 0 | 1* | 1 | 1 | 1 | 1 | 0 | 9 | III |
| 10 | 0 | 1 | 0 | 0 | 1 | 0 | 0 | 0 | 1* | 1 | 1* | 0 | 5 | V |
| 11 | 0 | 0 | 0 | 0 | 0 | 0 | 1 | 1 | 1 | 0 | 1 | 1* | 5 | V |
| 12 | 0 | 1 | 1 | 0 | 0 | 0 | 1 | 1 | 1* | 1 | 1 | 1 | 8 | IV |
| Dependence power | 6 | 11 | 8 | 6 | 8 | 6 | 11 | 11 | 5 | 11 | 12 | 6 | 101 | |
| Level | IV | II | III | IV | III | IV | II | II | V | II | I | IV | | |

Note: 1* Entries are included to incorporate transitivity

## 3.5   Partitioning of the FRM

To make sure the construction of digraph is smooth and easy, the FRM is extracted by level partitioning. The factors of reachability set are defined as the factor that is related or influenced by other factors. Whereas, the factors of the antecedent set are defined as the factors which are influenced by other factors. The intersection set was derived from the intersection of the reachability set and antecedent set. The partition of FRM was illustrated in Table 5. It is observed that the "resistance to change" is at Level-I. Therefore, it would be placed at the top of the ISM.

**Table 5.** Partition on final reachability matrix

| Factor | Reachability set | Antecedent set | Intersection set | Level |
|--------|------------------|----------------|------------------|-------|
| 11 | 7, 8, 9, 11, 12 | 1, 2, 3, 4, 5, 6, 7, 8, 9, 10, 11, 12 | 7, 8, 11 | I |
| 2 | 1, 2, 3, 6, 7, 8, 10, 11, 12 | 1, 2, 3, 4, 5, 6, 7, 8, 9, 10, 12 | 2, 10 | II |
| 7 | 1, 2, 3, 4, 6, 7, 8, 10, 11 | 1, 2, 3, 4, 5, 6, 7, 8, 9, 11, 12 | 2, 10 | II |
| 8 | 2, 4, 5, 6, 7, 8, 9, 10, 11, 12 | 1, 2, 3, 4, 5, 6, 7, 8, 9, 11, 12 | 2, 10 | II |
| 10 | 2, 5, 9, 10, 11 | 1, 2, 3, 4, 5, 6, 7, 8, 9, 10, 12 | 2, 10 | II |
| 3 | 1, 2, 3, 4, 5, 7, 8, 10, 11 | 2, 3, 4, 5, 6, 7, 9, 12 | 3, 5 | III |
| 5 | 2, 3, 4, 5, 6, 7, 8, 10, 11 | 1, 3, 4, 5, 6, 8, 9, 10 | 3, 5 | III |
| 1 | 1, 2, 5, 7, 8, 10, 11, 12 | 1, 2, 3, 4, 7, 9 | 1 | IV |
| 4 | 1, 2, 3, 4, 5, 6, 7, 8, 10, 11, 12 | 3, 4, 5, 6, 7, 8 | 4, 6 | IV |
| 6 | 2, 3, 4, 5, 6, 7, 8, 10, 11 | 2, 4, 5, 6, 7, 8 | 4, 6 | IV |
| 12 | 2, 3, 7, 8, 9, 10, 11, 12 | 1, 2, 4, 8, 11, 12 | 12 | IV |
| 9 | 1, 2, 3, 5, 7, 8, 9, 10, 11 | 8, 9, 10, 11, 12 | 9 | V |

## 3.6   Formation of the Structural Model

The final ISM based model for readiness factors that influence healthcare personnel for TeleRehab is demonstrated in Fig. 2.

This model is constructed from the final reachability matrix shown in Table 5, where all the twelve (12) factors are summarized into five (5) levels. The different levels are identified using a level partitioning process, which shows the driving and dependence power of a factors and how they are connected at the same level and with the factors at the next level above. It is observed from Fig. 2 that "e-Healthcare knowledge" appearing at Level-V is a very significant factor in influencing healthcare personnel for TeleRehab, as this factor becomes the base of the ISM hierarchy.

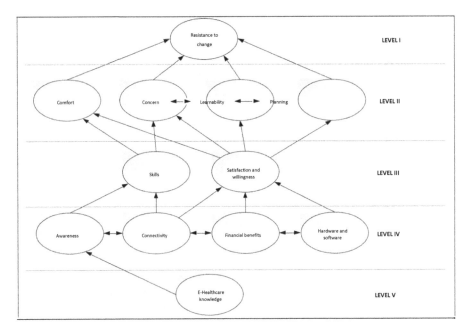

**Fig. 2.** Proposed ISM model on readiness for TeleRehab

### 3.7 MICMAC Analysis

The aim of MICMAC analysis is to analyze the driving power and dependence power of elements [29]. The factors can be grouped into four (4) clusters - autonomous, dependent, linkage, and independent.

(1) **Autonomous factor:** This cluster includes factors have weak driving power and weak dependence power. They are relatively disconnected from the system, with which they have only few links, which may be strong. These factors were represented in quadrant I.

(2) **Dependent factor:** In this quadrant, factors have weak driving power but strong dependence power. These factors were classified in quadrant II.

(3) **Linkage factor:** In this cluster, factors have strong driving power as well as and strong dependence power. These factors were placed in quadrant III. They are also unstable, so any action on them will influence the others and will affect themselves.

(4) **Independent factor:** In this quadrant, factors have strong driving power but weak dependence power. These factors were categorized in quadrant IV.

Figure 3 shows the driving power and dependence of each of the factors.

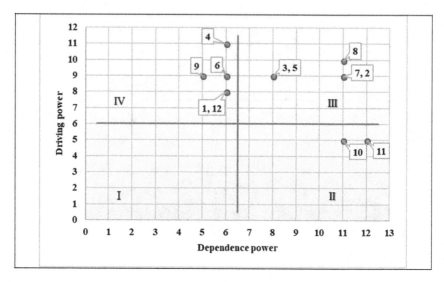

**Fig. 3.** Driving power and dependence power diagram. Note: Quadrant * (I) Autonomous factor; (II) Dependent factor; (III) Linkage factor; and (IV) Independent factor

## 4 Findings

From the ISM in Fig. 2, the empirical investigation suggests that the most fundamental consideration for factor influencing readiness of healthcare personnel for TeleRehab is "e-Healthcare knowledge". e-Healthcare knowledge is the knowledge aboute-Healthcare and its contribution to the healthcare domain [12]. The factor is located in Level V of the model shows the greatest effect on the factor in the upper levels which is "awareness". The awareness of healthcare personnel towards existing technology, new technology, and advantage and disadvantage of TeleRehab are affected by their knowledge in healthcare. The exposition of the healthcare personnel to e-Healthcare knowledge allows them to be always up-to-date or aware of the current and new innovations in the field. This knowledge indirectly allows the acceptance of healthcare personnel towards new innovation of TeleRehab and at the same time fixing the weaknesses of the current technologies.

Besides "awareness", other factors present at Level IV are "financial benefits", "connectivity", and "hardware and software" can impact some factors at the same level and Level III directly and indirectly. For instance, the "awareness" influences "financial benefits" are at the same level and also influence skills factor at level above. The identification and understanding of "financial benefits" of the new innovation are vital before implementing any costly innovation such as TeleRehab. This factor has a link with cost factor because the variables such as initial cost, continuing cost, and loss returns cost needed to be considered in order to adopt new innovation [23]. TeleRehab as new innovation will benefit the patients due to the cost reduction for rehabilitation service for the long term which also allows them to be aware, accept, and use it [6, 24]. The "awareness" links with the "skills" since in adopting new intelligence innovation, high skills are needed to allow the healthcare personnel to adopt and use it easily [18]. Next, "financial benefits" influences "satisfaction and willingness". One of the variables that lead healthcare personnel to satisfy and willing to adopt new innovation such as TeleRehab to replace current technology is the benefits of financial to patients [23]. Besides, connectivity factor linked to all another factor at Level IV (i.e., "awareness", "financial benefits", and "hardware and software") and "satisfaction and willingness", and "skills" at Level III. The good connectivity allows the healthcare personnel to keep aware towards current and new innovations evolving in the health field. The enhancement of behavior change can be affected by strong and secure internet connectivity [17]. The "connectivity" also affected the "financial benefit" since good connectivity allows TeleRehab to be adopted well to the targeted patients [9, 16]. In addition, "connectivity" is linked to "hardware and software" factor because both of them are the main elements in TeleRehab project and to ensure the project can be run thoroughly [4, 17]. Other than the relationship between factors at the same level, "connectivity" also impacts the "satisfaction and willingness" of healthcare personnel in accepting new innovations. The secure internet connection is one of the elements needed for healthcare personnel who seek for the improvement from current technology used in healthcare organization [14]. The "connectivity" influences other factors at Level III which is "skills". The strong connection with good computer skills is significant in order to use a computer and related tools efficiently [16]. Overall, these factors at Level IV of ISM are related to each other and considered impact the readiness of healthcare personnel in receiving TeleRehab service.

Level III consist of the "satisfaction and willingness", and "skills", which affect the second level of the ISM model directly. The significant factors at this level is "satisfaction and willingness" because it has links to all the factors at the Level II and "skills" at the same level. The "satisfaction and willingness" influenced by "skills" due to the level of skills especially in handling hardware (i.e., computer, printer) and software (i.e., TeleRehab application) affect the satisfaction and willingness of healthcare personnel to learn and adopt new innovation [9, 13, 14]. Moreover, "comfort" is the state which the individual is ready to accept innovation and practice it [9, 13, 14]. The comfortability of healthcare personnel of adopting new innovation affecting their dissatisfaction with current technology used and willingness to adopt a new innovation. In addition, the "satisfaction and willingness" also influence "concern" in determining the quality of medical practice. The healthcare personnel tends to be ready and is willing to adopt new innovation if they can deliver better rehabilitation service to the patients. Therefore, the quality of the medical practice is in the best possible condition. Next, "satisfaction and willingness" affect "planning".

The dissatisfaction towards current technology applied encourages the healthcare personnel to come up with ideas for improvement. It starts with the idea followed by the participants of healthcare personnel for planning new innovation [9, 14, 20]. Finally, "satisfaction and willingness" also influence "learnability". At the same level, the "skills" effects the "comfort", "concern", and "learnability" factors. The good "skills" available for every healthcare personnel allow them to feel "comfortable" to accept and practice new innovation [9]. The healthcare personnel are also "concerned" about their "skills" in handling the assigned patients. The skillful healthcare personnel is needed in handling TeleRehab application. In addition, the "skills" also affects the "learnability" of the healthcare personnel. The good skills allow the healthcare personnel to be able to learn the new innovation more efficiently and have the belief that they are more productive using it [14, 22].

The factors available at Level II are "comfort", "concern", "planning", and "learnability". The healthcare personnel needs to be "concerned" of their healthcare knowledge to ensure it is the same level or beyond the need of new innovation. Therefore, the healthcare personnel should always continue learning and upgrading their knowledge. Next, the "concern" factor also affects the idea and "planning" of the new innovation. The adoption of new innovation such as TeleRehab needs a big investment. Thus, the effective champion or the responsible individual needs to make sure that that there is a good plan in place [14]. In addition, the good "planning" of new innovation encourages healthcare personnel to prepare themselves with knowledge to implement the new innovation.

Finally, top-level variable reveals strong factor among other factors. "Resistance to change" is the state the healthcare personnel is not ready to accept change [14]. In term of this study, the change refers to the TeleRehab service. If the healthcare personnel are faced with issues to adopt and use TeleRehab, they tend to be resistant. From the case study, one of the issues faced by healthcare personnel is the appropriateness of the planned innovation towards patients and the possible acceptance among the patients. Therefore, these possible issues should be identified and resolved to enable TeleRehab to be adopted in this Malaysia.

## 5 Discussion and Conclusion

This research has examined the readiness of healthcare personnel for TeleRehab. The study presented a model of readiness that encapsulated factors and showed the relationships between them that identified during the interviews conducted with healthcare personnel. Twelve (12) factors were found to be associated with TeleRehab. Five (5) factors were found to have both strong driving and dependence powers, thus classifying them as linkage factors that should be considered as relatively unstable. Here, factors of "comfort", "satisfaction and willingness", "skills", "concern" and "planning" will have an effect to others as well as feedback on themselves. This indicates that healthcare personnel in the case study are struggling to make sense of TeleRehab to be adopted in their institution. Findings of the case study also showed that other five (5) factors including "awareness", "connectivity", "hardware and software", "e-Healthcare knowledge", and "financial benefits", will have strong driving power but weak dependence. This is supported from the ISM in Fig. 2, where all these factors are located at the bottom level of the model with "e-Healthcare knowledge" has the highest driving power. Hence, the top management should focus on this issue by giving more knowledge related with e-Healthcare to all healthcare personnel (i.e., physician, therapist and nurse) in the healthcare institution so as to enable them to ready and adopt TeleRehab. Further, the MICMAC analysis also shows that there are two (2) factors, "learnability" and "resistance to change" which have low driving power and high-dependence and termed as result factors, as both are influenced by driving factors of the matrix. There are no factors which have weak driving and weak dependence powers.

Although the case study of this research work is restricted to one Malaysian healthcare institution, the model can be generalized to other healthcare institutions in the country. The ISM presented provides significance of the readiness of healthcare personnel in adopting TeleRehab. The factors that form the basis of the hierarchy must be given utmost consideration by the top-management leaders of healthcare institutions. Finally, in this work, an interrelationship model among the readiness factors of TeleRehab has been developed using the ISM approach. The model was obtained based on the team healthcare personnel' opinion by judging the contextual relationship between the factors, but it was not validated statistically. It is suggested for future study to conduct a combination of quantitative study along with qualitative study by means using questionnaire survey approach in collecting the data, and then the structural equation modeling technique be clubbed to get new insights of ISM.

**Acknowledgment.** The author wants to appreciate the Editor and anonymous referees for their constructive comments and criticism. This work was supported by the International Grant USIM/INT-NEWTON/FST/IHRAM/053000/41616 under Newton-Ungku Omar Fund.

# References

1. Marzano, G., Lubkina, V., Stafeckis, G.: Some reflections on designing effective social telerehabilitation services for older adults. Int. J. Telerehabilitation @BULLET **85195**(210), 3–8 (2016)
2. Tinelli, F., Cioni, G., Purpura, G.: Development and implementation of a new telerehabilitation system for audiovisual stimulation training in hemianopia. Front. Neurol. **8**(Nov), 1–10 (2017)
3. Brennan, D.M., Lum, P.S., Uswatte, G., Taub, E., Gilmore, B.M., Barman, J.: A telerehabilitation platform for home-based automated therapy of arm function. In: Proceedings of Annual International Conference IEEE Engineering Medicine Biology Society EMBS, pp. 1819–1822 (2011)
4. Rezai-Rad, M., Vaezi, R., Nattagh, F.: E-health readiness assessment framework in Iran. Iran. J. Public Health **41**(10), 43–51 (2012)
5. Mars, M., Scott, R.E.: Being spontaneous: the future of telehealth implementation? Telemed. e-Health **23**(9), 1–7 (2017)
6. McCue, M., Fairman, A., Pramuka, M.: Enhancing quality of life through telerehabilitation. Phys. Med. Rehabil. Clin. N. Am. **21**(1), 195–205 (2010)
7. Mars, M.: Telerehabilitation in South Africa – is there a way forward? Int. J. Telerehabilitation **3**(1), 11–18 (2011)
8. Jafni, T.I., Bahari, M., Ismail, W., Radman, A.: Understanding the implementation of telerehabilitation at pre-implementation stage: a systematic literature review. Procedia Comput. Sci. **124**, 452–460 (2017)
9. Khoja, S., Scott, R.E., Casebeer, A.L., Mohsin, M., Ishaq, A.F.M., Gilani, S.: e-Health readiness assessment tools for healthcare institutions in developing countries. Telemed. J. e-health Off. J. Am. Telemed. Assoc. **13**(4), 425–431 (2007)
10. Légaré, É., et al.: Developing and validating the French-Canadian version of the practitioner and organizational telehealth readiness assessment tools. J. Telemed. Telecare **16**(3), 140–146 (2010)

11. Scharwz, F., Ward, J., Willcock, S.: E-health readiness in outback communities: an exploratory study. Rural Remote Health **14**(3), 1–12 (2014)
12. Justice, E.: E-healthcare/telemedicine readiness assessment of some selected states in Western Nigeria. Int. J. Eng. Technol. **2**(2), 195–201 (2012)
13. Chipps, J., Mars, M.: Readiness of health-care institutions in KwaZulu-Natal to implement telepsychiatry. J. Telemed. Telecare **18**(3), 133–137 (2012)
14. Kgasi, M.R., Kalema, B.M.: Assessment E-health readiness for rural South African areas. J. Ind. Intell. Inf. **2**(2), 131–135 (2014)
15. Hebert, M.A., Korabek, B.: Stakeholder readiness for telehomecare: implications for implementation. Telemed. J. E. Health **10**(1), 85–92 (2004)
16. Chattopadhyay, S., Li, J., Land, L., Ray, P.: A framework for assessing ICT preparedness for e-health implementations. In: 2008 10th IEEE International Conference e-Health Networking, Applications Services Health, pp. 124–129 (2008)
17. Khatun, F., Heywood, A.E., Ray, P.K., Hanifi, S.M.A., Bhuiya, A., Liaw, S.: Determinants of readiness to adopt mHealth in a rural community of Bangladesh. Int. J. Med. Inform. **84** (10), 847–856 (2015)
18. Li, J., Land, L.P.W., Ray, P., Chattopadhyaya, S.: E-health readiness framework from Electronic Health Records perspective. Int. J. Internet Enterp. Manag. **6**(4), 326–348 (2010)
19. Hogenbirk, J.C., et al.: Framework for Canadian telehealth guidelines: summary of the environmental scan. J. Telemed. Telecare **12**(2), 64–70 (2006)
20. Snyder-Halpern, R.: Indicators of organizational readiness for clinical information technology/systems innovation: a Delphi study. Int. J. Med. Inform. **63**, 179–204 (2001)
21. Aziz, K., Yusof, M.M.: Measuring organizational readiness in information systems adoption. In: Proceedings of Eighteenth Americas Conference Information Systems, 9–12 August, pp. 1–8 (2012)
22. Parmanto, B., Lewis Jr., K.M., Graham, A.N., Bertolet, M.H.: Development of the telehealth usability questionnaire (TUQ). Int. J. Telerehabilitation **8**(1), 3–10 (2016)
23. Ross, J., Stevenson, F., Lau, R., Murray, E.: Factors that influence the implementation of e-health: a systematic review of systematic reviews (an update). Implement. Sci. **11**(146), 1–12 (2016)
24. Benvenuti, F., et al.: Community-based exercise for upper limb paresis: a controlled trial with telerehabilitation. Neurorehabil. Neural Repair. **28**(7), 611–620 (2014)
25. Li, J., et al.: e-Health preparedness assessment in the context of an influenza pandemic: a qualitative study in China. BMJ Open **3**(3), 1–9 (2013)
26. Pramuka, M., Van Roosmalen, L.: Telerehabilitation technologies: accessibility and usability. Int. J. Telerehabilitation **1**(1), 25–36 (2015)
27. Jayant, A., Azhar, M.: Analysis of the barriers for implementing green supply chain management (GSCM) practices: an interpretive structural modeling (ISM) approach. Procedia Eng. **97**, 2157–2166 (2014)
28. Talib, F., Rahman, Z., Qureshi, M.N.: An interpretive structural modelling approach for modelling the practices of total quality management in service sector. Int. J. Model. Oper. Manag. **1**(3), 223–250 (2011)
29. Al Sagheer, F.A., Al-Sughayer, M.A., Muslim, S., Elsabee, M.Z.: Extraction and characterization of chitin and chitosan from marine sources in Arabian Gulf. Carbohydr. Polym. **77**(2), 410–419 (2009)

# An Ontological Model for Analyzing Liver Cancer Medical Reports

Rim Messaoudi[1,2]([⊠]), Taher Labidi[1,4], Antoine Vacavant[3],
Faiez Gargouri[1,6], Manuel Grand-Brochier[3], Ali Amouri[5],
Hela Fourati[5], Achraf Mtibaa[1,4], and Faouzi Jaziri[3]

[1] MIRACL Laboratory, University of Sfax, Sfax, Tunisia
rimmessaoudii@gmail.com, faiez.gargouri@isimsf.usf.tn
[2] CRNS Laboratory, University of Sfax, Sfax, Tunisia
[3] Institut Pascal, Université Clermont Auvergne, Clermont-Ferrand, France
{antoine.vacavant, manuel.grand-brochier,
faouzi.jaziri}@uca.fr
[4] National School of Electronic and Telecommunications, University of Sfax,
Sfax, Tunisia
taherlabidi@gmail.com, achraf.mtibaa@enetcom.usf.tn
[5] CHU Hédi Chaker, Sfax, Tunisia
ali_amouri@yahoo.fr, fouratihelal5@gmail.com
[6] Higher Institute of Computer Science and Multimedia, University of Sfax,
Sfax, Tunisia

**Abstract.** The rapid adoption of Electronic Health Record (EHR) systems requires advanced enactment strategies for analyzing medical reports. Indeed, the information presented in these reports is difficult to access and it is onerous to analyze it by medical decision support systems. Medical reports characterize full descriptions of the patient diagnosis process. They bring together information about exam steps such as applied techniques, results, synthesis and medical conclusions. In this paper, we propose a medical report modeling and analyzing approach that aims to analyze medical reports for Magnetic Resonance Imaging (MRI) exams. Ontological model is dedicated to represent information from radiological reports in order to make them comprehensible and machine readable. Moreover, reasoning techniques are used to treat a large amount of clinical data. This provides an analyzing system allowing user to be informed about the evolution of the patient state. The proposed system was successfully applied to a set of Hepatocellular Carcinoma (HCC) medical reports from University Hospital of Clermont-Ferrand (CHU), France.

**Keywords:** Ontology · MRI reports · Liver cancer · Reasoning rules

## 1 Introduction

Electronic health record (EHR) systems contain a big amount of clinical data that potentiates the clinical decision. Among these data, medical reports (i.e. radiology reports and doctor reports) represent key documents that facilitate the exploration of diseases. Each disease has specific diagnostic tools and requires specific treatments [11,

© Springer Nature Switzerland AG 2019
M. Themistocleous and P. Rupino da Cunha (Eds.): EMCIS 2018, LNBIP 341, pp. 369–382, 2019.
https://doi.org/10.1007/978-3-030-11395-7_29

12]. In this work, we focus on liver cancer disease as part of the CIRRHOSE[1] project. Moreover, our work tends to concentrate on MRI image technique that provides multi-parametric information [9].

The medical report consists of a set of physical or computerized documents that contain mainly radiological observations and notes about patient state, disease, and laboratory results. This medical document includes all information that contribute to diagnosis, treatment or prevention actions. It contains especially exams results, consultation records, medical interventions and therapeutic prescriptions. This report can be exchanged between doctors, radiologists or healthcare professionals. Medical reports are used in the diagnosis and monitoring of liver tumors which are one of the most aggressive diseases that attack hepatic cells (i.e. hepatocytes). Liver tumors are evaluated generally in a damaged liver caused by chronic effects (i.e. HCC, Cholangiocarcinoma, Angioma). The diagnosis process of liver tumors is the most critical phase. It is achieved through radiological observations [7]. To attempt diagnosis part, some tools are used, namely, MRI, Scanner, physical exams, biopsy, etc. Indeed, various causes could be deduced for liver cancer such as alcohol, tobacco, hereditary diseases, and obesity. Regarding applied treatments, we find ablation, chemo-embolization, surgery, and transplantation.

The large volume of medical reports and their unstructured textual formats make the medical data ambiguous. Consequently, medical data exploration becomes increasingly difficult. Thus, the first challenge is to make these documents as clear and understandable as possible. Moreover, medical decision support systems require tools that assist in analyzing medical reports. This requires advanced analysis strategies, especially when we are faced a sheer amount of medical reports. In this paper, we present a medical reports modeling and analyzing approach for liver cancer. Our approach assists user, such as doctors, radiologists or laboratory technicians, to analyze medical reports with the aim of describing the evolution of the patient state. For this reason, we study the benefit of semantic representation and reasoning aspects in ontology. This knowledge engineering technique is used actually in several research areas such as biology [3, 8], medicine [1, 4, 18, 19], cloud computing [15, 16] and physics [2]. It paves the way to communicate automatically with clinical data. Subsequently, this paper seeks to address the problem of applying semantic techniques to represent, store and retrieval clinical patient information from clinical reports. Additionally, we want to concentrate on integrating reasoning rules to query data semantics through the ontology. On the one hand, ontology allows the modeling of medical reports to be readable and comprehensible. On the other hand, it allows deducing new knowledge about the liver cancer, its stage and its advanced degree through inference. Our aim is to analyze medical reports for MRI patient exams by considering the semantic meaning of reports data and taking profit from the power of reasoning techniques.

---

[1] CIRRHOSE project (Classification d'Images Rpartie pour la Reconnaissance de lsions Hpatiques, avec des OntologieS, et grande Echelle). It focuses on liver tumors diagnosis and treatment and it takes into account in particular HCC diseases.

The remaining of this paper is structured as follows: Sect. 2 survey the state of the art. In Sect. 3, we provide our medical reports modeling and analyzing approach for liver cancer. Afterwards, in the Sect. 4, we describe the different aspects of our implementations. Finally, conclusions will be drawn in Sect. 5.

## 2 Related Work

Nowadays, a good medical reports structuring is imperative in medical decision support systems. Various research works applied several techniques to deal with this type of topics. Moreover, medical information extraction from narrative texts or from clinical reports is treated and explained in several works [21].

In the field of using Natural Language Processing (NLP) techniques for clinical purposes, Xu et al. [22] proposed "MedEx" system to organize and select medical information from clinical narratives. This system allows transforming free-text recorders to a structural format representation. Also, it applies new technologies (i.e. sequential tagger, combined parser) to analyze medical texts. These technologies remove terms ambiguities and offer a regular system dedicated essentially to solve several complicated expressions. Jensen et al. [13] applied NLP to allow medical research, clinical care, and patients phenotypes description using EHR. This work gives also an overview about the useful frameworks in this domain challenge. It is used to remove knowledge omissions and assist in the clinical data decision. Then, it focuses on integrating medical terminologies for diversity healthcare purposes. Hahn et al. [10] proposed a natural language processor called MEDSYNDIKATE. It offered semantic interpretation taken from medical documents. It interested on building a text knowledge base which will be used later as data information sources. In [6], Chapman et al. suggested an algorithm named "ConText" to maintain text mining from clinical narratives and to allow their reliability in several data types.

Medical reports are also treated using ontological model. Chan et al. [5] used the Systematized Nomenclature of Medicine (SNOMED) [19] to model clinical reports finding. They tacked into account essentially the medical image finding. In addition, they followed the strategy of mapping clinical terms with SNOMED ontology in order to detect HCC diseases. Starlinger et al. [20] focused on organizing Germen medical documents in order to surpass obstacles related to clinical data extraction. To this end, semantic representations are integrated to achieve clinical terms recognition and standardization. Moreover, progressing medical search methods in clinical routines is also mentioned in this work. Thus, Marwede et al. [17] developed an ontology based approach dedicated for radiology reporting tasks. They generated a prototype "RadiO" allocated for image features extraction. In this context, Kokciyan et al. [14] designed a semantic model for liver Computerized Tomography (CT) images. They gathered information from medical reports in order to design similar diseases cases.

To sum up, few researchers have addressed the problem of integrating ontologies to treat clinical reports for liver cancer. The majority has focused only on applying NLP techniques to extract information. Despite the importance of the presented works, MRI reports have not been deeply treated compared to CT exams. Other works have only used existing ontologies as they are structured without appending other supporting information. On one hand, they did not provide user interaction machine, so there are no implemented means or tools that can achieve human control or communicate with the proposed model. On the other hand, these works did not outline reasoning rules to validate the usefulness of their proposed semantic models. Also, they did not address clearly the problem of liver cancer reports analyzing. Subsequently, one of the main purposes of our work is integrating semantic aspects to model radiologist's observations. We try to apply semantic techniques to ensure textual reports formalization. To this end, this paper outlines knowledge engineering techniques by using reasoning rules to treat, organize and interrogate several MRI reports.

## 3   Medical Reports Modeling and Analyzing Approach

Modeling the wealth of information that exists in patient medical reports is performed by an ontology which forms the core of our approach. Ontology allows sharing knowledge and maintaining semantic information. It characterizes a structural representation format by offering a large amount of terms and concepts related to a specific domain. Ontology contains also semantic relations, attributes and instances that are used to maintain a shareable referential vocabulary. In our work, we would like to take advantage of this knowledge engineering technique in order to model medical data reports. We introduce semantic representation to analyze patient information. Also, we include reasoning rules to extract clinical observations from real patient reports.

Our proposed approach is composed of two phases as shown in Fig. 1. Firstly, the reports modeling step includes a Medical Reports Ontology (MROnt) that aims to make the patient medical reports comprehensible and machine readable. Then, the report analyzing step contains an analyzing system allowing users (doctors, radiologists or laboratory technicians) to be informed about the evolution of the patient state. Steps of our approach are improved and enhanced with semantic aspects. These improvements allow getting an automatic medical reports processing, where appropriate methods are taken to analyze patient state.

### 3.1   Populating Knowledge Base

The large volume of medical reports and their unstructured textual formats may result in ambiguous and complex medical data. In order to minimize this complexity, we propose the MROnt ontology. It contains main concepts of the patient medical reports, their properties and their relationships and allows a better medical report representation. MROnt takes into account MRI patient reports describing especially HCC cases. Figure 2 illustrates an overview of MROnt ontology using OntoGraf[2] plugin.

---

[2] https://protegewiki.stanford.edu/wiki/OntoGraf.

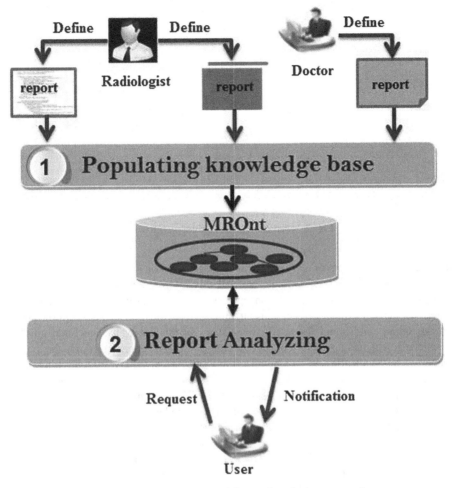

**Fig. 1.** Medical reports modeling and analyzing approach

The proposed ontology is defined in accordance with real medical reports structure. We used Protege[3] framework and the Ontology Web Rule (OWL[4]) language to develop MROnt model.

MROnt model is composed of the required concepts assisting the disease detection during the diagnosis process. The "Radiologist" concept refers to the person who realizes the MRI exam and notes its descriptions as "Observations". The concept "Report" refers to the medical exam that contains all information about the patient state. This concept is linked to "Radiologist" through the relation "elaboratedBy". "Patient" refers to the person who undergoing medical examination and following a

---

[3] https://protege.stanford.edu/.

[4] https://www.w3.org/.

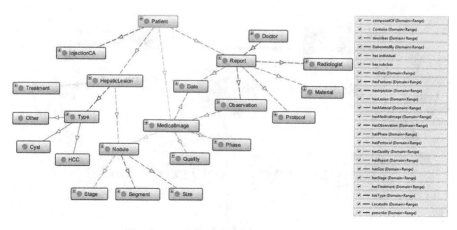

**Fig. 2.** Medical Report Ontology (MROnt)

specific treatment type or surgery. This concept contains all fundamental patient information such as name, sex, age, etc. All this information is solved as data type properties. Thus, "MedicalImage" concept describes medical image used by the radiologist to make medical observations. It aims to provide a visual description about strange organs and about the whole liver state. In this work, we are interesting in hepatic medical images. This concept is connected to "Patient" through the object property "hasMedicalImage". "HepticLesion" presents a variety of liver tumors. It characterizes abnormalities inside liver tissue. "Nodule" concept describes the detected hepatic mass. It is characterized essentially by its abnormal format. The relation "composedOf" is used to link these two concepts. It explains that the hepatic lesion can be composed of one or more nodules. Other object properties are defined to carry out relationships between concepts and individuals. In our model, "observedIn" is used as object properties to link "Nodule" and "Report" concepts. "hasReport" relation connects "Patient" and "Report". Table 1 highlights a description of the used concepts.

**Table 1.** MROnt concepts definition

| Concept | Definition |
|---|---|
| Patient | Refers to the individual who is medically examined or given treatment. This concept is identified by ID, name, sexe, age, birth date, etc |
| Radiologist | Represents a specialist in radiology domain who applies medical techniques to perform patient diagnosis using X-rays and reports notes after the exam. He is identified by his name |
| Doctor | Prescribes MRI exams and analyzes radiology reports |
| Report | Represents a narrative text noted by the radiologist in order to offer information about the patient state, the disease detected and the treatment applied |

*(continued)*

**Table 1.** (*continued*)

| Concept | Definition |
|---|---|
| Protocol | Identifies techniques used by the radiologist to realize the medical exam, such as signal T1, T2, T2 FS, etc |
| HepaticLesion | Represents the hepatic mass detected in MRI sequences. It can be HCC, Cyst or other Type of lesion. It is characterized by its stage, size and localization |
| Type | Represents the liver cancer type detected through the medical observation. It can be HCC, Cyst or other type (i.e. Angioma) |
| HCC | Designs a malignant hepatic lesion. It is developed frequently in a damaged liver and it attacks rapidly its cells |
| Cyst | Designs a benign liver cancer type |
| Other | Refers to hepatic diseases other than HCC and Cyst types |
| Nodule | Characterizes the hepatic lesion detected in the medical image. It is identified by size and number. The hepatic lesion can be constituted by one or more nodules |
| Segment | Represents liver composition parts. There are 7 segments in the liver; Segment I, Segment II, Segment III, Segment IV, Segment V, Segment IV and Segment IIV |
| Observation | Represents visual and clinical interpretations of the radiologist or the doctor during diagnosis process |
| Stage | Provides information about the hepatic lesion stage |
| Size | Represents the size of the hepatic lesion detected in the MRI image |
| Treatment | Represents the suitable treatment to be applied after the diagnosis process |
| InjectionAC | Refers to contrast agent that injects the patient before the MRI exam |
| Date | Refers to the date when the patient had made the medical exam |
| Material | Represents the materials applied to realize the MRI exam |
| Quality | Represents the quality of the MRI image |
| Phase | Represents the MRI exam phase (i.e. portal, late) |

## 3.2    Report Analyzing

Analyzing medical reports is an essential step to support medical decision systems. Our purpose is to facilitate analyzing multiple medical reports and to duly provide the required information to the user. Therefore, we semantically link MROnt concepts in run time. This is important since we have many medical reports of various patients.

Thus, inference rules characterize another advantage of the ontology. In fact, to ensure a good exploitation of MROnt, a reasoning step is essential. We de ne some inference rules using the Semantic Web Rule Language[5] (SWRL). A rule of the SWRL has a semantic meaning by expressing the relation between an antecedent and a consequent in order to infer or deduce new knowledge from a set of implicit data. An antecedent represents a conjunction of atoms defining the conditions that must be met.

---

[5] http://www.w3.org/Submission/SWRL/.

However, the consequent determines the fact to do in case of achievement of the antecedent. SWRL rules are based on SWRL built-ins (e.g. swrlb:equal) or SQWRL queries (e.g. sqwrl:select). SWRL built-ins include mathematical operators and functions for string manipulations. Thus, SQWRL[6] queries can be seen as SQL operations used to exploit the knowledge inferred by SWRL rules [16].

We make some simulations in Protege to ensure the proper functioning of the created inference rules. Thus, we populate our ontology with individuals, de ne object properties and data type properties related to those individuals and execute the inference engine. We de ne various inference rules to analyze medical reports.

For instance, in Rule 1, we used the SQWRL language to return information about the nodule. More precisely, we return the size, the segment and the stage of each nodule defined in our ontological model MROnt.

### Rule 1: Select Size, Segment and Stage of Nodule

$Patient(?p) \land HepaticLesion(?h) \land hasLesion(?p,?h) \land Nodule(?n) \land composedOf(?h,?n) \land Size(?size) \land hasSize(?n,?size) \land Segment(?segment) \land locatedIn(?n,?segment) \land Stage(?stage) \land hasStage(?n,?stage) \rightarrow sqwrl : select(?size) \land sqwrl : select(?segment) \land sqwrl : select(?stage)$

Rule 2 is used to evaluate the detected nodule state. In particular, we check the observation list using the defined built-in "swrlb:equal". If all required observations are founded, we can deduce a HCC liver cancer and classify the nodule instance as HCC.

### Rule2: Deduce HCC

$Patient(?p) \land HepaticLesion(?h) \land hasLesion(?p,?h) \land Nodule(?n) \land composedOf(?h,?n) \land MedicalImage(?i) \land contains(?i,?n) \land describes(?a,?i) \land Observation(?a) \land swrlb : equal(?a,"dysmorphic liver") \land Observation(?b) \land swrlb : equal(?b,"hypertrophy segment I") \land describes(?b,?i) \land Observation(?c) \land swrlb : equal(?c,"hypertrophy segment II") \land describes(?c,?i) \land Observation(?d) \land swrlb : equal(?d,"micronodular architecture") \land describes(?d,?i) \land Observation(?e) \land swrlb : equal(?e,"no portal dilation") \land describes(?e,?i) \land Observation(?f) \land swrlb : equal(?f,"no portal thrombose") \land describes(?f,?i) \land Observation(?g) \land swrlb : equal(?g,"portal washout") \land describes(?g,?i) \land Observation(?j) \land swrlb : equal(?j,"hypersignal T1") \land describes(?j?i) \rightarrow HCC(?h) \land ClassifiedAs(?n,?h)$

In order to show the result of Rule 2 and to better explain the deduced case, we compare in Fig. 3 the evolution of our MROnt ontological model before and after executing Rule 2. We can determine the Hepatic Lesion type (HCC in our case) and create a new object property "ClassifiedAs" between the nodule and the HCC instances.

---

[6] https://github.com/protegeproject/swrlapi/wiki/SQWRL.

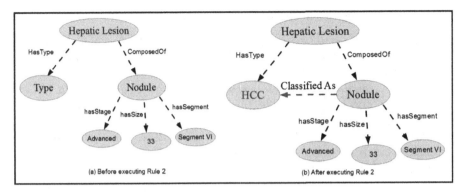

**Fig. 3.** SWRL rule for MROnt analyzing system (a) Before execution and (b) After execution

Rule 3 allows deducing that the patient disease is not HCC. This is explained by the fact that the observations founded do not justify a liver cancer.

**Rule 3: Deduce Not HCC**

$Patient(?p) \land HepaticLesion(?h) \land hasLesion(?p, ?h) \land Nodule(?n) \land$
$composedOf(?h, ?n) \land MedicalImage(?i) \land contains(?i, ?n) \land describes(?a, ?i) \land$
$Observation(?a) \land swrlb : equal(?a, "dysmorphic\ liver") \land Observation(?b) \land$
$swrlb \quad : \quad equal(?b, "periferic \quad rehaussement") \land describes(?b, ?i) \land$
$Observation(?c) \land swrlb : equal(?c, "no\ arterialization") \land describes(?c, ?i) \land$
$Observation(?d) \land swrlb \quad : \quad equal(?d, "micronodular \quad architecture") \land$
$describes(?d, ?i) \land Observation(?e) \land swrlb : equal(?e, "no\ hepatic\ sus") \land$
$describes(?e, ?i) \quad \land \quad Observation(?f) \quad \land \quad swrlb \quad :$
$equal(?f, "no\ portal\ thrombose") \land describes(?f, ?i) \land Observation(?g) \land swrlb :$
$equal(?g, "no\ cliac\ abnormalities") \land describes(?g, ?i) \land Observation(?h) \land$
$swrlb : equal(?h, "hypersignal\ T2") \land describes(?h, ?i) \land Observation(?j) \land$
$swrlb \quad : \quad equal(?j, "hypersignal \quad FAT \quad SAT") \land describes(?j, ?i) \land$
$Observation(?k) \land swrlb \quad : \quad equal(?k, "hypersignal \quad diffusion") \land$
$describes(?k, ?i) \rightarrow Other(?h) \land ClassifiedAs(?n, ?h)$

Rule 4 provides information about the nodule state compared to precedent MRI exams. It takes into account precedent exam observations related to the same patient then it gives details about lesion progression such as change in size, appearance of another tumor, stage detection and lesion type extraction. For the example below, we create the property "value" to show that the detected HCC nodule has undergone changes in size from 20 mm to 22 mm.

**Rule 4: Tumor Progression Check**

$Patient(?p) \land HepaticLesion(?h) \land hasLesion(?p,?h) \land Nodule(?n) \land$
$composedOf(?h,?n) \land MedicalImage(?i) \land contains(?i,?n) \land describes(?a,?i) \land$
$Observation(?a) \land swrlb : equal(?a,"dysmorphic\ liver") \land Observation(?b) \land$
$swrlb\ :\ equal(?b,"periferic\ rehaussement") \land describes(?b,?i) \land$
$Observation(?c) \land swrlb : equal(?c,"no\ arterialization") \land describes(?c,?i) \land$
$Observation(?d) \land swrlb\ :\ equal(?d,"micronodular\ architecture") \land$
$describes(?d,?i) \land Observation(?e) \land swrlb : equal(?e,"no\ hepatic\ sus") \land$
$describes(?e,?i) \qquad \land \qquad Observation(?f) \qquad \land \qquad swrlb \qquad :$
$equal(?f,"no\ portal\ thrombose") \land describes(?f,?i) \land Observation(?g) \land swrlb :$
$equal(?g,"no\ cliac\ abnormalities") \land describes(?g,?i) \land Observation(?h) \land$
$swrlb : equal(?h,"hypersignal\ T2") \land describes(?h,?i) \land Observation(?j) \land$
$swrlb\ :\ equal(?j,"hypersignal\ FAT\ SAT") \land describes(?j,?i) \land$
$Observation(?k) \land swrlb\ :\ equal(?k,"hypersignal\ diffusion") \land$
$describes(?k,?i) \land hasSize(?n,?v) \land value(?v,20) \land ClassifiedAs(?n,HCC) \rightarrow$
$hasSize(?n,?v) \land value(?v,22)$

## 4 Implementation

In this section, we test our approach with real patient cases. Figure 4 represents the architecture we follow for the implementation of medical report analyzing services. First, we parse medical report documents using parsing techniques such as Eclipse Modeling Framework (EMF[7]). Then, we populate our MROnt ontology with real MRI patient exams using Jena API[8]. This package is used to built semantic java applications. It offers the possibility to interrogate medical data tacked from the medical reports. Later, we test our SWRL and SQWRL rules to show our analyzing system efficiency in deducing disease cases.

### 4.1 Data Source Approval

The data used for this article has taken from University Hospital of Clermont-Ferrand (CHU), France. Medical reports, acquired by doctors and radiologists, have been first anonymized and stored in a secured way in servers located in CHU. The patients delivered their personal data and signed an informed consent. They must be able to understand and willing to sign the written informed consent so that medical images and other data can be used for any research issue. The first set of analyses, investigated in our work, is composed of 28 medical reports for patients who were diagnosed with liver cancer. These reports characterize various patients disease states. They describe the whole medical exam steps starting by general information until giving specific details about the clinical interpretations.

---

[7] https://www.eclipse.org/modeling/emf/.

[8] https://jena.apache.org/.

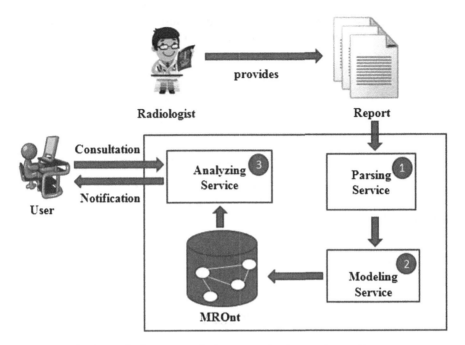

**Fig. 4.** Medical reports analyzing system implementation architecture

## 4.2 Medical Report Analyzing System

Our medical report analyzing system allows populating MROnt ontology with real MRI exams. It brings together all information and includes it in MROnt. First, it takes into account general information about the patient (i.e. ID, name, sex, age, birth date, etc.). Later, it focuses on radiological interpretation which starts by the applied techniques to realize the MRI exam. This interpretation describes the liver state (i.e. dysmorphic state, irregular contours) and the hepatic lesion (i.e. size, localization, nodule number). In addition, our system checks if there is any anomaly related to the whole hepatic system and other organs including pancreas or reins observations. Also, it introduces other data for MRI signals such as T1, T2 and T2 FAT SAT that can be visualized after patient contrast injection. These data can be for example hyposignal T1, hypersignal T2 or portal washout. Finally, our medical report analyzing system provides a conclusion, in which a radiologist notes its decision about the nodule type (HCC, Cyst or other type of hepatic diseases).

All the above mentioned steps are performed throughout the execution of SWRL and SQWRL rules. These rules pave the way to realize high-level reasoning process. For example, SQWRL rules are used to interrogate clinical data tacked from the medical reports. We present in this section a case of SQWRL rule execution. The example below selects the observations related to the medical exam identified by MI124589. This medical exam describes the patient's observations. Among the selected observations, we find (i.e. dysmorphic liver, hypertrophy of the segment I, micronodular architecture, no portal thrombose, portal washout, hypersignal T1).

Figure 5 shows the SQWRL rule example and the result of execution via Protege. These results are used later to extract the disease type.

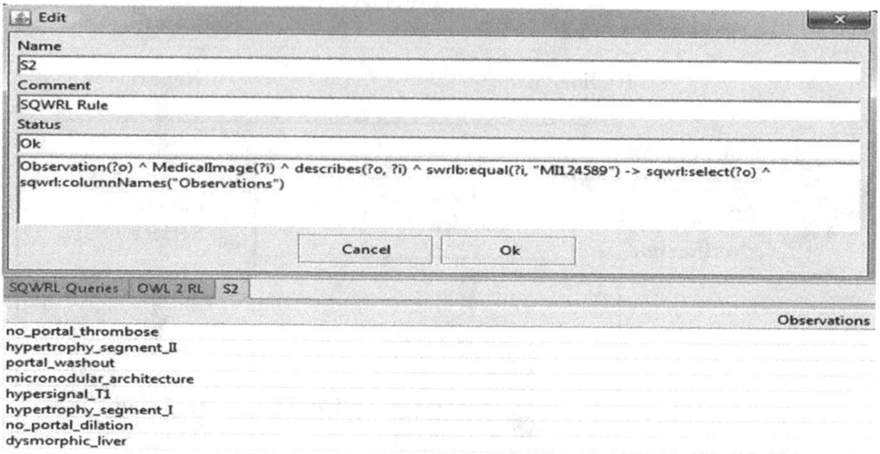

**Fig. 5.** SQWRL rule execution

Figure 6 represents the list of observations deduced for the patient identified by "P3534533". The patient exam, tacked in this example, is characterized by various observations that can be applied to deduce the hepatic lesion type. Among these observations, we find portal washout, portal thrombose, micronodular architecture, hypersignal T1, and a lesion with a size of 21 mm located in segment III of the liver. When applying our analyzing system, we can deduce that this patient is affected by HCC.

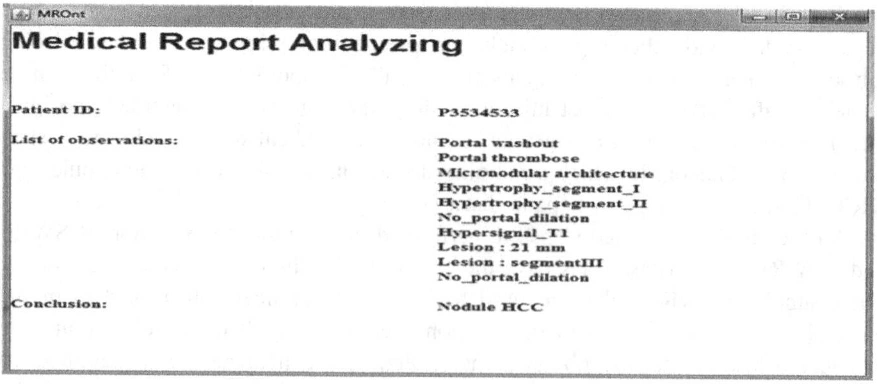

**Fig. 6.** Analyzing medical report interface

# 5   Conclusion

An effective medical reports processing is the key to improve medical decision support systems. Due to the large volume of medical reports and their unstructured textual formats, the use of these documents is affected by heavy treatments that greatly influence the patient state monitoring. In this paper, we present medical reports modeling and analyzing approach for liver cancer. We use the benefits of representation and inference of ontologies to clearly determine the evolution of the patient state. We tested our approach with a set of liver lesions medical reports from CHU - University Hospital of Clermont-Ferrand. The obtained findings show the applicability of the proposed work in liver cancer analysis.

As future work, we aim enlarging our ontology in order to support other liver diseases types. Also, we aim testing the proposed approach on other medical datasets to increase its performance level. Additionally, we focus on enhancing the quality of search methods by appending further studies, which take into account large report datasets.

**Acknowledgements.** This work was financially supported by the "PHC Utique" program of the French Ministry of Foreign A airs and Ministry of higher education and research and the Tunisian Ministry of higher education and scientific research in the CMCU project number 18G139.

# References

1. Alfonse, M., Aref, M., Salem, A.B.M.: Ontology-based knowledge representation for liver cancer. In: International eHealth: Telemedicine and Health ICT Forum for Educational, Networking and Business, pp. 821–825 (2012)
2. Abdi, A., Idris, N., Ahmad, Z.: QAPD: an ontology based question answering system in the physics domain. Soft. Comput. **24**, 1–18 (2016)
3. Bertolaso, M., Ratti, E.: Conceptual challenges in the theoretical foundations of systems biology. In: Bizzarri, M. (ed.) Systems Biology. MMB, vol. 1702, pp. 1–13. Springer, New York (2018). https://doi.org/10.1007/978-1-4939-7456-6_1
4. Bodenreider, O.: The unified medical language system (UMLS): integrating biomedical terminology. Nucleic Acids Res. **37**, 267–270 (2004)
5. Chan, L., et al.: Association patterns of ontological features signify electronic health records in liver cancer. J. Healthc. Eng. **2017**, 9 (2017)
6. Chapman, W., Chu, D., Dowling, J.: Context: an algorithm for identifying contextual features from clinical text. In: BioNLP (2007)
7. Darby, S., et al.: Mortality from liver cancer and liver disease in haemophilic men and boys in UK given blood products contaminated with hepatitis C. Lancet **350**, 1425–1431 (1997). UK Haemophilia Centre Directors' Organisation
8. Gao, W., Baig, A., Ali, H., Sajjad, W., Farahanic, M.: Margin based ontology sparse vector learning algorithm and applied in biology science. Saudi J. Biol. Sci. **24**, 132–138 (2017)
9. Haacke, E., Brown, R., Thompson, M., Venkatesan, R.: Magnetic Resonance Imaging: Principles and Sequence Design. Wiley, Hoboken (2014)
10. Hahn, U., Romacker, M., Schulz, S.: MEDSYNDIKATE-a natural language system for the extraction of medical information from findings reports. Int. J. Med. Inf. **67**, 63–74 (2002)

11. Hoerbst, A., Ammenwerth, E.: Electronic health records. A systematic review on quality requirements. Methods Inf. Med. **49**, 320–336 (2010)
12. Häyrinen, K., Saranto, K., Nykänen, P.: Definition, structure, content, use and impacts of electronic health records: a review of the research literature. Int. J. Med. Inform. **77**, 291–304 (2008)
13. Jensen, P., Jensen, L., Brunak, S.: Mining electronic health records: towards better research applications and clinical care. Nat. Rev. Genet. **13**, 395–407 (2012)
14. Kokciyan, N., Turkay, R., Uskudarli, S., Yolum, P., Bakir, B., Acar, B.: Semantic description of liver CT images: an ontological approach. IEEE J. Biomed. Health Inform. **18**, 1363–1369 (2014)
15. Labidi, T., Mtibaa, A., Brabra, H.: CSLAOnto: a comprehensive ontological SLA model in cloud computing. J. Data Semant. **5**, 179–193 (2016)
16. Labidi, T., Mtibaa, A., Gaaloul, W., Tata, S., Gargouri., F.: Cloud SLA modeling and monitoring. In: IEEE International Conference on Services Computing (SCC), pp. 338–345 (2017)
17. Marwede, D., Fielding, M., Kahn, T.: Radio: a prototype application ontology for radiology reporting tasks. In: AMIA Symposium Proceedings, vol. 37, pp. 513-517 (2007)
18. Ben Salem, Y., Idoudi, R., Saheb Ettabaa, K., Hamrouni, K., Solaiman, B.: Ontology based possibilistic reasoning for breast cancer aided diagnosis. In: Themistocleous, M., Morabito, V. (eds.) EMCIS 2017. LNBIP, vol. 299, pp. 353–366. Springer, Cham (2017). https://doi.org/10.1007/978-3-319-65930-5_29
19. Spackman, K., Campbell, K., Côté, R.: SNOMED RT: a reference terminology for health care. In: Proceedings of the AMIA Annual Fall Symposium, pp. 640–644 (1997)
20. Starlinger, J., Kittner, M., Blankenstein, O., Leser, U.: How to improve information extraction from German medical records. IT - Inf. Technol. **59**, 171–179 (2016)
21. Wang, Y., et al.: Clinical information extraction applications: a literature review. J. Biomed. Inform. **77**, 34–49 (2017)
22. Xu, H., Stenner, S., Doan, S., Johnson, K., Waitman, L., Denny, J.: MedEx: a medication information extraction system for clinical narratives. J. Am. Med. Inform. Assoc. **17**, 19–24 (2010)

# The Road to the Future of Healthcare: Transmitting Interoperable Healthcare Data Through a 5G Based Communication Platform

Argyro Mavrogiorgou[1(✉)], Athanasios Kiourtis[1], Marios Touloupou[1], Evgenia Kapassa[1], Dimosthenis Kyriazis[1], and Marinos Themistocleous[1,2]

[1] Department of Digital Systems, University of Piraeus, Piraeus, Greece
{margy, kiourtis, mtouloup, ekapassa, dimos, mthemist}@unipi.gr
[2] University of Nicosia, Nicosia, Cyprus
themistocleous.m@unic.ac.cy

**Abstract.** Current devices and sensors have revolutionized our daily lives, with the healthcare domain exploring and adapting new technologies. The rapid explosion of digital healthcare happened with the help of current 4G LTE technologies including innovations such as the continuous monitoring of patient vitals, teleporting doctors to a virtual environment or leveraging Artificial Intelligence to generate new medical insights. The arised problem is that current 4G LTE based communication platforms will not be able to keep up with the exploding connectivity demands. This is where the new 5G technology comes, expected to support ultra-reliable, low-latency and massive data communications. In this paper, an end-to-end approach is being provided in the healthcare domain for gathering medical data, anonymizing it, cleaning it, making it interoperable, and finally storing it through 5G network technologies, for their transmission to a different location, supporting real-time results and decision-making.

**Keywords:** 5G network · Data integration · Data anonymization
Data cleaning · Data quality · Data interoperability · Healthcare

## 1 Introduction

In recent years, there has been a lot of focus on how medical and health-monitoring devices, clinical wearables, and remote sensors can contribute to better health for patients and a more efficient healthcare that can drive better systems, population, and patient outcomes [1]. Currently, healthcare is one of the fastest industries to adopt the Internet of Things (IoT) technologies, which help in personalized services, reducing operating costs, and improving patient care and quality of life. However, for most patients and providers, the vague promises of the IoT has not yet led to dramatic changes in how patients experience healthcare [2].

It is undeniable that what is needed is faster connection speeds that will be transforming the healthcare providers - patients relationship, integrating electronic communications into medical care, which can be achieved through the arrival of the

© Springer Nature Switzerland AG 2019
M. Themistocleous and P. Rupino da Cunha (Eds.): EMCIS 2018, LNBIP 341, pp. 383–401, 2019.
https://doi.org/10.1007/978-3-030-11395-7_30

5G networks [3]. From the comfort of their homes, patients will wear remote medical sensors, transmitting their vital signs to healthcare providers that will allow doctors and caregivers to monitor an array of vitals, dynamically manage treatment plans, and conduct a consult or intervention over webcam. To this context, 5G networks will take this recent medical trend to the next level and provide a significant economic boost to the medical community. According to IHS Market, 5G will enable more than $1 trillion dollars in products and services for the global healthcare sector [4], while by 2020, around 50 billion connected devices and 212 billion connected sensors are expected to be supported by the 5G network [5]. For healthcare, this means the birth of entire digital ecosystems that can aid medical research, diagnose conditions, and provide treatment at ever-increasing rates. Hence, 5G represents a completely new way for accomplishing digital networking and upgrading the healthcare experiences, by delivering a holistic personalized view of the patients anytime and anywhere.

However, apart from this challenge, additional problems remain concerning the transmission of the medical data, since 5G networks are providing solutions on 'how' data will be transmitted, and not on 'what' kind of data will be transmitted. Consequently, the problem is not only the difficulty of data exchange between systems, but also the devices' data incompatibility. More particularly, IoT medical devices are typically characterized by a high degree of heterogeneity, in terms of having different capabilities, functionalities, etc. In such a scenario, it is necessary to provide abstractions of these heterogeneous devices and manage their interoperability so as to finally collect medical data out of them [6]. However, existing integration technologies lack of sufficient flexibility to adapt to these changes, as their techniques are both static and sensitive to new or changing device implementations [7].

Even if some researches have overcome this problem, the next problem that arises is that the collected data is difficult to be anonymized due to its inherent heterogeneity, and therefore preventing the sharing of data for secondary purposes (e.g. data analysis, research). At the same time, anonymization and pseudo-anonymization techniques have been heavily debated in the ongoing reform of EU data protection law [8]. Thus, the main question that arises is how to implement anonymization in such a way that will protect individual privacy, but will still ensure that the data is of sufficient quality [9].

Nevertheless, the problem does not stop there. Even if it has become feasible to manage thousands of heterogeneous IoT devices, collect data out of them, and anonymize it, the quality of these devices, as well as their derived data are of dubious quality. Henceforth, the next challenge that emerges is the identification of the devices' quality levels, in conjunction with their derived data that need to be qualitative in the maximum degree. The quality evaluation of the devices, as well as of their produced data are mainly treated as black boxes in the IoT domain, and not much thought is given to their quality when integrated into larger systems [10]. Using such devices without proper quality evaluations may have serious implications in the health domain, whilst the absence of data quality could reduce the grade of the successful interpretation of the out coming results and findings [11].

On top of all these, data heterogeneity is one of the most fundamental challenges in the healthcare domain, as medical devices are rapidly expanding, producing tons of heterogeneous data. In this context, interoperability is the only sustainable way to enable healthcare entities acting in various locations, and using distinct information systems from different vendors, to collaborate and deliver quality healthcare. A study estimated that savings of approximately $78 billion could be achieved annually if data exchange standards were utilized across the healthcare sector [12]. Multi-site healthcare provisioning and research requires electronic health records (EHRs) data to be restructured into a common format and standard terminologies, linked to other data sources, which is currently delivered through the HL7 FHIR standard [13].

Taking into consideration all of the aforementioned challenges, in this paper an end-to-end approach is being introduced in the healthcare domain for gathering medical data, anonymizing it, processing it, making it interoperable, and finally storing it, through 5G network technologies. In short, an approach is proposed for the dynamic integration of both known and unknown heterogeneous medical devices during runtime, by providing a Dynamic Data Acquisition API for efficiently collecting their data. In order to anonymize this data, an anonymization part is added to the approach, by implementing k-Anonymity techniques for impeding re-identification, and removing some information, letting concurrently the data to be intact for future use, protecting both individual privacy, and making sure that the data is of sufficient quality.

On top of this, in order to assess the quality of the selected heterogeneous devices in conjunction with their derived data, the proposed approach facilitates the devices' reliability, in combination with the quality estimation of their provided data, by firstly cleaning all the acquired data. As soon as the devices' reliability is being completed, and as a result only the reliable devices are kept connected to the platform in conjunction with their corresponding gathered cleaned data, the interoperability of the latter occurs. For that reason, a filtering mechanism is proposed for defining EHRs and medical data as ontologies, which are used to provide a semantic model for representing definition rules of multiple medical standards that are being finally transformed into HL7 FHIR format. All the aforementioned, are being performed through the implementation of a 5G communication network, as well as an enhanced 5G platform with fully virtualized infrastructure, that are likely to change the way that personalized healthcare is currently provided, for both patients and caregivers.

The rest of this paper is organized as follows. Section 2 presents the state of the art regarding the related work in the healthcare context with regards to the 5G networks, data transmission, security, devices and data heterogeneity comparing them with our approach. Section 3 describes the proposed approach of the interoperable data transmission through the proposed eHealth 5G platform, while Sect. 4 analyzes our conclusions and future goals.

## 2  Related Work

### 2.1  5G Networks

While many things on the road to 5G are uncertain, it is easy to envision the emergence of new and innovative use cases. This new technology allows a significantly higher data capacity and extremely fast response times, opening up completely new potential applications for a fully connected society. Especially in the healthcare domain this constitutes a prerequisite, as faster and more accurate results are needed. Consequently, the industry is facing a new wave of digitalization, referred as Healthcare 4.0 [14]. Healthcare 4.0 is a vision of care delivery that is distributed and patient-centered, and there is already evidence of a shift towards virtualization and individualization of care. Virtualization in the healthcare domain comes with the emergence of next generation mobile network strategies (5G) as foundation, in order to complete the transition to personalized care [15]. The delivery of such virtualized care needs to be executed in real time and based on real time data collection, which can be delivered anywhere, anyhow and at any time. Thus, 5G will be a catalyst to trigger innovation of new products and services in the health care domain, by integrating networking, computing and storage resources into one unified infrastructure.

As the 5G Infrastructure Public Private Partnership (5G-PPP) emphasized in [16], the new 5G network should facilitate the integration with the service layer and enable an effective network resource negotiation (i.e. QoS, latency, speed, reliability). Especially in the healthcare domain, various researches have been conducted trying to cover the different aspects of 5G. In more details, in [17] a summary of the benefits offered by 5G to eHealth is presented, pointing out the new imaging techniques and the possibility of a second opinion thanks to the high-speed transmission of X-rays or scans, the telemonitoring that helps to obtain better diagnostics, and the data mining applied to medical data that helps to adjust the treatment among others. Also, an architecture with 5G for a typical Wireless Body Area Network was presented in [18], while in [19] the 5G-Health is introduced as the next generation of eHealth, discussing the possibilities of medical video streaming, thanks to the high speed reached in 5G networks. To that concept, [20] described how 5G technologies will enable new ways of instant exchange of information in order to deliver personalized healthcare data in real time, as well as how to provide more effective and efficient therapeutic approaches. Additional research included in [21], where the authors introduced systems of wearable medical devices and sensors for monitoring physiological recorded signals, within a 5G infrastructure. Finally, in [22] a potential 5G network and machine-to-machine communication is presented for developing and evolving mobile health applications.

## 2.2 Data Integration

Data integration is considered a key component and, especially in the healthcare domain, where in most of the cases it is considered as a prerequisite in nearly every systematic attempt to achieve integrated care. In the context of healthcare, data integration is a complex process of combining multiple types of data from different heterogeneous sources into a single system/platform [23]. Henceforth, regardless of the way in which devices are connected to each platform, they should be able to be uniformly discoverable and integrated with different platforms, in order for the latter to have access to the sources' medical data.

To this concept, various IoT infrastructures have been proposed in the literature, especially in the healthcare domain, putting their efforts on the integration of heterogeneous medical devices in order to be interoperable and pluggable to different platforms, while offering their data. In more details, the authors in [24] proposed a system to automate the process of collecting patient's vital data via a network of sensors connected to legacy medical devices and deliver this information to the medical center's cloud for storage, processing, and distribution. Moreover, the authors in [25] proposed an ontology-based cognitive computing eHealth system, aiming to provide semantic interoperability among heterogeneous IoT fitness devices and wellness appliances in order to facilitate data integration, sharing and analysis. In the same notion, in [26] the ContQuest was proposed, a framework that among its functionalities, defined a development process for integrating new data sources including their data description and annotation, by using the Ontology Web Language (OWL) [27] to model and describe data sources. In the same concept, the proposed approaches in [28–31] coped with the frequent modification of data source's schemas, by providing homogeneous views of various data sources based on a domain ontology [7]. In addition, the authors in [32] presented an ontology based on data integration architecture within the context of the ACGT project, where emphasis was given to resolve syntactic and semantic heterogeneities when accessing integrated data sources. Finally, the authors in [33] proposed an IoT based Semantic Interoperability Model (IoT-SIM) to provide semantic interoperability among heterogeneous IoT devices in healthcare domain.

### 2.3 Data Anonymization

In the healthcare domain, privacy issues must be taken into consideration, as eHealth services offer efficient exchange of the patients' data between different entities [34]. Hence, all this medical data that is exchanged and shared among them must be fully anonymized, overcoming the various security issues that may arise. Therefore, in order to comply with these issues, healthcare stakeholders seek to use personal data protection solutions, using mainly data anonymization [35]. More particularly, data anonymization refers to the process of modifying personal data in such a way that individuals cannot be re-identified and no information about them can be learned [36], ensuring that even if anonymous data is stolen, it cannot be used in violation of the law. Especially in the healthcare domain, all the data that can identify a patient must be removed together with any other information, which in conjunction with other data held by or disclosed to the recipient, could identify the patient [37].

Hence, in order to achieve this kind of anonymization, k-anonymity [38] is most widely implemented, ensuring that each record in a dataset has at least k-1 indistinguishable records. To this context, various researches have been conducted, focusing mainly on data privacy preserving in cloud networks [39, 40], while most of them are mainly using k-anonymity. Apart from this, the authors in [41] adopted the (a, k)-anonymity model as a privacy detection scheme to collect data and propose a new privacy preserving data collection method based on anonymity for healthcare services. Moreover, in order to avoid privacy leakage, the authors in [42] adopted k-anonymity to protect data from re-identification, proposing a semantic-based linkage k-anonymity (LA) to de-identify record linkage with fewer generalizations and eliminate inference disclosure through semantic reasoning, whilst the authors in [43] proposed the LA through which only obfuscated individuals in a released linkage set are required to be indistinguishable from at least k-1 other individuals in the local dataset.

## 2.4   Data Cleaning

Data cleaning plays a significant role in a broad variety of scientific areas, being responsible for detecting and removing errors and inconsistencies from data, improving its quality [44]. Therefore, data cleaning routines shall be applied to clean the data by filling in missing attributes and values, smoothing and leveling noisy data, identifying and removing outliers, as well as determining and settling inconsistencies [45]. Thus, preparing and cleaning data prior to analysis is a perennial challenge in data analytics, and especially in the healthcare domain, where the produced data is of major importance given that they drive medical decision making.

For that reason, over the last two decades data cleaning has been a key area of research, and many authors have proposed algorithms for data cleaning to remove inconsistencies and noises out of data. The most common inconsistency type has to do with the missing data, for which various algorithms have been proposed so far (i.e. constant substitution, mean attribute value substitution, random attribute value substitution [46]). However, apart from these approaches, there have been proposed several other solutions regarding the different data cleaning problems that may occur. In [47] a method is implemented for managing data duplications, where duplication detection is done either by detecting duplicate records in a single database or by detecting duplicate records in multiple other databases. In the same concept, in [48] a two-step technique that matches different tuples to identify duplicates and merge the duplicate tuples into one is proposed. What is more, to compensate the complexity of data expression, many data cleaning methods are using heuristic rules and user guidance, such as [49–52], which require manual labor for the cleaning process. Hence, in [53] an ontology-based data cleaning solution is implemented, using existing technologies to understand and differentiate the contents of the data, and performing data cleaning without the need of human supervision. Apart from these, in [54] the authors proposed a solution for detecting and repairing dirty data, by offering a commodity data cleaning system that resolves errors like inconsistency, accuracy, and redundancy, by treating multiple types of quality rules holistically. In this context, in [55] a rule-based data cleaning technique is proposed, whereby a set of domain specific rules define how data should be cleaned.

## 2.5   Sources Reliability

A great attention has been given to the reliability challenge, confronting system reliability as a fundamental requirement of IoT devices. In more details, reliability is a measure of the ability that a system operates as expected under predefined conditions for a predefined time [56]. According to [57] reliability is a technical effort made to ensure that a developed system is free from any fault that can result to failure during operation. It entails that the system is highly dependable and functions maximally at any given time or condition over the period it is created or developed to serve.

To this context, various reliability methods have been proposed in the literature regarding the IoT world, and especially the healthcare domain, putting their efforts on measuring the reliability of the IoT devices that are being used for various health purposes. More particularly, in [58] the authors presented a new methodology for estimating hardware and software reliability given uncertain use conditions, so as to derive probabilistic estimates for overall system reliability. In the same notion, in [59] a probability-based concept is proposed for measuring the reliability of IoT devices, investigating the proposed model from the perspectives of consumer world, by using things link analysis. Furthermore, in [60] the evaluation of the inter-device reliability of activity monitors was discussed, while in the same concept, in [61] the authors examined the reliability of consumer activity trackers for measuring step count in both laboratory and free-living conditions. The study in [62] evaluated the criterion-related reliability of field-based leg stiffness devices in different testing approaches, by measuring the coefficient of variation, the intraclass correlation coefficient, and the standard error of measurement of these devices. Moreover, in [63] the intra and interrater reliability were evaluated upon the point-of-care nerve conduction device in patients with diabetes and a broad spectrum of nerve injury, while in [64] several criteria and methods presented for assessing reliability of medical equipment.

## 2.6    Data Interoperability

Interoperability is considered a necessity in electronic healthcare systems. At the same time, the development of medical standards has significantly evolved, yet bearing unsolved challenges with clinical data distributed among heterogeneous sources [65]. The Health Level Seven International (HL7) organization provides the development and the framework of standards, of which the most commonly used is the HL7 v2.x [66], however, HL7 FHIR [13] is the latest standard created by the HL7 organization for the exchange of clinical information, whose main motivation was to simplify and reduce the complexity of the mechanisms and structures defined by it, avoiding the mistakes made in its previous standards (HL7 v3 [67], CDA [68]).

To this context, various researches have been developed for covering the different standards that exist for confronting data interoperability. In more details, the Detailed Clinical Models (DCM) [69] have been used for defining clinical information independently of a specific clinical standard, but aiming to offer the possibility of being transformed into other medical standards. Another approach of data harmonization was the 5-year strategy of NHS Wales focusing on developing an open platform across a fully integrated electronic patient record with the core of the clinical terminology Systematized Nomenclature of Medicine Clinical Terms (SNOMED CT) [70]. A process based on HL7 standard and SNOMED CT vocabulary from the biomedical domain and the latest semantic web technologies has been developed and tested within the framework of EURECA EU research project [71], aiming to homogenize the representation and normalization of clinical data. Moreover, in [72] the interoperability among different healthcare systems was reached by annotating the Web Service messages through archetypes defined in OWL, whereas the same researchers presented an approach [73] based on archetypes, ontologies and semantic techniques for the interoperability between HL7 CDA and ISO 13606 systems, which were represented in OWL. Finally, the work of [74] must be mentioned, where the authors presented a solution based on the Enterprise Service Bus that was translated into the healthcare domain using the ideals of HL7 V3 and SNOMED CT.

Taking into consideration all the aforementioned approaches that have been proposed for dealing with the different challenges that exist concerning 5G networks, data integration, anonymization, cleaning, reliability, as well as interoperability in the healthcare domain, we can conclude that our approach is extremely innovative. More particularly, compared with the existing 5G platforms, the proposed eHealth 5G Platform provides simple and powerful access to the medical devices, along with high system capacity, great speed and ultra-high reliability. Apart from this, all the researches that have been made for integrating heterogeneous devices, lack of sufficient flexibility and adaptability to solve challenges arisen from dynamically integrating both known and unknown devices during runtime, a scenario that is fully supported by the data integration part that is developed in our approach. Regarding data anonymization, no innovation is being proposed, as we simply make use of the k-anonymity algorithm. Regarding data cleaning, the existing surveys have presented different approaches for it, lacking an end-to-end iterative data cleaning process, a problem that is totally eliminating in our approach, where an end-to-end iterative data cleaning process is implemented, being capable of cleaning data deriving from both known and unknown devices. As for devices reliability, all the researches that have been proposed so far for characterizing devices' reliability are based only upon the devices' reliability itself, without considering data reliability issues, thus not stating a combined approach, which is crucial for any application in the healthcare domain. Henceforth, the devices reliability part of our approach is considered innovative, as it confronts devices' reliability in combination with their derived data quality. Finally, considering data interoperability, several solutions have been proposed enabling the access to the existing medical data for specific clinical organizations, lacking however to be applied to different medical standards and incoming data, thus not providing a generic approach being able to address heterogeneous healthcare data. To address this gap and confront the interoperability issues, our approach includes a generalized mechanism that employs several matching operations to the HL7 FHIR standard.

## 3  Proposed Approach

In our approach, an innovative mechanism is proposed for gathering medical data from numerous heterogeneous IoT medical devices, anonymizing this data, cleaning it, making it interoperable, and finally storing it through 5G communication technologies. More specifically, the proposed approach consists of the six (6) main stages: (i) 5G Communication Network, (ii) Data Integration, (iii) Data Anonymization, (iv) Data Cleaning, (v) Devices Reliability, and (vi) Data Interoperability, accompanied with Data Storage, as illustrated in Fig. 1.

**5G Network.** The architecture of the used 5G Network consists of two (2) major steps related to the 5G communication and integration. Initially, the collection of the data takes place at high reliable edge-nodes, in order to allow the connection of the physical world (i.e. biological system) and the virtual world (i.e. 5G infrastructure). In order to achieve this, the deployment of the edge node in each medical device is being connected through a 5G Radio Access Network (5G RAN) [75], enabling finally the

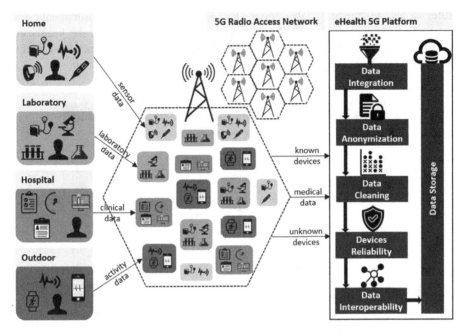

**Fig. 1.** Architecture of the proposed approach

analysis of the information inside the eHealth 5G Platform through the appropriate integration of different Virtual Network Functions (VNFs) [76].

In more details, in the first step the identification of the available heterogeneous IoT medical devices takes place, through the established 5G RAN communication network. Due to the diverse and extreme requirements of the healthcare data, as well as the eHealth services, the 5G RAN designed to operate in a wide range of spectrum bands, with diverse characteristics, such as channel bandwidth and propagation conditions. The challenge in 5G RANs is how to dynamically assign the foreseen wide range of services with diverse requirements to the many spectrum bands, usage types and radio recourses. Therefore, the proposed approach comes to resolve this challenge by using the Radio Access Network as a Service (RANaaS) [77], by partially centralizing the functionalities of the RAN depending on the actual needs, as well as the network characteristics, being able to handle huge amounts of data, in high-speed with low-cost, providing on-demand resource provisioning delay-aware storage, and high network capacity wherever and whenever needed. Thus, through this established connection, all the data of the connected health devices are being gathered, containing information about the used devices' APIs (i.e. source code) that is assumed that is written in the same programming language, accompanied with the devices' specifications (i.e. hardware and software) that contain the same semantics in terms of specifications' descriptions and measurement units. To this end, it should be noted that the gathered data comes from different entities and systems, referring that is coming either from (i) medical devices that are used by the patients for their in-home monitoring, or (ii) medical devices, EHRs, PHRs that are used by the patients and the healthcare professionals in medical laboratories for keeping patients' measurements, or (iii) medical devices, EHRs, PHRs that are used by the patients and the healthcare professionals in hospitals for recording and keeping patients' measurements, or finally (iv) medical devices that are used by the patients for their outdoor activities.

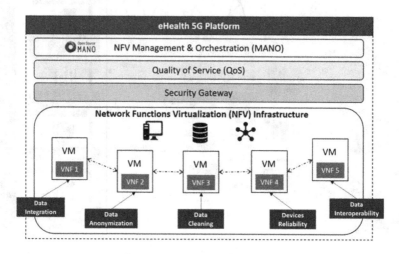

**Fig. 2.** 5G enhanced platform

As soon as all this data has been collected, the second step occurs, where the 5G architecture of the eHealth platform is being developed, using the technologies of Network Function Virtualization (NFV) [78] and Software Defined Network (SDN) [79]. The value of the 5G SDN (especially in conjunction with NFV and virtualized networking) is its ability to provide network virtualization, automation and creation of new services over virtual resources, affording an extremely manageable and cost-effective architecture, making it ideal for the dynamic, high-bandwidth nature of eHealth. Furthermore, VNFs move individual network functions out of dedicated hardware devices into software that runs on commodity hardware, while it is worth saying that VNFs can run as virtual machines (VMs). In the current approach, we adapted the ongoing 5GTANGO's Service Platform [80], which consists mainly of three (3) discrete blocks: (i) the Service Development Kit, (ii) the Validation and Verification, and (iii) the Service Platform that will be parameterized in our approach. As shown in Fig. 2, the proposed eHealth 5G platform consists of several components which support the whole lifecycle of the VNFs, by the time that they are developed until the time that they are instantiated. Initially, through the NFV Infrastructure all the data management mechanisms that are provided through the eHealth 5G platform (i.e. data integration, data anonymization, etc.) are constructed in the form of VNFs. This transformation is a prerequisite for the efficient operation of the platform, providing it with quite flexibility, cost-efficiency, and scalability, being able to be virtualized in different eHealth platforms running in different entities (i.e. hospitals, health clinics etc.). As soon as all the mechanisms are being transformed into VNFs, the Security

**Data Integration**

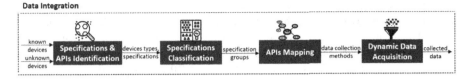

**Fig. 3.** Data integration process

Gateway component is being implemented, which is responsible for controlling the privileges and the users' access to the platform, by validating the corresponding requests. This is of crucial importance in the context of open 5G ecosystems, where entry barriers are disruptively lowered, without decreasing security [81]. Apart from this, it is of crucial importance to guarantee Quality of Service (QoS) of the developed eHealth 5G platform. For that reason, we create an integrated view of the healthcare applications, the interconnection infrastructure support, and the operational support with common services. Finally, on top of all these, the eHealth 5G platform provides the NFV Management & Orchestration component that uses the MANO framework [82], which is responsible for managing the lifecycle of all the VNFs requests and instances by orchestrating the available infrastructure.

**Data Integration.** In this stage the data integration occurs, for easily and rapidly integrating heterogeneous IoT medical devices during runtime, concerning both known and unknown devices, so as to be able to collect data out of them. Therefore, this stage contains the first data mechanism of the eHealth 5G platform, while it consists of four (4) discrete substages (Fig. 3), following the work conducted in [83].

In the first substage of the mechanism, as soon as all the devices have been connected to the eHealth 5G platform, these are categorized into either known (in terms of devices of known type, containing predefined APIs methods) or previously unknown devices (in terms of devices of unknown type, containing undefined APIs methods). Afterwards, through the established 5G network connection, information is gathered concerning both devices' specifications (i.e. hardware and software) and APIs (i.e. multiple methods). Thus, information is gathered about (i) both known and unknown devices' specifications, (ii) known devices' APIs in terms of source code and of what exactly each method in the API represents, and (iii) unknown devices' APIs in terms of source code, as the significance of each method in the API is unknown.

Afterwards, in the second substage the classification of the devices' specifications occurs, following the approach proposed in [84]. By knowing (i) the device type of the known devices as well as their specifications, and (ii) the specifications of the unknown devices, their classification occurs, considering the known devices' types and the similar specifications that all these devices may have with the unknown devices. Based on the classification outcomes, the identification of the unknown devices' type takes place, assuming that the devices with the same specifications are of the same type (e.g. all the spirometers will have approximately the same specifications). As a result, all the devices of unknown type are considered as known.

In the third substage, the mapping of the devices' APIs methods occurs. More particularly, in the first substage of Data Integration, knowledge about known devices'

APIs methods was acquired in terms of source code and of what exactly each method in the API represents. However, with regards to the unknown devices' APIs methods, the acquired knowledge referred only to the source code, as the significance of each method in the API was unknown. Henceforth, in this substage it becomes feasible to map the known devices' APIs methods with those of the unknown devices, by comparing the API methods of the devices of the same type (e.g. all the spirometers). In order to achieve this mapping, for each one of these devices a Generic API Ontology (GAO) is constructed, based on the approaches proposed in [7, 85], in order to identify and model a hierarchical tree of the different classes and sub-classes of the semantics of the devices' APIs methods. In more details, each GAO contains different ontologies for each different method of each device's API, thus a hierarchical tree is being created for each API, allowing us to understand and probabilistically map the similar methods. In our case, the mechanism has to identify and map the method that is responsible for gathering the unknown devices' data, thus the method that has been assigned with higher probability levels, is automatically assigned as the most appropriate method.

Finally, as soon as this mapping is completed, in the fourth substage the implementation of the Dynamic Data Acquisition API occurs. More particularly, the latter constitutes of a unified API that merges into a single unified data method all the different devices APIs' data methods that are responsible for collecting data, and thus the collection of devices' data takes place.

**Data Anonymization.** In this stage the data anonymization occurs, where the collected data is pre-processed through k-Anonymity using data suppression and data generalization, following two (2) different substages, as depicted in Fig. 4.

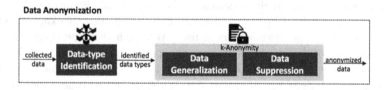

**Fig. 4.** Data anonymization process

In the first substage, the data-type identification of the collected data takes place, through which we are able to identify whether an individual value of an attribute can be anonymized through the data suppression or the data generalization method, by identifying the data type of each value. It should be mentioned that only the personal data (i.e. data that identify a person) are being filtered through this mechanism.

Therefore, in the second substage, the anonymization of the collected data occurs, where k-Anonymity is being implemented, applying data generalization and/or data suppression, depending on the results of the data-type identification. In more details, through the data suppression method, certain values of the attributes are replaced by a hashtag '#', according to their semantics and to what they represent. Regarding the data generalization method, individual values of attributes are replaced with a broader category, being given a range where the anonymized value can be found in between.

Consequently, implementing the corresponding method upon the collected data, we result into the fully anonymization of it, taking into consideration that the numeric values are being anonymized through the data generalization method, while all the other types of values are anonymized through the data suppression method.

**Data Cleaning.** In this stage, the cleaning of the anonymized data takes place, which is received as an input in conjunction with the device type that gathered this data, maintaining the data model of each device type. Within this data model, the elements of the data are defined in addition to a set of constraints, predefined rules for the corrective actions, and the automated data filling. Therefore, for each dataset four (4) discrete substages are followed sequentially, as illustrated in Fig. 5.

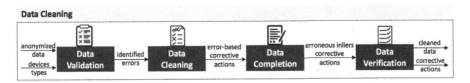

**Fig. 5.** Data cleaning process

In the first substage, the data validation occurs that identifies all the errors associated with the conformance to a set of predefined rules, such as data type (i.e. integer, string, etc.), range constraints (i.e. minimum and maximum values), uniformity (i.e. data format), predefined values (i.e. values selected from a predefined list), and mandatory fields. Hence, a variety of validity checks is performed aiming to safeguard the accuracy and the consistency of the data by ensuring the conformance both to the specified constraints on the data model for this device type and the identified duplicates.

In the second substage, the data cleaning occurs that eliminates the errors identified in the previous substage, where based on the set of the predefined rules, corrective/removal actions are applied on the identified erroneous records of the data.

Sequentially, in the third substage the data completion takes place that safeguards the appropriateness and completeness of the data, especially referring to erroneous inliers, where the conformance to mandatory fields and required non-empty attributes of the data is ensured based on the predefined conformance rules of the data model.

Finally, in the fourth substage, the data verification occurs that executes the evaluation of the undertaken actions in the previous substages, ensuring the accuracy and consistency of the cleaned data. Thus, the final results are produced, indicating the undertaken total corrective actions in combination with the derived cleaned data.

**Devices Reliability.** In this stage the devices reliability takes places, in combination with the quality estimation of their provided data, as depicted in Fig. 6. This stage is of major importance, as it is not sufficient to keep all the derived data and use it for further analysis, as many of it may have derived either from unreliable devices, or from reliable devices being uncleaned and faulty. For that reason, it is necessary to measure and evaluate the quality of both the connected devices and their produced data, so as to finally keep only the reliable data that comes from only reliable devices. In our case, for measuring devices' reliability we captured the metric of the availability of the connected devices, an important metric for assessing the quality of the devices [57]. Therefore, we measure each device's availability by getting the corresponding values, setting a timestamp in order to measure how often each device communicates with the platform and provides its data. However, it is not sufficient to measure only the devices' availability for deciding whether the latter is being considered as reliable or not, but it is more effective to measure also the data quality of these devices. For that reason, we use as an input from the Data Cleaning stage the number of the undertaken actions that were applied upon the collected datasets, in order to correlate it with the availability results of the corresponding devices that produced these datasets, and finally decide whether each device, and as a result its derived data, are considered as reliable or not.

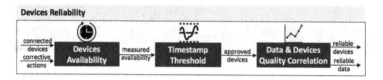

**Fig. 6.** Devices reliability process

**Data Interoperability.** In this stage, the final transformation of the data takes place. Thus, the data interoperability process occurs, including an automated way for transforming the ingested data into HL7 FHIR format in terms of structure (Fig. 7).

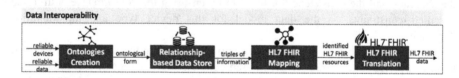

**Fig. 7.** Data interoperability process

In the first substage, ontologies are created for the source data by transforming the provided data into an ontological form. Thus, this substage delivers the means so that the different relationships, classes and instances are discovered, providing a way for easily classifying these categories, enabling easier manipulation for the next substages.

Afterwards, the second substage provides a relationship-based data store for storing the identified relationships, classes, and instances, making it easier to perform queries through the collected data that can possibly contain information concerning one or more of the stored information. Through this substage it is easier to probabilistically identify faulty or missed relationships among different classes/instances, through a relationship matching mechanism that contains a functionality for identifying missing values, and re-assigning the relationships that have a larger degree of association to a specific class.

Sequentially, the third substage provides a mechanism that offers the capability of understanding and interpreting the semantic meaning of the different classes that have already been stored into the previous substage. Afterwards, this substage is incorporating a mechanism that iterates and scans through the different HL7 FHIR resources, in order to probabilistically map the semantics of the stored classes with a specific HL7 FHIR resource. In the end, the HL7 FHIR resource with higher probability levels of correspondence is automatically assigned to the identified class.

Finally, the fourth substage provides a mechanism for setting the final HL7 FHIR-based form of the classes. Hence, the classes along with their identified HL7 FHIR resources are obtained, including the name of the HL7 FHIR resource along with the specific attribute that the class may belong to, translating them using the HL7 FHIR-based formatting (i.e. *Resource.attribute*). Thus, all the data is translated into a common format, being finally stored into the eHealth 5G platform's database.

# 4   Conclusions

While current devices have revolutionized our daily lives in multiple domains, the quantity of available healthcare data is rising rapidly, far exceeding the capacity to deliver personal or public health benefits from analyzing this data. Hence, a substantial overhaul of methodology is required to address the real complexity of health. In this paper, an innovative end-to-end approach was proposed for gathering medical data, anonymizing it, cleaning it, making it interoperable, and finally storing it through 5G network technologies. Therefore, it combined core technologies that are crucial in the healthcare domain, for delivering results of high-reliability and efficiency. Even though there have been proposed several techniques for addressing the aforementioned data domains, most of these have been designed to give a solution to specific problems, with low flexibility and adaptability. Contrariwise, our approach promises faster results of high accuracy, merging multiple innovative data manipulation techniques.

Nevertheless, the proposed approach still has to be compared with multiple mechanisms that provide similar services, and evaluated with datasets of different nature and size, and in multiple systems, so as to have better interpretable results. Our future work includes that the mechanism will be also evaluated by testing it with a huge amount of heterogeneous IoT medical devices of different types. We also plan to extend the list of the supported data cleaning constraints including more advanced and sophisticated constraints, while we aim to configure the data anonymization mechanism by testing it with additional data anonymization algorithms. Finally, we plan to evaluate our approach with multiple healthcare data, including formats of unknown nature.

**Acknowledgements.** A. Mavrogiorgou and A. Kiourtis would like to acknowledge the financial support from the "Hellenic Foundation for Research & Innovations (HFRI)". Moreover, part of this work has been partially supported by the 5GTANGO project, funded by the European Commission under Grant number H2020ICT-2016-2 761493 through the Horizon 2020 and 5G-PPP programs (http://5gtango.eu).

# References

1. Population health outcomes. http://www.healthcatalyst.com/population-health-outcomes-3-keys-to-drive-improvement
2. The role of IoT in the healthcare industry. https://hackernoon.com/the-role-of-internet-of-things-in-the-healthcare-industry-759b2a1abe5
3. Healthcare needs 5G. https://www.chilmarkresearch.com/healthcare-needs-5g/
4. How will 5G impact different industries? http://prescouter.com/2018/01/5g-impact-different-industries
5. The Journey to 5G. http://www.healthcareitnews.com/news/journey-5g
6. Pires, F., et al.: A platform for integrating physical devices in the Internet of Things. In: Embedded and Ubiquitous Computing (EUC), pp. 234–241. IEEE (2014)
7. Gong, P.: Dynamic integration of biological data sources using the data concierge. Health Inf. Sci. Syst. **1**, 1–19 (2013)
8. GDPR requirements. https://www.delphix.com/white-paper/gdpr
9. El Emam, K., Arbuckle, L.: Anonymizing Health Data: Case Studies and Methods to get you started, 2nd edn, p. 1005. O'Reilly Media Inc., Newton (2013)
10. Kruger, P., Hancke, G.: Benchmarking internet of things data sources. In: 12th IEEE International Conference on Industrial Informatics (INDIN). IEEE (2014)
11. Macfarlane, S., Tannath, T., Scott, J., Kelly, V.: The validity and reliability of global positioning systems in team sport: a brief review. JSCR **30**(5), 1470–1490 (2016)
12. Mead, C.: Data interchange standards in healthcare IT-computable semantic interoperability. JHIM **20**, 71–78 (2006)
13. HL7 FHIR. https://www.hl7.org/fhir/
14. HEALTHCARE 4.0: A NEW WAY OF LIFE? http://www.vph-institute.org/news/healthcare-4-0-a-new-way-of-life.html
15. A new Generation of eHealth Systems Powered by 5G. http://www.wwrf.ch/files/wwrf/content/files/publications/outlook/Outlook17.pdf
16. 5G on eHealth. https://5g-ppp.eu/wp-content/uploads/2016/02/5G-PPP-White-Paper-on-eHealth-Vertical-Sector.pdf
17. INTERNET OF THINGS & 5G REVOLUTION. http://www.astrid-online.it/static/upload/stud/studio-i-com_internet_5g_.pdf
18. Mishra, A., Agrawal, P.: Continuous health condition monitoring by 24 × 7 sensing and transmission of physiological data over 5G cellular channels. In: ICNC, pp. 584–590 (2015)
19. Banaee, H., et al.: Data mining for wearable sensors in health monitoring systems: a review of recent trends and challenges. Sensors **13**(12), 17472–17500 (2013)
20. Ryan, M., et al.: Facilitating health behaviour change and its maintenance: interventions based on self-determination theory. Eur. Health Psychol. **10**, 2–5 (2008)
21. Oleshchuk, V., Fensli, R.: Remote patient monitoring within a future 5G infrastructure. Wirel. Pers. Commun. **57**, 431–439 (2011)
22. Mattos, W., Gondim, P.: M-health solutions using 5G networks and M2M communications. IT Prof. **18**(3), 24–29 (2016)
23. Leventer-Roberts, M., Balicer, R.: Data integration in health care. In: Amelung, V., Stein, V., Goodwin, N., Balicer, R., Nolte, E., Suter, E. (eds.) Handbook Integrated Care, pp. 121–129. Springer, Cham (2017). https://doi.org/10.1007/978-3-319-56103-5_8
24. Rolim, C.O., et al.: A cloud computing solution for patient's data collection in health care institutions. In: Second International Conference on ETELEMED 2010. IEEE (2010)
25. Carbonaro, A., Piccinini, F., Reda, R.: Integrating heterogeneous data of healthcare devices to enable domain data management. JeLKS **14**(1), 45–56 (2018)

26. Pötter, B., Sztajnberg, A.: Adapting heterogeneous devices into an IoT context-aware infrastructure. In: Software Engineering for Adaptive and Self-Managing, pp. 64–74. ACM (2016)
27. OWL. https://www.w3.org/TR/owl-guide/
28. Globle, C., et al.: Transparent access to multiple bioinformatics information sources. IBM Syst. J. **40**, 534–551 (2001)
29. Donelson, L., et al.: The BioMediator system as a data integration tool to answer diverse biologic queries. In: Proceedings of MedInfo, pp. 768–772 (2004)
30. Philippi, S.: Light-weight integration of molecular biological databases. Bioinformatics **20**, 51–57 (2004)
31. Eckman, B., Lacroix, Z., Raschid, L.: Optimized seamless integration of biomolecular data. In: IEEE International Conference on Bioinformatics and Biomedical Engineering, pp. 23–32 (2001)
32. Martín, L., et al.: Ontology based integration of distributed and heterogeneous data sources in ACGT. In: HEALTHINF, pp. 301–306 (2008)
33. Jabbar, S., et al.: Semantic interoperability in heterogeneous IoT infrastructure for healthcare. Wirel. Commun. Mobile Comput. (2017)
34. Truta, T., Vina, B.: Privacy protection: p-sensitive k-anonymity property. In: 22nd International Conference on Data Engineering Workshops, Atlanta (2006)
35. El Emam, K.: Data anonymization practices in clinical research. a descriptive study. University of Ottawa (2006)
36. El Emam, K., et al.: A systematic review of re-identification attacks on health data. PLoS One **6**(12), e28071 (2011)
37. Zhong, S., et al.: Privacy-enhancing k-anonymization of customer data. In: PODS 2005, pp. 139–147 (2004)
38. Sweeney, L.: k-anonymity: a model for protecting privacy. Int. J. Unc. Fuzz. Knowl. Based Syst. **10**(5), 557–570 (2002)
39. Benjamin, E., et al.: Systematic literature review on the anonymization of high dimensional streaming datasets for health data sharing. Procedia Comput. Sci. **63**, 348–355 (2015)
40. Dubovitskaya, A., Urovi, V., Vasirani, M., Aberer, K., Schumacher, M.I.: A cloud-based eHealth architecture for privacy preserving data integration. In: Federrath, H., Gollmann, D. (eds.) SEC 2015. IAICT, vol. 455, pp. 585–598. Springer, Cham (2015). https://doi.org/10.1007/978-3-319-18467-8_39
41. Li, H., et al.: (a, k)-anonymous scheme for privacy-preserving data collection in IoT-based healthcare services systems. J. Med. Syst. **42**(3), 56 (2018)
42. Lu, Y., Sinnott, R.O., Verspoor, K.: A semantic-based k-anonymity scheme for health record linkage. Stud. Health Technol. Inform. **239**, 84–90 (2017)
43. Lu, Y., Verspoor, K., Sinnott, R.O., Parampalli, U.: Effective preservation of privacy during record linkage. In: School of Computing and Information Systems, p. 25 (2017)
44. Fatima, A., Nazir, N., Gufran, K.: Data cleaning in data warehouse: a survey of data pre-processing techniques and tools. JITCS **9**, 50–61 (2017)
45. Rahm, E., Do, H.: Data cleaning: problems and current approaches. IEEE Bull. Tech. Comm. Data Eng. **23**(4), 2000–2012 (2000)
46. Krishnan, S., Haas, D., Franklin, M., Wu, E.: Towards reliable interactive data cleaning: a user survey and recommendations. In: HILDA, California (2016)
47. Dallachiesa, M., et al.: NADEEF: a commodity data cleaning system. In: ACM SIGMOD International Conference on Management of Data, New York (2013)
48. Dagade, A., Mali, M., Pathak, N.: Survey of data duplication detection and elimination in domain dependent and domain-independent databases. IJARCSMS **4**(5), 238–243 (2016)

49. Benjelloun, O., et al.: Swoosh: A Generic Approach to Entity Resolution. Stanford InfoLab, Stanford (2005)

50. Bohannon, P., Fan, W., Flaster, M., Rastogi, R.: A cost-based model and effective heuristic for repairing constraints by value modification. In: ACM SIGMOD (2005)

51. Cong, G., Fan, W., Geerts, G., Jia, X., Ma, S.: Improving data quality: consistency and accuracy. In: The 33rd International Conference on Very Large Data Bases, Vienna (2007)

52. Fan, W., et al.: Towards certain fixes with editing rules and master data. VLDB J. **21**(2), 213–238 (2012)

53. Yakout, M., et al.: Guided data repair. Proc. VLDB Endowment **4**(5), 279–289 (2011)

54. Cheng, K., Hong, J.: A novel data cleaning with data matching. Adv. Sci. Technol. Lett. **136**, 161–169 (2016)

55. Gohel, A., et al.: A commodity data cleaning system. Int. Res. J. Eng. Technol. **4**(5), 1011–1014 (2017)

56. Joseph, W.: Quantifying test-retest reliability using the intraclass correlation coefficient and the SEM. J. Strength Cond. Res. **19**(1), 231 (2005)

57. Toporkov, A.: Criteria and methods for assessing reliability of medical equipment. Biomed. Eng. **42**(1), 11–16 (2008)

58. Mudasir, A.: Reliability models for the internet of things: a paradigm shift. In: IEEE International Symposium on ISSREW. IEEE (2014)

59. Zin, T.T., et al.: Reliability and availability measures for Internet of Things consumer world perspectives. In: 5th Global Conference on Consumer Electronics. IEEE (2016)

60. Ryan, R., et al.: Validity and reliability of Fitbit activity monitors compared to ActiGraph GT3X+ with female adults in a free-living environment. J. Sci. Med. Sport **20**(6), 578–582 (2017)

61. Kooiman, T., et al.: Reliability and validity of ten consumer activity trackers. BMC Sport. Sci. Med. Rehabil. **7**(1), 24 (2015)

62. Ruggiero, L., et al.: Validity and reliability of two field-based leg stiffness devices: implications for practical use. J. Appl. Biomech. **32**(4), 415–419 (2016)

63. Justin, L., et al.: Reliability and validity of a point-of-care sural nerve conduction device for identification of diabetic neuropathy. PLoS One **9**(1), e86515 (2014)

64. Misra, P., et al.: An interoperable realization of smart cities with plug and play based device management (2015)

65. Rastegar-Mojarad, M., et al.: Need of informatics in designing interoperable clinical registries. Int. J. Med. Inform. **108**, 78–84 (2017)

66. Introduction to HL7 Standards. http://www.hl7.org/implement/standards/

67. HL7 v3. https://www.hl7.org/fhir/comparison-v3.html

68. The HL7 Clinical Document Architecture. https://www.ncbi.nlm.nih.gov/pmc/articles/PMC130066/

69. Goossen, W., et al.: Detailed clinical models. Healthc. Inform. **16**, 201–214 (2010)

70. Wardle, M., Spencer, A.: Implementation of SNOMED CT in an online clinical database. Futur. Hosp. J. **4**(2), 126–130 (2017)

71. EURECA EU project. https://www.dceureca.eu/

72. Dogac, A., et al.: Artemis: deploying semantically enriched web services in the healthcare domain. Inf. Syst. **31**, 321–339 (2006)

73. Schulz, S., Udo, H.: Part-whole representation and reasoning in formal biomedical ontologies. AI Med. **34**(3), 179–200 (2005)

74. Ryan, A., Eklund, P.: A framework for semantic interoperability in healthcare. Stud. Health Tech Inform. **136**, 759 (2008)

75. Marsch, P., et al.: 5G radio access network architecture: design guidelines and key considerations. IEEE Commun. Mag. **54**(11), 24–32 (2016)

76. VNF. https://searchsdn.techtarget.com/definition/virtual-network-functions
77. Ferreira, L., et al.: An architecture to offer cloud-based radio access network as a service. In: European Conference on Networks and Communications. IEEE (2014)
78. Network Functions Virtualisation. http://www.etsi.org/technologies-clusters/technologies/nfv
79. SDN. https://www.opennetworking.org/sdn-definition/
80. 5G Development and Validation Platform for global Industry-specific Network Services and Apps. http://5gtango.eu/
81. Parada, C., et al.: 5GTANGO: A Beyond-MANO Service Platform (in press)
82. Open Source MANO. http://www.etsi.org/technologies-clusters/technologies/nfv/open-source-mano
83. Mavrogiorgou, A., Kiourtis, A., Kyriazis, D.: Plug'n'play IoT devices: an approach for dynamic data acquisition from unknown heterogeneous devices. In: Barolli, L., Terzo, O. (eds.) CISIS 2017. AISC, vol. 611, pp. 885–895. Springer, Cham (2018). https://doi.org/10.1007/978-3-319-61566-0_84
84. Mavrogiorgou, A., Kiourtis, A., Kyriazis, D.: A comparative study of classification techniques for managing IoT devices of common specifications. In: Pham, C., Altmann, J., Bañares, J.Á. (eds.) GECON 2017. LNCS, vol. 10537, pp. 67–77. Springer, Cham (2017). https://doi.org/10.1007/978-3-319-68066-8_6
85. Kiourtis, A., et al.: Aggregating heterogeneous health data through an ontological common health language. In: DeSE 10th International Conference. IEEE (2017)

# IT Governance

# Agile Requirement Engineering Maturity Framework for Industry 4.0

Samaa Elnagar[✉], Heinz Weistroffer, and Manoj Thomas

Virginia Commonwealth University, Information Systems, Richmond, VA, USA
{elnagarsa, hrweistr, mthomas}@vcu.edu

**Abstract.** *Industry 4.0 (I4.0)* is changing business models and processes. I4.0 uses innovative trends such as *Big Data, Cloud Computing*, and *Internet of things (IOT)* to maximize economic benefits and return on investments. However, developing an I4.0 project may be costly, complex and risky for some companies. Therefore, careful requirements definition and mature *Requirement Engineering (RE)* processes are necessary. Undeveloped RE processes and poorly defined business requirements will often result in an inferior or a cancelled project. In addition, to ensure agility and allow for iterative changes in developing projects for I4.0, *agile* methodologies should be applied and prudently assessed. Unfortunately, most of existing assessment models are narrow focused and lack theoretical foundation and proper validation. This research proposes a comprehensive maturity framework called *agile Requirement Engineering Maturity Model for Industry 4.0* (ARE-MMI4.0). The framework provides assessment of the minimum maturity levels to start a project for I4.0. The framework integrates an I4.0 maturity model with RE and agile maturity models to ensure the ultimate maturity assessment for the business processes.

**Keywords:** Industry 4.0 · Agile · Requirements engineering
Maturity models integration

## 1 Introduction

The term *Industry 4.0* (I4.0) or the fourth industrial revolution was introduced by the German government [1, 2]. I4.0 aims to enhance productivity an operational efficiency with high levels of process automation. It forms a new kind of intelligent, networked and agile value chain [3]. Moreover, it helps companies reduce cost, enhance customer satisfaction and improve the relation with business partners [4]. I4.0 encompasses many different technologies and new paradigms such as *cloud-based* manufacturing and *enterprise resource planning* (ERP) [5]. Pfeiffer [6] suggests that for companies to compete efficiently in global markets, they should reshape their business processes and business models in the direction of I4.0 through the digitization of their current products and systems. Digitization is no longer limited to certain departments in the company, but rather, it takes place throughout the entire value chain [7].

The characteristics of I4.0 include: horizontal integration across whole value networks, strong vertical integration within the company, and digital transparency of engineering across the entire value chain [8]. I4.0 requires careful specification of the

© Springer Nature Switzerland AG 2019
M. Themistocleous and P. Rupino da Cunha (Eds.): EMCIS 2018, LNBIP 341, pp. 405–418, 2019.
https://doi.org/10.1007/978-3-030-11395-7_31

changing production requirements, and it is strongly related to agile methodologies [9]. I4.0 is ongoing with cyber physical systems (CPS), which is based on heterogeneous data and knowledge integration. CPS and I4.0 aim to fulfill the agile and dynamic requirements of production and improve the effectiveness and efficiency of the entire industry [10]. In addition, the concept of agile factory has emerged as a result of I4.0 manufacturing processes [11]. The agile factory transfers agile software engineering techniques to the domain of manufacturing that accepts customer changes during assembly time.

Unfortunately, many challenges face projects that target I4.0. Most software development models are gravely hampered by immature practices, lack of a sound, widely accepted theoretical basis, and lack of credible experimental evaluation and validation [12]. Moreover, 40–50% of software development effort is dedicated to rework [13]. This percentage may be very costly and exhaustive for I4.0 projects because it impacts the entire value chain. I4.0 affects mainly large companies, as small- and medium-sized enterprises (SMEs) consider it too complex, expensive, risky and not relevant [8]. In addition, studies show that many companies have serious problems grasping the overall idea of I4.0, because they cannot readily apply it to their specific domain and their particular business strategy. Another problem is that companies cannot easily assess their state-of-development, and therefore they are not able to identify tangible fields of action, programs and projects [14].

Hence, to avoid uncertainty, reduce application cost, and minimize risk with respect to applying I4.0, a company must accurately define the technical and organizational requirements beforehand, and assess the maturity of all the processes involved in any project targeting I4.0. Maturity models are widely used instruments that measure the maturity of an organization's processes concerning specific target states based on a more or less comprehensive set of criteria [15]. Since I4.0 processes are agile in nature [16], the maturity of the processes should not only be measured with regards to I4.0 but also with regard to requirement engineering maturity and level of agility.

This research aims to develop an assistive framework that is applicable across many business domains to guide companies in safely migrating to or developing projects for I4.0, with minimum effort, risk and cost. The framework integrates I4.0, requirement engineering (RE), and agile maturity models to assess the minimum level of processes maturity and iteratively evaluate the readiness of the processes to migrate to I4.0.

The rest of this paper is organized as follows: in the next section we provide a review of the literature on applicable maturity frameworks. The following section describes the methodology used in developing the framework. Next is the actual design of our framework, followed by discussion the framework's application. Finally, a summary of the research and future work are presented in the conclusion.

## 2  Literature Review

The first question to be answered to build this maturity framework is how to conduct a comprehensive literature review to select the best maturity models and learn how to integrate more than one model. The precision of the selection criteria will help build a robust reliable framework and facilitate integration of different models. In early stages to apply I4.0 principles to requirements engineering, Berre et al. [17] developed the ATHENA project, which is able to fulfill users' requirements in an entire industry. ATHENA's interoperability framework (AIF) coordinates the solutions and methodologies involved in enterprise applications and software systems. It consists of conceptual integration, applicative integration, and technical integration. Conceptual integration deals with concepts, meta-models, languages, and model relationships. Applicative integration is about methodologies, standards, and domain models. Technical integration concerns technical development and information and communication technology (ICT) environments. ATHENA offers a holistic approach to deal with interoperability, heterogeneity, and complexity of developing enterprise applications.

Glazer et al. [18] integrated the agile approach with capability maturity model integration (CMMI) to offer organizations developing Web software the opportunity to build quality systems, while keeping their ability to change flexibly. I4.0 technologies are based on Web software development. Using an agile approach to reach a certain CMMI maturity level in a Web environment will keep the ability of agile methods to quickly respond to changes. The absence of a consistent and detailed agile approach that could help an organization developing Web systems achieve a certain CMMI maturity level is seen as a main gap in today's "state-of-the-art" that requires further research [19].

Based on review of different maturity models in RE, agile, and I4.0, a comparison was done to select the best models from each topic, as shown in Table 1. The general criteria for selection are whether the model was evaluated or not. Unevaluated models cast doubt on their applicability and validity in business environments. Moreover, implemented models provide ready tools to be used in real life, especially if they are used by different companies in terms of scale, focus, and culture. One of the main drawbacks of existing maturity models is that they neither adequately capture domain specific issues and complexities, nor are they built and evaluated based on scientific IS theories. Moreover, while there are many maturity models with broad applications, there is little documentation on how to develop a maturity model that is rigorously tested and widely accepted [15].

Models that can be applied across many domains and that are based on IS theories would seem more credible and reliable. Another common problem with maturity models is that most of them focus on either only the organizational or only the technical aspect of a project or an organization. A more powerful maturity model should assess both aspects of an organization. In addition, the selected maturity model should be scalable to different organizational sizes, cultures, and foci. The measurement tools and processes should be clear and feasible. Finally, the selected maturity models should be applicable to web environments as I4.0 technologies are all web-based.

In Table 1, the criteria were applied to five popular RE models. The model of Sommerville et al. [20] didn't match the criteria as it is not built nor evaluated based on any theory. Moreover, the measurement instrument is complex. The model of Niazi et al. [21] matched the criteria but it didn't built the model as a tool. The models of Beecham et al. [22] and Gorschek et al. [23] weren't implemented. In addition, their models target only the technical side of the RE processes. Beecham model has a main design flaw as there is a weak link between process improvement goals and customer expectations. The model by Kang et al. model [13] has not been implemented nor evaluated.

**Table 1.** Comparison of maturity models.

| Category | Model | Evaluated | Implemented | Based on a theory | Aspects | Problems |
|---|---|---|---|---|---|---|
| RE | [20] | Yes | Yes | No | Org./Tech. | Confusing measurement process |
| | [21] | Yes, case studies | Yes | TAM | Org./Tech. | No calculation tool |
| | [22] | Yes | No | No | Tech. | Only 2 level process maturity |
| | [23] | Yes | No | No | Tech. | Targets project assessment |
| | [13] | No | No | No | Org./Tech. | Need implementation and evaluation |
| Agile | [24] | Yes | Yes | Yes | Org./Tech. | Not feasible for web systems |
| | [25] | Yes | Yes | No | Org./Tech. | Cannot be scaled |
| | [26] | Yes | Yes | Yes | Org./Tech. | Limited evaluation |
| I4.0 | [8] | No | No | No | Org./Tech. | Needs evaluation and implementation |
| | [3] | Yes | Yes | Yes | Org./Tech. | Needs more evaluation |
| | [12] | Yes | Yes | No | Org./Tech. | Targets large organizations with established strategy |
| | [27] | Yes | Yes | Yes | Tech. | For readiness only |

For agile models, the Team model [24] matched the selection criteria but it is not designed to fit web environments which is essential for Industry 4.0 applications. The Sidky et al. model [25] has not been evaluated and cannot be scaled. Despite the fact that the Stojanov et al. [26] model has only limited evaluation, it does match the selection criteria. For I4.0 models, the Leyh et al. model [8] is not evaluated nor implemented. The Schumacher et al. [3] model best fits the selection criteria. The Comuzzi and Patel model [12] is limited in scale to large companies. The Lichtblau et al. model [27] was used only for readiness assessment but the proposed framework should be able to assess the processes before and after applying I4.0.

The three selected maturity models that satisfy our criteria for the best maturity models are shown in Table 2. A maturity model incorporates a set of practices or processes or activities (we use these terms interchangeably) in the form of questions that help define its maturity. The maturity of the processes is assessed according to defined maturity levels [28] (e.g. maturity levels can start from initial to optimized or advanced). These practices are also categorized into certain dimensions or aspects that describe the focus of the maturity model [15].

The I4.0 model selected is the Schumacher et al. [3] model which followed the principles developed by Roblek et al. [1] and Posada et al. [29] of: digitization, optimization, and customization of production; automation and adaptation; human machine interaction (HMI); value-added services and businesses, and automatic data exchange

**Table 2.** Selected maturity models from I4.0, agile and RE.

| Maturity model | Dimensions | Levels | Practices |
|---|---|---|---|
| I4.0 maturity model [3] | 1. Technology<br>2. Governance<br>3. Products<br>4. Customers<br>5. Operations<br>6. Strategy<br>7. Leadership<br>8. Culture<br>9. People | 1. Basic<br>2. Cross-departmental<br>3. Horizontal and vertical<br>4. Full digitization<br>5. Optimized | 62 practices |
| RE maturity measurement framework (REMMF) [21] | 1. Approach<br>2. Deployment<br>3. Results | 1. Initial<br>2. Repeatable<br>3. Defined | 66 practices |
| Scaled agile framework (SAFe) [26] | 1. Team<br>2. Program<br>3. Portfolio | 1. Collaborative<br>2. Evolutionary<br>3. Effective<br>4. Adaptive<br>5. Encompassing | 24 practices |

and communication. These principles were translated into nine dimensions of *products, customers, operations,* and *technology,* (to assess the basic enablers), plus *strategy, leadership, governance, culture,* and *people* (to allow for including organizational aspects into the assessment). The model has been transformed into a practical tool and tested by several companies. The model validation showed its transparency, easiness of use and proved its applicability in real production environments.

The second model selected is developed by Niazi et al. [21] who proposed a new RE maturity measurement framework (REMMF) based on Sommerville's model [20]. REMMF is based on the *technology Acceptance Model* (TAM) theory and offers an effective measure of the maturity of the RE processes. The framework consists of 66 requirements practices, classified as basic, intermediate and advanced for the seven phases of RE which are: requirements documentation, elicitation, analysis, description, system modelling, validation, and management. The framework evaluation only focused on the perceived usefulness and perceived ease of use of REMMF. The instrument used for the evaluation of the framework is Motorola's instrument on three different dimensions.

The third selected model is scaled agile framework (SAFe) [26] for adopting agile and software development. The authors extended the SAMI agile maturity model with practices that are key to scaling agile practices for SAFe. The five principles of SAFe are: embrace change to deliver customer value, plan and deliver software frequently, human centricity, technical excellence, and customer collaboration. The model is developed and refined using a Delphi study to assess the maturity level of the organization in adopting agile.

# 3    Research Methodology – Development of ARE-MMI4.0

We adopted a design science approach to develop our *agile requirement engineering maturity model for Industry 4.0* (ARE-MMI4.0). Following the design science principles of [30], the framework development process passed through three phases: Identifying the problem, designing the artifact, and evaluation of the artifact. To identify the main problems that face enterprises trying to migrate to I4.0, we performed an extensive systematic literature review. The problems we found that our framework tries to address are: the ambiguity regards I4.0, the unawareness of I4.0 benefits and outcomes, and the lack of guidance to assess the required capabilities to migrate to I4.0. In the design phase of the framework, the basic concepts of I4.0 were taken into consideration such as the vertical and horizontal integration of manufacturing systems across the entire value chain. The design of the ARE-MMI4.0 framework followed a thorough development strategy based on the integration and modification of existing RE, agile, and I4.0 maturity models. Those models were selected from a comparison held between different maturity models according to predefined criteria as discussed in the previous section. Several components of those models were combined and modified according to I4.0 requirements.

Guided by [15, 28] and [31] generic models for developing maturity model, we developed our framework. These generic models combined the development process of the *business process maturity model* (BPMM) and *knowledge management capability assessment* (KMCA) and suggest four basic steps of development: *scope, design, populate, and evaluate*. According to these steps, the *scope* of the ARE-MMI4.0 framework is I4.0, and the target audiences are stakeholders, IT, and management of a company. For the *design* step, we selected the method of application to be third party assisted by an I4.0 consultant company. The driver of application to be both internal and external and the application domain to be across single entity/multiple region. In the *populate* step, a company should define its domain components and sub components. The domain components of the framework are: the nine dimensions of the I4.0 model, the eight phases of the RE Model and the five principles of the agile model as shown in Fig. 2. The sub components are the practices of these three models. These components are mutually inclusive and collectively exhaustive. The basic model for the framework is the I4.0 model because it shares four dimensions with the De Bruin et al. [15] model of *strategic alignment, governance, technology, and people*.

To integrate the framework components, we followed the soft systems methodology [32] approach to integrate maturity models which is used extensively to analyze complex situations in their real-world settings. The first phase of integration is the *reflection* phase where we understand the relation between the dimensions of the three maturity models and how assessing a model dimension can assess another model dimension. The second phase is *planning* where we modify and combine the three models' practices, where each practice defines the maturity of one or more dimension of the framework. The third phase is *action and observation* where these practices are modified, tested, and evaluated.

## 4   ARE-MMI4.0 Design

Maturity models are descriptive, prescriptive or comparative [15]. The descriptive model assesses the as-is situation while a prescriptive model indicates how to approach maturity improvement in order to positively affect business value i.e. enable the development of a road-map for improvement. A comparative model compares similar practices across organizations to evaluate the maturity within different industries. ARE-MMI4.0 is a prescriptive model as it assesses the required maturity levels for a company before and after developing a project for I4.0.

The components of the ARE-MMI4.0 framework is shown in Fig. 1. The framework integrates the three selected maturity models from Table 2. The framework is used mainly for readiness assessment which measures whether a company is ready to migrate to I4.0. The base model in the framework is the I4.0 model which defines the minimum maturity level needed before building a project for I4.0. The instrument used for measurement is a set of questions integrated from the practices of the three models and modified to fit the ARE-MMI4.0 purpose. The framework can be evaluated based on *task-technology fit* (TTF) [33] and TAM [34] theories.

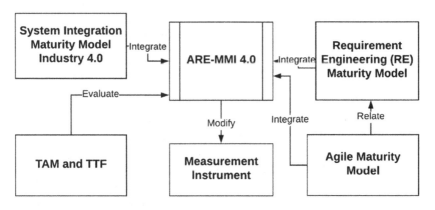

**Fig. 1.** The ARE-MMI4.0 components

Following the steps suggested by Karokola et al. [35] for integrating maturity models, the ARE-MMI4.0 architecture is described in Fig. 2. The readiness assessment is based mainly on the nine dimensions of the I4.0 model. Each of these dimensions is assessed by a set of maturity items with one question per item with a score on a Likert scale from 1 to 5. In addition, each dimension contributes to one or more agile stages and RE phases. The I4.0 model has five maturity levels from basic to optimized as shown in Table 2. The model has a total of 62 maturity practices grouped into nine dimensions and each maturity practice has a *weighting factor* from 1 to 4 depending on its importance. The maturity level of a dimension is the weighted average of its maturity practices. The overall maturity level needed for migration is determined by the average of the maturity levels of the nine dimensions. Each dimension can define some practices in the RE sub-model and agile sub-model.

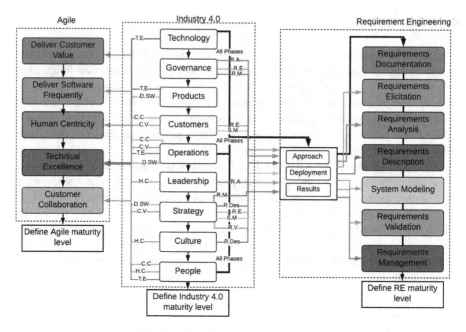

**Fig. 2.** The ARE-MMI4.0 architecture

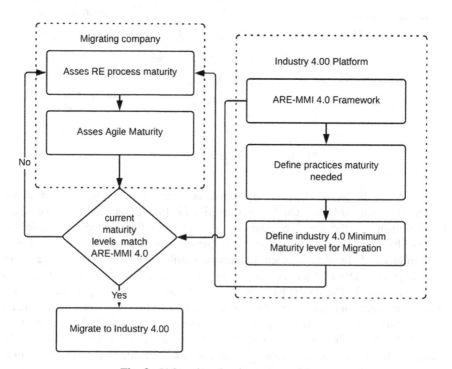

**Fig. 3.** I4.0 project development workflow

The migration process is summarized in Fig. 3. The workflow starts from ARE-MMI4.0 framework. The framework defines the minimum maturity levels required for I4.0, then the estimated maturity of practices for RE and agile are calculated based on maturity level of I4.0 dimensions. From the migrating company side, the current state of RE and agile practices maturity are assessed, then they are compared to the estimated maturity levels of ARE-MMI4.0. If they match, the company is ready for migration. If they don't, they should be enhanced first to meet I4.0 levels.

## 5  Discussion

ARE-MMI4.0 is a prescriptive model that provides assessment for companies to build projects for I4.0. Migration to I4.0 is inevitable for companies to remain competitive in the market. ARE-MMI4.0 integrates three maturity models, one each for RE, agile and I4.0. The I4.0 model is the base model, which has nine dimensions that are needed for building an I4.0 project from the organizational and technical aspects. The assessment of each I4.0 dimension corresponds to defining other dimensions in RE, agile. For example, the technology, operations and people dimensions contribute in defining the maturity of all RE phases as shown in Fig. 2. In other words, each RE or agile practice is partially assessed by the maturity of I4.0 dimensions.

The RE model consists of eight phases and each phase has its practices. These practices are evaluated across three dimensions of approach, deployment and result. The score of each maturity practice is the average of the scores in the three dimensions. The Agile model has five principles and each principle has a set of practices and defined by one or more I4.0 dimensions. For example, the *strategy* dimension defines the *"deliver value to customer"* and *"deliver software frequently"* phases of Agile maturity model. Moreover, this dimension defines five phases of *requirement elicitation, requirement description, system modeling, requirement validation, and requirement management* in the RE maturity model as shown in Fig. 2. In other words, defining a dimension maturity level in I4.0 model, corresponds in defining the maturity of related phases in the other two models. For example, the maturity level of strategy dimension also contributes in defining the maturity of some RE and Agile phases.

### 5.1  Illustrative Example

Company A begins the assessment process by answering the questionnaire to assess the maturity level of the I4.0 nine dimensions needed to build a project for I4.0. It has scored 3 in technology dimension, 2.5 governance, 3 in operation, and 2 in people. These four dimensions contribute in defining the maturity of the *requirements analysis* phase practices in the RE maturity model as shown in Fig. 2. The *requirements analysis* phase consists of five basic practices. The maturity of each practice is represented as a percentage of the maturity of the four dimensions of technology, governance, operation, and people as shown in Table 3. The contribution of each dimension across the *requirements analysis* practices is shown in the radar chart in Fig. 4. The chart shows that the operation dimension is nearly equally distributed along the basic *requirements analysis* practices.

In Table 3, The minimum maturity level needed for each practice is the sum of the four dimensions maturity levels times their contribution percentage, e.g. RA1 minimum maturity level = $(0 * 3) + (.4 * 2.5) + (.4 * 3) + (.2 * 2) = 2.6$. However, when company A tried to assess its current RA1 maturity level it scored 2 which is less than the minimum level required. So, company A needs to enhance the maturity of RA1. In other words, company A has to redefine its system boundaries to meet the minimum level required. The minimum maturity level for the entire *requirements Analysis* phase is the average of its practices. Although the current maturity level of the *requirements Analysis* is higher than the minimum level, RA1 and RA3 needs enhancement because their current maturity levels are less than the minimum level needed.

**Table 3.** Dimensions contribution to requirements analysis practices

| Requirements analysis and negotiation basic practices | | Techno. | Govern. | Operate | People | Min. maturity | Current maturity |
|---|---|---|---|---|---|---|---|
| RA1 | Define system boundaries | 0 | 0.4 | 0.4 | 0.2 | 2.6 | 2 |
| RA2 | Use checklists for requirements analysis | 0.2 | 0 | 0.5 | 0.3 | 2.7 | 3 |
| RA3 | Provide software to support negotiations | 0.6 | 0 | 0.3 | 0.1 | 2.9 | 2.5 |
| RA4 | Plan for conflicts and conflict resolution | 0 | 0.3 | 0.3 | 0.4 | 2.45 | 3.25 |
| RA5 | Prioritize requirements | 0.2 | 0.1 | 0.5 | 0.2 | 2.75 | 3.75 |
| Average | | | | | | 2.68 | 2.9 |

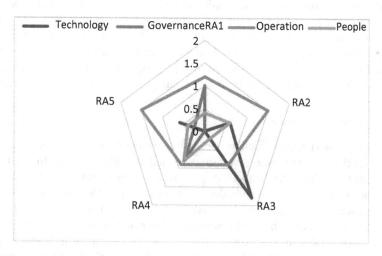

**Fig. 4.** Requirements analysis practices scores across four I4.0 dimensions

# 6  Future Work

The framework presented in this research is considered a first version of ARE-MMI4.0. The framework is currently at phase three *"populate"* according to the general model of De Bruin et al. and at phase *"planning"* in integration steps developed by Checkland et al. The next phases are the *"evaluation"* in developing the framework and the *"action and observation"* in integrating the maturity models. The evaluation phase consists of three stages: test, deploy and maintain. In the test stage, the framework is tested for relevance and rigor through case studies incorporated with surveys and interviews. The steps of the testing stage are as described below.

The **first step** is conducting expert interviews in several companies that already use industry 4.0. These interviews aim to test the validity of process integration e.g. test if the requirements analysis practices are really percentages of the four dimensions shown in Table 3. We may adjust the framework based on the interviews findings if necessary. To avoid threats to external validity, the interviews should be tested in companies with different scale, business focus, culture, business strategies, management styles, and business operations to ensure the generalizability of the model across situations and people.

The **second step** is modifying the measurement instruments of the three maturity models to fit the objectives of the framework. These instruments will be used for two purposes: first to assess the current maturity level of a company, and second to calculate the minimum maturity level needed to build a project for Industry 4.0.

The **third step** is grouping the maturity models' practices into a survey questionnaire and send the surveys to different companies. We plan to select companies that are already migrated to industry 4.0 and companies that need to migrate to Industry 4.0. The companies that use Industry 4.0 already should have current maturity levels greater than or equal to the minimum maturity levels needed. However, the companies that haven't migrated yet would most likely have maturity levels less than the needed levels. This process will test the validity of the measurement instrument for the two purposes. After testing the framework, it should be deployed to companies that target industry 4.0. The deployment will ensure the practicability of the framework in the real world. The deployment process should be applied to small projects to reduce the risks and cost of experimenting with the framework. Later, the framework can be applied to bigger projects to test if it can successfully be applied to different scales. This stage also fulfills the *action and observation* phase requirements.

Finally, the model should be evaluated for user perception and technical excellence using instruments based on TAM and TTF theories. TAM evaluates user satisfaction and ease of use; and TTF evaluates data quality, locatability of data, authorization to access data, data compatibility, production timeliness, and systems reliability. To achieve this target, we are planning to use structural equation modeling (SEM), as it focuses on latent constructs such as ease of use and user satisfaction. SEM would be used to investigate the relationships between TAM, TTF variables and the measurements taken from companies.

# 7 Conclusion

I4.0 is an evolutionary technology that changes business processes and value chains. As more companies migrate their production processes to I4.0, more companies perceive I4.0 as complex and expensive. Therefore, careful assessment of process maturity must be conducted to reduce the application cost and build trust in I4.0. Moreover, the requirements needed for migration must be specified beforehand and the maturity of requirement engineering processes must be also assessed. I4.0 projects are agile in nature, so the assessment of the agility of the migrating company processes is vital. This paper presented a comprehensive framework that help companies migrate to I4.0 with minimum cost and risk by assessing the minimum maturity levels needed for migration and compare them to current maturity levels. The framework integrates existing I4.0, agile, and RE maturity models and uses the maturity levels of the I4.0 model dimensions to specify the minimum required maturity levels for agile, and RE. The main future work is to implement this framework and test it through case studies, interview, and surveys. In addition, we are planning to evaluate the framework based on TTF and TAM theories to test the practicability and usefulness of the framework.

# References

1. Roblek, V., Meško, M., Krapež, A.: A complex view of industry 4.0. SAGE Open **6**, 2158244016653987 (2016)
2. Vogel-Heuser, B., Hess, D.: Guest editorial industry 4.0–prerequisites and visions. IEEE Trans. Autom. Sci. Eng. **13**, 411–413 (2016)
3. Schumacher, A., Erol, S., Sihn, W.: A maturity model for assessing industry 4.0 readiness and maturity of manufacturing enterprises. Proc. CIRP **52**, 161–166 (2016)
4. Thames, L., Schaefer, D.: Software-defined cloud manufacturing for industry 4.0. Proc. CIRP **52**, 12–17 (2016)
5. Schlick, J., Stephan, P., Loskyll, M., Lappe, D.: Industrie 4.0 in der praktischen Anwendung. In: Bauernhansl, T., ten Hompel, M., Vogel-Heuser, B. (eds.) Industrie 4.0 in Produktion, Automatisierung und Logistik, pp. 57–84. Springer, Wiesbaden (2014). https://doi.org/10.1007/978-3-658-04682-8_3
6. Pfeiffer, S.: Robots, industry 4.0 and humans, or why assembly work is more than routine work. Societies **6**, 16 (2016)
7. El Sawy, O.A., Malhotra, A., Park, Y., Pavlou, P.A.: Research commentary—seeking the configurations of digital ecodynamics: it takes three to tango. Inf. Syst. Res. **21**, 835–848 (2010)
8. Leyh, C., Bley, K., Schäffer, T., Bay, L.: The application of the maturity model SIMMI 4.0 in selected enterprises (2017)
9. Lu, Y.: Industry 4.0: a survey on technologies, applications and open research issues. J. Ind. Inf. Integr. **6**, 1–10 (2017)
10. Lukac, D.: The fourth ICT-based industrial revolution "Industry 4.0", HMI and the case of CAE/CAD innovation with EPLAN P8, pp. 835–838 (2015)
11. Scheuermann, C., Verclas, S., Bruegge, B.: Agile factory-an example of an industry 4.0 manufacturing process. In: 2015 IEEE 3rd International Conference on Cyber-Physical Systems, Networks, and Applications (CPSNA), pp. 43–47. IEEE (2015)

12. Comuzzi, M., Patel, A.: How organisations leverage big data: a maturity model. Ind. Manag. Data Syst. **116**, 1468–1492 (2016)
13. Kang, S., et al.: A general maturity model and reference architecture for SaaS service. In: Kitagawa, H., Ishikawa, Y., Li, Q., Watanabe, C. (eds.) DASFAA 2010. LNCS, vol. 5982, pp. 337–346. Springer, Heidelberg (2010). https://doi.org/10.1007/978-3-642-12098-5_28
14. Erol, S., Schumacher, A., Sihn, W.: Strategic guidance towards industry 4.0–a three-stage process model. In: International Conference on Competitive Manufacturing (2016)
15. De Bruin, T., Freeze, R., Kaulkarni, U., Rosemann, M.: Understanding the main phases of developing a maturity assessment model (2005)
16. Bondar, S., Hsu, J.C., Pfouga, A., Stjepandić, J.: Agile digital transformation of system-of-systems architecture models using Zachman framework. J. Ind. Inf. Integr. **7**, 33–43 (2017)
17. Berre, A.J., et al.: The ATHENA interoperability framework. In: Gonçalves, R.J., Müller, J. P., Mertins, K., Zelm, M. (eds.) Enterprise Interoperability II. Springer, London (2007). https://doi.org/10.1007/978-1-84628-858-6_62
18. Glazer, H., Dalton, J., Anderson, D., Konrad, M.D., Shrum, S.: CMMI or agile: why not embrace both! (2008)
19. Torrecilla-Salinas, C., Sedeño, J., Escalona, M., Mejías, M.: Agile, web engineering and capability maturity model integration: a systematic literature review. Inf. Softw. Technol. **71**, 92–107 (2016)
20. Sommerville, I., Ransom, J.: An empirical study of industrial requirements engineering process assessment and improvement. ACM Trans. Softw. Eng. Methodol. (TOSEM) **14**, 85–117 (2005)
21. Niazi, M., Cox, K., Verner, J.: A measurement framework for assessing the maturity of requirements engineering process. Softw. Qual. J. **16**, 213–235 (2008)
22. Beecham, S., Hall, T., Rainer, A.: Software process improvement problems in twelve software companies: an empirical analysis. Empir. Softw. Eng. **8**, 7–42 (2003)
23. Gorschek, T., Svahnberg, M., Tejle, K.: Introduction and application of a lightweight requirements engineering process. In: Ninth International Workshop on Requirements Engineering: Foundation for Software Quality (2003)
24. C.P. Team: CMMI for development, version 1.2 (2006)
25. Sidky, A., Arthur, J., Bohner, S.: A disciplined approach to adopting agile practices: the agile adoption framework. Innovations Syst. Softw. Eng. **3**, 203–216 (2007)
26. Stojanov, I., Turetken, O., Trienekens, J.J.: A maturity model for scaling agile development. In: 2015 41st Euromicro Conference on Software Engineering and Advanced Applications (SEAA), pp. 446–453. IEEE (2015)
27. Lichtblau, K., et al.: Studie: industrie 4.0 readiness (2017)
28. Becker, J., Knackstedt, R., Pöppelbuß, J.: Developing maturity models for IT management. Bus. Inf. Syst. Eng. **1**, 213–222 (2009)
29. Posada, J., et al.: Visual computing as a key enabling technology for industrie 4.0 and industrial internet. IEEE Comput. Graph. Appl. **35**, 26–40 (2015)
30. Hevner, A.R., March, S.T., Park, J., Ram, S.: Design science in information systems research. MIS Q. **28**, 75–105 (2004)
31. Pöppelbuß, J., Röglinger, M.: What makes a useful maturity model? A framework of general design principles for maturity models and its demonstration in business process management. In: ECIS, p. 28 (2011)
32. Checkland, P., Scholes, J.: Soft systems methodology: a 30-year retrospective. Wiley, Chichester (1999)
33. Goodhue, D.L., Thompson, R.L.: Task-technology fit and individual performance. MIS Q. **19**, 213–236 (1995)

34. Davis, F.D., Bagozzi, R.P., Warshaw, P.R.: User acceptance of computer technology: a comparison of two theoretical models. Manag. Sci. **35**, 982–1003 (1989)
35. Karokola, G., Kowalski, S., Yngstrom, L.: Secure e-government services: towards a framework for integrating IT security services into e-government maturity models. In: Information Security South Africa (ISSA), pp. 1–9. IEEE (2011)

# Exploring Determinants of Enterprise System Adoption Success in Light of an Ageing Workforce

Ewa Soja[1]([⊠]) and Piotr Soja[2]

[1] Department of Demography, Cracow University of Economics,
Kraków, Poland
Ewa.Soja@uek.krakow.pl
[2] Department of Computer Science, Cracow University of Economics,
Kraków, Poland
Piotr.Soja@uek.krakow.pl

**Abstract.** The main goal of this exploratory study is to investigate the role of employees' age in the perception of factors having an influence on enterprise systems (ES) adoption process. In doing so, the current study draws from opinions of 75 ES practitioners collected during an exploratory research conducted in Poland. The gathered data was analyzed following the grounded theory approach and incorporating open and axial coding. In consequence, a two-level taxonomy of elements including determinants and determinant categories was worked out. Then, the distribution of respondent opinions among different age groups, i.e. younger, middle-aged, and older, was analyzed. The main findings imply that project schedule and employees' attitudes and involvement are the fundamental determinants emphasized regardless of respondent age. At the same time, older respondents perceived implementation process-related determinants to a greater extent, while the youngest particularly highlighted determinants associated with technology.

**Keywords:** Enterprise systems · Adoption · Determinants
Age-diverse workforce · Ageing · Poland

## 1 Introduction

Population ageing is a global demographic phenomenon and will be aggravating in the future. This, among other things, results in labor force shrinking and ageing [10]. Furthermore, older adults in the workforce are and will be working until later ages [5, 7]. Such a situation calls for an effective management of an age-diverse workforce [30]. In this respect, research in the field of work psychology and organizational behavior indicates that several age-related characteristics have to be considered, such as decrease of cognitive and physical capacities as people age [22], age-related changes in psychological variables affecting organizational outcomes e.g. work attitudes [35], or intergenerational differences in values and attitudes which can contribute to conflict in the workplace [31]. The proposed solutions should aim at accommodating and

© Springer Nature Switzerland AG 2019
M. Themistocleous and P. Rupino da Cunha (Eds.): EMCIS 2018, LNBIP 341, pp. 419–432, 2019.
https://doi.org/10.1007/978-3-030-11395-7_32

leveraging age differences, for instance by considering job design from a lifespan perspective to improve work attitudes such as job satisfaction and involvement [30, 35].

Information and communication technology (ICT) is an integral component of contemporary businesses and its use is obligatory for more and more employees. An example of a widely used technology whose usage is mandatory within organizations are enterprise systems (ES) [12]. ES are very complex systems that support management and integration of the whole company and offer inter-organizational integration with company's clients and suppliers [33]. ES implementation and use involves many stakeholders representing several organizations. Prior research suggests that ES adoption success might be determined by various factors, including considerations related to both technology and employees' involvement [9, 25]. Taking into considerations changes in labor supply and the fact that attitudes toward computers tend to be more negative with age [34], it appears important to investigate to what extent the perceptions of ES adoption determinants depend on employee age. Therefore, we formulated the following research question which guided our exploratory study:

- What is the role of employee age in perceiving determinants of ES adoption successfulness?

The remainder of the paper is organized as follows. In the next section, presenting research background, we focus on implications of workforce ageing and we outline main determinants of ES adoption successfulness reported by prior research. Next we reveal our research approach and present our results. We then discuss our findings and explain implications for practice. The study ends with concluding remarks.

## 2 Background

Ageing of the population is inevitable and will be deepening in the future. According to demographic projections, the share of the population aged 65 and more years in high-income countries will increase, while the percentage of population aged 20–64 representing potential labor force will decrease [5, 10]. At the same time, it is also foreseen that the participation rate of older people (55–64) will increase due to the projected impact of pension reforms and societal trends affecting women participation rates [5]. This means that in the future potential labor force will not only shrink but also gradually age.

The consequences of population ageing will be a particular challenge for companies not only because of the changing age composition of the workforce, but also due to the changes of the working environment related to the growing digitization of the economy [19]. Work and organizational psychology researchers indicate that due to automation of physical work and computerization of cognitive work, the emphasis should not only be put on problems with cognitive and physical capacities of workers as they age [22], but also how their personal preferences or attitudes can change and further develop over time, and how these changes can impact on work in a way that compensates for potential decreases in performance capacity and employability [21, 22]. For example, upward trends in agreeableness across the life span bode well for interpersonal relationships among older adults, who, on average when compared to younger adults, are perceived as being more psychosocially mature and as having greater emotional control [21]. In this context, it is also important to take into account the relationship between the different generations in an organization [22] and possible tensions arising among generations, stemming from perceptions of generational differences in values and behaviors [31] and perceptions of technological advances [8].

Prior research shows that as age increases, attitudes toward computers tend to be more negative [34] and technology anxiety increases [16]. As ICT-based solutions are widely used by today's businesses, therefore, in light of an ageing workforce, implementation of advanced ICT solutions might present a challenge to adopting organizations. This especially refers to the process of ES adoption in an organization, which is complex, risky, and associated with numerous considerations. Complexity and riskiness of ES adoption call for an investigation of factors that affect the successful implementation of such systems, i.e. determinants of ES adoption [4]. In other words, determinants capture various organizational, human, and managerial considerations that are associated with ES project successfulness, which plays the role of a dependent variable in this relationship [2, 18].

Extant research on determinants of ES adoption suggests a variety of influential factors. In particular, Holsapple et al. [11] emphasize the importance of so called fitness factors (i.e. compatibility and task relevance) and the critical role of user education. In a similar vein, Lech [14] advocated that determinants of ES success may include personnel skills and attitudes, and also suggested the critical importance of top management support and sound project management. Pan and Jang [18] illustrated the significance of technology readiness, company size, perceived barriers, and production and operations improvement for the adoption of ES. In general, prior research suggest that determinants of ES adoption may comprise a great many various issues associated with adoption process, people involved in this process, and employed technology [27].

The introduction of an enterprise system into the organization provides new conditions with a multitude of impacts. In particular, ES influences the behaviors of people, which in turn changes how systems are used, or not used in the case of user resistance and workarounds. Therefore, communication, change management, education, and user involvement are critical for the successful use of the ES, and to successfully guide ES adaptation and evolution in later phases [9]. Based on research into critical success factors of ES adoption, these determinants can be supplemented by a number of influential factors, such as top management commitment and support, training and job redesign, project team composition, consultant selection and relationship, and project champion [6].

ICT-related complexity of ES, multifaceted considerations of ES adoption process, and many stakeholders involved in such projects suggest a vital need to examine ES projects from the perspective of multiple stakeholders. In particular, in light of an ageing workforce it appears necessary to investigate ES adoption determinants from an employee age standpoint. Exploring age-related differences in the perception of ES adoption determinants should allow us to understand how to better use employees' potential. This, in turn, might yield some implications for ES practitioners related to, for instance, better cooperation within age-balanced project teams and adaptation of implementation process to an ageing workforce.

## 3  Method

In order to answer our research question, we employed a qualitative research approach and we turned to practitioners to learn what are their views concerning determinants of successful ES implementation projects. To obtain data on determinants, the respondents were asked an open-ended question related to their perception of the most important issues having an influence on ES implementation project successfulness. The respondents were asked to provide opinions on the basis of their prior experience and participation in ES implementation projects. Such a data-driven approach was believed to help in gathering a broad range of respondent opinions allowing us to perform an in-depth investigation of the phenomenon in question.

As a result of data gathering process, respondent opinions expressed in natural language have been collected. We then performed the process of open and axial coding, following the grounded theory approach [3]. In the first step, during the process of open coding, we analyzed and compared the respondent opinions in search of similarities and differences. In consequence, the respondent statements were given conceptual labels and preliminary categories and subcategories were created. Next, the process of axial coding was performed, during which the relationships between the previously defined categories and subcategories were tested against data and verified. As a result, the categorization of the reported determinants was worked out and agreed upon by the authors.

In the next step of the data analysis process, the distribution of determinants and determinant categories across different respondent age ranges has been elaborated. Such an examination was performed in order to investigate the role of employee age in perceiving determinants of successful ES adoption. While defining the age groups, we adopted chronological age, which is one of the work-based age measures based on Sterns and Doverspike's five conceptualizations of age: chronological, functional, psychosocial, organizational, and lifespan [1, 28]. The chronological age is determined by the calendar and is linked with predictable changes across a number of domains that involve health, work, family, and life changes; however, it is only a general marker of becoming "older" [1].

While no generally accepted cut-off exists, for practical purposes, most organizations define "older workers" as those individuals either 40, 45, or 50 years and older [13]. We decided to choose the age cutoff of 50 years because most organization decision markers in Poland refer to older workers as 50 years and older [24, 29]. A similar definition of older employee was adopted by van Dalen et al. [32] in their investigation into potential of ageing workers. Van Dalen et al. also defined younger workers as those not older than 35 years. In consequence, the following age groups were defined: Age1 – less than 35 years (Younger), Age2 – between 35 and 49 years (Middle-aged), and Age3 – 50+ years (Older).

In total, 75 respondents expressed their opinions as regards perceived determinants of successful ES adoption. During data gathering we made an attempt to reach a broad range of respondents holding various organizational positions and different roles played in the ES adoption projects. We also made an effort to achieve a proper representation of the defined age groups. The distribution of respondents by age groups and their organizational age, i.e. the length of career stage in the current workplace, is presented in Table 1. The table also displays the distribution of respondents by their role in the implementation process and organizational position.

**Table 1.** Sample demographics

|  | Overall | Younger | Middle-aged | Older |
|---|---|---|---|---|
| *Median age* | | | | |
| Chronological age | 40 | 31 | 40 | 55 |
| Organizational age* | 8 | 4 | 10 | 19 |
| *Organizational position* | | | | |
| Specialist | 26 | 10 | 8 | 8 |
| Manager | 24 | 10 | 7 | 7 |
| Director | 15 | 3 | 6 | 6 |
| Top management | 10 | 2 | 4 | 4 |
| *Role in the implementation process* | | | | |
| Member of the project team | 20 | 7 | 7 | 6 |
| None | 15 | 5 | 4 | 6 |
| Supervisor/steering committee | 13 | 4 | 5 | 4 |
| Project manager | 12 | 4 | 4 | 4 |
| Provider's representative/consultant | 9 | 3 | 3 | 3 |
| User | 6 | 2 | 2 | 2 |

Note: *length of career stage in the current workplace

# 4 Results

On the basis of empirical data analysis, three main categories of determinants were extracted. They include factors associated with people involved in (or affected by) the implementation project (category "People"), elements related to implementation process (category "Process"), and reported determinants associated with technology-related issues concerning the system and the adopting organization (category "Technology"). The resulting categorization of determinants into People-Process-Technology framework is consistent with prior research in various fields, such as ES adoption research (e.g. [23]) and product development and operations management [17]. The categories of determinants and individual determinants indicated by the respondents are described in the following subsections.

## 4.1 Category "People"

The category "People" is the most popular category in respondent opinions. It includes determinants associated with different stakeholders holding various organizational positions and responsibilities within a company, such as employees, management personnel, and members of the implementation team. The related determinants refer first and foremost to employees' positive attitudes towards the ES adoption project such as commitment, determination to succeed, and acceptance. Next, the respondents emphasized the crucial role of company's top management, whose members should be determined to implement the system, ought to support the adoption project, and should be involved in the project. Then, the respondents highlighted the importance of the composition of the project team, who should consist of carefully selected people possessing relevant experience and knowledge.

The next determinant refers to the role of management personnel, who should be involved in the adoption process, ought to reveal positive attitudes towards the project, and should exert pressure on employees to complete the project successfully. The respondents also emphasized the role of the project team performance, highlighting the importance of efficient teamwork and project team members' commitment and cooperation. The next determinant refers to the role of project manager, who should be experienced in ES implementation and should know the adopted system. The last determinant within the category "People" refers to employees' skills related to their professional qualifications and experience gained in previous implementation projects.

## 4.2   Category "Process"

The category "Process" is the second most popular category in respondent opinions; however, it contains the greatest number of individual determinants. The process-related determinants refer first and foremost to project definition, which should include a carefully planned implementation strategy and project schedule allocating adequate time for the adoption process. The second most important process-related determinant refers to project management, which should put emphasis on documentation of project tasks, cost control, timeliness, problem solving, and motivating project participants. The next important determinants refer to the system and implementation services provider and project preparation. The provider-related issues include commitment and competence of provider's consultants, and also good cooperation between the provider and adopter companies. The project preparation-related issues mainly boil down to conducting a pre-implementation analysis and a careful selection of implementation partner and the new enterprise system solution.

The next determinant refers to cooperation during the ES adoption project, which should involve various stakeholders. In particular, good cooperation is needed between the company's departments and between employees and the project team. The respondents also highlighted the importance of communication, which should be established within the project team and also between the project team and the company's management and employees. The next determinant highlights the importance of visible benefits from the system adoption occurring relatively soon and being noticed by employees, such as the improvement of work conditions and effectiveness. Next, the respondents emphasize the importance of company's condition, which refers to the questions if the company is well organized and has a development strategy. The last but one process-related determinant refers to trainings and highlights the importance of adequate trainings during the ES project and their role in convincing employees of the system usefulness. Finally, the last determinant emphasizes the importance of business process reengineering performed during the ES project.

### 4.3 Category "Technology"

The category "Technology" includes just two determinants: system and fit. The former refers to the enterprise system quality and highlights its reliability, user friendliness, and possibility to extend its functionality. The latter, in turn, is associated with the idea of fit between the system functionality and company requirements. In this respect, the respondents highlight the necessity of adjusting the enterprise system to the company needs.

## 5 Data Analysis and Discussion

### 5.1 Perceptions of Determinants by Age

The results of data analysis from the employee age perspective are presented in Table 2. The table shows the distribution of reported determinants across the three age groups. While presenting the data we used the symbols ●, ◓, ◑, and ◔ for high, medium, low, and very low importance of perceived determinants. The levels of importance were defined on the basis of the percentage of responses provided by the respondents from an individual age group declaring a given determinant.

Taking into consideration the respondents' age, we can notice that the older and middle-aged respondents attach the greatest importance to the category Process, and then, to a smaller extent, to the category People. The younger respondents emphasize the importance of both abovementioned categories; however, they also highlight technology-related issues as possible determinants of ES adoption success. In addition, it should be noted that only the oldest respondents indicated all determinants with the category People, the middle-aged practitioners declared all elements within the Process category, and the youngest indicated all determinants within the category Technology.

Taking into consideration the category People, we may notice that the older respondents first and foremost emphasize the importance of the attitudes of employees, management personnel, and top management. Other factors important to the older respondents include knowledge and skills possessed by the implementation team members and company employees. The middle-aged respondents emphasize to the greatest extent the project team members' involvement and performance. However, they do not indicate the importance of knowledge and experience gained by the project team members. The younger respondents, in turn, seem to value experience, knowledge, and involvement of the project team members to the greatest extent. They also perceive employees' attitudes as a strong determinant of ES success.

Summing up, all respondents, regardless of age, strongly emphasize the importance of involvement; however, the oldest perceive its meaning in the broadest context, pointing out at employees, management personnel, and project team. The middle-aged emphasize the project team members' skills resulting in the team operation, while the project team experience appears the most important for the youngest respondents.

**Table 2.** Determinants of ES adoption by age

| Determinant\Age group | Younger | Middle-aged | Older |
|---|---|---|---|
| *People* | | | |
| Employees' attitudes | ◑ | ◒ | ● |
| Top management support | ◑ | ◑ | ◐ |
| Project team composition | ● | | ◑ |
| Management personnel | ◓ | ◑ | ◐ |
| Project team performance | ◓ | ◐ | ◓ |
| Project manager | | ◓ | ◓ |
| Employee skills | ◓ | | ◓ |
| *Process* | | | |
| Project definition | ◑ | ◐ | ◐ |
| Project management | ◑ | ◑ | ◐ |
| Provider | ◐ | ◓ | ◐ |
| Preparation | ◓ | ◑ | ◑ |
| Cooperation | ◑ | ◑ | ◓ |
| Communication | ◓ | ◑ | ◓ |
| Visible benefits | | ◓ | ◑ |
| Company condition | | ◑ | ◓ |
| Trainings | | ◓ | ◑ |
| Business process change | ◓ | ◓ | |
| *Technology* | | | |
| System | ◑ | | ◓ |
| Fit | ◑ | ◓ | |

Note: ● – very high, ◐ – high, ◑ – medium, ◓ – low level of importance

Among the six most important determinants from the category Process (indicated by all respondent groups), the perception of three elements appear to grow with respondent age. They are: project definition, project management, and preparation. For these determinants, interestingly, individual aspects describing the factors (except for the issue "schedule" describing the determinant "project definition") were indicated by respondents from only a single age group.

In the case of project definition, the oldest perceived to the greatest extent the importance of project schedule and, to a lesser extent, stressed the significance of project documentation, financing, and project scope. The middle-aged respondents equally to the importance of project schedule stressed the significance of the roll-out strategy. The youngest respondents, in turn, apart from emphasizing the importance of project schedule, to a lesser extent highlighted the significance of goal definition. In the case of project management, the most important aspects include the necessity of control (indicated by the oldest), documentation-related issues (reported by the middle-aged), and working according to schedule (appreciated by the youngest respondents). In the case of project preparation, the oldest focused mainly on the problem of system choice, the middle-aged concentrated on the provider choice, and the youngest emphasize the pre-implementation analysis.

Among the three remaining determinants within the category Process reported by all respondent groups, provider was perceived to the greatest extent by the youngest and oldest respondents, while good communication was highlighted to the smallest degree by these groups. At the same time, their perception of cooperation decreased with age. In the case of the three determinants being discussed, the middle-aged respondents highlighted the importance of the external cooperation and cooperation with provider, the oldest highlighted the significance of provider's involvement and support, while the youngest reported the importance of internal cooperation and the significance of provider's involvement and competence.

In addition, there are three determinants within the category Process not perceived by the youngest respondents but reported by the two remaining groups of respondents. For such determinants, those associated with trainings and visible benefits appeared important to the oldest respondents, while the middle-aged appreciated the impact of company condition, emphasizing the role of company strategy.

Determinants system and fit, making up the Technology category, were perceived as important by the youngest respondents. In general, the oldest and middle-aged respondents perceived the category Technology to a limited extent, paying attention to single determinants within this category, i.e. system in the case of the oldest, fit in the case of the middle-aged respondents.

## 5.2   Implications

The results of the current study suggest a number of implications for ES adoption projects improvements in light of an ageing workforce. They are associated with team building, cooperation and involvement, project schedule, project management, and change management.

Our findings suggest that in order to better use the employees' potential during the ES adoption project it is beneficial to establish an age-balanced project team. The results, illustrating that the middle aged and older respondents attach special importance to the implementation process, imply that employees at middle and older age can be especially helpful during the ES adoption process. This can be explained by their greater accumulated experience and knowledge about the company and cognitive changes associated with a so called crystallized intelligence. Crystallized intelligence is the ability to use the skills, knowledge, and experience that one has accumulated over one's life. It increases until older ages during one's forties; further, age-related declines begin to occur in our 60s, according to longitudinal research [1, 7]. It appears that older employees' potential might be used to a greater extent if they are being assigned tasks where they can apply their accumulated skills, do challenging work, and have some degree of autonomy [30]. Therefore, it might be suggested that with age the positions being held by the employees should evolve towards supervisory or managerial posts.

As new technologies are an integral part of ES adoption, the project team should also include younger employees, as they possess greater experience and knowledge of ICT. This is related to the fact that the younger, as "digital natives", represent the first generations to grow up with this new technology [20]. Our investigation also illustrated this relationship as the youngest respondents emphasized the technology-related determinants to the greatest extent, pointing out considerations associated with both the system and its fit. Additionally, younger employees possess better cognitive abilities associated with fluid intelligence (which reflects working memory capacity, processing speed, and episodic memory), which is considered to be somewhat independent from knowledge and education [1]. To the extent that these cognitive processes decline with age, tasks that require e.g. higher levels of information-processing may be more difficult for older workers to perform compared with younger workers [7].

Age-related diversity of the project team is associated with cooperation between people at different age. In the case of the youngest employees, it appears that their involvement will be growing when they have an opportunity to perform many diverse tasks. This is related to the fact that task variety provides them the opportunity to accumulate the job skills that they need to advance in their careers. On the other hand, the involvement of middle-aged and older employees will be growing if they are able to use their experience in mentoring [30, 35]. The role of the middle-aged employees appears especially important due to possible occurrences of tensions among older and younger generations. In this context, Urick et al. [31] emphasize the need for a person who would manage such situation successfully for better cooperation, motivation and key task results. The middle-aged employees might fit for such a role as they strongly emphasized the importance of good communication and cooperation during the ES adoption process.

Our results suggest that special attention should be paid to the project schedule, which ought to be aligned with the company's workforce age structure and its diversity. In general, in the case of an older workforce, the amount of time needed to complete implementation tasks becomes especially important. Haste or too restricted time might have a negative impact on the quality of tasks completed by the older employees. In this respect, prior research indicates that when the older employees perform activities which require knowledge-based judgments, they should not be under time pressure [15]. Taking into consideration younger employees, it appears beneficial to assign them a wide range of different tasks in the project schedule. Such a job design can improve their work satisfaction and involvement [30, 35]. Our findings correspond to this proposition, revealing that working according to schedule is the most important aspect of project management for the youngest respondents.

While defining the project schedule, it appears beneficial to plan regular meetings designed for monitoring of the project run, current problem solving and fostering cooperation. In the case of an older age composition of the project team, it appears important to plan important meetings in the morning, which is the most beneficial solution for older employees due to cognitive task performance [21].

Our findings suggest that in the case of a company with an older workforce, ensuring a strong support and involvement of top management and management personnel appears especially important. It is also essential to ensure an effective project management and the presence of strong and determined project manager. Such suggestions can be drawn from the respondent opinions, illustrating that with age employees' expectations of people managing the company and project are growing.

The results imply that the importance of change management is growing with employee age. In the context of ES implementation, our results suggest that with age employees might be less and less open to communication and cooperation. In addition, older respondents did not appear to perceive the need for company reorganization.

In this context, drawing from our findings, we might suggest two main instruments helping older employees to go through the process of changes. These are: alignment of training time with the workforce age structure and managing the project in such a way that partial benefits from ES adoption appear as early as possible. While aligning the training schedule with older employees, as mentioned earlier, it is beneficial to schedule the trainings in the morning and allocate sufficient time for training sessions. It also appears that older employees can be encouraged to cooperate when their potential is acknowledged by creating an environment where they may be helpful in mentoring younger team members and sharing insights gained from years of work experience.

### 5.3   Limitations and Future Research

The main limitation of the current analysis stems from its exploratory character and the fact that the study was based on the data gathered in one country, i.e. Poland. Prior research suggests that Poland, being a transition economy, may experience different ICT-related considerations than well-developed economies [26]. Therefore, the application of the current study's findings to more developed economic settings should be done with caution. Nevertheless, as similar changes in workforce structure are taking place in other European Union countries [5], the current study's findings might be applied, to a certain extent, to other countries within the EU.

The current study's limitations suggest that one of the interesting avenues of future research might be a cross-country research aiming at an in-depth comparison of age-related considerations between transition and well-developed economies. In particular, an interesting research issue is related to the investigation into the proposed solutions considering job design for older worker such as autonomy [30] in a transition economy setting. In this respect, a specific question arises if older workers, pointing out the important role of management personnel, reveal their need for autonomy, or rather if such a perception results from considerations typical of transition economy, such as low level of trust in relationships. The latter seems to be partially supported by our findings, i.e. the older respondents' strong emphasis put on determinants related to control in project management.

## 6   Conclusion

The current study examined the role of employee age in the perception of factors having an influence on enterprise system (ES) implementation success and built on the experience of ES practitioners from Poland. Using a data-driven approach, the discovered determinants were divided into three main categories: People, Process, and Technology. In order to analyze the role of respondent age in determinant perception, we identified the following age groups: younger, middle-aged, and older. The analysis of determinant distribution by respondent age allowed us to conclude that the respondents regardless of age emphasized the importance of employees' attitudes, involvement, and project schedule. The results also suggest that older employees perceived process-related determinants to a greater extent, while the youngest highlighted determinants associated with technology to a large extent. Our findings suggest that one of the most important determinants, employees' involvement, might be fostered by an appropriate job design. In the case of older employees, this is related to assignments requiring accumulated experience (e.g. mentoring), while younger workers should benefit from allocation of many diverse tasks. Such propositions should be incorporated into the project schedule, taking care of an extended time allocated for activities assigned to older workers. The results achieved might help practitioners in fostering use of employees' potential and working out change management programs adapted to the age-diverse workforce in the organization.

**Acknowledgments.** This research has been financed by the funds granted to the Faculty of Management, Cracow University of Economics, Poland, within the subsidy for maintaining research potential.

# References

1. Cleveland, J.N., Hanscom, M.: What is old at work? Moving past chronological age. In: Parry, E., McCarthy, J. (eds.) The Palgrave Handbook of Age Diversity and Work, pp. 17–46. Palgrave Macmillan UK, London (2017)
2. Cohen, J.F.: Contextual determinants and performance implications of information systems strategy planning within South African firms. Inf. Manag. **45**, 547–555 (2008)
3. Corbin, J., Strauss, A.: Grounded theory research procedures, canons, and evaluative criteria. Qual. Sociol. **13**(1), 3–21 (1990)
4. DeLone, W.H.: Determinants of success for computer usage in small business. MIS Q. **12**, 51–61 (1988)
5. European Commission: The 2015 Ageing Report. Economic and budgetary projections for the 28 EU Member States (2013–2060). European Economy 3 (2015)
6. Finney, S., Corbett, M.: ERP implementation: a compilation and analysis of critical success factors. Bus. Process Manag. J. **13**(3), 329–347 (2007)
7. Fisher, G.G., Chaffee, D.S., Tetrick, L.E., Davalos, D.B., Potter, G.G.: Cognitive functioning, aging, and work: a review and recommendations for research and practice. J. Occup. Health Psychol. **22**(3), 314–339 (2017)
8. Foster, K.: Generation and discourse in working life stories. Br. J. Sociol. **64**, 195–215 (2013)
9. Grabski, S.V., Leech, S.A., Schmidt, P.J.: A review of ERP research: a future agenda for accounting information systems. J. Inf. Syst. **25**(1), 37–78 (2011)
10. Harper, S.: Economic and social implications of aging societies. Science **346**(6209), 587–591 (2014)
11. Holsapple, C.W., Wang, Y.-M., Wu, J.-H.: Empirically testing user characteristics and fitness factors in enterprise resource planning success. Int. J. Hum. Comput. Interact. **19**(3), 323–342 (2005)
12. Keong, M.L., Ramayah, T., Kurnia, S., Chiun, L.M.: Explaining intention to use an enterprise resource planning (ERP) system: an extension of the UTAUT model. Bus. Strat. Ser. **13**(4), 173–180 (2012)
13. Kooij, D.T.A.M., DeLange, A.H., Jansen, P.G.W., Dikkers, J.S.E.: Older workers' motivation to continue to work: five meanings of age. J. Manag. Psychol. **23**(4), 364–394 (2008)

14. Lech, P.: Time, budget, and functionality?—IT project success criteria revised. Inf. Syst. Manag. **30**(3), 263–275 (2013)
15. Maertens, J.A., Putter, S.E., Chen, P.Y., Diehl, M., Huang, Y.-H.: Physical capabilities and occupational health of older workers. In: Hedge, J.W., Borman, W.C. (eds.) The Oxford Handbook of Work and Aging, pp. 215–235. Oxford Library of Psychology, Oxford (2012)
16. Meuter, M.L., Ostrom, A., Bitner, M.J., Roundtree, R.: The influence of technology anxiety on consumer use and experiences with self service technologies. J. Bus. Res. **56**, 899–906 (2003)
17. Morgan, J.M., Liker, J.K.: The Toyota Product Development System: Integrating People, Process and Technology. Productivity Press, New York (2006)
18. Pan, M.-J., Jang, W.-Y.: Determinants of the adoption of ERP within the technology–organization–environment framework: Taiwan's communications industry. J. Comput. Inf. Syst. **48**, 94–102 (2008)
19. Parry, E., Strohmeier, S.: HRM in the digital age – digital changes and challenges of the HR profession. Empl. Relat. **36**(4) (2014)
20. Prensky, M.: Digital natives, digital immigrants part 1. Horizon **9**(5), 1–6 (2001)
21. Rizzuto, T.E., Cherry, K.E., LeDoux, J.A.: The aging process and cognitive capabilities. In: Hedge, J.W., Borman, W.C. (eds.) The Oxford Handbook of Work and Aging, pp. 236–255. Oxford Library of Psychology, Oxford (2012)
22. Schalk, R., et al.: Moving European research on work and ageing forward: overview and agenda. Eur. J. Work Organ. Psychol. **19**(1), 76–101 (2010)
23. Soja, E., Soja, P.: Exploring root problems in enterprise system adoption from an employee age perspective: a people-process-technology framework. Inf. Syst. Manag. **34**(4), 333–346 (2017)
24. Soja, E., Stonawski, M.: Zmiany demograficzne a starsi pracownicy w Polsce z perspektywy podmiotów gospodarczych. In: Kurkiewicz, J. (ed.) Demograficzne uwarunkowania i wybrane społeczno-ekonomiczne konsekwencje starzenia się ludności w krajach europejskich, pp. 173–210. Wydawnictwo Uniwersytetu Ekonomicznego w Krakowie, Kraków (2012)
25. Soja, P.: Reexamining critical success factors for enterprise system adoption in transition economies: learning from polish adopters. Inf. Technol. Dev. **22**(2), 279–305 (2016)
26. Soja, P., Cunha, P.R.: ICT in transition economies: narrowing the research gap to developed countries. Inf. Technol. Dev. **21**(3), 323–329 (2015)
27. Soja, P., Themistocleous, M., Cunha, P.R., Silva, M.M.: Determinants of enterprise system adoption across the system lifecycle: exploring the role of economic development. Inf. Syst. Manag. **32**(4), 341–363 (2015)
28. Sterns, H.L., Doverspike, D.: Aging and the retraining and learning process in organizations. In: Goldstein, I., Katzel, R. (eds.) Training and Development in Work Organizations, pp. 229–332. Jossey Bass, San Francisco (1989)
29. Stypińska, J.: Starszy pracownik na rynku pracy w Polsce: 40+? 50+? Czy tylko "plus"? Stud. Socjologiczne **217**(2), 143–165 (2015)
30. Truxillo, D.M., Cadiz, D.M., Rineeret, J.R.: The aging workforce: implications for human resource management research and practice. In: Hitt, M.A., Jackson, S.E., Carmona, S., Bierman, L., Shalley, C.E., Wright, D.M. (eds.) The Oxford Handbook of Strategy Implementation, pp. 179–237. Oxford University Press, Oxford (2014)
31. Urick, M.J., Hollensbe, E.C., Masterson, S.S., Lyons, S.T.: Understanding and managing intergenerational conflict: an examination of influences and strategies. Work Aging Retire. **3**(2), 166–185 (2016)
32. Van Dalen, H.P., Henkens, K., Schippers, J.: Productivity of older workers: perceptions of employers and employees. Popul. Dev. Rev. **36**(3), 309–330 (2010)

33. Volkoff, O., Strong, D.M., Elmes, M.: Understanding enterprise systems-enabled integration. Eur. J. Inf. Syst. **14**, 110–120 (2005)
34. Wagner, N., Hassanein, K., Head, M.: Computer use by older adults: a multi-disciplinary review. Comput. Hum. Behav. **26**, 870–882 (2010)
35. Wille, B., Hofmans, J., Feys, M., De Fruyt, F.: Maturation of work attitudes: correlated change with big five personality traits and reciprocal effects over 15 years. J. Organ. Behav. **35**(4), 507–529 (2014)

# Limiting the Impact of Statistics as a Proverbial Source of Falsehood

Yiannis Kiouvrekis[1,3], Petros Stefaneas[1], Angelika Kokkinaki[2(✉)],
and Nikos Asimakis[1]

[1] Department of Mathematics, National Technical University of Athens,
Herron Polytechniou 9, 15780 Zografou, Greece
yiannisq@central.ntua.gr, petros@math.ntua.gr
[2] Department of Management and MIS, University of Nicosia, Nicosia, Cyprus
kokkinaki.a@unic.ac.cy
[3] Medical Informatics and Physics Lab, University of Thessaly,
41110 Larissa, Greece

**Abstract.** This paper presents an early version of a decision-making "eco" system. We refer to it as an "eco" system because it is primarily based on mathematical logic and combines concepts and principles from the fields of statistics, decision theory, artificial intelligence and modeling of human behavior. The primary goal of the proposed approach is to address errors that occur resulting from the misuse of statistical methods. In practice, such errors often occur either owning to the use of inappropriate statistical methods or wrong interpretations of results. The proposed approach relies on the LPwNF (Logic Programming without Negation as Failure) framework of non-monotonic reasoning as provided by Gorgias. The proposed system enables automatic selection of the appropriate statistical method, based on the characteristics of the problem and the sample. The expected impact could be twofold: it can enhance the use of statistical systems like R and, combined with a Java-based interface to Gorgias, make non-monotonic reasoning easy to use in the proposed context.

**Keywords:** Gorgias · Decision theory · Mathematical logic · Information
AI · Health care

## 1 Introduction

In this paper we propose an information system that uses argumentation logic, specifically the LPwNF framework provided by Gorgias [8, 9, 12, 14], to augment and enhance use of statistical methods. The information system supports automatic selection of the proper method, based on the problem at hand, features of the statistical sample and the applicability of the statistical method according to previously defined parameters. The proposed approach aims to limit errors related to statistics applicability by users who often lack knowledge and/or skills in this domain. Some of the errors include conceptual misrepresentations, inappropriate use of statistical analytics software, or faults in the interpretation of results [1–7].

© Springer Nature Switzerland AG 2019
M. Themistocleous and P. Rupino da Cunha (Eds.): EMCIS 2018, LNBIP 341, pp. 433–442, 2019.
https://doi.org/10.1007/978-3-030-11395-7_33

The main advantage of the proposed system is derived by the proof procedure employed by Gorgias; more specifically, to explain the answer in relation to logical rules employed and to provide data that lead to a more appropriate answer. In this way, the proposed system provides correct answers and over a period of repetitive use the system trains the user with regards to proper use of statistical methods.

Furthermore within the proposed system, it is still possible to express the logical rules that define its behavior in alignment with the relevant mathematical theorems of statistical analysis, which leads towards the verification of employed rules. This is possible because one can trace the logical rules that drive the program and interpret the result through Gorgias' functionality [11, 17]. Within this framework, a fully developed system could be used to provide verifiable answers in a similar manner like a mathematician would do. The system could be used in many different domains and provide valuable support to a large user base. To demonstrate its potential, we are going to examine common errors in applied statistics and statistical software and explain how LPwNF framework provided by Gorgias can limit occurrence of such errors. A special purpose interface has been developed in Java to integrate Gorgias, which is based on SWI-Prolog and the system R so that the full benefits of argumentation logic in statistical analysis may be outlined.

## 2  Problem Recognition and Specification

Mathematicians have developed numerous theories about human behavior modeling, including but not limited to gaming theory, mathematical logic, artificial intelligence and predictive behavior.

The existence of such numerous attempts may be explained by the fact that although constructed theories are consistent, still aspects of human behavior remain elusive. An enlightening example comes from gaming theory. Assume that we play a game. We have to write a number from 0 to 100 on a piece of paper. The winner will be the person who writes the number that is equal to half the maximum number that all the players write. For example, if there are five players and they write the numbers 20, 30, 32, 40, and 60, the winner would be the player who wrote the number 30. In theory, if all players behave rationally, then each should write 0 on the paper, since 0 is the Nash equilibrium of this game. But as research [16] has shown, this is rarely the case.

It has been documented in the literature [1, 6, 7] that proper methodology in statistical analysis has not been always followed and various errors occur in all levels of the research process. Errors appear in the initial stages, such as during the literature review in order to specify the basic research questions. Errors related to p-values, statistical tests, usage of statistical symbols as well as failure to summarize the data and demonstrate the findings mathematically, [4, 7] all occur frequently during the important statistical/mathematical stages. Such errors highlight the need for developing system that supports all aspects of the research process. The system ought to support researchers through the entire data analysis process by guiding them through the necessary thorough apprehension of statistics without necessarily being an expert in the field.

# 3  System Design

## 3.1  Logic

In logical systems, such as propositional logic and first order logic, if a theory contains a contradiction, it is then inconsistent. Furthermore, in the standard logical systems, the proof system is monotonic, i.e. if, in the linear path of a proof, types $\varphi$, $\neg\varphi$ occurs, then the theory is inconsistent. We can overcome this by using non-monotonic logic, which manages in a completely different way the simultaneous presence of a proposition and its negation.

We use a system like Logic Programming without Negation as Failure (LPwNF) [9]. In the context of logical programming without negation as failure (LPwNF), logical programs are non-monotonous theories where each program is treated as a collection of propositions from which we must choose an appropriate subset, called an "extension". Propositions in a logical program are written in an ordinary logical language, although standard negation is used but not refusal as a failure.

*Example 1* [9]. Consider the follow program - set of rules:

$$\texttt{bird}(x) \rightarrow \texttt{fly}(x) \tag{1}$$

$$\texttt{penguin}(x) \rightarrow \neg\texttt{fly}(x) \tag{2}$$

$$\texttt{penguin}(x) \rightarrow \texttt{bird}(x) \tag{3}$$

$$\texttt{bird}(Tweety) \tag{4}$$

From this set of rules we can conclude $\texttt{fly}(Tweety)$ because we can extract it from the first rule and there is no way to extract $\neg\texttt{fly}(Tweety)$.

If we add $\texttt{penguin}(Tweety)$ as a statement then we can derive $\texttt{fly}(Tweety)$ and $\neg\texttt{fly}(Tweety)$ from the rules of the program. This example may seem basic, but it is fundamentally important to our work. In essence, we described mathematically what everyone understands: although birds usually fly, penguins, which are also birds, do not fly. Such reasoning is not invalid, because we are used to the exceptions to the rules, but when we go about modelling it with in a rigid monotonic logical system, we will face a problem.

We can assume that the non-expert can understand that the previous system of rules-propositions allows for contradiction, and it thus constitutes an inconsistent set of propositions, in the framework of standard logical systems. This could lead to confusion if one does not take into account that the logical system is non-monotonic. In this way, we allow a set of rules to be consistent and at the same time to prove a proposition and its negation. In standard logical systems, we define only the consistent set of formulas, but in our underlying logic there are new definitions, such as "acceptable", "weak conclusion" and "strong conclusion" [8–10].

# 4  System Implementation

## 4.1  Gorgias

Gorgias [13, 14] is a general framework of argumentation theory. It can form the basis dynamic policy framework, despite incomplete information. Gorgias' syntax is based on Prolog. The predicates of Gorgias are divided into three categories:

- abducibles
- defeasible
- background (non-defeasible).

The literals are represented by Prolog terms: A negation literal is called `neg(L)`. Futhermore, the language for the representation of the theories is defined by the rules below:

```
rule(Signature, Head, Body).
```

where

- `Head` is a literal
- `Body` is a list of literals
- `Signature` is a compound term consisting of name of the rule along with selected variables from `Head` and the `Body` of the rule.

The special predicate `prefer/2` is used to locally codify the relative priority of the theory's rules. For example, the following means that the rule with signature `Sig1` has higher priority than the rule with signature `Sig2`, if the conditions in `Body` apply:

```
rule(Signature, prefer(Sig1,Sig2), Body).
```

Abducible literals are declared using the special predicate `abducible/2`, for example:

```
abducible(Literal, Preconditions).
```

Finally, the statement `conflict (Sig1, Sig2)` indicates that the rules with signatures `Sig1` and `Sig2` collide. In many cases `conflict (Sig1, Sig2)` are true if they are `Head` of the `Sig1` and `Sig2` they are literally opposite.

## 4.2  Representation of Knowledge and Belief

To declare the rules, conflicts and preferences between them, we will normally use Prolog terms using the predicates of the Gorgias system as we have previously defined.

*Example 2.* To say something flies when it is a bird and that something does not fly when it is penguin we write:

```
rule (r1 (X), fly (X), [bird (X)]).
rule (r2 (X), neg (fly (X)), [penguin (X)]).
```

In this example, it is clear that these two rules are in conflict when something is both a penguin and a bird:

```
rule (f1, bird (tweety), []).
rule (f2, penguin (tweety), []).
```

To solve the conflict, we use the special hypothesis `prefer/2`. Therefore, for in our example we have:

```
rule (pr1 (X), prefer (r2 (x), r1 (x)), []).
```

## 5 Review and Maintenance

### 5.1 Chi Square Test Implementation

For calculating the statistics we will use the language R. Our information system will choose the appropriate statistical test depending on the characteristics of the sample, and if the conditions are satisfied, it will then use Gorgias to interpret these results and then to test hypotheses.

This architecture is chosen because:

- R is the basic scientific data analysis tool and provides many ready-made statistical functions.
- The underlying logic of the interpretation is concentrated in a Gorgias rule file, and it fully corresponds to what is reported in statistics literature. If in the future a part of the rules need to be corrected or extended, then the code does not need to be changed for the set of the software.
- The user, who is often not a expert, will be trained in statistical methods and will use the tools of statistical methods correctly.

In order to show that our system works, we will conduct a statistical test to check if there is dependence between two attributes: *A* and *B*. One way we can do this is to use a $\chi^2$ independent test. To apply this test, we typically represent the data from one sample size *n*, in the form of a $2 \times 2$ **contingency table** (Table 1). This matrix is a frequency table where we have them two subpopulations (attribute categories *B*) and their columns successes and failures (*A* attributes). The user usually considers that the conditions of the Central Limit Theorem apply, which in our case translates into the condition: all the expected frequencies being $\geq 5$. The programming language R supplies us with the appropriate functions, such as the `chisq.test ()`     and

**Table 1.** $2 \times 2$ contingency table

|                      | Success  | Failure  | Total |
|----------------------|----------|----------|-------|
| First subpopulation  | $n_{11}$ | $n_{12}$ | $n_1$ |
| Second subpopulation | $n_{21}$ | $n_{22}$ | $n_2$ |
| Total                | $n_1$    | $n_2$    | $n$   |

`fisher.test ()` - which implements the Fisher's exact test when the conditions of Central Limit Theorem do not apply.

Then the user uses standard statistical analysis software to check the appropriate conditions to see whether two features of the population are independent. This process can answer questions such as, "Is the level of respondents' exercise in a statistical survey independent of whether they are smokers?", or "Is the rate of defective items independent of the line production?".

Such an approach, it is not necessary for the user to know all the "details" of mathematical statistics. The program will work as a "mathematician" and will suggest answers. This can help to avoid errors that may occur when non-experts use statistical tools, for example in medicine.

### 5.2 Implementing a Java Interface with R

To enable Java to communicate with R, we will use rJava to supply R with the Java interface library. This allows us have the results as a Java variable. We will implement - using the JRI – the `Statistics.java` class that contains the relevant functions. The next step is to apply the independence test $\chi^2$ or Fisher's exact test using the `chisq ()` and `fisher ()` functions. The results of these tests are stored in a different variable for each contingency table, therefore we can retrieve them with several functions (Fig. 1).

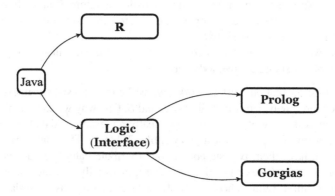

**Fig. 1.** The basic structure of our system

## 5.3    Policy for Statistics in Gorgias

In the previous section, we described the `Statistics`  class that is responsible for the handling of R and the collection of statistical results. Based on what we said in the introduction, interpretation of these results will be made in our system using the functions of interface `Logic.` We will utilize the underlying logic of Gorgias, which allow us to express our reasoning, as a mathematician would. Furthermore, through the production of the acceptable argument made by Gorgias, we can inform the user of what rules and data have led to this answer.

We have thus managed to use Gorgias as a knowledge database of the characteristics of a population. Maybe in the future this knowledge database can be extended to include additional queries. Also the policy defined by the Gorgias rules avoids calling functions that will not be needed. For example, the Fisher's test is running only when $\chi^2$ test is invalid. Finally, thanks to the ability to set preferences between the rules and higher order preferences (as described in the chapter of Gorgias), the extension of the rules and the introduction of new rules is easy without need to change the old ones, and we can use tools such as Gorgias-B and SoDA development methodology (Software Development for Argumentation).

## 5.4    Example Usage

To show the use of the application and the format of the results, we will try three different context tables for the $A$ and $B$ features from samples of four different populations. Tables [15] of relevance are:

**Table 2.**  Contingency table data1

|  | Defective products | Non-defective products |
|---|---|---|
| First production process | 12 | 288 |
| Second production process | 20 | 380 |

**Table 3.**  Contingency table data2

|  | Defective products | Non-defective products |
|---|---|---|
| Third production process | 12 | 288 |
| Fourth production process | 100 | 380 |

The final application response and hypothesis testing with the help of Gorgias is: (Table 5)

```
Cannot reject null hypotheses, data1 are independent
Why? [[h0_is_not_rejected(data1)]]

Null hypotheses rejected, data2 are codependent.
Why? [[f1, f6, f5, chisq_is_valid(data2), f5, chisq_rejects_h0(data2)]]

Cannot reject null hypotheses, data3 are independent
Why? [[h0_is_not_rejected(data3)]]

Null hypotheses rejected, data4 are codependent.
Why? [[f1, f17, f16, fisher_rejects_h0(data4)]]

Gorgias state
-------------
consult(stats.pl).
rule(f1,significance(0.050000000000000044),[]).
rule(f2,chisq(data1),[]).
rule(f3,chisq_pvalue(data1,0.6570195719690067),[]).
rule(f4,chisq_minexpected(data1,13.714285714285714),[]).
rule(f5,chisq(data2),[]).
rule(f6,chisq_pvalue(data2,1.386470999319574E-10),[]).
rule(f7,chisq_minexpected(data2,43.07692307692308),[]).
rule(f9,chisq_pvalue(data3,0.22674842690343286),[]).
rule(f10,chisq_minexpected(data3,4.2),[]).
rule(f11,fisher(data3),[]).
rule(f12,fisher_pvalue(data3,0.24022012054762612),[]).
rule(f14,chisq_pvalue(data4,0.05485393990013243),[]).
rule(f15,chisq_minexpected(data4,4.125),[]).
rule(f16,fisher(data4),[]).
rule(f17,fisher_pvalue(data4,0.030221989999279542),[]).
```

**Table 4.** Contingency table data3

|        | No smoker | Semi-smoker | Smoker |
|--------|-----------|-------------|--------|
| Man    | 28        | 8           | 22     |
| Woman  | 26        | 2           | 14     |

**Table 5.** Contingency table data4

|                          | Defective products | Non-defective products |
|--------------------------|--------------------|------------------------|
| Fifth production process | 1                  | 10                     |
| Sixth production process | 14                 | 15                     |

By interpreting these results, we see that, for Table 2, a $\chi^2$ test was valid but insufficient evidence was found and the null hypothesis $H_0$ was rejected. In Table 3, the result of the $\chi^2$ test provided sufficient data to reject the null hypothesis, and this is reflected in the accepted argument. For Table 4, the Fisher's exact test had to be applied because the expected frequencies that resulted from `chisq.test ()` made $\chi^2$ invalid.

## 6 Conclusions

We have claimed that the framework of logic programming without negation as failure (LPwNF) provided by Gorgias can be applied to the use of existing statistical packages like R and provide ease of use and correctness. More specifically a common source of errors in the use of statistics in various fields, like medical and business cases, stems from the misuse of statistical methods and misinterpretation of the results since the researchers are often not experts in the field of statistical analysis. The system that we suggest acts as an intelligent agent that solves this problem by automatically selecting the appropriate method and interpreting the result like a mathematician while also explaining to the user the answer with references to the relevant rules and conditions. Furthermore, by keeping the logic of Gorgias rule file, and taking advantage of custom ordering relation of rules and default reasoning (abduction), there are development benefits like increased encapsulation, easier extensibility without disrupting current functionality and verification of correctness due to the natural mapping of rules to the relevant mathematical theorems.

The information system we presented is in its early state. Additional work is needed to integrate other basic parametric and non-parametric statistical tests and to integrate the process of selecting the correct statistical test. The last one requires the creation of a specialized knowledge base, but the creation and integration of such knowledge base will be a matter of routine since the fundamental structure of our cognitive bases has been described successfully. Finally the methodology we described can bring the benefits of non-monotonic logic to different fields, like legal reasoning, business cases, and combine existing software packages that use different technologies with Gorgias and thus augment their use.

**Acknowledgements.** This research is funded in the context of the project "MIS5005844" under the call for proposals "Supporting researchers with emphasis on new researchers" (EDULLL 34). The project is co-financed by Greece and the European Union (European Social Fund-ESF) by the Operational Programme Human Resources Development, Education and Lifelong Learning 2014–2020.

## References

1. Strasak, A.M., Zaman, Q., Pfeiffer, K.P., Göbel, G., Ulmer, H.: Statistical errors in medical research–a review of common pitfalls. Swiss Med. Wkly. **137**(3–4), 44–49 (2007)
2. Murphy, J.R.: Statistical errors in immunologic research. J. Allergy Clin. Immunol. **114**(6), 1259–1263 (2004)

3. Young, J.: Statistical errors in medical research – a chronic disease? Swiss Med. Wkly. **137**, 41–43 (2007)
4. Ercan, I., et al.: Misusage of statistics in medical research. Eur. J. Gen. Med. **4**(3), 4 (2007). https://doi.org/10.29333/ejgm/82507. ISSN 1304-3897
5. Hanif, A., Ajmal, T.: Statistical errors in medical journals (A critical appraisal). Ann. King Edward Med. Univ. **17**, 178–182 (2011)
6. Clark, G.T., Mulligan, R.: Fifteen common mistakes encountered in clinical research. J. Prosthodont. Res. **55**(1), 1–6 (2011). https://doi.org/10.1016/j.jpor.2010.09.002. ISSN 1883-1958
7. Holmes, T.H.: Ten categories of statistical errors: a guide for research in endocrinology and metabolism. Am. J. Physiol. Endocrinol. Metab. **286**(4), E495–E501 (2004)
8. Kakas, A.C., Mancarella, P., Dung, P.M.: The acceptability semantics for logic programs. In: Van Hentenryck, P. (ed.) Proceedings of the Eleventh International Conference on Logic Programming, pp. 504–519. MIT Press, Cambridge (1994)
9. Dimopoulos, Y., Kakas, A.: Logic programming without negation as failure. In: Proceedings of the Fifth International Logic Programming Symposium, ILPS 1995, pp. 369–384. MIT Press (1995)
10. Kakas, A., Toni, F., Mancarella, P.: Argumentation logic. In Proceedings of the 5th International Conference on Computational Models of Argument, COMMA, pp. 12–27 (2014)
11. Spanoudakis, N.I., Constantinou, E., Koumi, A., Kakas, A.C.: Modeling data access legislation with Gorgias. In: Benferhat, S., Tabia, K., Ali, M. (eds.) IEA/AIE 2017. LNCS, vol. 10351, pp. 317–327. Springer, Cham (2017). https://doi.org/10.1007/978-3-319-60045-1_34
12. Kakas, A.C., Mancarella, P.: On the semantics of abstract argumentation. J. Log. Comput. **23**(5), 991–1015 (2013). https://doi.org/10.1093/logcom/exs068
13. Gorgias: An Argumentation System with Abduction. http://www.cs.ucy.ac.cy/nkd/gorgias/
14. Gorgias-B Argumentation Tool. http://gorgiasb.tuc.gr/
15. Fouskakis, D.: Data Analysis using R (2013). ISBN 9786188074156
16. Fudenberg, D., Levine, D.K.: The Theory of Learning in Games. Levine, D.K. Levine's Working Paper Archive 2 (1996)
17. Kiouvrekis, Y., Stefaneas, P., Kokkinaki, A.: An argumentation-based statistical support tool. In: Proceedings of the International Workshop on Applied Methods of Statistical Analysis, Nonparametric Methods in Cybernetics and System Analysis, Krasnoyarsk, The Russian Federation, 18–22 September 2017 (2017)

# Comparison of the Non-personalized Active Learning Strategies Used in Recommender Systems

Georges Chaaya[1]([⊠]), Jacques Bou Abdo[2], Elisabeth Métais[1],
Raja Chiky[3], Jacques Demerjian[4], and Kablan Barbar[4]

[1] CEDRIC Laboratory, CNAM, Paris, France
gchaaya@ndu.edu.lb
[2] Faculty of Natural and Applied Sciences, Notre Dame University,
Deir El Kamar, Lebanon
[3] LISITE Laboratory, ISEP, Paris, France
[4] LARIFA-EDST Laboratory, Faculty of Sciences, Lebanese University,
Fanar, Lebanon

**Abstract.** The study of recommender systems is essential nowadays due to its great effect on businesses and customer satisfaction. Different active learning strategies were previously developed to gain ratings from the users on specific items, and this enables the system to have more information and consequently make more accurate recommendations. In previous studies, these strategies were evaluated using a different selection of metrics in each work, and the experimentations were done on different datasets. In this paper, we solve these weaknesses by comparing the main ten non-personalized strategies on a fair ground, by simulating them against two datasets and using seven of the mostly agreed upon metrics. This gives more trust and less biased results when comparing their performances. Also, the analysis of the computation time and the elicitation efficiency is added.

**Keywords:** Recommender systems · Collaborative filtering · Active learning
Cold-start problem · Non-personalized strategies · Accuracy metrics

## 1 Introduction

The increase use of the Web as a medium for business transactions, and the need for companies to know more about their customers' preferences in order to provide them with a more efficient service, were the main reasons for developing recommender systems. Items are suggested by the recommender system based on the users' preferences, and this is done by several approaches such as content-based [1, 2], demographic [3, 4], knowledge-based [5, 6], collaborative filtering [7–9], and hybrid approaches [10–12].

Collaborative filtering recommender systems rely on items' ratings provided by the users. They analyze the previous ratings, the similarities between users, and recommend items that are not yet rated but that are most likely to be enjoyed by the user. The power of a recommender system lies in having accurate predictions in order to give the

© Springer Nature Switzerland AG 2019
M. Themistocleous and P. Rupino da Cunha (Eds.): EMCIS 2018, LNBIP 341, pp. 443–456, 2019.
https://doi.org/10.1007/978-3-030-11395-7_34

most specific recommendations. A major problem that arises is the cold-start problem [30]; it refers to a new user or a new item added to the system, having few or no ratings at all. Different "active learning" techniques were used in previous studies to deal with this problem. The active learning process consists of giving the new user a certain number of items to rate, and these ratings will eventually enable the system to provide better recommendations [13, 14]. It is important to design an active learning strategy that selects a small number of items that are the most informative to the system. The important active learning strategies can be non-personalized or personalized [15], depending on whether the selected items given to the users for rating are different for each user or not. In this paper, we limit our study to the non-personalized strategies, being an essential element in the choice of the first item in some personalized strategies.

The previous evaluations, existing until today, present some weaknesses. First, no previous research compared all the non-personalized strategies against the same metrics and over a unified dataset [16–21]. This doesn't provide a decisive conclusion that classifies the strategies from best to worst, and makes the results biased. Moreover, in most of the studies, the main methods for evaluating the strategies relied only on the used metrics, while the number of elicited items was mentioned in very few researches, with-out giving attention to other important factors that can affect the results and performance.

In this work, a clear and exhaustive comparison between the main ten non-personalized strategies is provided: the study is performed on two different datasets to better validate the results, and seven different predictive and classification accuracy metrics are used to calculate the accuracy of all these strategies. This would provide more certainty and credibility to the result of the evaluation. In addition to that, we analyze the elicitation efficiency (which gives an importance to the number of ratings gained by the system at each iteration), and the computation time.

The remainder of the paper is organized as follows: Sect. 2 reviews some of the previous studies done on non-personalized strategies. Section 3 shows the implementation details: it states the tested strategies, the datasets and metrics used, and the algorithm used for splitting the dataset and implementing the strategies. Section 4 shows and discusses the experimental results, and finally a conclusion and some future work are shown in Sect. 5.

## 2 Background and Related Work

In this section, we present an overview of the strategies, datasets and metrics that will be evaluated in this paper, along with some details about the previous experiments done in the literature on the non-personalized strategies.

### 2.1 Strategies

Different non-personalized strategies were presented in previous research, and they were divided into single-heuristic and combined-heuristic [1]. The non-personalized single-heuristic strategies are divided into three main types other than the random strategy: uncertainty based (which includes variance, entropy, and entropy0), error reduction (greedy extend and representative-based), and attention based (popularity and co-coverage), whereas the combined-heuristic are a static combination of two single-heuristic strategies, and they include: random-popularity, log(popularity)*entropy, sqrt (popularity)*variance, and HELF [16–21]. The explanation of these strategies can be found in our previous work [33]. The main goal is to decide which items should be selected and given to the user to rate.

The work in this paper was limited to the non-personalized strategies as a first step.

These strategies will be compared to the personalized strategies in an upcoming study.

## 2.2 Metrics

In the previous studies that tackled the non-personalized strategies [16–21], different metrics were used to evaluate each of the strategies. The accuracy metrics are divided into three major classes [27, 28]:

- Predictive accuracy metrics: they measure how close the ratings estimated by a recommender system are to the true user ratings. They are usually used to evaluate non-binary ratings. The most popular metrics in this category are Mean Absolute Error (MAE), Mean Absolute User Error (MAUE), and Root Mean Squared Error (RMSE) [25, 32].
- Classification accuracy metrics: they ignore the exact rating or ranking of items, and measure only the correct or incorrect classification. The most used metrics in this category are precision and recall, inverse precision, inverse recall, and F1 measure. For more information about these metrics, the reader can refer to [26].
- Rank accuracy metrics: they measure how much the recommender system is able to estimate the correct order of items with respect to the user's preferences [32].

A major problem with the frequently used classification accuracy metrics is that they can include great biases. This issue can be solved by the Matthews correlation coefficient introduced by Powers [29], which is considered as a balanced measure since it involves values of all the four quadrants of a confusion matrix:

$$
\begin{aligned}
& Matthews\, Correlation = \\
& \pm \sqrt{Precision + InversePrecision - 1).(Recall + InverseRecall - 1)}
\end{aligned}
\tag{1}
$$

## 2.3 Previous Implementations

Many studies dealt with non-personalized strategies, whether to present these strategies, or to use some of them as a baseline to be compared to a new strategy. In the following we present these studies, focusing on which strategies, which metrics, and which datasets are used in each of them.

In [16], the authors proposed strategies based on variance and entropy. They worked on two different datasets, Active WebMuseum and EachMovie, and the evaluation was done using MAE.

In [17], the authors tested a new algorithm by introducing the influence criterion which measures the effect that rating an item has on the approximated values of other unrated items. The concepts of uncertainty and coverage were combined, and the proposed strategy was tested against the random, variance, entropy, popularity, and Log(Popularity)*Entropy strategies. The experimentations were done on the Movie-Lens dataset by randomly selecting 100 users that have each rated at least 100 items, and the MAE was also used as an evaluation metric.

In [18], the authors tested the entropy, random, popularity, Popularity*Entropy, Log(Popularity)*Entropy, along with other personalized strategies on a version of the MovieLens dataset containing 7335 users, 4117 movies and around 2.7 million ratings (by considering users who have at least 200 ratings). Also the MAE was calculated to compare these strategies.

In [19], entropy0 was suggested, and it was compared to popularity, entropy and Harmonic mean of Entropy and Logarithm of Frequency (HELF), along with other personalized algorithms. The experiments were conducted on a version of the MovieLens dataset having about 11000 users, 9000 movies, and 3 million ratings (by considering only the users who have rated at least 20 movies and logged in at least twice). In addition to the MEA, the "Expected Utility" metric was used in order to penalize false positives more than false negatives, since MEA has a limitation of considering only absolute differences.

In [20], most of the single-heuristic non-personalized strategies were conducted on the Netflix dataset and by using 200 items as a seed set. The methods were evaluated using the RMSE metric. In [21], the representative-based strategy was introduced, and it was compared to the random and popularity strategies. This method was tested on three datasets, Netflix, 10M MovieLens, and last.fm, and it was evaluated using Precision at K (Pre@K) and MAP. In [31], six non-personalized single-heuristic strategies were compared and evaluated on the 100K MovieLens dataset using different predictive accuracy metrics and classification accuracy metrics.

In most of the previous studies, offline simulation was employed, in addition to few online testing in some of them. MAE was mostly used to evaluate strategies, but it is also important to use other metrics that can provide more information. Since these methods were tested on different datasets, and using different metrics, we cannot generalize the results and draw a decisive conclusion concerning their importance. In addition to that, more factors need to be taken into consideration when deciding about the validity of a certain method. Therefore, it would be very useful to implement these methods on the same datasets, and to evaluate them using a greater number of metrics that will give a better understanding of the differences between the strategies.

# 3    Implementation Environment

In this section, we present the implementation details taken into consideration in this study. We explain the used algorithm, the programming language, the selected strategies, along with the datasets and metrics.

### 3.1    Algorithm

To implement each of the strategies explained previously, a version of the algorithm suggested by Elahi et al. was implemented [23], and it was explained and presented in our previous work [31]. In this paper, we perform 10 iterations for each strategy.

### 3.2    Selected Strategies

As mentioned before, different non-personalized active learning strategies were implemented in previous studies. Since error reduction strategies are not widely used (presented in one study each), and they are not relied on in the available combined-heuristic strategies, and since they mostly cannot be applied in practice, we will focus our study on implementing the other strategies: random, variance, entropy, entropy0, popularity, co-coverage, random-popularity, log(popularity)*entropy, sqrt(popularity) *variance, HELF [16–21].

### 3.3    Selected Datasets

In this paper, we consider two datasets: the 100K MovieLens dataset which contains 100000 ratings of 1682 movies made by 943 users, and the 1M MovieLens dataset which contains 1 million ratings of 3900 movies made by 6040 users [22, 24].

We use the file "ratings.dat" which contains ratings and is in the following format: UserID::MovieID::Rating::Timestamp

The ratings are made on a 5-star scale (whole-star ratings only), and each user has at least 20 ratings.

### 3.4    Selected Metrics

In this study, we use the predictive accuracy metrics and the classification accuracy metrics mentioned in Sect. 2.3. The rank accuracy metrics will not be used in this paper since we are working on movie recommendations, and in this specific application we are not interested in predicting the ranking of the items. These metrics can be used in other applications and employed in the evaluation of the strategy similarly to the way the other metrics are employed in this study.

## 4    Experimental Results

Since we are considering in this study two different datasets, each was divided randomly into three datasets as follows: The 100000 ratings were divided to 557 ratings in S, 68806 ratings in Q, and 30637 ratings in E. The 1 million ratings were divided to 5493 ratings in S, 690366 ratings in Q, and 304350 ratings in E.

In the following, we provide a comparison of all the strategies.

## 4.1 Performance Using Predictive Accuracy Metrics

We start by analyzing the performance of the ten strategies for the first 10 iterations since the datasets are not very large, which causes the strategies to behave similarly after a certain period. In addition to that, it helps in getting a better view of the differences between the strategies since most users tend to rate few items, so we are basically interested in the first stages of elicitation. Figure 1 shows the progress of the predictive accuracy metrics' values (MAE, MAUE and RMSE) for the different strategies on both the 100K and 1M datasets and for the first 10 iterations.

Starting by the 100K dataset, the first observation is that the random strategy is the worst, since the selection of the items is not being done based on any logical factor. For the other strategies, it can be seen that no definite conclusion can be drawn, since the dataset is sparse and almost all strategies except the random strategy will lead sooner or later to very close results.

After the first iteration, and when using MAE or RMSE, popularity, entropy0 and HELF had the best performance with a slight difference between them; and random, rand-pop and co-coverage were clearly worse. When considering MAUE, the difference slightly increases between HELF and the other two, with an advantage for the popularity and entropy0 strategies. After the second iteration, entropy, entropy0, log (pop)*entropy, and HELF have the best performance, with a slightly better result for entropy0.

As the number of iterations increases, the differences between MAE values for most strategies become very small. At the 9th iteration, variance, entropy, log(pop)*ent and sqrt(pop)*var start having the exact same values for MAE. It is at this stage that these strategies become identical in behavior, since they will always be selecting the same items (in increasing order of MovieID). This is mainly caused by the sparsity of the dataset. These patterns are the same for all predictive accuracy metrics.

The reason why this happened is that whenever we have a tie in the value of the parameters used for selection, we selected the items based on their MovieId ordering, i.e. taking the items that have the smaller MovieId. Since at the beginning we don't have many ratings in S (the dataset is sparse), many items will have the same value when using variance or entropy or log(pop)*ent or sqrt(pop)*var at the 9th iteration (after eliciting 90 items for each user). Therefore, we will be selecting the same items for elicitation regardless of the strategy used. For larger datasets where S has more ratings, there will be a difference between these strategies even if the choice of the items on tie is done in increasing order of movieID.

Although the differences are very small for the 100K dataset, the results are different for the 1M dataset where there exists more users, movies and ratings. This helps to show in a better way the performance of each strategy.

For the 1M dataset, MAE was initially equal to almost 1.735. After the first iteration, the popularity strategy performs the best improvement, with a drop of the MAE to 1.095, and the entropy0 and HELF strategies come directly after it. For the first two iterations (20 ratings requested from each user), popularity and entropy0 have the best performance. It is observable that random, rand-pop, variance, entropy and co-coverage behave worse than the other strategies.

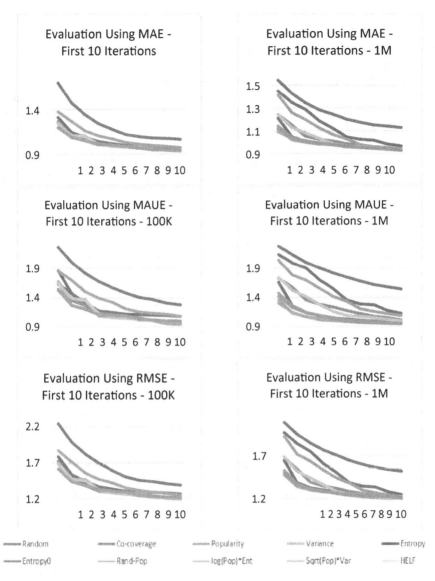

**Fig. 1.** Comparison of the predictive accuracy metrics for the first 10 iterations on the 100K and 1M datasets

## 4.2 Performance Using Classification Accuracy Metrics

Figure 2 shows the performance of the ten strategies on the 100K and 1M datasets using the classification accuracy metrics. As can be seen from the figure, during the first

8 iterations the value of the metrics is not stable, it performs small changes, and then starts increasing but at a very low rate. After the $8^{th}$ strategy, the entropy0 is the best in terms of classification accuracy, enabling the system to recommend more preferred items to the user.

No conclusion can be drawn concerning which strategy performs better in terms of classification accuracy. As it can be seen from the graph of the 100K dataset, all strategies have precision values bounded between 61% and 64%, recall between 56% and 57.5%, F1-measure between 58.4% and 60.4%, and Matthews Correlation between 14% and 19%. Moreover, these values do not follow a logical trend, they increase and decrease randomly. This observation also applies to the first 10 iterations of the 1 M dataset. This is due to the sparsity of the dataset, and might be related to the formula used in calculating the similarity between the users, and to the fact that we calculate the predicted ratings with respect to a comparison with all the users, not only K neighbors. The improvement in performance is observable when using the predictive accuracy metrics since any small change to the predicted value can cause an improvement in the metrics, but when using the classification accuracy metrics we are only taking into consideration the top 10 predicted items for each user, and a small change in the predicted value is not able to move a certain item in or out this list. These values most probably will increase in the next iterations on the 1M dataset.

## 4.3    Number of Elicited Items

It is important to observe the number of items added to S after each iteration using each strategy. This reflects the number of items known to the users among all items presented to them for rating. The importance of this factor lies in the care of the businesses to gain customers, and it is extremely useful to give to the new users the items they have had experience with. The results of the elicitation efficiency on the 100K dataset are shown in Fig. 3 in terms of the cumulative number of ratings obtained after specific iterations, and the number of ratings at each iteration. The random and rand-pop strategies are the worst, while the other strategies have somehow close values.

When using a larger dataset, the results give a clearer idea about the differences between the strategies. As shown in Fig. 4, the popularity strategy acquires the most ratings when using the MovieLens 1M dataset, and this behavior is expected since this is the main purpose of this strategy. Entropy0 comes next, and HELF in the $3^{rd}$ place. This behavior is identical to the one observed when using the 100K dataset. The random and rand-pop strategies are the worst. It can be seen that the cumulative number of ratings for almost all strategies increases in a linear way, with an emphasis that the first iteration always leads to the highest number of acquired ratings.

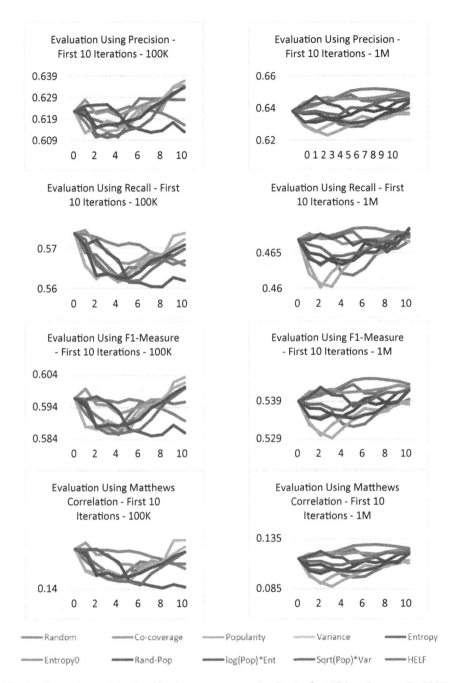

**Fig. 2.** Comparison of the classification accuracy metrics for the first 10 iterations on the 100K and 1M datasets

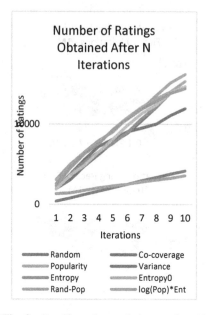

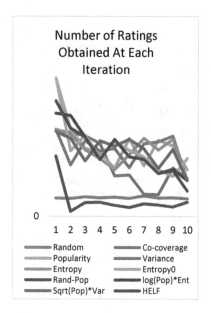

**Fig. 3.** Specific and cumulative number of ratings obtained at each iteration – 100K dataset

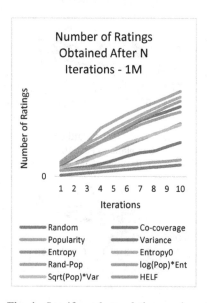

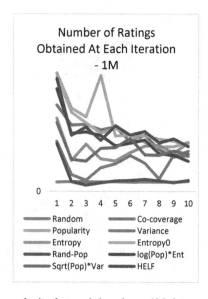

**Fig. 4.** Specific and cumulative number of ratings obtained at each iteration – 1M dataset

## 4.4    Computation Time

Besides the accuracy and the number of elicited items, an important factor to consider is the time complexity of each of these strategies. As a general pattern, the computation time increases with each iteration since the number of ratings involved in calculating the similarity and the predicted ratings increases as the number of iterations increases. In the following, we consider the total iteration time, which includes the elicitation time, the prediction calculation time, and the accuracy calculation time. Figure 5 shows the total computation time for the 10 iterations on the 100K dataset. The popularity strategy takes the longest time, followed by entropy0. Although these two strategies have a high computation time, they give the most accurate results.

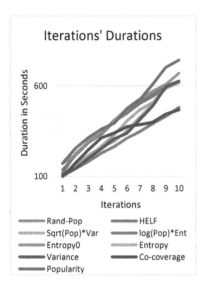
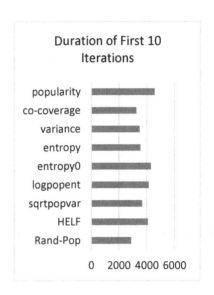

**Fig. 5.** Durations of the iterations when applying each strategy to the 100K dataset

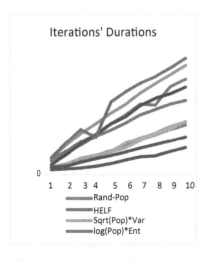
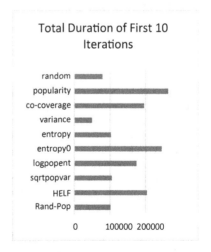

**Fig. 6.** Total duration of the iterations when applying each strategy on the 1M dataset

Figure 6 shows the total computation time (in seconds) when applying the strategies to the 1M dataset, and it considers the duration of each iteration and the total time of all 10 iterations. The duration of all the strategies is increasing linearly, with a bit of pattern violation in the popularity and HELF strategies. Variance is the fastest strategy, followed by random and rand-pop (since these two strategies are selecting the items randomly – no need to do any calculation before selecting the items). The popularity and entropy0 strategies, which were shown to have a good performance when evaluating them with the accuracy metrics, are the slowest strategies to elicit ratings, predict the values of the missing ratings and calculate the metrics.

## 5   Conclusion and Future Work

As previously discussed, the evaluation of the non-personalized active learning strategies in earlier studies had some limitations and was biased. In this paper, we were able to provide a better comparison between the existing mostly used non-personalized strategies (random, popularity, co-coverage, variance, entropy, entropy0, random-popularity, log(pop)*entropy, sqrt(pop)*variance, HELF) using seven metrics. The study was done on the 100K and 1M MovieLens datasets, and the results of the comparison were analyzed. Moreover, we added two more factors to the study: the elicitation efficiency and the computation time.

In the future, this comparison will be performed on a larger dataset (10M, or 20M MovieLens), and on datasets from other domains, in order to have more accurate results. Also, these strategies will be compared against other personalized strategies to provide a more general overview, and a new strategy that outperforms all the studied strategies can be proposed. A new comparative evaluation method that includes different important factors will be suggested.

## References

1. Lops, P., de Gemmis, M., Semeraro, G.: Content-based recommender systems: state of the art and trends. In: Ricci, F., Rokach, L., Shapira, B., Kantor, P.B. (eds.) Recommender Systems Handbook, pp. 73–105. Springer, Boston (2011). https://doi.org/10.1007/978-0-387-85820-3_3
2. de Gemmis, M., Lops, P., Musto, C., Narducci, F., Semeraro, G.: Semantics-aware content-based recommender systems. In: Ricci, F., Rokach, L., Shapira, B. (eds.) Recommender Systems Handbook, pp. 119–159. Springer, Boston, MA (2015). https://doi.org/10.1007/978-1-4899-7637-6_4
3. Wang, Y., Chan, S.C.-F., Ngai, G.: Applicability of demographic recommender system to tourist attractions: a case study on trip advisor. In: Proceedings of the 2012 IEEE/WIC/ACM International Joint Conferences on Web Intelligence and Intelligent Agent Technology, WI-IAT 2012, vol. 03, pp. 97–101. IEEE Computer Society, Washington, DC (2012)
4. Beliakov, G., Calvo, T., James, S.: Aggregation functions for recommender systems. In: Ricci, F., Rokach, L., Shapira, B. (eds.) Recommender Systems Handbook, pp. 777–808. Springer, Boston, MA (2015). https://doi.org/10.1007/978-1-4899-7637-6_23
5. Burke, R.: Knowledge-based recommender systems (2000)

6. Felfernig, A., Friedrich, G., Jannach, D., Zanker, M.: Constraint-based recommender systems. In: Ricci, F., Rokach, L., Shapira, B. (eds.) Recommender Systems Handbook, pp. 161–190. Springer, Boston, MA (2015). https://doi.org/10.1007/978-1-4899-7637-6_5
7. Adomavicius, G., Tuzhilin, A.: Toward the next generation of recommender systems: a survey of the state-of-the-art and possible extensions. IEEE Trans. Knowl. Data Eng. 17(6), 734–749 (2005)
8. Koren, Y., Bell, R.: Advances in collaborative filtering. In: Ricci, F., Rokach, L., Shapira, B. (eds.) Recommender Systems Handbook, pp. 77–118. Springer, Boston (2015). https://doi.org/10.1007/978-1-4899-7637-6_3
9. Desrosiers, C., Karypis, G.: A comprehensive survey of neighborhood-based recommendation methods. In: Ricci, F., Rokach, L., Shapira, B., Kantor, P.B. (eds.) Recommender Systems Handbook, pp. 107–144. Springer, Boston, MA (2011). https://doi.org/10.1007/978-0-387-85820-3_4
10. Burke, R.: Hybrid recommender systems: survey and experiments. User Model. User-Adap. Inter. 12(4), 331–370 (2002)
11. Degemmis, M., Lops, P., Semeraro, G.: A content-collaborative recommender that exploits wordnet-based user profiles for neighborhood formation. User Model. User-Adap. Inter. 17(3), 217–255 (2007)
12. Adomavicius, G., Kwon, Y.: Multi-criteria recommender systems. In: Ricci, F., Rokach, L., Shapira, B. (eds.) Recommender Systems Handbook, pp. 847–880. Springer, Boston, MA (2015). https://doi.org/10.1007/978-1-4899-7637-6_25
13. Elahi, M., Ricci, F., Repsys, V.: System-wide effectiveness of active learning in collaborative filtering. In: Bonchi, F., Buntine, W., Gavald, R., Gu, S. (eds.) International Workshop on Social Web Mining, Co-located with IJCAI, Universitat de Barcelona, Spain, p. 1 (2011)
14. Kutty, S., Yu, F.: Recommendations and predictions with ET greedy active learning. Technical report, Electrical Engineering and Computer Science Department of University of Michigan (2009)
15. Elahi, M., Ricci, F., Rubens, N.: A survey of active learning in collaborative filtering recommender systems. Comput. Sci. Rev. 20, 29–50 (2016)
16. Kohrs, A., Merialdo, B.: Improving collaborative filtering for new users by smart object selection. In: Proceedings of International Conference on Media Features, ICMF (2001)
17. Rubens, N., Sugiyama, M.: Influence-based collaborative active learning. In: Proceedings of the 2007 ACM Conference on Recommender Systems, RecSys 2007, pp. 145–148. ACM, New York (2007)
18. Rashid, A.M., et al.: Getting to know you: learning new user preferences in recommender systems. In: Proceedings of the 7th International Conference on Intelligent User Interfaces, IUI 2002, pp. 127–134. ACM, New York (2002)
19. Rashid, A.M., Karypis, G., Riedl, J.: Learning preferences of new users in recommender systems: an information theoretic approach. ACM SIGKDD Explor. Newsl. 10, 90–100 (2008)
20. Golbandi, N., Koren, Y., Lempel, R.: On bootstrapping recommender systems. In: Proceedings of the 19th ACM International Conference on Information and Knowledge Management, CIKM 2010, pp. 1805–1808. ACM, New York (2010)
21. Liu, N.N., Meng, X., Liu, C., Yang, Q.: Wisdom of the better few: cold start recommendation via representative based rating elicitation. In: Proceedings of the 2011 ACM Conference on Recommender Systems, RecSys 2011, Chicago, IL, USA, pp. 37–44 (2011)
22. Harper, F.M., Konstan, J.A.: The MovieLens datasets: history and context. ACM Trans. Interact. Intell. Syst. 5(4), 19 (2015)

23. Elahi, M., Repsys, V., Ricci, F.: Rating elicitation strategies for collaborative filtering. In: Huemer, C., Setzer, T. (eds.) EC-Web 2011. LNBIP, vol. 85, pp. 160–171. Springer, Heidelberg (2011). https://doi.org/10.1007/978-3-642-23014-1_14

24. Resnick, P., Iacovou, N., Suchak, M., Bergstrom, P., Riedl, J.: GroupLens: an open architecture for collaborative filtering of netnews. In: Proceedings of the 1994 ACM Conference on Computer Supported Cooperative Work, CSCW 1994, pp. 175–186. ACM, New York (1994)

25. Massa, P., Avesani, P.: Trust metrics in recommender systems. In: Golbeck, J. (ed.) Computing with Social Trust, pp. 259–285. Springer, London (2009). https://doi.org/10.1007/978-1-84800-356-9_10

26. Schröder, G., Thiele, M., Lehner, W.: Setting goals and choosing metrics for recommender system evaluations. In: UCERSTI2 Workshop at the 5th ACM Conference on Recommender Systems, Chicago, USA (2011)

27. del Olmo, F.H., Gaudioso, E.: Evaluation of recommender systems: a new approach. Expert Syst. Appl. 35(3), 790–804 (2008)

28. Herlocker, J.L., Konstan, J.A., Terveen, L.G., Riedl, J.T.: Evaluating collaborative filtering recommender systems. ACM Trans. Inf. Syst. 22(1), 5–53 (2004)

29. Powers, D.M.: Evaluation: from precision, recall and f-factor to roc, informedness, markedness and correlation. Technical report, School of Informatics and Engineering, Flinders University Adelaide, South Australia (2007)

30. Hossein, M., Shahraki, N., Bahadorpour, M.: Cold-start problem in collaborative recommender systems: efficient methods based on ask-to-rate technique. J. Comput. Inf. Technol. - CIT 22(2), 105–113 (2014)

31. Chaaya, G., Metais, E., Bou Abdo, J., Chiky, R., Demerjian, J., Barbar, K.: Evaluating non-personalized single-heuristic active learning strategies for collaborative filtering recommender systems. In: 16th IEEE International Conference on Machine Learning and Applications, Cancun, Mexico (2017)

32. Shani, G., Gunawardana, A.: Evaluating recommendation systems. In: Ricci, F., Rokach, L., Shapira, B., Kantor, Paul B. (eds.) Recommender Systems Handbook, pp. 257–297. Springer, Boston, MA (2011). https://doi.org/10.1007/978-0-387-85820-3_8

33. Chaaya, G., Bou Abdo, J., Demerjian, J., Chiky, R., Metais, E., Barbar, K.: An improved non-personalized combined-heuristic strategy for collaborative filtering recommender systems. In: IEEE Middle East & North Africa COMMunications Conference, MENA-COMM (2018)

# Board Interlocking and IT Governance: Proposed Conceptual Model

Allam Hamdan[1]([⊠]), Abdalmuttaleb Musleh Al-Sartawi[1],
Reem Khamis[2], Mohammed Anaswah[3], and Ahlam Hassan[1]

[1] Ahlia University, Manama, Bahrain
{ahamdan,ahassan}@ahlia.edu.bh,
amasartawi@hotmail.com
[2] Brunel University, London, UK
reem.Hamdan@brunel.ac.uk
[3] Mutah University, Maan, Karak, Jordan
msanaswah@yahoo.com

**Abstract.** This paper seeks to present a new dimension to the dimensions of IT governance; it proposes a model for the board interlocking and the IT governance. This conceptual model is based primarily on the Resource Dependence theory and tries to interpret the relationship between the board interlocking and the IT governance. This paper has theoretically reviewed the existing literature of the board interlocking; it has also added to the real gap in the literature of corporate governance which has not explained the importance of the board interlocking with IT governance. The researchers hope to provides a solid foundation for IT governance in order to supply companies with information about the IT environment surrounding it, the operating procedures, and the effective monitoring of the information systems, the challenges they face, the opportunities they may have, and to provide members of the board of directors with neutral opinion about these opportunities and challenges. The paper presents several contributions at both theoretical and practical levels; it paves the way for researchers to discuss the board interlocking with IT governance which contributes to the development of the theories governing the work of these concepts. It also draws the attention of the companies' administration to one of the most important practices in forming and structuring the board, i.e. the necessity of connecting the board of directors with managers who are qualified with practical experience in information systems.

**Keywords:** Board interlocking · IT governance · Board of director's
Board independence

## 1 Introduction

Board interlocking is defined as the case in which directors are also members of board of directors in other Firms (Al- Mussali and Ismail 2012). Board interlocking is considered one of the commonest management practices because it is a reliable and inexpensive tool of communication that makes use of experiences (Hannschild 1993). In general, the work of members of board of directors in other corporations provides them with more

© Springer Nature Switzerland AG 2019
M. Themistocleous and P. Rupino da Cunha (Eds.): EMCIS 2018, LNBIP 341, pp. 457–463, 2019.
https://doi.org/10.1007/978-3-030-11395-7_35

experience in management, specifically in issues related to strategic planning (Riberio and Colauto 2016). The literature (Dooley 1969; Allen 1974; Fich and White 2005) viewed this practice from the perspective of firm's endeavors to attract experiences by employing members of board of directors of other firms, or the reason might be the absence of distinguished directors. Thus, companies try to attract them to their boards (Santos and Silveira 2007). Board interlocking is also regarded a way by which it can have an access to sources of knowledge, ideas, and capitals of other firms (Hermalin and Weisbach 2003; Weisbach 2003). Board interlocking is also considered a communication channel of knowledge transfer among firms (Shropshire 2010). Riberio and Colauto (2016) outline that in: getting external material, getting foreign support, giving a legislative status to the organization, and creating significant communication channels among organizations. Some of the other benefits of board interlocking is the ability of firms to get to the best trade partners, in addition to having an access to the strategies of certain competitive firms (Gales and Kesner 1994). There are two trends in literature: the first led by Mol (2001) assures that board interlocking enriches firms with adequate experiences and provides it with a competitive advantage through firm's information on sources of competitive companies, its creditors creativity, and development plans. Even if all this was not used to achieve the competitive advantage, it would be inevitably used to develop firm techniques and organizational environment. The second trend led by (Fich and Shivadasani 2006) sees that board interlocking has a negative impact on the market value of the company and its performance, due to the deterioration of corporate governance associated with this interlocking.

Explaining board of director's behavior depends on two main theories which are: Agency Theory and Resource Dependence Theory. Agency theory explains the role of board of directors in controlling and monitoring corporate decisions in order to mitigate agency conflicts among stakeholders of a firm (Fama and Jensen 1983). While, Resource Dependence theory explains how board of directors serves as a resource for the firm in order to reach external resources as well (Ribeiro and Colauto 2016). The majority of the literature relies on agency theory to understand board of directors, however researchers such as Eisenhardt (1990) argues that agency theory is unable to provide sufficient practical explanation due to the environmental complexities faced by board of directors in a specific environment. Due to such inability, resource dependence theory sheds the light on the importance of board of directors in reducing uncertainties found in the environment.

## 2 Literature Review and Developing Conceptual Model

### 2.1 Board Interlocking

From resource dependence perspective, firms tend to hire board directors to serve as human capital that provides the firm with effective relations that develop the firm (Hermalin and Weisbach 2003). It is also considered to be a technique to manage external resources, reducing uncertainties surrounding the firm, reducing transaction costs and linking the firm to its external environment. (Pfeffer and Salancik 1978; Williamson 1984). Board members use their reputation and personal relations to bring necessary external resources to the firm where they serve as a board director in. Despite the power and resources found in any firm, it will always need a third party that mitigates the access to external resources. That's why many firms tend to hire board members who serve in other boards. In addition to the fact that, firms need to work together to be able to protect their shared interests (Zald 1969). Corporations will always look for board members who serve their interests in other organizations, in order to increase their capital from a third party (Hermalin and Weisbach 2003) such as: the ability of the firm to gain facilitated loans with discounted interest rates due to the relations they have with financial institutions which may lead to enhance performance eventually. Davis in (Davis 1991) discovered that, during the eighties of last century, 40 American companies had board members in seven other firms at least. In Canada, it was found that between 19640–1977 there were 1600 interlocking between companies (Ornstein 1982). (Santos and Silveira 2007) tested 230 companies in Brazil between 2003–2005 and found that approximately 74% in 2003 and in 2005 69% of members had relations with other councils in Brazil. In 1997 there was 61% of interlocking among 200 big companies in Hong Kong; 69% in England and 64% in the U.S.A during the same period (Au et al. 2000). The effect of board interlocking on firm performance was handled by researchers, such as: Kim (2005) who cleared out that Korean firms has acceptable level of board interlocking which enhance firm performance, however increasing that level might harm firm performance.

Board interlocking does not only enhance firm performance, but also enhances the relation between the firm and civil society and improves firm image in the society as well. Ribeiro and Colauto (2016) mentioned that interlocking enhances the firm's relationship with societal and environmental pressure groups. Moreover, some corporations tend to hire members of such groups in the boards in order to suppress any counter act from these groups against them or getting to know their point of views early. Such action tends to improve the firms' societal image. Ribeiro and Colauto (2016) considered board interlocking as a continuous method of learning as it contributes in improving board members skills and experience and transferring knowledge in an informal way which reflects positively on their own and firm performance.

This learning, might not be always in a positive way. As some creative and unethical practices may be transferred between corporations, such as earnings management. (Chiu et al. 2013; Ribeiro and Colauto 2016) indicated that board interlocking facilitates sharing practices among corporations such as earnings smoothing. However, this might not be generalized as some studies found a positive effect for board interlocking in reducing such practices like Mindzak (2013) in his study among Canadian firms. In general, comprehending board interlocking leads to the understanding of several phenomena related to companies work. For example, Haunschild (1993) noticed that mergers and acquisitions behavior between companies is related in a way or another to board interlocking. He conducted a study on 32 firms in the U.S and noticed that processes of merging or acquisition among companies are strongly related to the relation between board of directors of such companies.

## 2.2 Board Interlocking and IT Governance

IT governance is defined as leadership, organizational structures, and control processes which ensure that the information technology of the company works to support and

expand the company and achieve its objectives (Li et al. 2007). In addition to organizational structures that support and monitor IT operations, the company needs an
external source that provides support and advice to IT operations and transactions; this
source is also considered as a independent source of the company that can often have a
neutral opinion. Consequently, the company's board of directors is linked to a highly
experienced external source in the field of information technology. This source is fully
informed about the latest developments in the world of information technology and has
the knowledge and experience in order to give various opinions and attitudes to the
board based on practical experience it owns in the field of information technology.
Figure 1 illustrates a model for two companies; the first company is specialized in
information technology development and management, and another is working in
health care. The link between the boards of directors of the two companies will benefit
both companies; the health care company will hire an independent board member from

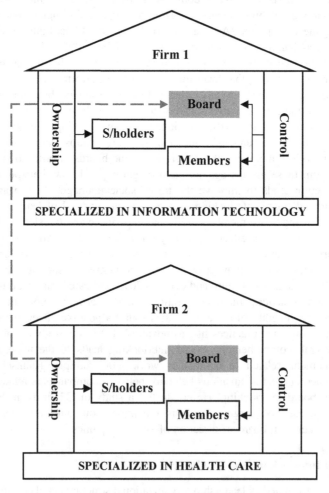

**Fig. 1.** Board interlocking

the other company who works in the field of information systems. This member can expert in this company and provides guidance and in the field of information systems, monitoring control, Operation procedures in addition to source of information latest be an advice and being a on the developments in the field of information systems, operations and control. For the health care company, this member will be an inexpensive source of continuing education that is supposed to provide an independent individual opinion that contribute to improving corporate governance, in general, and information systems governance, in particular. On the other hand, the company which specializes in information systems will be able to access administration files and databases of the companies that consume its products and systems in order to understand their needs and understand their decision-making powers, thus achieving a competitive edge.

The current paper investigates the relationship between board interlocking and IT governance; it is based primarily on the resource dependence theory, without dispensing the Agency theory that interprets the relationship between IT governance and the board of directors. The agency theory explains the traditional functions of the board of directors and controls the nature of its role in running the company and its operation. It includes many characteristics of the board such as the size of the board, its members' experience and the number of its meetings they hold. The resource dependence theory interprets and explains the independence of members of the board of directors as well as the interlocking between the board of directors and other boards of directors of other companies. The interlocking between the boards of directors must be deliberate and orderly, not arbitrary; the company must choose its board of directors carefully so as to provide the board of directors with the experts who are able to rationalize the decisions of the board and improve the performance of the company in general.

## 3 Conclusion

The interlocking among the board of directors is a common practice in companies; it works to connect the company to its external environment and provides information about the environment; it also works to identify the opportunities and risks surrounding its work. The interlocking among the board of directors is also a common practice in companies that work as suppliers and providing other companies with raw materials in addition to banks, credit and insurance institutions. However, the boards interlocking with the IT companies has not received attention despite its huge importance in providing the company with the most important developments in the world of technology, on the one hand, and providing them with specialists within its board of directors to give them neutral technical opinion on the adoption and operation of systems information as well as providing them with neutral opinions away from the administration's interests. This paper adopts a new framework for information technology governance that links the company's board of directors to the IT governance councils within the framework of the resource dependence theory through hiring independent board members who represent IT companies; the paper also invites researchers and people interested in corporate governance and IT governance to deeply research mechanisms of applying and adopting board interlocking with the IT companies, the paper of the specific factors that lead to this, in addition to the variables and the factors affecting it. Finally, interested researchers are invited to investigate the various elements that may have an impact on the performance of the company and its internal control systems and information systems.

# References

Allen, M.: The structure of interorganizational elite cooptation: interlocking corporate directorates. Am. Sociol. Rev. **39**(3), 393–406 (1974)

Al-Musalli, M., Ismail, K.: Intellectual capital performance and board characteristics of GCC banks. Procedia Econ. Financ. **2**(1), 219–226 (2012)

Au, K., Peng, M.W., Wang, D.: Interlocking directorates, firm strategies and performance in Hong Kong: towards a research agenda. Asia Pac. J. Manag. **17**(1), 29–47 (2000)

Chiu, P.C., Teoh, S.H., Tian, F.: Board interlocks and earning management contagion. Account. Rev. **88**(3), 915–944 (2013)

Davis, G.: Agents without principles? The spread of the poison pill through the intercorporate network. Adm. Sci. Q. **36**(1), 583–613 (1991)

Dooley, P.: The interlocking directorate. Am. Econ. Rev. **59**(2), 314–323 (1969)

Eisenhardt, K.: Speed and strategic choice: how managers accelerate decision making. Calif. Manag. Rev. **32**(3), 39–54 (1990)

Fama, E., Jensen, M.: Separation of ownership and control. J. Law Econ. **26**(4), 301–325 (1983)

Fich, E.M., Shivdasani, A.: Are busy boards effective monitors? J. Financ. **61**(2), 689–724 (2006)

Fich, E.M., White, L.: Why do CEOs reciprocally sit on each other's boards? J. Corp. Financ. **11** (1/2), 175–195 (2005)

Gales, L., Kesner, I.: An analysis of board of director size and composition in bankrupt organizations. J. Bus. Res. **30**(3), 271–282 (1994)

Haunschild, P.: Interorganizational imitation: the impact of interlocks on corporate acquisition activity. Adm. Sci. Q. **38**(3), 564–592 (1993)

Hermalin, B.E., Weisbach, M.: Boards of directors as an endogenously determined institution: a survey of the economic literature. Econ. Policy Rev. **9**(1), 7–26 (2003)

Kim, Y.: Board network characteristics and firm performance in Korea. Corp. Gov. Int. Rev. **13** (6), 800–808 (2005)

Li, C., Lim, J., Wang, Q.: Internal and external influences on IT control governance. Int. J. Account. Inf. Systems **8**, 225–239 (2007)

Mindzak, J.: Interlocked boards of directors, voluntary disclosures and earnings quality. In: Proceedings of the Canadian Academic Accounting Association Annual Conference, Montreal, Quebec, Canada, vol. 37 (2013)

Mol, M.: Creating wealth through working with others: interorganizational relationships. Acad. Manag. Exec. **15**(1), 150–152 (2001)

Ornstein, M.D.: Interlocking directorates in Canada: evidence from replacement patterns. Soc. Netw. **4**(4), 3–25 (1982)

Pfeffer, J., Salancik, G.R.: The External Control Of Organizations: A Resource Dependence Perspective. Harper & Row, New York (1978)

Ribeiro, F., Colauto, R.: The relationship between board interlocking and income smoothing practices. R. Cont. Fin. **27**(70), 55–66 (2016)

Santos, L., Silveira, A.: Board interlocking no Brasil. Revista Brasileira de Finanças 5(2), 125–163 (2007)

Shropshire, C.: The role of the interlocking director and board receptivity in the diffusion of practices. Acad. Manag. Rev. 35(2), 246–264 (2010)

Williamson, E.: The Economic Institutions of Capitalism: Firms, Markets, Relational Contracting. Free Press, New York (1984)

Zald, M.: The power and functions of boards of directors. Am. J. Sociol. 5(4), 97–111 (1969)

# Business Model Representations
# and Ecosystem Analysis: An Overview

Alejandro Arreola González[1]([⊠]), Matthias Pfaff[1],
and Helmut Krcmar[2]

[1] fortiss GmbH, Guerickestr. 25, 80805 Munich, Germany
{gonzalez, pfaff}@fortiss.org
[2] Technical University of Munich, Boltzmannstr. 3, 85748 Garching, Germany
krcmar@in.tum.de

**Abstract.** Some approaches to represent business models can support the analysis of value creation in platform ecosystems and its impact on the business models involved, by improving the understanding of roles, structure and, ideally, risks. This work contributes by providing an integrated overview of business model representations and examines if ecosystem risk analysis is supported, thus providing researchers and practitioners with a deeper insight into suitable tools for understanding digital platform ecosystems and the business models involved.

**Keywords:** Business model · Ecosystem strategy · Digital platform

## 1 Motivation

Digital platforms co-create value directly or indirectly and form complex networks of innovation, where business models intersect and interoperate across different players, calling for richer models that delineate interdependent ecosystems [1]. The complexity of platform ecosystems calls for models and software tools to better understand their structure and dynamics, as well as their impact on business models [2]. Previous works in different domains have proposed business model representations (BMR) to understand business models and ecosystems. Some BMR allow for the analysis of ecosystem roles and structure. However, an ecosystem strategy also includes a view on ecosystem risks [3]. Previous comprehensive literature reviews on this topic have provided a synthesizing framework and overview of existing BMR [4] as well as classified these according to the cognitive functions and the phases of the business innovation process they support [5]. However, BMR haven't been held up against criteria for analyzing ecosystems. Thus, the purpose of this work is, apart from updating and extending previous reviews on BMR and integrating both existing classification frameworks, to examine if existing BMR allow the analysis of ecosystem risks (i.e. research question). To achieve the latter, we derive criteria from [3] and find that despite the many BMR available, only one partially meets the criteria proposed.

M. Themistocleous and P. Rupino da Cunha (Eds.): EMCIS 2018, LNBIP 341, pp. 464–472, 2019.
https://doi.org/10.1007/978-3-030-11395-7_36

## 2  Theoretical Background

As many industries have moved towards value creation in value networks, the modeling tools used by practitioners and researchers have evolved to analyze the increased amount of firms involved in value creation [6]. Researchers use BMR to model and analyze ecosystems as well as understand the business models involved. BMR are a mix of textual and graphical elements, or a (more or less) formalized ontology [7]. BMR are tools for improving understanding [8], analysis [9], experimentation [10, 11] and for defining underlying information systems requirements [9, 11]. Classification frameworks for BMR have been proposed for ontologies [12], to provide a comprehensive overview [4], to differentiate between environmental and internal concepts [13], to differentiate types of value [14], flows and decision variables, and to differentiate content views and graphical forms [5]. [15] describes ecosystems as interacting organizations and individuals which coevolve their capabilities and roles, and tend to align themselves with the direction set by one or more central companies that enable members to move toward shared visions to align their investments, and to find mutually supportive roles. Also, [16] describe a shift in different industries from hierarchical, integrated supply chains to fragmented networks of strategic partnerships. More recently, [3] argues that for an ecosystem to be successful (i.e. Pareto equilibrium) partners need to be aligned and that strategies to approach alignment should not only be defined by structure and roles but also around ecosystem risks, namely co-innovation and adoption chain risks. In information systems literature, value creation in ecosystems is described in the context of IT enabled business models (e.g. [17]) and, in particular, multisided digital platforms. [1] argue that companies such as Google, Apple or Facebook use multisided business models to capture value from information involving the coordination of business models in networks of developers and content providers.

[18] also shows how cross-boundary industry disruptions can shift digitally enabled value networks to multisided platforms. In particular, a platform ecosystem is comprised by the core technical platform and the apps that complement it [2, 19].

## 3  Research Approach

To identify BMR, we build on the literature review carried out by [4] and perform a forward and a backward search. Querying Scopus, we went forward by searching for articles that cited the articles identified in [4]. Then we went backwards by reviewing the articles cited in the ones identified in the forward search. To narrow down the results, the keywords identified by [20] "business model representation", "business model ontology", "business modeling", and "conceptual model" were searched for in the abstracts. The query was limited to the subject areas of computer science, business, management and accounting as well as engineering and decision sciences. Although Scopus' results encompass only conference papers and journal articles, the backward search performed on query results led us to include cited books and dissertations in our review as well. The classification framework used provides an overview of BMR by integrating two previous frameworks used to classify BMR. [4] provide a comprehensive classification framework with the dimensions of reach, perspective, notation principle and tool support of BMR. The reach differentiates between layers: strategy, business model and process layer. The perspective can be either a single view or multiple views depending on specific aspects of a business model. The notation principle can be either map-based, like a spatially structured template, or network based, with different graphical notations depending on the concept. Finally, the BMR can be either just a formalization, or already implemented as a design or even a financial evaluation tool. Since we are not only interested in financial evaluation, but rather in experimentation-enabled innovation in general, we additionally categorize using the term "other evaluation" to include other types of analyses as well. [5] review BMR from a cognitive perspective. The authors propose a classification framework according to the information transmitted (content) and the graphic form of BMR, to identify which ones are more suitable, depending on the phase in the business model innovation process. The dimension content is categorized in an elements', transaction and a causal view. The dimension graphic form is, in turn, categorized in brainstorming webs, conceptual maps and graphic organizers. The business model innovation phases ideation, initiation and integration, [5] argue, are best supported, respectively, by brainstorming webs with an elements view, by conceptual maps with causal or transactional views, and by graphic organizers with an elements view. Further, firms in ecosystems define their ecosystem strategy around a vision of structure, roles, and activity-based risks that arise from the partners' ability to undertake new activities (co-innovation) and from their willingness to adopt an innovation (adoption chain) [3]. The novelty of this work is therefore to introduce a new dimension to complement the previous synthesizing frameworks. This dimension aims at assessing the usefulness of a BMR in evaluating ecosystem risks and thus analyzing ecosystems. We categorize this dimension in activity configuration, to examine if partner dependence is explicit at this level, as well as co-innovation and adoption risks. Next, we only focus our analysis and discussions on those BMR that have been implemented as an analysis software tool, which is needed to deal with the complexity, reduce uncertainty and enable experimentation.

## 4  Analysis and Discussion

Table 1 shows the identified BMR that have been implemented as software tools, sorted chronologically. Although the table shows few BMR have software tool support for design and financial analysis, and limited possibilities to evaluate ecosystem strategy as proposed by [3], it allows to identify BMR that could be used to analyze of digital platform ecosystems. Only SimulValor [14] allows a financial evaluation that considers also strategic decisions. This BMR is suitable for the initiation phase of business model innovation. We expected that, as platform ecosystems and the way the firms involved strategically approach it, have become increasingly relevant for the business models involved, ecosystem risks would somehow be supported by existing BMR. To find out if BMR can be effectively used in a context such as digital platform ecosystems or not, we built on recent theory developments that point at ecosystem risks as one of the main components of ecosystem strategy. [4] had already shown which

**Table 1.** Business model representations with software tool, classified following [3–5].

| | Layer reach | | | Perspective | | Content view | | Notation | | | Graphic form | | Software tool support | | | | | Ecosystem risks | | |
|---|---|---|---|---|---|---|---|---|---|---|---|---|---|---|---|---|---|---|---|---|
| | Strategy | Business | Process | Single view | Multiple view | Elements | Transactional | Causal | Map | Network | Graph. orgzr. | Brainst. web | Concept. map | Formalization | Design | Fin. eval. | Other eval. | Interfirm act. | Co-innov. | Adptn. chain |
| e3-value [22] | X | X | | X | | X | X | | | X | | | X | X | X | X | X | | | |
| Eriksson-Penker business extensions [11] | | X | X | | X | X | X | | | X | | | X | X | X | X | | | | |
| Description model for internet-based business models [23] | | X | | X | | X | X | | X | X | X | | X | X | X | | | | | |
| SimulValor [21] | | X | | | X | X | | X | | X | | | X | X | X | X | X | | | |
| Reference ontology for business models [24] | X | X | | | X | X | | X | | X | | | X | X | X | | | | | |
| Strategic business model ontology [25] | X | X | | | X | X | | X | | X | | | | X | X | | | | | |
| Business model system dynamics modules [26] | | X | | | X | X | | X | | X | | | X | X | | | X | | | |
| Business models for e-government [27] | X | X | | X | | X | X | | X | | | | X | X | X | X | X | | | |

(continued)

**Table 1.** (*continued*)

| | Layer reach | | | Perspective | | Content view | | Notation | | | Graphic form | | | Software tool support | | | | Ecosystem risks | | |
|---|---|---|---|---|---|---|---|---|---|---|---|---|---|---|---|---|---|---|---|---|
| | Strategy | Business | Process | Single view | Multiple view | Elements | Transactional | Causal | Map | Network | Graph. orgzr. | Brainst. web | Concept. map | Formalization | Design | Fin. eval. | Other eval. | Interfirm act. | Co-innov. | Adpln. chain |
| Service value network structure [28] | | | | | | | | | | | | | | | | | | | | |
| Dynamic structure of business models [29] | | X | | X | | | | X | | X | | | X | X | X | X | X | | | |
| Business model canvas [30] | | X | | X | | X | | | X | | X | | | X | X | | | | | |
| Resource-event-agent [31] | | X | | | X | | X | | | X | | | X | X | X | | | | | |
| [moby] Business Model Ontology [32] | | X | | | X | X | | X | | X | X | | X | X | X | X | | | | |
| e3-value + Real Options [20] | | X | | X | | X | X | | | X | | | X | X | | X | X | | | |
| DYNAMOD [33] | | X | | X | | | | X | X | | | | X | X | | | X | | | |
| Modified SimulValor [14] | X | X | | X | | X | X | X | | X | | | X | X | X | | X | X | | |

(*continued*)

**Table 1.** (*continued*)

| | Layer reach | | | Perspective | | Content view | | Notation | | | Graphic form | | | Software tool support | | | | Ecosystem risks | | |
|---|---|---|---|---|---|---|---|---|---|---|---|---|---|---|---|---|---|---|---|---|
| | Strategy | Business | Process | Single view | Multiple view | Elements | Transactional | Causal | Map | Network | Graph. orgzr. | Brainst. web | Concept. map | Formalization | Design | Fin. eval. | Other eval. | Interfirm act. | Co-innov. | Adptn. chain |
| Business model magic triangle [34] | | X | | X | | X | | | X | | X | | | X | X | | | | | |
| Business model extract in the system dynamics notation [35] | | X | | | X | X | | X | X | X | | | X | X | | X | X | | | |
| Dynamic business model canvas [36] | | X | | | X | X | X | X | X | X | X | | X | X | X | | X | | | |
| Value-based process model design [37] | | X | X | | X | X | X | | | X | | | X | X | X | X | X | | | |

BMR could be used for structure and roles, while [5] showed which ones to use when in the business model innovation process. Ecosystem risks could be either explicit concepts in each BMR, or one could make them so, if dependencies to partners were explicit at the activity or transaction level. This is currently only partly supported by the modifications made to SimulValor [21] by [14] in the form of explicit activity-level partner interdependence.

## 5  Summary and Outlook

We believe modified SimulValor [14] could serve as a conceptual basis to incorporate ecosystem risk analysis, maybe in combination with other BMR. Also, the overview provided can be used to identify BMR that best suit a certain alignment or innovation phase, to conceptually extend it, or even implement ecosystem risk analysis as a software tool. In order to assess ecosystem risks, existent BMR could be enhanced, maybe based on the logic proposed by [14]. Possible candidates from an alignment perspective could be business extensions [11], business engineering meta model [38] or e3-value [22] (already extended by [20, 37, 39]). Future research could extend existing concepts of a BMR such as e3-value to include ecosystem risk analysis. This kind of ecosystem analysis, complementary to structure and roles analysis, can be used to better assess the impact of business model designs on a platform ecosystem and vice versa. Therefore, we propose that ecosystem risks be included as a new determinant of the performance of a business model (representation) in the case of a digital platform. Software tools that support the analysis of the impact of interdependence on profit or value could be implemented using simulation methods such as system dynamics, discrete event or agent-based simulation. Simulation methods could thus be used to analyze alignment between firms. BMR can support the analysis at the strategy, business model and business processes level. From an ecosystem perspective, ecosystem roles can be analyzed using some of the ontologies underlying BMR. Ecosystem structure can be analyzed using positions and links of BMR in the graphic form of conceptual maps. While the analysis of roles and positions can help to identify gaps in partner expectations, the analysis of ecosystem risks could improve ecosystem analysis and therefore the odds of success in aligning the partners, thus creating the necessary conditions for an ecosystem to thrive. Nevertheless, An important limitation of this work is the fact that we heavily rely on the work of [3] for the criteria against which we hold up the BMR we identified, even though other authors (e.g. [19]) also see the need to deal with these same risks. This means further criteria to assess the suitability of BMR for platform ecosystem risks, or further analyses, could be used. This could extend current theory on digital platform ecosystems and contribute to their understanding. The extension of the ontology of a BMR could be a first, rather formal step in this direction. As mentioned above, most of the approaches are informal, semi-formal at best. So, formal semantics, theorems and proofs are still needed to increase rigor with axioms.

# References

1. Bharadwaj, A., El Sawy, O.A., Pavlou, P.A., Venkatraman, N.: Digital business strategy: toward a next generation of insights. MIS Q. **37**, 471–482 (2013)
2. de Reuver, M., Sørensen, C., Basole, R.C.: The digital platform: a research agenda. J. Inf. Technol. **33**, 1–12 (2017)
3. Adner, R.: Ecosystem as structure: an actionable construct for strategy. J. Manag. **43**, 39–58 (2017)
4. Kundisch, D., John, T., Honnacker, J., Meier, C.: Approaches for business model representation: an overview. In: Mattfeld, D.C., Robra-Bissantz, S. (eds.) Multikonferenz Wirtschaftsinformatik, pp. 1839–1850. TU Braunschweig, Braunschweig (2012)
5. Täuscher, K., Abdelkafi, N.: Visual tools for business model innovation: recommendations from a cognitive perspective. Creat. Innov. Manag. **26**, 160–174 (2017)
6. Krcmar, H., Böhm, M., Friesike, S., Schildhauer, T.: Innovation, Society and Business: Internet-Based Business Models and their Implications. Berlin (2012)
7. Zott, C., Amit, R., Massa, L.: The business model: recent developments and future research. J. Manag. **37**, 1019–1042 (2011)
8. Osterwalder, A.: The Business Model Ontology a Proposition in a Design Science Approach (2004)
9. Gordijn, J., Akkermans, J.M.: Value-based requirements eengineering: exploring innovative e-commerce ideas. Requir. Eng. **8**, 114–134 (2003)
10. Chesbrough, H.: Business model innovation: opportunities and barriers. Long Range Plann. **43**, 354–363 (2010)
11. Eriksson, H., Penker, M.: Business Modeling with UML (2000)
12. Gordijn, J., Osterwalder, A., Pigneur, Y.: Comparing two business model ontologies for designing e-business models and value constellations. In: Proceedings of 18th Bled eConference eIntegration in Action, Bled, p. 17 (2005)
13. Burkhart, T., et al.: A comprehensive approach towards the structural description of business models. In: Proceedings of the International Conference on Management of Emergent Digital EcoSystems, pp. 88–102. ACM (2012)
14. Daaboul, J., Castagna, P., Da Cunha, C., Bernard, A.: Value network modelling and simulation for strategic analysis: a discrete event eimulation approach. Int. J. Prod. Res. **52**, 5002–5020 (2014)
15. Moore, J.F.: The Death of Competition: Leadership and Strategy in the Age of Business Ecosystems. HarperCollins, New York (1996)
16. Bitran, G., Gurumurthi, S., Sam, S.L.: The Need for Third-Party Coordination in Supply Chain Governance (2007)
17. Rai, A., Tang, X.: Information technology-enabled business models: a conceptual framework and a coevolution perspective for future research. Inf. Syst. Res. **25**, 1–14 (2014)
18. Pagani, M.: Digital business strategy and value creation: framing the dynamic cycle of control points. MIS Q. **37**, 617–632 (2013)
19. Tiwana, A.: Platform Ecosystems: Aligning Architecture, Governance, and Strategy. Morgan Kaufmann, Waltham (2014)
20. Kundisch, D., John, T.: Business model representation incorporating real options: an extension of e3-value. In: 2012 45th Hawaii International Conference on System Sciences, Hawaii, pp. 4456–4465. IEEE (2012)
21. Elhamdi, M.: Modélisation et Simulation de Chaînes de Valeurs en Entreprise – Une Approche Dynamique des Systèmes et Aide à la Décision: SimulValor (2005)

22. Gordijn, J., Akkermans, H.: e3-value: design and evaluation of e-business models. IEEE Intell. Syst. **16**, 11–17 (2001). https://doi.org/10.1109/5254.941353
23. Breuer, S.: Beschreibung von Geschäftsmodellen Internetbasierter Unternehmen - Konzeption, Umsetzung, Anwendung (2004)
24. Andersson, B., et al.: Towards a common ontology for business models. In: CEUR Workshop Proceedings 200 (2006). https://doi.org/10.1007/11901181
25. Samavi, R., Yu, E., Topaloglou, T.: Strategic reasoning about business models: a conceptual modeling approach. Inf. Syst. E-Bus. Manag. **7**, 171–198 (2008)
26. Grasl, O.: Business Model Analysis - Method and Case Studies (2009)
27. Peinel, G., Jarke, M., Rose, T.: Business models for egovernment services. Electron. Gov. An Int. J. **7**, 380–401 (2010)
28. Kijl, B., Nieuwenhuis, B.: Deploying a telerehabilitation service innovation: an early stage business model engineering approach. In: 43rd Hawaii International Conference on System Sciences (2010)
29. Lerch, C., Selinka, G.: Dynamics of business models: long-ranging impact assessment of business models in the capital goods industry. In: The 28th International Conference of the System Dynamics Society, Seoul, p. 13 (2010)
30. Osterwalder, A., Pigneur, Y.: Business Model Generation. Wiley, New York (2010)
31. Sonnenberg, C., Huemer, C., Hofreiter, B., Mayrhofer, D., Braccini, A.: The REA-DSL: a domain specific modeling language for business models. In: Mouratidis, H., Rolland, C. (eds.) CAiSE 2011. LNCS, vol. 6741, pp. 252–266. Springer, Heidelberg (2011). https://doi.org/10.1007/978-3-642-21640-4_20
32. Weiner, N., Weisbecker, A.: A business model framework for the design and evaluation of business models in the internet of services. In: Annual SRII Global Conference, San Jose, pp. 21–33 (2011)
33. Zutshi, A., Grilo, A., Jardim-Goncalves, R.: DYNAMOD: a modelling framework for digital businesses based on agent based modeling. In: 2013 IEEE International Conference on Industrial Engineering and Engineering Management, pp. 1372–1376 (2013)
34. Gassmann, O., Frankenberger, K., Csik, M.: The St. Gallen business model navigator. Int. J. Prod. Dev. **18**, 249–273 (2013)
35. Groesser, S.N., Jovy, N.: Business model analysis using computational modeling: a strategy tool for exploration and decision-making. J. Manag. Control **27**, 61–88 (2016)
36. Cosenz, F.: Supporting start-up business model design through system dynamics modelling. Manag. Decis. **55**, 57–80 (2017)
37. Hotie, F., Gordijn, J.: Value-based process model design. Bus. Inf. Syst. Eng. **59**, 18 (2017)
38. Österle, H., Blessing, D.: Business engineering modell. In: Österle, H., Winter, R. (ed.) Business Engineering, pp. 65–85. Springer, Heidelberg (2003). https://doi.org/10.1007/978-3-642-19003-2_4
39. Weigand, H., Johannesson, P., Andersson, B., Bergholtz, M., Edirisuriya, A., Ilayperuma, T.: Strategic analysis using value modeling-the c3-value approach. In: 2007 40th Annual Hawaii International Conference on System Sciences, p. 175c (2007)

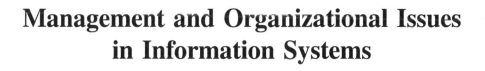

# Management and Organizational Issues
# in Information Systems

# Strategy in the Making: Assessing the Execution of a Strategic Information Systems Plan

José-Ramón Rodríguez[✉], Robert Clarisó,
and Josep Maria Marco-Simó

Universitat Oberta de Catalunya (UOC), Barcelona, Spain
{jrodriguezber, rclariso, jmarco}@uoc.edu

**Abstract.** Recent research on IT Strategy is in a phase of renewal, after a long period of static formal comprehensive planning. Currently, more importance is given to incremental continuous planning, program implementation and organizational learning, what has been labeled as strategy as practice. However, less attention has been paid to the evaluation of the implementation process and results.

In this paper, we introduce an exploratory approach for assessing the implementation of IT Strategic planning, based in the combination and iteration of different methods. It is grounded in an Action Design Research exercise recently made up at a leading on-line European university.

The assessment includes three major dimensions (strategy, performance and governance), extracted from the academic and professional research. Its application to this context through a varied scaffolding of methods, tools and techniques, that is summarized in the article, seems robust, able to work out with the business and IT senior stakeholders and allows a quick deployment, even in a complex institutional environment.

We propose further research in order to extend and validate this model through its implementation and evaluation in different contexts, selecting new variables and metrics, developing improved maturity frameworks and repeating the exercise on a periodical basis.

**Keywords:** Strategic information systems plan · IT strategy evaluation
IT strategy implementation · Higher Education

## 1 Introduction

IT Strategy formulation (more specifically Strategic Information System Planning or SISP) is living a period of far reaching renewal, both in its content and in the processes of strategy making [53]. This is due to the convergence of business and IT strategies in a new brand Digital Transformation [11] and to the consolidation of the "strategy as practice" school [43, 61]. Strategy is now considered an ongoing social process and literature has experienced a shift towards "the realities of strategy formation" [31] (p. 372), such as incremental planning, program implementation, strategy evaluation and organizational learning. But, over this evolution not much interest has been paid to

© Springer Nature Switzerland AG 2019
M. Themistocleous and P. Rupino da Cunha (Eds.): EMCIS 2018, LNBIP 341, pp. 475–488, 2019.
https://doi.org/10.1007/978-3-030-11395-7_37

IS strategy implementation by itself, let alone the evaluation of the implementation process and results [3, 55].

This article is a part of a broader practice-oriented research on the process of Strategy making in the Universitat Oberta de Catalunya (UOC), a foremost European on-line institution. The implementation of its SISP (named Information Systems Master Plan or ISMP) [46] has been recently evaluated and the Plan is being updated nowadays. The researcher is a member of the leading team of the project, in an Action Design Research mode [50]. The piece presented here collects the process, methods and outcomes of the evaluation phase (we prefer the term "assessment").

Our working hypothesis is that evaluating the implementation of the strategy planning on a periodical basis, if properly conducted, executed and communicated, is crucial (a) to attain the results of the intended strategies, (b) to adapt and update them to emerging threats and opportunities, (c) to ensure common understanding and ownership of information systems between business and IT and (d) to ensure organizational learning and transformation, this latter being one of the most compelling challenges in an academic institution [10]. Our aim is to validate existing models of IT Strategy evaluation in complex organizations, to provide novel insights and to contribute to the development of better approaches and methods.

On the following pages we summarize in Sect. 2 relevant research in the field of assessment of the execution of a SISP. Section 3 provides basic information of the setting of the research, i.e., the institution and the status and contents of the ISMP. Section 4 presents the research approach, methods and tools and Sect. 5 highlights the main results of the evaluation process. Finally, Sect. 6 concludes with discussion and proposals for researchers and practitioners.

# 2 Related Research

The study of SISP has attracted considerable scholar attention since the 1980s. On the grounds of reported lack of implementation or severe implementation problems of IT Strategy planning, some papers were issued intended to identify prescriptions and critical factors for better strategy formulation [19, 23, 27, 36, 39, 51, 54]. Nevertheless, much less interest has been paid to IS strategy implementation by itself, and even less to the evaluation of the implementation process and results, which is the focus of this work [12, 13, 15, 16, 20, 22, 24, 37, 48, 55, 59].

In 2008, Teubner and Mocker [55] studied a sample of 434 papers published in major MIS journals between 1977 and 2001. Of those, only 21 were related to implementation. Although with a different methodology, in 2013, Amrollahi et al. [3] found 9 papers on implementation and 8 papers on evaluation, out of 102 papers on SISP published between 2000 and 2009. Following this thread, we retrieved and analyzed some more recent ones. Most of them describe comprehensive SISP methods put into practice in individual settings, with a special consideration to implementation and evaluation issues as compared to former literature constructs: they thoroughly document the development phases, process and techniques, people and organizational interactions and, to a lesser extent, the measurement of success [4, 33, 62].

**Table 1.** Dimensions of assessment

| Dimension | Key concepts | Main references |
|---|---|---|
| Strategy | Alignment | Henderson and Venkatraman [28], Chan and Reich [14], Juiz and Toomey [32] |
| | Intended and realized strategies | Mintzberg and Waters [41], Chan et al. [13], Vaara and Whittington [58] |
| Performance | Benefits realization | Ambrosini et al. [2], Parker et al. [42], Ashurts et al. [5], Hunter et al. [29], Ward and Daniel [60] |
| | Program execution | Thiry [56], Meskendahl [40], Kopmann et al. [35] |
| Governance | Stakeholders satisfaction | Galliers [22], DeLone and McNeal [17, 18], Gable et al. [21], Petter et al. [44] |
| | Program management and governance | Bartenschlager et al. [8], Thiry [56], Isaca [30] |

Interestingly, some of the latest are Case and Action Research studies in the Higher Education industry [7, 34, 52].

Salmela and Spil [47] proposed a framework of "cycles" and "choices" of planning that could be flexibly adapted to the needs, the context ant the maturity of each organization and could be improved and refined over time. Taking that approach, we selected from the analysis of the academic and professional literature and discussed with the Customer[1], a model of assessment aimed to evaluate the main achievements and pitfalls over the execution of the Plan, to update the Plan accordingly with new business priorities and to improve its governance. From these considerations and other of practical nature (available information, coordination costs, time-frame), we chose three major dimensions of analysis and two categories of key concepts for each dimension (Table 1). The application of these concepts into specific methods is shown in Sects. 4 and 5 of this article.

# 3 Research Setting

The UOC is the oldest fully online University in the world. Founded in 1995, it now enrolls 75.000 students, 300 full-time professors and 3.000 associate part-time professors, provides 57 graduate programs and runs a budget of 98.8 M€. It operates within a public-private funding and governance regime, in a highly-regulated environment. The current governing board, appointed in 2013, designed an ambitious growth and transformation strategy [57], of which the ISMP for the period 2014 to 2018 was an instrumental part. The annual budget allocated to the Plan is about 3 M€, out of a total IT budget of 7.8 M€. The IS department (reporting to the Chief Operations Officer) has 49 internal and 79 external full-time employees.

---

[1] In this context, "Customer" is the usual term used in Action Research [9].

The IT expenditure vs. revenue and the weight of the strategic or transformational projects within the portfolio of IT assets is remarkable and could be well compared with the figures of digital industries [26], such as software and Internet services. The fact of being a pure digital player makes critical for the UOC the effective exploitation of information technologies in the global and rapidly evolving market of Higher Education and long life learning [1, 6, 25, 38, 45, 49].

The ISMP was structured in 10 strategic initiatives (meaning collections of programs and projects aimed to a single business objective) and 42 individual projects to be deployed over a period of 4 years (2015–2018). Since its inception, the ISMP was designed as (a) a top-down transformation program, (b) addressed to renovate the core business applications and the technology infrastructure base, (c) ruled by the top management and (d) led and executed by the CIO (Chief Information Officer), (e) with the support of a Program Office [46]. Table 2 shows the major strategic initiatives that make up the Plan.

**Table 2.** Content of the Information Systems Master Plan (ISMP)

| | |
|---|---|
| 1 | Customer and community relationships management |
| 2 | Learning management environment and learning applications |
| 3 | Mobile first: responsive web site and mobile apps environment |
| 4 | Enterprise data management |
| 5 | Student information system |
| 6 | Administration support (finance, human capital, other) |
| 7 | Technology architecture and migration to the cloud |
| 8 | User experience transformation |
| 9 | Digital empowerment and change management |
| 10 | Security and data privacy |

The assessment process studied in this paper was carried out in the Summer of 2017. To conduct this effort and to prepare a proposal for the Executive Board of the University, a Steering Committee (SC) and a project team (PT) were settled. A researcher in IS was commissioned by the University as the project co-leader, took part in most of the workshops and meetings and carried out personally individual interviews with prominent members of the management and the faculty. This latter commission was made explicit, both as a support to the management and as an Action Research exercise. The researcher was able to work with scientific rigor, freedom of action and independence but his proposals regarding the method had to be adapted to the available information and the organizational context, within a demanding time-frame. An organization chart of the project is shown in Table 3.

**Table 3.** Project organization

| Group | Role | Members |
|---|---|---|
| Steering committee (SC) | Discuss and approve final and intermediate outcomes Raise proposals to the executive board of the university | CEO, Vice-chancellor of learning, COO, CFO, dean of the computer science school, leader of the PMO, researcher |
| Project team (PT) | Gather and analyze data and documents, prepare and lead meetings and workshops, summarize conclusions and write reports and presentations | Project office of the ISMP (PMO), IT demand manager, researcher |
| Project sponsors | Secure time and resources Communicate and act in favor of the project | COO, CIO |
| Project co-leaders | Plan, monitor and execute tasks Prepare final deliverables | Head of the PMO, researcher |
| Researcher | Proposes methods and professional and scientific references Co-leads the project team Runs top individual interviews | Lecturer and researcher in IS management at the computer science department |

# 4   Research Methods

The overall framework of this research is an Action Design Research [50] approach. Under this paradigm, a toolkit combining different techniques and tools methods was proposed for the deployment of the assessment. For example, a case study stance was taken to better understand the original ISMP and the changes produced over time. A quantitative and qualitative independent survey was ordered to better capture the satisfaction and feedback of the major stakeholders. The different work streams are correlated and the process works through a number of iterations. The timing, the content and the setting of individual and group interactions over the project were critical, as it was their preparation through previous analysis of the bulk of materials produced by the Program office and the project leaders. A summary of this toolkit is shown in Table 4. The assessment was completed in ten weeks. Forty two people of different ranks (mainly top and middle managers) took part, with an estimated effort of 800 man hours.

To complete our research purposes, an additional round of in-depth reflective interviews with members of the PT, the sponsors and the SC were conducted between October and December of 2017.

# 5   Results

Next, we will show the main results of the assessment process, arranged according the different dimensions (Table 1) and work streams (Table 4).

**Table 4.** Research methods

|  | Strategy | Performance | Governance |
|---|---|---|---|
| Key concepts | Alignment. Deliberate and emergent strategies | Program and project execution Benefits realization | Satisfaction of key stakeholders Program and IT Governance |
| Input and sources | Business strategic plan (2014–2020) Original IS Master Plan case study PMO execution reports | PMO execution reports KPI standard inventories of IT impact Management reporting | Online survey to managers and key users (115 respondents) Individual interviews to executives (23) (Source: report by external evaluator) |
| Process | Qualified impact matrix Overall analysis (2 iterations) Semi-structured interviews with top management (11) | Structured workshops with executives and managers for feedback and analysis (12) Lessons learned workshop (1) and individual reports | Results included for discussion and refinement in top management interviews and workshops Internal discussion with sponsors and project steering committee |
| Participants | Members of the Project Steering Committee Members of the board of executive directors | Business executives and managers (28) IT Project Leaders (15) | All |
| Outcome | Summary of conclusions | Individual summary per project (10) Prioritized issue map for project leaders Summary of conclusions | Summary of key values and major qualitative Conclusions |
| Timeframe | June 15$^{th}$–July 30th 2017 | July 15$^{th}$–Sept. 30th 2017 | Survey: Feb. 2017 Further analysis: Sept. 2017 |

## 5.1   Strategy

**Strategic Alignment:** The main business objectives were grouped into six categories, and rated in five levels of compliance, according to the potential vs. actual impact of each IT strategic initiative against each category. An impact matrix was prepared and discussed with the project team and the results were presented in a radar chart. The most successful initiatives were related with "process standardization", "productivity and collaboration" and "flexibility to compete", as compared to lower results in "excellence in research" and "student orientation" (Fig. 1). Actually, those project related with the academic and academic support units show lower level of execution and higher deviations than the rest.

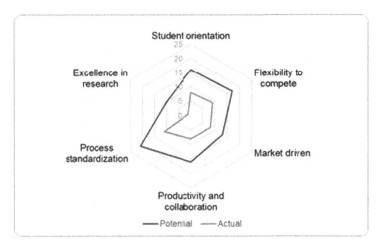

**Fig. 1.** Strategic alignment

It may be said that the most relevant contribution of IT over this period has been to enable growth and provide scale advantages, by delivering technical infrastructure and business process support to serve more than double the number of students enrolled and almost triple the program offering, keeping constant the operational fixed costs. This seemed more than satisfying to the opinion of the SC.

**Intended and Realized Strategies:** This dimension is related with the difference between the projects included in the plan and the ones which were effectively executed. The difference amounts to 2.1 M€ in a list of nine large projects, out of a total expenditure of 8.3 M€ in 23 large projects. Two of those unplanned schemes are related to major business shifts, as the change of the branding concept and image and the new multimedia format of learning materials. Those decisions were made by the Board of Executive Directors. Some other changes were related with mandatory legal issues or management style and preferences of newly arrived top executives. It may be said that the organization showed flexibility to adapt to major strategic changes, at the expense of a significant budgetary deviation and a lower execution of some planned projects. This observation deserved mixed judgment among the members of the SC.

## 5.2    Performance

**Program Execution:** We applied here the conventional "iron triangle" that compares the baselines of scope, time and cost with the realized outcomes. It explains the deviations within each planned project, not the emergence of new projects, that was explained in the former paragraph. For the scope dimension we broke down each major program into individual projects and each project into separate phases and milestones. The results showed an execution level of 89.0% in scope. The deviation in budget was of 14.2%. Major factors affecting execution were discussed within the team and with

**Table 5.** Factors affecting execution

| Positive | Negative |
|---|---|
| Well defined business strategy and needs | Slow public tendering procedures |
| Strong and dedicated leadership of business managers | Large cross departmental projects, especially those involving the faculty |
| Clear technological solution | Underestimation of integration and migration costs |

the project leaders. Results are shown in Table 5. The execution of the planned projects of the ISMP seemed very satisfying for the SC.

**Benefits Realization:** Of all the dimensions of analysis, this one was the least familiar and most difficult to acquire for the teams, be IT or business. It was also the most interesting to share with mid-level managers, since it allows to improve the quality and effectiveness of the dialogue between the two parties.

For its preparation, we first took several libraries of standard benefits coming from professional and academic sources (see Table 1), then selected a list for each major project and asked the IT project leaders to make a first review. Later we went to the administrative and faculty management teams to provide them with feedback on the program execution and open a discussion on the realization of benefits or specific performance impact and its measurement. In some cases, it was easy to identify key value indicators, find figures and establish a relationship with the program effectiveness. In others, it was not that easy. Table 6 provides some samples, separating those indicators which are suitable and measure value (left) versus those that only measure effort or activity (right).

### 5.3   Governance

**Key Stakeholder's Satisfaction:** The Customer ordered a quantitative and qualitative survey in February 2017 to an external provider, as a proxy to understand the awareness, acceptance and commitment of executives, managers and key users (senior referrals of IT in every functional area) about the ISMP. This survey was used as an input for discussion in the various forums of the project. The main results are summarized in Table 7.

Respondents, mainly among the facullty, show a relative low level of awareness of the design and execution of the program. Contribution to the corporate strategy gets better scores than the response to individual needs. The major complaints from mid-level management were related with lack of information and lack of response to demands of incremental improvements (evolutionary maintenance) of the current legacy systems. In our interviews, top business and IT management accepted these results as "expected", since the focus of the ISMP was precisely to renovate the core of the enterprise IT and to better respond to the corporate business strategy as compared to individual user demands. In any case, they acknowledged the risks of losing adherence to the ISMP among users, mainly academicians.

**Table 6.** Suitability of the definition of Key Performance Indicators (samples)

| KPIs measuring value | KPIs measuring effort/activity |
|---|---|
| Productivity and conversion rate of the call center | User experience improvements |
| Enrolments from target countries | Availability and accessibility of new services at the classroom |
| Increased multilingual portfolio | New mobile apps |
| Personnel per student ratio | New management dashboards |
| Regular users of Google Apps | Files managed with the new academic administration application |
| Time for processing the payroll | |
| Malicious IP addresses intercepted | Expenditure in cloud infrastructure |
| IT expenditure per student/personnel | Training sessions and tutorials |
| | New contingency platform |

**Table 7.** Key stakeholders satisfaction with the ISMP

| | Areas | | |
|---|---|---|---|
| Question | Administration | Teaching & research | Average |
| Awareness of the ISMP | 4.43 | 3.69 | 4.06 |
| Contribution of the ISMP to the corporate strategy | 5.07 | 4.50 | 4.78 |
| Contribution of the ISMP to the different functional areas | 5.02 | 4.05 | 4.53 |
| Contribution of the ISMP to | 4.64 | 3.88 | 4.26 |
| Information about the execution of the ISMP | 4.09 | 3.52 | 3.80 |
| Overall rating | 4.64 | 3.88 | 4.26 |

Values between 1 and 6 (higher is better). Respondents: 115. Response rate: 65%

**Program Governance and Management:** The execution of the ISMP was governed by a small Steering Committee, chaired by the Managing Director of the UOC. The Vice-Chancellor of Teaching participated in some sessions. The executive leadership was charged to a Program Office of two people and ten project leaders from the IT department, with a variable business counterpart for every project. The original governance model envisioned a broader picture with stronger involvement of the faculty. Nevertheless, during the implementation straight execution was preferred to greater participation. The satisfaction survey and individual and group interviews voiced complaints about lack of information regarding the priority setting mechanisms and the overall progress of the Plan.

When performing the "lessons learned" exercises with the IT project leaders, they highlighted lack of resources, lack of business involvement and resistance to change as the major pain issues. Table 8 shows the main conclusions.

**Table 8.** Lessons learned according to the IT project leaders

| Order | Issue | Value |
| --- | --- | --- |
| 1 | Lack of project leaders and managers | 15 |
| 2 | Lack of planning of business resources allocated to projects | 10 |
| 3 | Lack of project quality control end to end | 9 |
| 4 | Lack of business sponsorship, especially in cross-departmental projects | 7 |
| 5 | Poor project definition | 7 |
| 6 | Resistance to change when business process transformation is required | 6 |

Finally, when discussing project management issues with top business managers, some expressed concerns on the quality of the project control mechanisms and proposed to select and develop project managers by their leadership and managerial skills, not so much by their technical capabilities.

### 5.4 Overall Balance

After this review and the discussions with the different involved groups, the following conclusions were drawn regarding the perception of the stakeholders:

1. The ISMP is a valuable tool for setting priorities to transform the IT base and to increase the IT effectiveness, ensuring alignment and providing value.
2. The level of execution and the agility to adapt the Plan to new business priorities is also considered satisfying overall and has allowed the institution to support its objectives of growth.
3. The focus on the ISMP has been at the expense of the day to day demands of improvement of the existing legacy applications and tools.
4. The improvement of the corporate governance of IT is perceived as compulsory, with a major involvement of the faculty management leaders.
5. Better prioritization mechanisms, communication policies and project management processes and metrics should be put in place, to ensure shared commitment of the different constituencies.

This feedback is being taken into consideration for the update of the Plan and its governance mechanisms. It is worth to mention that some of the negative perceptions were considered predictable results and unavoidable collateral effects of the intended primal strategy as designed on the original ISMP.

## 6    Conclusions and Discussion

IT Strategy making, now in the form of building Digital Strategies, is a major concern for IT and business executives and managers. Implementation issues have been the common pitfalls of the practice and the focus of a part of the research. The current paradigm advocates for an ongoing social process of strategy formation or strategy as practice. This paper adheres to this stance. However, academic and professional literature has paid less attention to the evaluation of the implementation of IT strategies and the way to integrate that evaluation within a continuous and more agile Strategy planning.

This article, after an Action Design Research exercise, contains some elements to build up a method or artifact to conduct these type of reviews. According to the process and results, it seems to be a quick, effective and efficient approach, in agreement with our initial working hypothesis and the literature.

We have suggested to select three main dimensions of analysis: (1) Strategy (that observes strategic alignment and the response to emergent business strategies); (2) Performance (in terms of benefits realization and program execution); and (3) Governance (including the perception of major stakeholders and the mechanisms of decision making).

The assessment occurs in a short time-frame through intensive individual and group interactions. The governance, preparation, content, setting and selection of participants are all crucial. Additional reflective interviews are undertaken to better understand the process, results and consequences. It may be said that the process is part of the product: the overall outcome seems to be an improved understanding and commitment (a buy-in) of the top and middle managers to the Plan.

Regarding future work, the selection of variables and indicators and their measurement should be improved through further research and effective implementation. We initially suggest that a specific dimension related with organizational learning and deep business transformation should probably be better developed and integrated in the model.

Furthermore, those variables related with benefits realization need to be worked out within each specific context. An examination of various contexts of application and improved maturity models could facilitate better choices of analysis and intervention for both practitioners and researchers. We also plan to repeat the exercise periodically, to validate and improve this approach.

As regards the specific results of the analysis and its comparison with reported cases, that was not the aim of this piece of the research, but it may be also considered an interesting working line.

**Acknowledgement.** The authors would like to thank Dr. Carlos Juiz (Univ. Illes Balears) and Dr. Joan Antoni Pastor (Univ. Politecnica de Catalunya) for their valuable advice; Clara Belena, Eva Gil and Daniel Caballe, UOC project team members, for their relentless commitment; and Rafael Macau (COO) and Emili Rubio (CIO) for their active sponsorship of the project.

# References

1. Altbach, P.G.: Global Perspectives on Higher Education. JHU Press, Baltimore (2016)
2. Ambrosini, V., Johnson, G., Scholes, K.: Exploring Techniques of Analysis and Evaluation in Strategic Management. Prentice Hall Europe, Hemel Hempstead (1998)
3. Amrollahi, A., Ghapanchi, A.H., Talaei-Khoei, A.: A systematic literature review on strategic information systems planning: insights from the past decade. Pac. Asia J. Assoc. Inf. Syst. **5**(2), 4:1–4:28 (2013)

4. Arvidsson, V., Holmstrm, J., Lyytinen, K.: Information systems use as strategy practice: a multi-dimensional view of strategic information system implementation and use. J. Strat. Inf. Syst. **23**(1), 45–61 (2014)
5. Ashurst, C., Doherty, N.F., Peppard, J.: Improving the impact of IT development projects: the benefits realization capability model. Eur. J. Inf. Syst. **17**(4), 352–370 (2008)
6. Barber, M., Donnelly, K., Rizvi, S., Summers, L.: An avalanche is coming. High. Educ. Revolut. Ahead **73** (2013)
7. Barn, B.S., Clark, T., Hearne, G.: Business and ICT alignment in higher education: a case study in measuring maturity. In: Linger, H., Fisher, J., Barnden, A., Barry, C., Lang, M., Schneider, C. (eds.) Building Sustainable Information Systems. Springer, Boston, MA (2013). https://doi.org/10.1007/978-1-4614-7540-8_4
8. Bartenschlager, J., Goeken, M.: IT strategy implementation framework-bridging enterprise architecture and IT governance. In: AMCIS, p. 400 (2010)
9. Baskerville, R., Wood-Harper, A.T.: A taxonomy of action research methods. Institut for Informatik og Økonomistyring, Handelshøjskolen i København (1996)
10. Bates, A.W., Bates, T., Sangra, A.: Managing technology in higher education: strategies for transforming teaching and learning. Wiley, Hoboken (2011)
11. Bharadwaj, A., El Sawy, O.A., Pavlou, P.A., Venkatraman, N.V.: Digital business strategy: toward a next generation of insights. MIS Q. **37**(2), 471–482 (2013)
12. Brown, I.T.: Testing and extending theory in strategic information systems planning through literature analysis. Inf. Resour. Manag. J. **17**(4), 20 (2004)
13. Chan, Y.E., Huff, S.L., Copeland, D.G.: Assessing realized information systems strategy. J. Strat. Inf. Syst. **6**(4), 273–298 (1997)
14. Chan, Y.E., Reich, B.H.: IT alignment: what have we learned? J. Inf. Technol. **22**(4), 297–315 (2007)
15. Chen, D.Q., Mocker, M., Preston, D.S., Teubner, A.: Information systems strategy: reconceptualization, measurement, and implications. MIS Q. **34**(2), 233–259 (2010)
16. da Cunha, P.R., de Figueiredo, A.D.: Information systems development as flowing wholeness. In: Russo, N.L., Fitzgerald, B., DeGross, J.I. (eds.) Realigning Research and Practice in Information Systems Development. ITIFIP, vol. 66, pp. 29–48. Springer, Boston, MA (2001). https://doi.org/10.1007/978-0-387-35489-7_3
17. DeLone, W.H., McLean, E.R.: Information systems success: the quest for the dependent variable. Inf. Syst. Res. **3**(1), 60–95 (1992)
18. DeLone, W.H., McLean, E.R.: The DeLone and McLean model of infor-mation systems success: a ten-year update. J. Manag. Inf. Syst. **19**(4), 9–30 (2003)
19. Doherty, N.F., Marples, C.G., Suhaimi, A.: The relative success of alternative approaches to strategic information systems planning: an empirical analysis. J. Strat. Inf. Syst. **8**(3), 263–283 (1999)
20. Earl, M.J.: Experiences in strategic information systems planning. MIS Q 1–24 (1993)
21. Gable, G.G., Sedera, D., Chan, T.: Re-conceptualizing information system success: the IS-impact measurement model. J. Assoc. Inf. Syst. **9**(7), 377 (2008)
22. Galliers, R.: Information systems planning in the United Kingdom and Australia: a comparison of current practice. Oxford University Press (1987)
23. Galliers, R.D.: Strategic information systems planning: myths, reality and guidelines for successful implementation. Eur. J. Inf. Syst. **1**(1), 55–64 (1991)
24. Gottschalk, P.: Strategic information systems planning: the IT strategy implementation matrix. Eur. J. Inf. Syst. **8**(2), 107–118 (1999)
25. Grajek, S., et al.: Top 10 IT Issues, 2018: The Remaking of Higher Education. Educause Review, January–February (2018)

26. Hall, L., Stegman, E., Futela, S., Gupta, D.: IT Key Metrics Data 2018: Key Industry Measures: Software Publishing and Internet Services Analysis: Multiyear. ID: G00341764. Gartner (2017)
27. Hartono, E., Lederer, A.L., Sethi, V., Zhuang, Y.: Key predictors of the implementation of strategic information systems plans. ACM SIGMIS: Database Adv. Inf. Syst. **34**(3), 41–53 (2003)
28. Henderson, J.C., Venkatraman, H.: Strategic alignment: leveraging information technology for transforming organizations. IBM Syst. J. **32**(1), 472–484 (1993)
29. Hunter, R., et al.: A Simple Framework to Translate IT Benefits Into Business Value Impact. ID: G00156986. Gartner (2008, 2016)
30. Isaca, C.: Cobit 5 A Business Framework for the Governance and Management of Enterprise IT, 2013 ISACA (2014). ISBN: 1963669381
31. Johnson, G., Whittington, R., Scholes, K., Angwin, D., Regnr, P.: Exploring Strategy: Text and Cases, 11th edn. Pearson Education, London (2016)
32. Juiz, C., Toomey, M.: To govern IT, or not to govern IT? Commun. ACM **58**(2), 58–64 (2015)
33. Kamariotou, M., Kitsios, F.: Information systems phases and firm performance: a conceptual framework. In: Kavoura, A., Sakas, D., Tomaras, P. (eds.) Strategic Innovative Marketing, pp. 553–560. Springer, Cham (2017). https://doi.org/10.1007/978-3-319-33865-1_67
34. Kirinic, V., Kozina, M.: Maturity assessment of strategy implementation in higher education institution. In: Central European Conference on Information and Intelligent Systems, p. 169. Faculty of Organization and Informatics, Varazdin (2016)
35. Kopmann, J., Kock, A., Killen, C.P., Gemnden, H.G.: The role of project portfolio management in fostering both deliberate and emergent strategy. Int. J. Proj. Manag. **35**(4), 557–570 (2017)
36. Lederer, A., Sethi, V.: The implementation of strategic information systems planning methodologies. MIS Q. 445–461 (1988)
37. Lederer, A.L., Sethi, V.: Key prescriptions for strategic information systems planning. J. Manag. Inf. Syst. **13**(1), 35–62 (1996)
38. Lowendahl, J.M., Thayer, T.B., Morgan, G., Yanckello, R.A.: Top 10 Business Trends Impacting Higher Education in 2018. ID Paper G00343300. Gartner (2018)
39. Mentzas, G.: Implementing an IS strategy - a team approach. Long Range Plan. **30**(1), 84–95 (1997)
40. Meskendahl, S.: The influence of business strategy on project portfolio management and its success - a conceptual framework. Int. J. Proj. Manag. **28**(8), 807–817 (2010)
41. Mintzberg, H., Waters, J.A.: Of strategies, deliberate and emergent. Strat. Manag. J. **6**(3), 257–272 (1985)
42. Parker, M.M., Benson, R.J., Trainor, H.E.: Information Economics: Linking Business Performance to Information Technology. Prentice-Hall, New Jersey (1988)
43. Peppard, J., Galliers, R., Thorogood, A.: Information systems strategy as practice: micro strategy and strategizing for IS. J. Strat. Inf. Syst. **23**(1), 1–10 (2014)
44. Petter, S., DeLone, W., McLean, E.: Measuring information systems success: models, dimensions, measures, and interrelationships. Eur. J. Inf. Syst. **17**(3), 236–263 (2008)
45. Pucciarelli, F., Kaplan, A.: Competition and strategy in higher education: managing complexity and uncertainty. Bus. Horiz. **59**(3), 311–320 (2016)
46. Rodríguez, J.-R.: El Master Plan (Plan Director) de Sistemas de Informacion de la UOC. Caso Practico. PID_00248250. FUOC. Barcelona (2017)
47. Salmela, H., Spil, T.A.: Dynamic and emergent information systems strategy formulation and implementation. Int. J. Inf. Manag. **22**(6), 441–460 (2002)

48. Sambamurthy, V., Venkataraman, S., DeSanctis, G.: The design of information technology planning systems for varying organizational contexts. Eur. J. Inf. Syst. **2**(1), 23–35 (1993)
49. Sarkar, S.: The role of information and communication technology (ICT) in higher education for the 21st century. Science **1**(1), 30–41 (2012)
50. Sein, M.K., Henfridsson, O., Purao, S., Rossi, M., Lindgren, R.: Action design research. MIS Q 37–56 (2011)
51. Segars, A.H., Grover, V.: Strategic information systems planning success: an investigation of the construct and its measurement. MIS Q 139–163 (1998)
52. Soares, S., Setyohady, D.B.: Enterprise architecture modeling for oriental university in Timor Leste to support the strategic plan of integrated information system. In: 5th International Conference on Cyber and IT Service Management (CITSM), pp. 1–6. IEEE (2017)
53. Sutherland, A.R., Galliers, R.D.: The evolving information systems strategy information systems management and strategy formulation: applying and extending the stages of growth concept. In: Strategic Information Management: Challenges and Strategies in Managing Information Systems, pp. 47–77, Routledge (2014)
54. Teo, T.S., Ang, J.S.: An examination of major IS planning problems. Int. J. Inf. Manag. **21**(6), 457–470 (2001)
55. Teubner, R.A., Mocker, M.: A literature overview on strategic information systems planning. European Research Center for Information Systems Working Paper No. 6 (2008). revised 2012
56. Thiry, M.: Program Management, Gower (2010)
57. Universitat Oberta de Catalunya: Strategic Plan 2014–2020 (2016). https://www.uoc.edu/portal/_resources/EN/documents/la_universitat/uoc-strategic-plan-2014-2020.pdf
58. Vaara, E., Whittington, R.: Strategy-as-practice: taking social practices seriously. Acad. Manag. Ann. **6**(1), 285–336 (2012)
59. Vitale, M.R., Ives, B., Beath, C.M.: Linking information technology and corporate strategy: an organizational view. In: ICIS, p. 30 (1986)
60. Ward, J., Daniel, E.: Benefits Management: How to Increase the Business Value of Your IT Projects. Wiley, Hoboken (2012)
61. Whittington, R.: Completing the practice turn in strategy research. Organ. Stud. **27**(5), 613–634 (2006)
62. Zelenkov, Y.: Critical regular components of IT strategy: Decision making model and efficiency measurement. J. Manag. Anal. **2**(2), 95–110 (2015)

# Information Flows at Inter-team Boundaries in Agile Information Systems Development

Scarlet Rahy$^{(\boxtimes)}$ and Julian Bass

School of Computing, Science and Engineering, University of Salford, Manchester, UK
S.Rahy@edu.salford.ac.uk, J.Bass@salford.ac.uk

**Abstract.** Agile software development methods are being used on larger projects thus the study of inter-team communication are becoming an important topic of interest for researchers. This research addresses inter-team communication by exploring the tools and three different boundaries, inter-team, team and customers, and geographically separated teams. In this research, we gathered data from semi-structured face-to-face interviews which were analyzed following the grounded theory approach. Our study reveals consensus from different teams on the importance of virtual Kanban boards. Also, some team members tend to adapt to other teams' preferred communication tool. We observed challenges around interdependent user stories among the different teams and highlighted the problems that rise at the different boundaries.

**Keywords:** Agile information system development ·
Inter-team communication · Agile team boundary · Communication
Agile methods · Cooperating agile teams

## 1  Introduction

Since the creation of the agile manifesto in 2001, agile methods enhanced the customer involvement, adaptability, and evolutionary delivery in software development [11]. Agile software development is growing horizontally within different organizations and deeply within the same organization [9]. Globalization is irreversible and so is the nature of the software development industry as a digital currency [15]. Multi-cultural and geographically distributed software development models are becoming more common. Thus rises the need to study how agile software development teams can work effectively in these geographically distributed settings [1].

Inter team communication is a crucial part to achieve the success of agile software development [10, 17, 25, 26]. Agile teams cannot work in isolation and thus coordination is a necessity. This study examines the means of communication used across the different teams through observing a case of a software development company spreading across two geographical locations, The Netherlands and Kenya. This study also addresses the issue of communication across three different boundaries, inter-teams, teams and customer, and geographically separated teams.

This paper is structured as follows. In the next section, an overview of the literature review is presented and includes an overview of agile and inter-team information flow

© Springer Nature Switzerland AG 2019
M. Themistocleous and P. Rupino da Cunha (Eds.): EMCIS 2018, LNBIP 341, pp. 489–502, 2019.
https://doi.org/10.1007/978-3-030-11395-7_38

in agile. Then the research method adopted is introduced providing information on the research site, data collection and data analysis. Then findings are presented and divided into main section, inter-team communication tools and communication at the boundaries. Finally at the end there is the discussion, recommendation, and conclusion.

## 2   Related Work

### 2.1   Overview of Agile

The Agile Manifesto has organized and made clear the application of agile in the software development industry. The agile methods are based on the values and philosophies developed in the Agile Manifesto [6]. It promotes people and social focused views on software development. The goal of agile application lies in adaptability, flexibility and responsiveness [14]. Agile adapts to the constantly changing word by learning through experimentation and introspection and adopting it as a problem solving method [14]. There are several agile methods that are applied in software development such as Lean Software Development [23], Scrum, and Extreme Programing.

Inter-team communication is highly related to the agile practices used. Furthermore, there are several agile practices that are adopted including Refactoring, Release Planning, Velocity, Iteration Planning, and Coding Standard [8]. The most used agile practice is the Daily Stand-up meetings, with 90% usage, followed by Sprint Planning, with 88% usage, and ranking third are the Retrospectives, with 85% usage [9] all of which demand effective communication skills. The Daily Stand up Meetings occur daily between the team members in a prearranged space and time to discuss what has been done, what is going to be done and impediments encountered, if any [27]. Sprint planning occurs when team members gather to share the details on user stories' complexity, utility, and dependency [7]. Retrospectives are devoted for the improvement of the agile software development process and for adaptation to changes that arise [18].

### 2.2   Inter-team Information Flow in Agile Software Development

Agile software development is based on inter-team collaboration and coordination [19, 25]. These teams and their members are known for the dynamic behavior that is able to adjust according to the customer's requirements; for customers are major influencers in the agile software development process [19, 24]. The identification and prioritization of customer requirements is conflicting in agile software development [5, 24]. Some team members do not accept criticism and perceive it as a personal offense and subsequently retreat and defend themselves rather than their ideas or work [17].

Agile team members are meant to be democratic, all team members are equal [17, 20]. Moreover, the Agile Manifesto guarantees that all team members have equal opportunity in the decision making process [6]. This enhances the self-organizing ability of teams and introduces it as a mean to achieve the best design, architecture, and customer requirements [6, 17]. Self-organizing teams in agile are characterized by communication, feedback, coordination, and collaboration [13]. But this collaborative nature introduces obstacles that team members face in relation to the decision making principles. A major obstacle is the unwillingness of team members to commit to a decision. Rather, team members tend to consider decision making as a burden rather than a privilege and rely on the Scrum Master for decision taking [13]. In these cases, Scrum Masters tend to choose either to take the decision and inform the team members, thus violating an agile principle, encourage team members and wait for their response, or use decision making support systems to aid in the process [4].

Effective inter-team knowledge sharing is highly important in agile software development. Santos and Goldman developed a theoretical model for inter-team knowledge sharing effectiveness. This model highlighted two influencing factors that are the organizational conditions and stimuli. Organizational conditions are identified as top management, team integration, environment and agile methods adopted. While stimuli are motivators that include common goals and incentives Dingsoyr et al. (2018) found a balance between the centralized behavior and the self-management agile driven behavior. Šmite et al. [26] highlighted the importance of networking and cultivating teams to practice cross team interaction. Also, boundary spanners act as coordinators who provide a source of information, a target for feedback [26], a mediator between different teams [29], and a sociomaterial assemblages [12].

There is extensive research on agile software development principles and practices [2, 3, 5, 16, 22] but less research is done on inter-team communication. Inter-team knowledge sharing in agile software development are still in the rise [10, 25, 26]. Inter-team communication is identified as an important topic in research [10]. Practices that are applied specifically for knowledge sharing in agile software development are still under study. Our study has added to the research in inter-team communication tools used and problems that rise at the boundaries between the different teams.

## 3   Method

The qualitative research methodology is adopted by this study. Specifically, qualitative research is used as a basis for implementing the grounded theory approach. Grounded theory was used since it enabled the suspension of preconceptions and the analysis of new concepts from the data. The three pillars of qualitative research include open ended interviews, direct observation, and written communication [21]. In this study, data was collected using semi-structured open ended interviews. The unit of analysis are employees [28] and product owners at this study's research site. An exploratory pilot study was conducted in the first phase to enable refinement and possible adjustments in the questions along with the familiarization with this type of research. In the second phase, a deductive synthesis of a series of interviews was done to enable analysis.

### 3.1   Research Sites

Data was obtained and analyzed from an international company providing services in software development. The company develops software using agile software development techniques and conducts administrative work also using agile. The international company has a main office in The Hague, Netherlands, 50 employees, and a partner office in Nairobi, Kenya, 15 employees. The company was chosen according to the snowball sampling technique; academic contact eased the connection. In the second phase, the professional contact provided access to study participants.

## 3.2    Data Collection

Participants were interviewed with different responsibilities and locations in the company. An overview of the participants' location, role, and responsibility are shown in Table 1. The data collected was obtained from semi-structured open-ended questions. All interviews were recorded after obtaining the practitioners' consent. Then interviews were transcribed manually since it ensures correct transcription and reminds the interviewer of the social and emotional aspects that occurred during the interview [28]. The most effective way to optimize the data collected from interviews is to record and transcribe data manually [2]. The conducted interviews followed a guide open-ended questions that enabled the participants to raise any issue that came up even if it wasn't mentioned in the guide.

**Table 1.** Participants' roles, responsibility, and location

| Participant | Role and responsibility | Location |
|---|---|---|
| Director-1 | Director of the company | Kenya |
| Director-2 | Director of the company and product owner | Netherlands/Kenya |
| Technical lead | Technical lead and product owner | Netherlands/Kenya |
| Public Relations (PR) | Public relations manager | Netherland |
| Sales | Sales coordinator | Netherlands |
| Designer | Designer and part of the public relations team | Netherlands |
| Developer-1 | Scrum master and developer | Kenya |
| Developer-2 | Front end developer | Netherlands |
| Human Resource (HR) | Human resources manager | Netherlands |

## 3.3    Data Analysis

The transcribed data was imported to an analyzing tool Nvivo 11. All interviews were coded, leading to deriving categories, high levels of abstraction, and concepts and patterns of behavior [2]. The categories where deduced solemnly from the transcribed interviews without inducing any preconceived ideas or thoughts. Significant points were highlighted form each interview and then compared with other interviews. This constant comparison technique was a key to identify concepts that were then grouped into categories that were coded.

Line-by-line open coding approach was used on the transcribed interviews. When coding line-by-line, data can be inspected and a special incident can be found in a word, a line, or through several lines [2]. This coding process was organized using the Nodes option in Nvivo. Each code was given a title and constant comparison method was used. The transcribed interviews were reviewed more than once and each time new categories emerged. This ensured that no data was left unnoticed. This process stopped when no new categories were created and theoretical saturation was reached.

The next step was the writing of the memos. After writing each memo roughly, the memos were revisited and written in a formal. This will ensure that memos are written in the "passion of the movement" [2] and guarantee that memos will be understood in the correct way through using correct and revised English. Also, constant comparison was applied to categories and the participants' responses from the two different geographical locations were compared. Thus, when a difference in opinion occurred, if any, it was indicated in the writing of the memos. Quotes from the interviews were used as evidence in the writing of memos.

# 4   Findings

The findings in this study are organized into two main parts. The first part discusses the inter-team tools that are used for communication such as team messaging tools, face-to-face, and virtual Kanban boards. The second part discusses the communication boundaries between teams inside the company, between teams and customers, and between teams that are located in separate geographical locations.

## 4.1   Inter-team Communication Tools

There are several forms of communication that are used to transfer information from one actor to another. These include team messaging tools, face-to-face, emails, virtual Kanban boards…

**Team Messaging Tools.** Team members use a messaging tool called Slack to chat inside the company. Slack is an application that works as a digital workspace for communication between the different members of the company.

During the interviews, we noticed a major difference in the point of views when it came to the usage of slack. The advocates and daily users of slack were mainly the developers; while the criticizers were the designers, sales, human resources and public relations team.

To begin with, the developers use slack daily as a way to communicate with the team members and other employees. Participants highlighted the different benefits of slack. The first benefit is that slack allows open communication between members of the same team, project, or the company as a whole. According to Developer-1:

> "In slack we are able to communicate to a group. A group can keep up with the communication and know what is going on in different aspects. Also they can chip in if they feel there is something they can input on any matter."

Also the Technical Lead highlighted the benefits of slack as a platform to ask for help when needed: "…we have channels for the teams on their own and we have channels for the project we have a channel were people can ask for help".

Second, slack has features, notifications, tags, and pins, which aid in simplifying and facilitating the communication process. Developer-1 said: "If we have a group that is *specific for a certain project I am able to tag the members of the team to draw their attention to something... everyone will get notified as soon as I post something".* Moreover, Developer-2 revealed how slack can be used as an updating tool when an employee is absent for a period of time: *"If we need to remember something for the next day we pin it on slack so we can see it the next day"*, and the Technical Lead agreed.

Third, developers use slack for archiving documents and saving conversation. Developer-2 indicated how slack can be used as a memory box: *"Everything that needs to be documented so we don't forget we just put it in [slack]".*

On the other hand, some other employees weren't that enthusiastic of slack and didn't use it that often. The non-developers used slack solemnly when communicating with the developers. The Designer said: *"I use slack in order to communicate but I mostly do that with developers".* The Sales person showed displeasure with the usage of slack: *"I use slack but not a lot...the only people I know who use slack are developers".* The Technical Lead said: *"It is more difficult for non-developers to actually express by text what they mean".* The dependence on verbal communication and neglecting slack highlights a tradeoff between the benefits of verbal communication and the availability of information for all the involved members. When information is transferred verbally between two members or more, it won't necessary reach all the involved members.

In addition, slack can be used to ask and answer small questions. For instance if a developer has a specific question about a certain color in the design or font this could be best transferred through slack. The Designer said: *"They [developers] always have short questions, like what is the color of this design, how big this should be... and many questions like that during the development process".*

**Face-to-Face.** Face-to-face communication is a mean to enhance collaboration and creativity in the workplace. When communicating face-to-face the information is not only limited to the words said, it also reveals the body language, tone, reactions and feelings. All the employees use face-to-face communication but some prefer it more than others. Director-2 said: *"When most people use a document we try to use an email. When most people use email we try to use chat message. When most people chat we try to talk to each other".* Face-to-face communication is used during daily standups, demos, retrospectives, and regularly during the day.

The PR, Sales, HR and designers tend to use face-to-face communication very often. This is their preferred form of communication. The Designer indicated that face-to-face communication is the first step toward creating the design of a certain project: *"Without face-to-face communication I cannot start with my design"*; the HR manager seconds that. Director-1 indicated the importance of body language in communication: *"I prefer face-to-face physical communication. Because communication is not just text it is also body language, tone facial expression which I think you lose most of it if you only type, text or email".*

One of the main challenges when communicating face-to-face rises when using Skype. For instance, when communicating between The Netherlands and Kenya, the main problem is the poor internet connection. The Designer indicated that *"sometimes in Kenya they are a bit slower and they have trouble with internet connection a lot. Sometimes the sprint would be affected by that"*; Developer-2 also indicated that.

**Virtual Kanban Board.** The uses of virtual Kanban boards are essential for software development companies implementing agile. The importance of virtual Kanban boards, in this case Trello boards, was recognized by all employees. Trello boards are used to keep track of everyone's work and daily activities. The Technical Lead stressed that Trello boards facilitates the managing process and helps managers and team leaders acquire a general overview of the work. The Technical Lead said: *"Trello keeps an overview of all the project, sprints, and teams at the same time".*

Moreover, Trello boards allows all members of the organization to check the status of work of different teams by simply examining the board of each team. Trello boards highlights the user stories' status. The Technical Lead said: *"we use Trello and this is where we set all the user stories for the teams....when you pass by you can see straight away what the status is of the sprint".*

### 4.2  Communication at the Boundaries

It has been discussed earlier how each person or team prefers a certain type of communication method. This along with other factors cause communication problems at the boundaries between teams, directors, product owners, and customers.

**Inter-team Boundaries.** One of the main issues in inter-team communication occurs when members do not respond to requests from other teams. Members tend to prioritize the tasks given by their own team leader or scrum master, and postpone the tasks or requests given to them by other team's leaders. The Sales describes an incident that occurred with one of the developers under that context:

> *"She started working at the customer but the screening wasn't completed yet and she needed to hand a document. I emailed her, called and she wasn't responding for several days and that was really frustrating. It took three days to complete that".*

Another issue that rises is how a team tends to assume that other teams know their status and if they are facing any setbacks. Developer 2 said: *"Teams are like, we know so the rest knows it as well. They are just assuming".* This brings up the role of the scrum master in inter-team communication. The scrum master is responsible to receive and send information to members in and outside his/her team. Developer-2 describes an incident where one team did not finish their sprint and another team was depending on the successful completion of that team's sprint to initiate their own. Developer said: *"If the scrum master had told the other team they could have done a new sprint planning. Now they were just waiting and two teams were set back by that".*

*Absence of Inter-team Communication in the Presence of Dependencies.* During a project, several sprints are interconnected. A sprint for Team A may be a prerequisite for the completion of the Team B's sprint. This reliability sometimes may cause problems especially if the work done by Team A's sprint was not complete on time or needed rework. Developer-2 explained a similar case:

> *"In the last sprint there was a team who picked up a bit too much, they under estimated their user stories and another team was dependent on what they were supposed to make but they weren't informed of the delay. So they were waiting for their sprint to start for some time."*

This case has occurred several times between the design team and the developing team. Since the developing team is highly dependent on the work of the design team and since the sprint of the design team are highly dependent on the customer's approval, the developing team has experienced incidences where they had idle time. The Designer described: *"If something goes wrong in my sprint then the developers don't have anything to do"*.

The Technical Lead suggested that: *"The delay can be caused by miscommunication"*. The lack of communication between teams can cause the delay of sprints and thus creating an idle time. This wait time could have been avoided if communication had occurred. Developer-2 said: *"So if they had told them [about the unfinished work] they could have done a new sprint planning and plan different stuff and finish other tasks"*.

**Team and Customer Boundaries.** Communication with customers through agencies, dealing with unclear customers' requirements, and reaction to customers' feedback are issues that rise at the team and customer boundary.

*Communicating with Customers through Agencies.* In an agile software development company, customer feedback directly reaches the employees. In cases where customers are contacted through agencies, the communication is faced with breakdowns. The Technical Lead said: *"when the development is through an agency, the communication is more difficult"*. First, These breakdowns can cause frustration for the employees especially with the involvement of several actors. Second, transfer of false information may occur. Third, employees will feel they have restrictions or limitations while performing their job which may lead to demotivation. The Technical Lead said: *"This becomes time consuming. This is something that we don't have control over. It is somehow frustrating"*.

*Unclear Customer Requirement.* Understanding the customer needs and building on their requests are of high importance. Lack of information and clarification may also lead to delay in delivery with respect to time. The PR manager said: *"Also the lack of information of the project we are doing is a factor that will negatively affect delivery time"*. Team members should be willing to ask questions at the beginning of the project before writing the user stories and planning the sprints. The Designer said: *"I ask a lot of questions make the story clear and make a proper sprint planning out of it"*. Director-1 highlights the importance of the scrum master's role in clarifying the customer's requirements: *"The scrum master can clarify the story or feature with the customer and product owner and communicate that to the team"*.

Unfortunately, sometimes the team members or the scrum master do not ask the correct questions and base the user stories and sprint planning solemnly on the customer's briefing. Director-2 said: *"I think the most common negative effect on the workload is the lack of clarity and understanding in what is required"*; the designer also agreed to that. Also some clients might not be involved in the process. Director-1said: *"The clients give the requirements but they don't get involved so much"*.

*Reaction to Customer's Feedback.* The customer feedback presented in the demo will directly affect the retrospective. Sometimes employees tend to express their feelings about the demo solemnly instead of expressing their feedback about the whole sprint and the demo. Director-2 indicated: *"In our last demo we had problem with the customer that resulted in negative feedback and then in the retro everybody put negative improvement stickys related to that particular incident"*. Some of the employees become directly affected by the customer feedback presented in the demo and it stretches further to affect not only the retrospective but also the performance in the coming day. The Technical Lead indicates that: *"It depends if they get affected with the customer's feedback"*. On one hand, some employees get affected by the feedback. As the Designer said: *"It [customer feedback] can discourage you especially. I think as a designer you know the feedback will always come up and it is never the way you thought it would be"*. Also Developer-2 talked about a recovery period: *"Usually the demo is on a Thursday and Friday is usually is a personal sprint day and Monday you can just start over. Friday would be like a day to recover"*.

On the other hand, some employees do not get affected by the feedback and understand that this is part of the job especially in the software development industry where clients tend to change their requirements frequently. Developer-1 indicated: *The scrum agile process is actually about making the software based on the customer's demand"*.

**Geographically Separated Inter-team Boundary.** During the first steps of agile implementation in Kenya, the Netherlands had a lot to offer and agile implementation was a challenge. The Kenyans were learning the agile process from the Dutch. Developer-1, based in Kenya, said: *"They were able to catch our weaknesses and give us a scrum agile implementation of a solution for the problems"*. But all throughout the implementation process, the people at the Netherlands, learned and enhanced the agile process. The Technical Lead said: *"After every sprint in Kenya we learned new things and we restarted the game"*.

First of all, the communication between the people in Netherlands improved after practicing long-distance communication with the Kenyans. Developer-2, having direct contact with the Kenyans, expressed:

> *"If you managed to communicate with people in Kenya every day for 10 sprints in a row then it is easier and becomes second nature to talk with people around you as well. Instead of calling them kilometers away you just walk the 5 meters to the next room and you talk with them".*

Other employees, who were not in contact with the Kenyans, saw this improvements in their colleagues and started enhancing their communication skills. The Technical Lead said: *"The whole company learned a lot about communication especially in the least two weeks...our communication improved immensely"*; Director-2 expressed the same.

Second, the Kenyans found a new way to design the Trello board and the office back in the Netherlands adopted this change. The Technical Lead said:

> *"In Kenya they came up with some ways to organize their Trello board for their office team, management team. And we adapted that and then we changed that for a more suitable way for our office".*

Third, the way user stories were written in the Netherlands also changed. After implementing agile in the Kenya, the need for detailed and descriptive user stories emerged. The Technical Lead explained:

*"Because we added extra description in Kenya, we found out that we need to give a little more information that they can look up afterwards instead of telling that in the sprint planning next to the user story".*

## 5  Discussion

This study responds to the call for further research on inter-team communication and customer involvement [10]. Thus our paper offers a case study that looks into inter-team communication, the methods used, and the difficulties that rise at the boundaries between different actors, employees and customers, and across diverse locations. In addition, our study reveals a combination of technology choices, organizational boundaries, and interfaces. Both aspects turned out to be a challenge in inter-team communication.

First, our findings show that employees fell into two groups when it came to inter-team communication means and preference. Developers, on one hand, preferred slack and recognized the importance of Trello boards and face-to-face. On the other hand, designers, sales, HR, and PR preferred face-to face communication while recognizing the importance of Trello boards and using Slack when communicating with developers. This reveals how people tend to adapt and improvise ways in order to enhance communication.

There was consensus among the participants in our reproach study that using virtual Kanban board is appropriate. Virtual Kanban boards are means to keep all employees up-to-date while highlighting the user stories without disturbing the flow of work. We observe that developers in this study are already benefiting from slack's features, tagging, pinning, and notifications while endorsing its usage in specific cases such as short clarifications, information storing platform when an employee is unavailable, and public information broadcasting. It is surprising that HR, PR, sales and designers are not seeing the benefits of slack but rather using it as means to communicate with developers. Maybe directors would see benefit in improving communication if they encourage face-to-face information sharing and networking behavior through offering communication skills training [26], giving cross team effective feedback, and encouraging ad-hoc conversations. 55/38/7 rule stresses on the importance of body language and tone and these can only be portrayed though face-to-face communication.

Second, we studied communication at the boundaries at three different levels: inter-team boundary, team and customer boundary, and geographically separated inter-team boundary. Previous literature has shown six informal roles in self-organizing agile teams that will smoothen the communication at the boundaries [17]. Our study reveals some of the problems at the boundaries while highlighting observations to enhance communication at the different boundaries. The figures below highlight the bottlenecks experienced and their respective results at the inter-team and geographically separated inter-team boundaries (Fig. 1) and team customer boundary (Fig. 2).

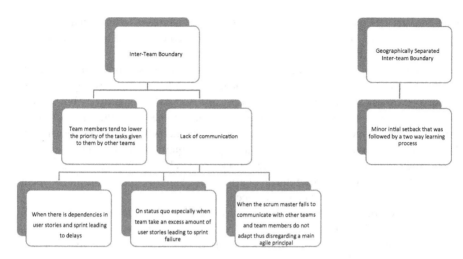

**Fig. 1.** Bottlenecks at inter-team and geographically separated inter-team boundaries

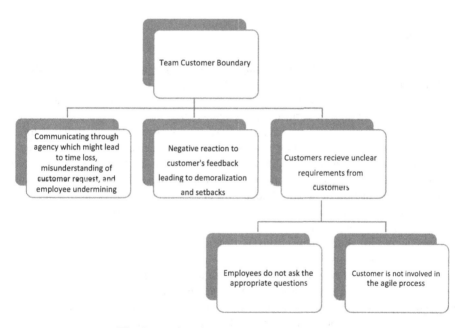

**Fig. 2.** Bottlenecks at team customer boundary

Smooth communication at the boundaries is hard to achieve [12, 29]. At the level of inter-team boundary, in addition to applying the communication tools mix provided earlier, team members may consider enhancing communication especially when user stories are interconnected, dependent, or are on the verge of failure. For example, this could be done by highlighting dependent user stories on the Trello board and ensuring the scrum masters involved conduct ad-hoc meeting to discuss updates. But if the scrum master failed to do so this may trigger the team members to jump in and perform the communication since in agile everyone is considered equal; and at the retrospective this can be highlighted, discussed, and resolved.

At the level of team and customer boundary, employees should understand that customer involvement and feedback is in the core of agile software development. Thus negative feedback should neither demoralize nor discourage employees but rather it should encourage them. This encouragement may come from the product owner especially while conducting the retrospective that should include constructive criticism. In addition, employees should learn to ask specific questions to the customers especially when the requirements are vague. Further research may involve creating general guidelines for customer requirement clarification. Moreover, the role of boundary spanners should be supported and enhanced.

At the level of the geographically separated inter team boundaries, unfamiliar tasks, lack of product knowledge, and cultural differences enhance communication and motivate particular networking behavior [26]. In addition, we observed that team members, having different levels of experience, exchange ideas leading to mutual benefits and learnings.

## 6   Conclusions

This study used the grounded theory approach to analyze inter-team communication tools at different boundaries. The study was focused on an agile software development company located in The Netherlands and Kenya and interviewed practitioners from different teams and later performed line-by-line coding, memoing, and constant comparison to the data to obtain two main findings. The first revealed the different tools used in inter-team communication and the difference in perceptions between practitioners about the three main tools, Slack, Trello, and face-to-face. The second revealed the problems faced at the levels of the boundaries, inter-teams, teams and customer, and geographically distributed teams. The contribution of this paper is to observe that communication has improved when people deliberately adopt somebody else's preferred communication mechanism.

We discovered different mechanisms that were used at the different boundaries. Teams learn how to benefit from the best of each type of communication tool and how to adapt to certain tools in order to enhance communication. Interdependent user stories may be highlighted on virtual Kanban boards and ensure information exchange about the status quo is achieved through encouraging ad-hoc meetings between scrum masters. In addition, boundary spanners play an important role in reducing the gap between different actors. Finally, geographically separated teams may use their differences in their favor in order to benefit and learn from each other.

# References

1. Aebert, C.: Global Software and IT: A Guide to Distributed Development, Projects, and Outsourcing. Ringgold Inc., Portland (2012)
2. Adolph, S., Hall, W., Kruchten, P.: Using grounded theory to study the experience of software development. Empirical Softw. Eng. **16**(4), 487–513 (2011)
3. Alahyari, H., Svensson, R.B., Gorschek, T.: A study of value in agile software development organizations. J. Syst. Softw. **125**, 271–288 (2017)
4. Rani, A., Vodanovish, S., Sundaram, D.: Ubiquitous decision making and SUpport: a framework and evaluation. In: European, Mediterranean & Middle Eastern Conference on Information Systems 2015, 1st–2nd June 2015 (2015)
5. Bass, J.M.: How product owner teams scale agile methods to large distributed enterprises. Empirical Softw. Eng. **20**(6), 1525–1557 (2015)
6. Beck, K., et al.: Manifesto for agile software development (2001)
7. Boschetti, M.A., Golfarelli, M., Rizzi, S., Turricchia, E.: A Lagrangian heuristic for sprint planning in agile software development. Comput. Oper. Res. **43**, 116–128 (2014)
8. Campanelli, A.S., Parreiras, F.S.: Agile methods tailoring – a systematic literature review. J. Syst. Softw. **110**, 85–100 (2015)
9. Collabnet and VersionOne: The 12th Annual State of Agile Report: Long Term Servey. VersionOne, Atlanta (2018)
10. Dingsøyr, T., Moe, N., Fægri, T., Seim, E.: Exploring software development at the very large-scale: a revelatory case study and research agenda for agile method adaptation. Empirical Softw. Eng. **23**(1), 490–520 (2018)
11. Dingsøyr, T., Nerur, S., Balijepally, V., Moe, N.B.: A decade of agile methodologies: towards explaining agile software development (2012)
12. Doolin, B.: Sociomateriality and boundary objects in information systems development. Eur. J. Inf. Syst. **21**(5), 570–586 (2012)
13. Drury, M., Conboy, K., Power, K.: Obstacles to decision making in Agile software development teams. J. Syst. Softw. **85**(6), 1239–1254 (2012)
14. Dyba, T., Dingsoyr, T.: What do we know about agile software development? IEEE Softw. **26**(5), 6–9 (2009)
15. Herbsleb, J.D., Moitra, D.: Global software development. IEEE Softw. **18**(2), 16–20 (2001)
16. Hoda, R., Noble, J., Marshall, S.: Developing a grounded theory to explain the practices of self-organizing Agile teams. Empirical Softw. Eng. **17**(6), 609–639 (2012)
17. Hoda, R., Noble, J., Marshall, S.: Self-organizing roles on agile software development teams. IEEE Trans. Softw. Eng. **39**(3), 422–444 (2013)
18. Jovanovic, M., Mesquida, A.L., Mas, A.: Process improvement with retrospective gaming in agile software development. In: O'Connor, R., Umay Akkaya, M., Kemaneci, K., Yilmaz, M., Poth, A., Messnarz, R. (eds.) EuroSPI 2015. CCIS, vol. 543, pp. 287–294. Springer, Cham (2015). https://doi.org/10.1007/978-3-319-24647-5_23
19. Lindvall, M., et al.: Empirical findings in agile methods. In: Wells, D., Williams, L. (eds.) XP/Agile Universe 2002. LNCS, vol. 2418, pp. 197–207. Springer, Heidelberg (2002). https://doi.org/10.1007/3-540-45672-4_19
20. Nerur, S., Mahapatra, R., Mangalaraj, G.: Challenges of migrating to agile methodologies. Commun. ACM **48**(5), 72–78 (2005)
21. Patton, M.Q.: Qualitative Research and Evaluation Methods, 3rd edn. SAGE, London (1945, 2002)

22. Petersen, K., Roos, P., Nyström, S., Runeson, P.: Early identification of bottlenecks in very large scale system of systems software development. J. Softw.: Evol. Process **26**(12), 1150–1171 (2014)

23. Poppendieck, M.: Lean Software Development: An Agile Toolkit. Addison-Wesley, London, Boston (2003)

24. Praby, R., Roland, W.: Can agile processes prevent spectacular information systems development failures. In: European, Mediterranean & Middle Eastern Conference on Information Systems EMCIS 2016, 23rd–24th June 2016 (2016)

25. Santos, V., Goldman, A., de Souza, C.: Fostering effective inter-team knowledge sharing in agile software development. Empirical Softw. Eng. **20**(4), 1006–1051 (2015)

26. Šmite, D., Moe, N.B., Šablis, A., Wohlin, C.: Software teams and their knowledge networks in large-scale software development. Inf. Softw. Technol. **86**, 71–86 (2017)

27. Stray, V., Sjøberg, D.I.K., Dybå, T.: The daily stand-up meeting: a grounded theory study. J. Syst. Softw. **114**, 101–124 (2016)

28. Vaivio, J.: Interviews – Learning the Craft of Qualitative Research Interviewing. Routledge, London (2012)

29. Yoo, Y.: The dynamics of IT boundary objects, information infrastructures, and organisational identities: the introduction of 3D modelling technologies into the architecture, engineering, and construction industry. Eur. J. Inf. Syst. **17**(3), 290–304 (2008)

# Critical Factors of Strategic Information Systems Planning Phases in SMEs

Maria Kamariotou[(⊠)] and Fotis Kitsios

Department of Applied Informatics, University of Macedonia,
Thessaloniki, Greece
tml367@uom.edu.gr, kitsios@uom.gr

**Abstract.** Strategic Information Systems Planning (SISP) supports business goals and business strategy, through the use of Information Systems (IS). Findings from previous surveys indicate that many managers make too much effort to SISP process while others too little. The implemented plans are not effective, successful and they do not meet the objectives. Researchers have noticed that family businesses focus on business's long-term sustainability, but they do not develop strategic planning. More attention is needed to be payed to and how they use IS and strategic planning in order to deal with the crisis. The purpose of this paper is to indicate the phases which contribute to a greater extent of success in order to provide conclusions regarding the implementation of this process in SMEs. Data were collected using questionnaires to IS executives in Greek SMEs. Factor Analysis is performed on the detailed items of the SISP process and success constructs.

**Keywords:** Strategic Information Systems Planning · Success
SMEs · IT strategy · Critical factors

## 1 Introduction

The current business environment is getting more and more complex and uncertain. Thus, businesses are obliged to deal with that environmental uncertainty. The use of Information Systems (IS) and Strategic Planning facilitate this effort. IS support business strategy, and accommodates decision making using management skills to increase competitive advantage [26]. The integration between IS and Strategic Planning is known as Strategic Information Systems Planning (SISP).

Researchers have paid attention to the process of SISP since 1970. SISP support business goals and business strategy, through the use of IS. IS help businesses to compete in a global market, to meet consumer needs and to reduce the product life cycles. Researchers claim that the use of technology could be a source of sustainable competitive advantage only if the IS strategy will be aligned with business strategy [17–19, 24]. The process of SISP involves five phases, named; Strategic Awareness, Situation Analysis, Strategy Conception, Strategy Formulation and Strategy Implementation Planning. These phases support businesses to define IS strategy as well as to develop IS [2, 3, 10–12, 14, 15].

M. Themistocleous and P. Rupino da Cunha (Eds.): EMCIS 2018, LNBIP 341, pp. 503–517, 2019.
https://doi.org/10.1007/978-3-030-11395-7_39

Previous surveys have studied the impact of these phases on SISP success in large firms [2, 3, 10–12, 14, 15]. Success was measured using the following dimensions: Alignment, Analysis, Cooperation and Capabilities [13, 14]. However, studies in Small-Medium Enterprises (SMEs), which compose the most important part of economy for each country, are limited [13].

SMEs are significant components of the national economy, because they constitute of a large number of businesses in a country. Nowadays they have been negatively affected by financial crisis. In order to face this, SMEs are obligated to gather information for their environment. This information should be appropriate in order to compete and face the environmental complexity, so the process of gathering information should be strategic. As SMEs try to compete in the current uncertain environment, so that it could be innovative and increase their growth, they need to align their business and Information Technology (IT) strategy [1]. The most important challenges which SMEs face which led to the failure of the alignment process are the lack of conscious planning, the lack of strategic decision making and sharing information [20]. Therefore, the purpose of this thesis is to indicate the phases which contribute to a greater extent of success and to provide conclusions regarding on the implementation of this survey in SMEs.

Researchers have suggested that more extensive planning would be more effective because it would support planners understand the impact of the environment and better respond to it. Therefore, the purpose of this paper is to indicate the phases which contribute to a greater extent of success and to provide conclusions regarding on the implementation of this survey in SMEs. Data were collected using questionnaires to IS executives in Greek SMEs in order to identify the phases that are more significant for them as well as the phases that need improvement to produce effective IS plans.

The structure of this paper is as following: after a brief introduction to this field, the next section includes the literature review in order to highlight the issues which are discussed in this paper. Section 3 describes the methodology, while Sect. 4 shows the results of the survey. Finally, Sect. 5 discusses the results and concludes the paper.

## 2   Theoretical Background

### 2.1   Information Systems and Strategic Planning in SMEs

In complex environments, SMEs tend to formalize processes using certain rules and procedures which support the limitation of environmental uncertainty. Formalization supports the development of aspects which encourage communication among the individuals and sharing of new information. Also, they transform the generation of new ideas through the inflicted structures into real plans, enhancing the growth of innovation. As the environment is getting more and more complex, the need for innovation is increasing if businesses are to be helped to be competitive so as to survive [4].

In Europe SMEs consist of 75% of all businesses. Despite the fact that family businesses focus on business's long-term sustainability, they do not develop strategic planning [22]. Specifically, Greece is a country which has a great extent of SMEs rather than other countries in Europe and the majority of them have been negatively influenced by the financial crisis [25].

Almost 80% of businesses have been highly influenced by the financial crisis. So, more attention should be paid to SMEs and how they realize and deal with the crisis. As SMEs play a significant role both in Greek and European competitive financial growth and as the world's economy is influenced by them be-cause they constitute 97% of businesses all over the world, it seems that formal processes in SMEs increase firm performance. These processes concern strategic management and information handling and require the support of managers in or-der to pay attention to strategies, structures and processes.

There is a lack of strategic planning and formal processes in SMEs and they use IS ineffectively because they cannot align business and IT strategy. Researches have thoroughly implemented in this research area so that managers could understand the relationship between strategic alignment and the business value of using IT. The results of these investigations show that researchers have determined the following types of alignment between business and IS strategy and structure. The first type presents business alignment between business strategy and structure. The second type concerns IS alignment and discusses issues such as alignment between IS strategy and structure. Finally, the third type is a cross-dimension alignment which involves either alignment between business structure and IS strategy either business strategy and IS structure. Researchers claim that the alignment between organizational perspectives such as strategy, structure, management processes, individual roles and skills with technology can help to increase value in businesses, IS effectiveness and business performance [23].

The accomplishment of a high degree of alignment between IT and organizational objectives has been mentioned as one of the important issues for IS managers [21]. In this view, both the organization and IT are consolidated, developing services with the support of IT so that businesses could effectively achieve their goals. Strategic IT alignment is unique for each business because it includes business and IT knowledge that are unique resources for each business in order to help business to achieve its objectives [5, 8, 9].

Researchers widely argue that the process of alignment is important for businesses for many reasons. First of all, alignment helps businesses to effectively identify the role of IT which efficiently helps the business to achieve its objectives. Second, another benefit is that alignment encourages businesses to improve both their business scope and their infrastructure by meliorating the relationship be-tween business aspects and IT. Researchers claim that the present alignment models are mostly business-driven rather than IT-driven. As a result, researchers should mostly focus on IT in order to determine the most suitable way in which technology can support the organization. Businesses require to know as well as to make their business strategy clear, so the use of IT can support this effort [24].

Although the contribution of alignment methodologies has been mentioned, the following challenges incommode many businesses to align IT with business strategy. First, many decisions about IT are made by business executives who are not aware about IT. This obstacle leads to the organization being misaligned. Another challenge concerns IT executives who are not aware about the business objectives and often cannot realize the needs of business decisions. Finally, business and IT executives are conflicted and they do not trust each other. This influences negatively their relationship and consequently the business competence [24].

## 2.2  Strategic Information Systems Planning and Success

The findings of surveys which study the influence of SISP phases on success conclude that IS executives focused their efforts on the Strategic Conception phase. Although planners concentrate their efforts on this phase, they cannot determine the suitable alternative strategies. As a result, their efforts do not positively influence SISP success. So, they cannot achieve their objectives. The most common problems which have been affected by the SISP process are the lack of involvement and the failure to apply strategic IS plans. Executives cannot be committed to the plan, consequently the members of the team have difficulties to implement the IS strategy. Moreover, results show that executives understand that the Implementation phase is difficult and significant, so they concentrate on this phase [9, 13, 14, 26].

Findings from previous surveys indicate that many managers put too many efforts to SISP process while others too little. When managers invest too many efforts, the process could be confused, delayed or its implementation is prevented. When managers avoid investing too much time into the process, the implemented plans could be inefficient so the objectives could not be achieved. Consequently, the assessment of the process is significant because managers can reduce these unsatisfactory results.

Findings conclude that managers concentrate more on Strategy Conception and Strategy Implementation and they do not invest time on Strategic Awareness and Situation Analysis and as a result the implemented plans are ineffective and unsuccessful and they do not meet the objectives [2, 13, 14]. Moreover, when managers concentrate on the implementation of the process, they may achieve shorter SISP horizons, but the strategic goals cannot be met. Executives do not focus on what strategic objectives really concern and how they can increase value to the business because they invest time on the horizon of the project and on minimizing its cost due to limited IT budget [2]. SISP phases and the relative activities are presented in Table 1.

The results indicate that executives should pay attention to implementing Situational Analysis with greater meticulousness, so that they can apply Strategy Conception and Strategy Implementation Planning with greater agility rather than now. Planners should analyze their current business systems, organizational systems, IS, as well as the business environment and external IT environment. If planners understand those elements, they can improve the result of the planning process excluding the increased time and cost which the process is needed. When executives understand the environment, they can determine important IT objectives and opportunities for improvement, they can evaluate them in order to define high-level IT strategies in their business' strategy conception [12]. SISP success dimensions are presented in Table 2.

Strategic Awareness should concentrate on the planning process on gaining appropriate knowledge about competitors, resources, customers and regulators. The understanding of that knowledge could be achieved through the careful organizing of the teams. Top management commitment provides greater organizational confidence and continued financial support for the process. Situation Analysis which focuses on the analysis of the business, organization and IS, would produce better knowledge about the organization's requirements. The analysis of external business and IT environments would help produce better knowledge about the effect of change and provide a better foundation for the plan, making it more possible to produce better results.

Strategy Conception, with recognition and assessment of opportunities, would provide more realistic alternatives. Recognition of IT objectives would enable the organization to align future IT and business objectives. Better alternatives and choices would support the plan produce better results. Strategy Formulation includes the identification of the plan itself as far as processes, architectures, and projects. When the identification of the plan is careful, it would make it more possible to meet planning objectives. Better prioritization would result in greater likelihood of implementation and a greater chance of meeting objectives. Finally, Strategy Implementation Planning, with more attention to change management and a better action plan, would be more possible to achieve good implementation. Better control would result in more of the plan being implemented and as a result better delivery of planning goals [12–14].

## 3    Methodology

A field survey was developed for IS executives. The instrument used five-point Likert-scales to operationalize two constructs: SISP phases and success. The SISP process constructs measured the extent to which the organization conducted the five planning phases and their tasks. The success constructs measured using four dimensions named alignment, analysis, cooperation and capabilities. The questionnaire was based on previous surveys regarding SISP phases [5–7, 11–14].

Four IS executives were asked to participate in a pilot test. Each one completed the survey and commented on the contents, length, and overall appearance of the instrument. A sample of IS executives in Greece was selected from the icap list [13, 14]. SMEs which provided contact details were selected as the appropriate sample of the survey. The survey was sent to 1246 IS executives and a total of 294 returned the survey. Data analysis was implemented using Factor Analysis.

As SMEs have been negatively influenced by the financial crisis, they try to align their business and IT strategy in order to compete in the current uncertain environment to be innovative and increase their growth [1]. Despite the fact that family businesses focus on business's long-term sustainability, they do not develop strategic planning [22]. There is a lack of strategic planning and formal processes in SMEs and they use IS ineffectively because they cannot align business and IT strategy [23]. Specifically, Greece is a country which has a great extent of SMEs rather than other countries in Europe and the majority of them have been negatively influenced by the financial crisis [25]. So, it was emergent to collect data during the economic crisis in Greek SMEs in order to examine the effectiveness of the SISP process and its success.

## 4    Results

The IS executive is typically seen as the most suitable person in the organization to provide data regarding SISP activities and success as defined in this study [13]. Respondents in this study were employed in a variety of industries, well educated, and experienced. 16% of them worked in agriculture and food, 11.3% in business services, 10.6% in retail and the rest in other industries. 35.2% had some postgraduate studies and 44.7% had a degree. They also had 16–25 years of IS experience. Tables 3, 4, 5, 6 and 7 show further respondent breakdown by industry, education and IS experience.

The internal consistency, calculated via Cronbach's alpha, ranged from 0.774 to 0.980, exceeding the minimally required 0.70 level [13, 16]. Factor analysis was implemented on the detailed items of the SISP process and SISP success constructs. Table 8 describes the reliability of SISP phases and success constructs.

Tables 9 and 10 present the principal component analysis using the Maximum Likelihood Estimate and the extraction of factors with Promax with Kaiser Normalization method. The factor loadings and cross loadings provide support for convergent and discriminant validity.

Findings indicate that IS executives are not aware of defining goals for the IS development. This finding is important because it confirms the negative consequences that SMEs face due to the lack of strategic planning. Furthermore, the new factor which was developed regarding to the understanding of the importance of SISP by managers is crucial. IS executives can define priorities, increase the cooperation among the IS team and provide guidelines regarding in order to support the effectiveness of IS plans.

Previous findings conclude that managers concentrate more on Strategy Conception and Strategy Implementation and they do not invest time on Strategic Awareness and Situation Analysis, as a result the implemented plans are not effective, successful and they do not meet the objectives [3, 13, 14]. Moreover, when managers concentrate on the implementation of the process, shorter SISP horizons are achieved but the strategic goals cannot be met. Executives do not focus on strategic objectives that really concern them and on how they can increase value to the business because they invest time on the horizon of the project and on minimizing its cost due to limited IT budget [3]. The results indicate that executives should pay attention to implementing Situational Analysis with greater meticulousness, so that they can apply Strategy Conception and Strategy Implementation Planning with greater agility rather than now. Planners should analyze their current business systems, organizational systems, IS, as well as the business environment and external IT environment. If planners understand those elements, they can improve the result of the planning process excluding the increased time and cost needed for the process.

When executives understand the environment, they can determine important IT objectives and opportunities for improvement and they can evaluate them in order to define high-level IT strategies in their business' strategy conception [12, 26].

## 5    Conclusion

So far, few academic researchers have paid attention to the effect of SISP phases on success. This paper examines the extent on which the phases of a formal process can be followed by IS executives and managers in order to plan and use the right IS and increase competitive advantage. The results of this survey indicate that they concentrate on Strategy Conception and Formulation, focusing on defining IT objectives and architectures. As a result, they might be planning inefficiently and ineffectively.

Findings show that IS executives do not concentrate on Strategic Awareness, Situation Analysis and Strategy Formulation phase. Also, problems have been created from the implementation of the process concerning the lack of managers' education, communication, participation and cooperation, alignment of business goals with IS and the support of the change. These factors have negatively affected the success of the process. Future research should examine how managers could focus more on these phases and how they could limit the negative effects of these factors on SISP success.

The results of this study contribute to IS executives' awareness of the strategic use of IS planning in order to increase competitive advantage. Understanding those phases may help IS executives concentrate their efforts on organizations' objectives and recognize the greatest value of the planning process in their business. Second, the results of this survey can increase their awareness of the phases of SISP. IS executives should be knowledgeable about the five phases and they should not ignore the tasks of each one because this might be an obstacle which presents the organization from achieving its planning goals and thus from realizing greater value. Finally, the findings contribute to IS executives in Greek SMEs who do not concentrate on strategic planning during the development of IS and they focus only on the technical issues. As a result, they should understand the significance of the SISP process in order to formulate and implement IS strategy which will be aligned with business objectives and increase the success of SMEs.

A limitation of this study stems from the fact that the survey was conducted only in Greece. Nevertheless, the results of an exploratory study will be summarized in an improved conceptual model for further research. Also, this survey is made for SMEs. Future researchers could examine and compare these results with relative ones from large companies. Apparently, future researchers may use different methodologies for data analysis, such as cluster analysis in order to compare the differences among organizations in each sector during the implementation of the SISP process.

# Annex

**Table 1.** SISP phases and activities.

| Phases | Activities | References |
|---|---|---|
| Strategic awareness | Determining key planning issues (SAw1) Determining planning objectives (SAw2) Organizing the planning team (Saw3) Obtaining top management commitment (SAw4) | [2, 3, 10–12, 14, 15] |
| Situation analysis | Analyzing current business systems (SA1) Analyzing current organizational systems (SA2) Analyzing current information systems (SA3) Analyzing the current external business environment (SA4) Analyzing the current external IT environment (SA5) | |

(continued)

**Table 1.**  (*continued*)

| Phases | Activities | References |
|---|---|---|
| Strategy conception | Identifying major IT objectives (SC1)<br>Identifying opportunities for improvement (SC2)<br>Evaluating opportunities for improvement (SC3)<br>Identifying high-level IT strategies (SC4) | |
| Strategy formulation | Identifying new business processes (SF1)<br>Identifying new IT architectures (SF2)<br>Identifying specific new projects (SF3)<br>Identifying priorities for new projects (SF4) | |
| Strategy Implementation Planning | Defining change management approaches (SIP1)<br>Defining action plans (SIP2)<br>Evaluating action plans (SIP3)<br>Defining follow-up and control procedures (SIP4) | |

**Table 2.**  Success dimensions.

| Dimensions | Items | References |
|---|---|---|
| Alignment | Maintaining a mutual understanding with top management on the role of IS in supporting strategy (AL1)<br>Understanding the strategic priorities of top management (AL2)<br>Identifying IT-related opportunities to support the strategic direction of the firm (AL3)<br>Aligning IS strategies with the strategic plan of the organization (AL4)<br>Adapting the goals/objectives of IS to changing goals/objectives of the organization (AL5)<br>Educating top management on the importance of IT (AL6)<br>Adapting technology to strategic change (AL7)<br>Assessing the strategic importance of emerging technologies (AL8) | [13, 14] |
| Analysis | Identifying opportunities for internal improvement in business processes through IT (AN1)<br>Maintaining an understanding of changing organizational processes and procedures (AN2)<br>Generating new ideas to reengineer business processes through IT (AN3)<br>Understanding the information needs through subunits (AN4)<br>Understanding the dispersion of data, applications, and other technologies throughout the firm (AN5)<br>Development of a "blueprint" which structures organizational processes (AN6) | |

*(continued)*

**Table 2.** (*continued*)

| Dimensions | Items | References |
|---|---|---|
| | Improved understanding of how the organization actually operates (AN7) | |
| | Monitoring of internal business needs and the capability of IS to meet those needs (AN8) | |
| Cooperation | Developing clear guidelines of managerial responsibility for plan implementation (CO1) | |
| | Identifying and resolving potential sources of resistance to IS plans (CO2) | |
| | Maintaining open lines of communication with other departments (CO3) | |
| | Coordinating the development efforts of various organizational subunits (CO4) | |
| | Establishing a uniform basis for prioritizing projects (CO5) | |
| | Achieving a general level of agreement regarding the risks/tradeoffs among system projects (CO6) | |
| | Avoiding the overlapping development of major systems (CO7) | |
| Capabilities | Ability to identify key problem areas (CA1) | |
| | Ability to anticipate surprises and crises (CA2) | |
| | Flexibility to adapt to unanticipated changes (CA3) | |
| | Ability to gain cooperation among user groups for IS plans (CA4) | |

**Table 3.** Respondents' industry.

| Primary business category | Respondents | Percentage |
|---|---|---|
| Agriculture & food | 47 | 16% |
| Business services | 33 | 11.3% |
| Chemicals, pharmaceuticals & plastics | 18 | 6.1% |
| Construction | 22 | 7.5% |
| Education | 4 | 1.4% |
| Electrical | 11 | 3.8% |
| Energy | 8 | 2.7% |
| IT, Internet, R&D | 24 | 8.2% |
| Leisure and tourism | 16 | 5.5% |
| Metals, machinery & engineering | 28 | 9.6% |
| Minerals | 3 | 1% |
| Paper, printing, publishing | 14 | 4.8% |
| Retail & traders | 31 | 10.6% |
| Textiles, clothing, leather, watchmaking, Jewellery | 14 | 4.8% |
| Transport & logistics | 20 | 6.8% |
| Total | 294 | 100 |

**Table 4.**  Education level

| Education level | Respondents | Percentage |
|---|---|---|
| 2 year college graduate | 59 | 20.1% |
| 4 year college graduate | 132 | 44.7% |
| Post graduate degree | 103 | 35.2% |
| Total | 294 | 100 |

**Table 5.**  Respondents' IS experience.

| Years | Respondents | Percentage |
|---|---|---|
| 0–5 | 22 | 7.5% |
| 6–15 | 81 | 27.6% |
| 16–25 | 118 | 39.9% |
| 26–35 | 61 | 20.8% |
| Total | 12 | 100 |

**Table 6.**  IS employees.

| Employees | Respondents | Percentage |
|---|---|---|
| 0–5 | 261 | 89.1% |
| 6–10 | 22 | 7.5% |
| 11–20 | 3 | 1% |
| 21–30 | 5 | 1.7% |
| 31–40 | 0 | 0 |
| 41–50 | 0 | 0 |
| >=51 | 2 | 0.7% |
| Total | 294 | 100 |

**Table 7.**  IS budges.

| IS budget | Respondents | Percentage |
|---|---|---|
| 0–50.000 € | 175 | 59.7% |
| 51.000–100.000 € | 64 | 21.8% |
| 101.000–150.000 € | 17 | 5.8% |
| 151.000–200.000 € | 12 | 4.1% |
| >=201.000 € | 25 | 8.5% |
| Total | 294 | 100 |

**Table 8.** Reliability analysis.

| Variables | Mean | S.D. |
|-----------|------|------|
| SAw1 | 3.820 | .9190 |
| SAw2 | 3.949 | .9130 |
| SAw3 | 3.752 | 1.0562 |
| SAw4 | 3.830 | 1.0540 |
| SA1 | 3.633 | 1.0258 |
| SA2 | 3.721 | .9147 |
| SA3 | 4.207 | .7932 |
| SA4 | 3.888 | .9443 |
| SA5 | 4.082 | .9384 |
| SC1 | 3.946 | .8608 |
| SC2 | 3.823 | .8952 |
| SC3 | 3.714 | .9420 |
| SC4 | 3.963 | .8677 |
| SF1 | 3.748 | .9299 |
| SF2 | 3.748 | 1.0920 |
| SF3 | 3.701 | .9486 |
| SF4 | 3.776 | .9035 |
| SIP1 | 3.765 | .9252 |
| SIP2 | 3.704 | 1.0004 |
| SIP3 | 3.415 | 1.0538 |
| SIP4 | 3.565 | .9953 |
| AL1 | 3.993 | .9347 |
| AL2 | 3.864 | .9502 |
| AL3 | 3.922 | .9185 |
| AL4 | 3.854 | .9469 |
| AL5 | 3.878 | .9303 |
| AL6 | 3.728 | 1.0552 |
| AL7 | 3.827 | .9350 |
| AL8 | 3.793 | .9462 |
| AN1 | 3.827 | .8388 |
| AN2 | 3.782 | .8667 |
| AN3 | 3.779 | .9212 |
| AN4 | 3.707 | .8721 |
| AN5 | 3.806 | .9740 |
| AN6 | 3.517 | .9589 |
| AN7 | 3.735 | .8885 |
| AN8 | 3.759 | .8702 |

(*continued*)

**Table 8.**  (*continued*)

| Variables | Mean | S.D. |
|-----------|------|------|
| CO1 | 3.639 | 1.0349 |
| CO2 | 3.415 | .9188 |
| CO3 | 3.687 | .9621 |
| CO4 | 3.551 | .9541 |
| CO5 | 3.622 | .9654 |
| CO6 | 3.476 | .9694 |
| CO7 | 3.554 | .9787 |
| CA1 | 3.711 | .9464 |
| CA2 | 3.571 | .9564 |
| CA3 | 3.670 | .9365 |
| CA4 | 3.840 | .9871 |

**Table 9.**  Factor loadings for SISP phases.

| Factors | Items | Loadings |
|---------|-------|----------|
| Strategy implementation planning | Evaluating action plans | .929 |
| | Defining action plans | .890 |
| | Defining change management approaches | .661 |
| | Defining follow-up and control procedures | .595 |
| Analysis of internal environment | Analyzing current information systems | .878 |
| | Analyzing the current external business environment | .728 |
| | Analyzing the current external IT environment | .639 |
| | Organizing the planning team | .635 |
| | Determining planning objectives | .472 |
| | Obtaining top management commitment | .329 |
| Strategy conception | Identifying opportunities for improvement | .925 |
| | Identifying major IT objectives | .846 |
| | Identifying high-level IT strategies | .556 |
| | Evaluating opportunities for improvement | .504 |
| Strategy formulation | Identifying new IT architectures | .906 |
| | Identifying new business processes | .500 |
| | Identifying priorities for new projects | .474 |
| | Identifying specific new projects | .351 |
| Analysis of external environment | Analyzing current business systems | .895 |
| | Analyzing current organizational systems | .711 |

**Table 10.** Factor loadings for success constructs.

| Factors | Items | Loadings |
|---|---|---|
| Cooperation | Identifying and resolving potential sources of resistance to IS plans | .835 |
| | Coordinating the development efforts of various organizational subunits | .814 |
| | Achieving a general level of agreement regarding the risks/tradeoffs among system projects | .800 |
| | Establishing a uniform basis for prioritizing projects | .772 |
| | Maintaining open lines of communication with other departments | .748 |
| | Developing clear guidelines of managerial responsibility for plan implementation Ability to anticipate surprises and crises | .688 |
| | Ability to anticipate surprises and crises | .523 |
| | Avoiding the overlapping development of major systems | .480 |
| | Ability to gain cooperation among user groups for IS plans | .471 |
| Analysis | Maintaining an understanding of changing organizational processes and procedures | .795 |
| | Generating new ideas to reengineer business processes through IT | .774 |
| | Improved understanding of how the organization actually operates | .773 |
| | Understanding the information needs through subunits | .746 |
| | Identifying opportunities for internal improvement in business processes through IT | .738 |
| | Monitoring of internal business needs and the capability of IS to meet those needs | .599 |
| | Understanding the dispersion of data, applications, and other technologies throughout the firm | .597 |
| | Ability to identify key problem areas | .562 |
| | Development of a "blueprint" which structures organizational processes | .522 |
| | Assessing the strategic importance of emerging technologies | .425 |
| | Flexibility to adapt to unanticipated changes | .323 |
| Strategic alignment | Understanding the dispersion of data, applications, and other technologies throughout the firm | .910 |
| | Aligning IS strategies with the strategic plan of the organization | .707 |
| | Identifying IT-related opportunities to support the strategic direction of the firm | .393 |
| Managers' understanding of IS | Maintaining a mutual understanding with top management on the role of IS in supporting strategy | .979 |
| | Understanding the strategic priorities of top management | .677 |

# References

1. Bourletidis, K., Triantafyllopoulos, Y.: SMEs survival in time of crisis: strategies, tactics and commercial success stories. Procedia - Soc. Behav. Sci. **148**, 639–644 (2014)
2. Brown, I.: Strategic information systems planning: comparing espoused beliefs with practice. In: ECIS 2010 Proceedings of 18th European Conference on Information Systems, pp. 1–12. South Africa (2010)
3. Brown, I.T.J.: Testing and extending theory in strategic information systems planning through literature analysis. Inf. Resour. Manag. J. **17**, 20–48 (2004)
4. Giannacourou, M., Kantaraki, M., Christopoulou, V.: The perception of crisis by Greek SMEs and its impact on managerial practices. Proc. - Soc. Behav. Sci. **175**, 546–551 (2015)
5. Kamariotou, M., Kitsios, F.: Strategic information systems planning. In: Khosrow-Pour, M. (ed.) Encyclopedia of Information Science and Technology 4th edn, Chap. 78, pp. 912–922. IGI Global Publishing (2018)
6. Kamariotou, M., Kitsios, F.: An empirical evaluation of strategic information systems planning phases in SMEs determinants of effectiveness. In: Proceedings of the 6th International Symposium and 28th National Conference on Operational Research, pp. 67–72 Greece (2017)
7. Kamariotou, M., Kitsios, F.: Strategic information systems planning: SMEs performance outcomes. In: Proceedings of the 5th International Symposium and 27th National Conference on Operation Research, pp. 153–157, Greece (2016)
8. Kearns, G.S., Lederer, A.L.: A resource-based view of strategic IT alignment: how knowledge sharing create competitive advantage. Decis. Sci. **34**, 1–29 (2003)
9. Lederer, A.L., Sethi, V.: Key prescriptions for strategic information systems planning. J. Manag. Inf. Syst. **13**, 35–62 (1996)
10. Maharaj, S., Brown, I.: The impact of shared domain knowledge on strategic information systems planning and alignment: original research. S. Afr. J. Inf. Manag. **17**, 1–12 (2015)
11. Mentzas, G.: Implementing an IS strategy- a team approach. Long Range Plan. **30**, 84–95 (1997)
12. Mirchandani, D.A., Lederer, A.L.: Less is more: information systems planning in an uncertain environment. Inf. Syst. Manag. **29**, 13–25 (2014)
13. Newkirk, H.E., Lederer, A.L., Srinivasan, C.: Strategic information systems planning: too little or too much? J. Strat. Inf. Syst. **12**, 201–228 (2003)
14. Newkirk, H.E., Lederer, A.L.: The effectiveness of strategic information systems planning under environmental uncertainty. Inf. Manag. **43**, 481–501 (2006)
15. Newkirk, H.E., Lederer, A.L., Johnson, A.M.: Rapid business and IT change: drivers for strategic information systems planning? Eur. J. Inf. Syst. **17**, 198–218 (2008)
16. Pai, J.C.: An empirical study of the relationship between knowledge sharing and IS/IT strategic planning (ISSP). Manag. Decis. **44**, 105–122 (2006)
17. Peppard, J., Ward, J.: Beyond strategic information systems: towards an IS capability. J. Strat. Inf. Syst. **13**, 167–194 (2004)
18. Premkumar, G., King, W.R.: Assessing strategic information systems planning. Long Range Plan. **24**, 41–58 (1991)
19. Premkumar, G., King, W.R.: The evaluation of strategic information system planning. Inf. Manag. **26**, 327–340 (1994)
20. Rathnam, R.G., Johnsen, J., Wen, H.J.: Alignment of business strategy and IT strategy: a case study of a fortune 50 financial services company. J. Comput. Inf. Syst. **45**, 1–8 (2004)
21. Reich, H., Benbasat, I.: Factors that influence the social dimension of alignment between business and information technology objectives. MIS Q. **24**, 81–113 (2000)

22. Siakas, K., Naaranoja, M., Vlachakis, S., Siakas, E.: Family businesses in the new economy: how to survive and develop in times of financial crisis. Procedia Econ. Financ. **9**, 331–341 (2014)
23. Suh, H., Hillegersberg, J.V., Choi, J., Chung, S.: Effects of strategic alignment on IS success: the mediation role of IS investment in Korea. Inf. Technol. Manag. **14**, 7–27 (2013)
24. Ullah, A., Lai, R.: A systematic review of business and information technology alignment. ACM Trans. Manag. Inf. Syst. **4**, 1–30 (2013)
25. Vassiliadis, S., Vassiliadis, A.: The Greek family businesses and the succession problem. Procedia Econ. Financ. **9**, 242–247 (2014)
26. Zubovic, A., Pita, Z., Khan, S.: A Framework for investigating the impact of information systems capability on strategic information systems planning outcomes. In: Proceedings of 18th Pacific Asia Conference on Information Systems, pp. 1–12, China (2014)

# Bargaining Between the Client and the Bank and Game Theory

Martina Hedvicakova and Pavel Prazak[✉]

Faculty of Informatics and Management, University of Hradec Králové,
Rokitanskeho 62, 500 03 Hradec Kralove, Czech Republic
{martina.hedvicakova,pavel.prazak}@uhk.cz

**Abstract.** Czech banking market is specific for its high percentage of earnings from bank charges as a total percentage of bank earnings. This article is focused on the problems associated with bargaining between bank clients and banking institutions in the Czech Republic. With most banks in the market, bank clients must pay monthly charges in order to maintain their bank accounts. The article describes the interaction between the bank and the client from the game theory perspective. Both bargaining parties have different goals and they encounter each other during the bargaining process about the price of bank charges. The game theory defines the pay-off function, the decision tree and the point of conflict. The result is a model of this interaction that appears as an extensive form game. The actual amount of charges that result from the bargaining is regularly ascertained by a national survey using the Client Index (Klientský index) for current accounts in the Czech Republic. The Client Index represents the quantification of average costs of maintaining a current account of individual respondents based on the monitoring of specific retail banking products and services according to fee schedules of individual banks and the behaviour of individual bank clients. The approximation of the value of this Client Index was used for the proposal of pay-off function in the model. The paper also deals with general theoretical bases of bargaining, particularly it focused on bargaining with a client. The cooperative and non-cooperative strategy towards the client are described. The reasons for bargaining with existing bank clients are presented as well. Finally the article also summarizes both the goals of clients and banks during bargaining.

**Keywords:** Bank · Game theory · Client · Client Index · Bargaining
Pay-off matrix · Decision tree · Bank charges

## 1 Introduction

The 21st century has seen continuous efforts to increase earnings and competitiveness. Banks have also been continuously trying to strengthen their market position and increase their earnings. The Czech banking market is specific for its high percentage of earnings from bank charges as a total percentage of bank earnings, see the Capgemini study [9].

The Government of the Czech Republic already had to address this problem when it issued a resolution in 2005 in which it agreed with the intention to:

© Springer Nature Switzerland AG 2019
M. Themistocleous and P. Rupino da Cunha (Eds.): EMCIS 2018, LNBIP 341, pp. 518–531, 2019.
https://doi.org/10.1007/978-3-030-11395-7_40

- Take active steps contained in the document, stated under point I/1 of this resolution, leading to improvement in the position of bank clients in the Czech Republic and to an increase in the transparency of the financial market in the Czech Republic, in compliance with standards and trends common in EU member states,
- Intensify the cooperation between representatives of the financial sector and consumer organisations in the sense of point II/1 of this resolution [18]. Note that the first paragraph of a section or subsection is not indented. The first paragraphs that follows a table, figure, equation etc. does not have an indent, either.

In spite of the Resolution by the Government of the Czech Republic and the supervision of the Czech National Bank, the banks still maintain high charges for maintaining accounts and charge high amounts for various "non-standard" products and services.

Moreover, the past six years have seen the entry of new low-cost banks (for ex. Air Bank, Equa Bank, ZUNO, mBank and others). Even though these banks are characterized by having low monthly costs for the administration of retail banking and they are slowly winning over clients of traditional big banks (for ex. Komerční banka, ČSOB, Česká spořitelna, etc.), there has been no decrease in bank charges with these big banks.

The recent financial crisis has shown that a liquidity risk plays an important role in the current developed financial system [31].

Customer satisfaction is an important factor in the performance and competitiveness of banks [4, 5, 19, 22, 23, 29]. Compliance with the consumers' needs and requirements [3], comprehensive customer care and the bank customers' satisfaction is currently at the center of attention of researchers and bankers (as it represents an important marketing variable for most of the companies [3, 24].

Bank clients are therefore left with no other option but to start actively bargaining with their banks.

Bargaining is the very thing that can be used in banking as well as in other sectors. However, there are several different views of bargaining.

## 2 The Aim and Methodology of the Paper

The aim of this paper is to analyze the amount of bank charges in the banking market in the Czech Republic with the calculation of the average price level using the Client Index for current accounts in the Czech Republic. The aim is to design a model that will characterize basic elements of a bank client's decision-making and that of the bank during the bargaining process about the amount of monthly charges in order to maintain a current account based on the quantification of real average costs for maintaining a current account. The model shall be formulated as an extensive form game.

Before the analysis itself, it is first necessary to define Income from charges and commissions that are kept in the profit and loss account. According to the Czech Statistical Office, these are the incomes and commissions gained from services related to accepted deposits, i.e. maintaining current and term accounts, opening and closing accounts, charges for withdrawing cash from ATMs, direct banking etc. Furthermore, this also includes commissions related to the granting of a loan, maintaining a loan account, maintaining credit cards, etc. (Czech Statistical Office, 2015).

Data about the amount of bank charges and commissions was acquired from publicly available data by the banks (fee schedules, yearly reports, management reports of banks and documents about the financial situation of the bank, etc.). Non-consolidated data from profit and loss accounts or from balances sheet were used to make calculations about Czech banks. For most parent banks, it was necessary to work with consolidated data for the given group. The data were also provided from www. bankov-nipoplatky.com, which runs a tool for comparing bank charges - Kalkulátor bankovních poplatků, [34], for which authors analyses bank charges in the Czech Republic. The Client Index was calculated based on these data.

The Client Index represents the quantification of average costs of maintaining a current account of individual respondents based on the monitoring of specific retail banking products and services according to fee schedules of individual banks and the behaviour of individual bank clients. The frequency of the individual items of the fee schedules is monitored based on a questionnaire (e.g. how many times clients use the given service and how much is charged for the service, what turnover and balance they have in their accounts, etc.) This is why a client who is active might have to pay hundreds of Czech crowns per month even in a bank that has average prices. If somebody uses the bank very little, they can pay under 100 CZK per month, even in a bank that is otherwise expensive.

Bank charges calculator with the Client Index differs from other calculators available in the market (e.g. www.chytryhonza.cz, www.finparada.cz etc.), which only follow average costs for maintaining a bank account. Calculator follows the clients' behaviour in great detail, more precisely, it captures the respondents' use of retail banking services.

After a verification and validation phase that filters out respondents who use retail products incorrectly (e.g. small entrepreneurs etc.), the calculations are carried out on a monthly basis from 2012 to 2013, and at the same time, since 2013, there has been quantification on a quarterly basis using the statistical software IBM PASW 18 and MS Excel 2013.

The methodology for calculating average costs of individual accounts is supported by information not only about the bank, but also about the specific accounts. The average costs of a specific account are established by the arithmetic average of clients who have chosen the monitored account computed by the Calculator. Data collection took place from 2012 until 2017. On average, 2000 respondents filled in the Calculator per month. For a more detailed description of the methodology, please see e.g. [13, 28].

# 3   Theoretical Bases

Earnings from bank charges were defined in the previous chapter. In addition, basic terms regarding bargaining shall be explained.

As mentioned in the introduction, there are several different points of view regarding the definition of bargaining. Fisher [15] defines bargaining as a discussion between two or more parties with different priorities who are trying to reach a mutual agreement. It serves the purpose of promoting one's own interests, usually with respect to the interests of the other party. One's attitude towards bargaining depends on the position in which the individual parties enter the discussion.

Bargaining is an interaction during which two or more individuals are trying to achieve a mutually acceptable consensus regarding the possible outcome [14]. Odell [25] uses a similar definition when he perceives bargaining as a sequence of actions in which two or more parties go through demands, suggestions and arguments with the advised view of reaching a consensus. The basic elements in bargaining include: time, information and power [12].

According to most authors, the criterion for dividing bargaining is whether the bargaining defends the position or interests of clients. There is a contrast in the terminology between the individual types of bargaining. For example, Plamínek [26] distinguishes between competitive, cooperative, virtual and principled bargaining. As early as six years later, the same author [27] only sets forth competitive, cooperative and principled bargaining. Holá [20] sets forth positional (competitive) bargaining and constructive (principled) bargaining [16].

## 3.1  Negotiation and Bargaining

In practice, the terms negotiation and bargaining are sometimes interchanged. Negotiation means targeted behaviour. The aim is to influence (change, maintain) a certain state or situation.

If we wish to define negotiation in banking, then we should say that it is a process of mutual interaction between the worker of the bank and the client that is related to the business goals of the bank and the financial needs of the client.

In practice, there can occur two basic situations during which a negotiation may take place:

- In a situation where differences of interests of the participating parties are not expressed (an example may be providing a service to the client based on business terms and conditions that had been previously set forth and accepted by the client – a negotiation in narrower terms).
- Or in situations where differences of interests are expressed (negotiating with a client regarding business conditions), or, alternatively, in a conflict situation (addressing claims).

On the other hand, bargaining is a targeted behaviour (acting) in a situation of conflict of interests. For example, 2 parties with different interests and goals are bargaining.

The process of negotiation about the conditions of a banking deal using means of communication may have two basic bargaining goals:

A congruent goal = making a deal between the bank and the client.

Incongruent goals = conditions of the deal. The goals of the participating parties concerning the conditions of the deal may be ambivalent or contradictory. This is when a conflict of interests arises, and we subsequently start bargaining about these interests. When we find a compromise between contradicting goals in order to attain more important congruent goals, then the bargaining is successful. In order to have successful bargaining, it is sometimes necessary to re-forge the differences in attitudes and standpoints.

## 3.2    Strategies Used During Bargaining with the Client

The bank uses a cooperative WIN – WIN strategy towards the client, because it prefers long-term cooperation to a one-off victory over the client (an instant advantage).

One-sided advantages attained by the bank by a WIN – LOSS strategy threaten the permanency of the business relationship and the loss of the client is impending.

The client may be expected to use a mixed strategy, sometimes a cooperative one, and at other times a competitive one (for example, a client's request for a change of conditions that had been settled right before signing).

Bankers should refrain from a victory over the client, because if the client is in need, they are forced to accept any contractual conditions that they consider to be at their loss and they will not ever forgive the bank for this. From a long-term perspective, this is a Pyrrhic victory for the bank, which can lose not only the client, but also a part of their image as well.

If the bank chooses a WIN – WIN strategy, but rewards based on a WIN-LOSE strategy, it contradicts the WIN-WIN relationship as a result. In a WIN-WIN solution, both sides win, for example, the bank gets higher bank charges for maintaining the account and the client gets quick and accessible services.

## 3.3    The Goals of Clients During Bargaining with a Bank

Each client is different and needs different services, has different financial means at their disposal and is in a different life situation. This is why it is possible to define the basic goals of clients during bargaining with a bank:

- Minimization of costs for maintaining current account.
- Full service for clients who do not want to take care of anything.
- Technologically advanced services. Above all, these clients demand high-tech technologies for internet banking and smart banking. The bank must offer platforms for their operating system and come up with the latest trends in banking.
- Non risk takers: These clients prefer the background of traditional big banks.
- Having a branch of the given bank close to their home or work. These clients can be called "branch" clients. They prefer carrying out financial operations right at the branch in spite of higher costs.
- Demanding clients need a broad range of services that online banks or smaller banks are not able to provide. These might include payments abroad or from abroad, etc.
- Certain clients demand a personal banker to advise them on financial operations, whether virtually or in person.
- Certain clients prefer bonuses and benefits for loyalty to the given bank or for using its products and services.

- Having everything with one bank. With growing competition, banks are gradually beginning to offer competitive products from different financial segments. For example loans, insurance, mortgages, etc. It might be convenient for clients to have everything with one bank.
- If the client is in need, he or she is willing to accept disadvantageous conditions and it is more important for him/her to get the product quickly or just plain get it.

### 3.4   Goals of the Bank

The following can be noted as the essential goals of banks:

- Maximizing earnings from provided products and services.
- Keeping existing clients at the expense of short-term earnings (a charge from a payment is better than not having the client at all).
- Acquiring new clients (the bank begins with lower income and it gradually convinces the client of the quality of its services in view of the fact that the client will be willing to pay more for services in the future).
- Targeting a certain segment or group in the market. For example, students who represent a source of income for the bank in the future, the working population, pensioners etc.
- Offering their clients as wide a range of products and services as possible, offering their clients product packages so that they are willing to have everything with one bank.
- These days, when most banks have an unnecessary amount of assets, focusing on providing loans to clients or assisting them in investing in stock exchanges or investment markets.
- If the client has, for example, a current account opened with the bank, the bank gains information about the client's financial operations. Using this information, it can offer the client products and services in a good way and it eliminates its risk, because it knows the movements and balances on the client's account.
- Reaching out to as wide a range of clients as possible via different competitions, promotions and events of the bank.

### 3.5   Reasons for Bargaining with Existing Bank Clients

Reasons for bargaining with existing bank clients include the following:

- Acquiring new clients is financially more demanding than keeping existing ones.
- There is tough competition in the Czech banking market and there is a range of tools to compare monthly costs for maintaining an account, which decreases the asymmetry of information in the banking market. It is also easy for the client to change banks using the banking code of conduct.
- The client's financial situation changes over time. Even though the client does not bring any earnings to the bank, he or she can turn into a very profitable client in the future.
- It is necessary for the bank to think of clients as partners, not adversaries. It should help the client and wish him or her success and growth, which is why it chooses a

cooperative strategy. It can help the client both through financial services and through advice.

- Moreover, the interest on current and savings accounts is nearly zero at the moment. The banks are slowly starting to speak of negative interest. This is why it is necessary to offer clients a whole wide range of services that the bank offers, for example, loans, mortgages, insurance, etc. If both the bank and the client bargain well, they may find several strategies during the bargaining process.
- A survey of GE Money Bank in January 2015 showed that 76% of the respondents had never received any reward from their bank, not even a one-off reward, or all they got was unneeded promotional merchandise. Seven per cent stated that their bank had given them a gift that really pleased them. Only 8% of the respondents had received a one-off financial sum from their bank. This, of course, does not concern interest on the balance of their accounts. "Our surveys reveal that clients are more and more demanding and if we really want to reward them for using their account actively, then the best way is a direct financial reward," says Štylerová, Director of Retail Products at GE Money Bank, [2].

## 4  Game Theory During the Bargaining Process Between the Bank and the Client

The relationship between the bank and its client regarding bank charges can be considered a conflict of two players in game theory. Game theory deals with the mathematical modelling of problems in which it is necessary to choose decision-making processes [8, 17, 30]. Each conflict in game theory can be characterized using four terms. These are game, players, strategy and pay-off. The term game generally means any conflict situation between two or more participants who are called players. It is usually assumed that the number of players is finite. Each of the players has a set of strategies at their disposal, out of which they choose individual strategies during the game according to values corresponding to the given strategies. These values are determined by the pay-off function of the given player or the pay-off and it may represent the utility, profit or win. However, the value of the pay-off does not depend solely on the strategy selected by one player, but also on the strategies selected by other players. This function is therefore defined on the Cartesian product of sets of strategies of all players. The strategy that secures the highest possible value of the pay-off function to the given player in the given game is called the optimum strategy. In some games, it is assumed that the player is intelligent. This means that he or she has all the information about the game and maximizes the value of his/her pay-off. Such an assumption shall be also made in the following model.

As has already been stated, in the game related to bank charges, which shall be labelled G, we will consider two players, the bank B and its client K. If the set of players is labelled by the symbol H, then H = {B, K}. The client K shall have two strategies available; he/she can be active or passive. In case of the active strategy A, he/she shall be interested in the amount of charges for the maintaining of his/her account with the bank, he/she shall demand a discount and in case the bank does not grant it, he/she will be ready to leave for another bank. In case of the passive strategy P, he/she shall not be actively interested in discounts for maintaining his/her bank account, however, he/she will not refuse them if they are offered and he/she will not be ready to change banks. Therefore, for the set of strategies XC of the client, XK = {A, P}. The bank B shall also have two strategies available; it can either offer cooperation or remain firm. In case of the cooperative strategy S, it shall offer its client a discount for maintaining the client's account or benefits. In case of firm strategy N, the bank shall not offer either any discount for maintaining the account or any benefits. Therefore, for the set of strategies of the client XB, XB = {S, N}. Let's label the pay-off functions of the client C, resp. bank B, fK(x, y), resp. fB(x, y), where x ∈ XK a y ∈ XB. These pay-off functions shall express the price for maintaining an account in CZK. The optimum strategy of the players can be found using the Nash equilibrium [8]. This is a game configuration that has the following property for each of the players: if all the other players use strategies from the given equilibrium, then the individual player cannot increase his or her pay-off by choosing a different strategy.

In our game with two players, the Nash equilibrium occurs when we find a coordinated pair (xo, yo), i.e. the strategy of the first and second player xo XK and yo XB for which the following holds: for each strategy x XK, it is true that fK (x, yo) ≤ fK (xo, yo) and at the same time, for each strategy y XB, it is true that fB(xo, y) ≤ fB(xo, yo). In other words, the point of equilibrium is a pair of strategies where neither player benefits from independently deviating from the equilibrium strategy. If we consider an antagonistic conflict, where one of the players wins what the other player loses, it holds that fK(x, y) + fB(x, y) = 0 and it is a zero-sum game. The values of the pay-off function of the bank fB(x, y) can therefore be summarised using the following Table 1.

**Table 1.** Values of the pay-off matrix of the bank

| client K/bank B | S | N |
|---|---|---|
| A | 50 | −185 |
| P | 120 | 185 |

Source: The author's own arrangement

The values of the pay-off function of the client fK(x, y) have the opposite sign, so it is not necessary to state them explicitly. The interpretation of these pay-offs may be, for example, as follows: fB(A, N) = −185 means that if the bank does not accede to the proposal of the active client, it loses an income of 185 CZK per month. Similarly, fB(P, N) = 185 means, that if the bank does not offer any discount to the passive client, it keeps a monthly income of 185 CZK. We shall further assume that it is a game with complete information where the players know the sets of their strategies and the amounts of their pay-offs. We shall characterize the game using a sequence of decisions by the client and the bank that follow one after another. We shall therefore suppose it is a game in an extensive form that can be illustrated using a game tree, see Fig. 1. The tree is a graph with a set of nodes and edges that is continuous and does not contain any circles [6]. If the initial node, called the root, is chosen, we get the root tree which usually has several final nodes. The nodes of the tree represent the decisions made by individual players and the final nodes characterize the pay-offs of the game. The nodes in which the player makes decisions are called decision nodes. The edges of the tree represent the strategies chosen by the players.

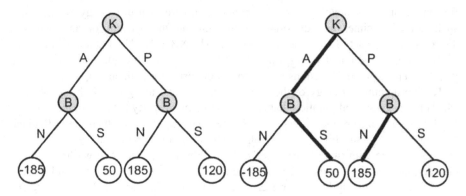

**Fig. 1.** On the left is the game tree with decision nodes K and B in which the client K, or the bank B make decisions and with final nodes that express the value of the game from the bank's point of view. On the right is the same game tree that demonstrates backward induction. Source: The author's own arrangement.

The game in an extensive form can be solved using the method of backward induction, [17], see also Fig. 1. Let's consider all the decision nodes whose edges lead to the final nodes of the game tree. In our case, these are two nodes of player B. In each of these decision nodes, we choose the edge that leads to the best final node from the perspective of the player to whom the node belongs, and we highlight it. We note the determined edge. For each decision node, we assign the pay-offs that correspond to the found best final node. We leave out all the edges stemming from the decision node, including their final nodes. This way there arises a new decision tree with new final points and their pay-offs. The whole procedure can now be repeated until we get to the root of the game tree. In our case, we finish after two steps and the rational client K chooses the edge that leads to a lower monthly charge for maintaining the account, i.e., he/she chooses the strategy of an active client A, see Fig. 1. This is how we found the Nash equilibrium $(x^\circ, y^\circ) = (A, S)$, which means that the bank client should be active during the bargaining process about the monthly price for his or her bank account. The bank should offer its client a discount so as not to lose him or her. It needs to be stressed that this result was obtained under the assumption that the game participants have complete information available, when the players know all the possible scenarios of the game. The requirement of an informed and active bank client is essential to achieve the found result of the game. The result leads us to the type of bargaining known as WIN-WIN, which was described in Sect. 3.2.

## 5  The Results of the Research of Bank Charges

In the 1st quarter of 2012, the value of the Client Index was 165.3 CZK. In the 1st quarter of 2012, clients paid 174 CZK on average in order to maintain their account. From this quarter, the value of the Client Index kept increasing (with the exception of the 1st quarter 2013, when there was a slight decrease of the value of the CI), up until the 3rd quarter of 2013, when the CI reached 180 CZK and its value turned steady. It can be seen from Fig. 2 that in the 1st quarter of 2015, there was growth to 184 CZK and in the 2nd quarter there was a decrease to 180 CZK. In the 3rd quarter, there was the most prominent increase in bank charges from the beginning of the measurement of the Client Index: an increase by 6 CZK. In the last quarter, there was another increase in average monthly costs by 2 CZK. In the next two years, amounted Client Index 184–189 CZK. The index reached the highest value in the fourth quarter 2017. (See Fig. 2). The increase in the Client Index happened repeatedly in the 4th quarter, and the authors attribute this to a more intensive activity by clients during Christmas holidays. Based on the analysis of data from the Calculator, there was particularly a higher number of withdrawals from ATMs and credit card payments (authors have been processing data for the server Bankovní poplatky [1] since the origin of the Calculator and these are their own calculations).

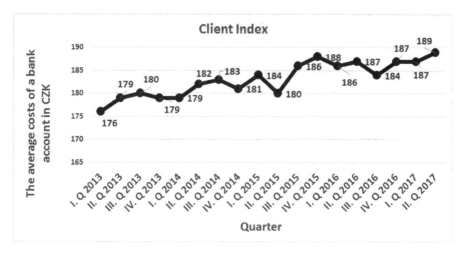

**Fig. 2.** The development of the Client Index: I. quarter 2013 – II. quarter 2017. (The average costs of a bank account in CZK. 1 EUR = 25,70 CZK.), Source: www.bankovnipoplatky.com, The author's own arrangement.

## 6  Discussion

It follows from the above research of the Client Index that the value of the Client Index increases on a year-to-year basis even though new low-cost banks that offer maintaining current accounts "for free" have entered the market. What is the reason for this increase? What are the reasons for the significant increase in the value of the Client Index in the last two quarters of 2017? Could it be higher activity by clients in the fourth quarter connected to Christmas shopping or, for example, an unwillingness of clients to bargain with their bank? Czech people are generally perceived as conservative clients not willing to change their customs and leave for another bank. On the other hand, the number of clients with newly-created low-cost banks keeps growing. With some banks, it is even a growth of tens of percentage points (e.g. Air bank, FiO banka, Equa banka, Hello bank etc.). Seven new bank has almost three million customers in January of 2018.

On the contrary, the highest year-on-year decrease in the number of clients can be seen with Česká spořitelna, which lost about 200,000 clients. "However, this is caused by abolishing the technical accounts for the sKarta," explains Marek Pšeničný from the press department. In spite of this, Česká spořitelna is slightly above the threshold of five million clients – it has 5,009,893. In the year-on-year comparison, it lost about 4% in the 1st quarter of 2015 [21]. Now Česká spořitelna has 4 670 000 clients in the beginning of 2018. ČSOB also saw a slight decrease. On the other hand, the number of clients of Komerční banka increased. The majority of clients have two or more accounts.

If we compare the current numbers of clients of the existing traditional banks and the ever growing numbers of clients of low-cost banks, we find out that the increase for these banks is not compensated by the decrease in the number of clients from traditional banks. According to Patrik Nacher from the server bankovnipoplatky.com which runs the Calculator of bank charges - Kalkulátor bankovních poplatků, [7, 34], the quick increase in the number of clients of smaller banks cannot be explained by a significant decrease in the number of clients from large banks. "The unbalanced increase and de-crease is currently given by the fact that clients do not automatically close their old account by opening a new one. However, I believe that the time when a client has several bank accounts for identical services is coming to an end," Nacher believes. Now, there are about 1.6 bank accounts per inhabitant of the Czech republic – towards the end of 2013, the Czech National Bank had 16.7 million accounts in its records.

## 7  Conclusion

The Czech Republic is characterized by high bank charges. Until 2011, there had been a growth in profits from charges and commissions, and these profits were the second highest right after profit from interest for banks in the Czech Republic. Over the past three years, there has been a slight decrease in income from charges and commissions and on the other hand, costs of making these incomes are increasing. The trend of the reduction in the volume of bank charges and commissions continued in the first quarter of 2015, when bank clients saved 281 million CZK on charges and banks saw an increase in the costs of bank charges and commissions by 95 million CZK. The banks are trying to make up for the decrease in profits from charges and commissions by increasing profits from other activities (e.g. profit from interest).

The overall profitability of banks in the Czech Republic is still growing. High bank charges are also of great importance for the stability of the banking sector in the Czech Republic. If we compare the development of the Client Index, we can see that there is an increase in spite of a slight decrease in income from bank charges and commissions. This trend has not changed after the entry of new low-cost banks in the Czech retail market. At the same time, the numbers of clients of these banks are growing by tens of percentage points per year.

However, this situation is not backed by a decrease in the number of clients of traditional big banks. The number of clients of Komerční banka increased by 1.8% in 2015 on a year-on-year basis compared to the preceding year 2014. Komerční banka has 1 664 000 clients in January 2018. If we consider the development of the number of current accounts per person in the Czech Republic, it follows that the number of accounts with low-cost banks is growing, but the clients keep their old account at the same time [19, 32, 33]. This is where there is space for bargaining with the current bank, which both banks and clients themselves should be interested in. Clients can get a free account, but in most cases they must meet the conditions given by the bank. In addition, it takes up their time and it is administratively demanding. Furthermore, it follows from the quoted pieces of research that the demandingness of Czech retail clients is growing. Both banks and clients can achieve interesting conditions with a suitable bargaining strategy and conclude more contracts for different products from the given bank.

Based on the quantification of average costs of maintaining a current account, we designed a model characterizing the essential elements of the decision-making process taken by the bank client and the bank when bargaining about the amount of monthly charges for maintaining a bank account. The model is formulated as game in an extensive form.

**Acknowledgement.** This paper is supported by specific project No. 2103 (2018) "Investment evaluation within concept Industry 4.0" at Faculty of Informatics and Management, University of Hradec Kralove, Czech Republic. In addition, the authors thank Martin Kral for his help with the project.

# References

1. Poplatky, B.: Analýza MPO (2012). http://www.bankovnipoplatky.com/analyza-mpo-porovnani-ceskych-bank-s-materskymi-bankami-17857.html. Accessed 9 Jan 2016
2. Bankovnictví: Elektronic newsletter of Journal Bankovnictví No. 04/ 27. 1. 2015. http://www.bankovnictvionline.cz/sites/de-fault/files/bank_2015_04_0.pdf. Accessed 30 Oct 2015
3. Belás, J., Lenka Gabčová, L.: The relationship among customer satisfaction, loyalty and financial performance of commercial banks. E&M Ekonomie a Manag. **19**(1), 132–147 (2016). https://doi.org/10.15240/tul/001/2016-1-010
4. Belás, J., Chochoľáková, A., Gabčová, L.: Satisfaction and loyalty of banking customers a gender approach. Econ. Sociol. **8**(1), 176–188 (2015). https://doi.org/10.14254/2071-789X.2015/8-1/14
5. Bilan, Y.: Sustainable development of a company: building of new level relationship with the consumers of XXI century. Amfiteatru Econ. J. **15**(7), 687–701 (2013)

6. Brualdi, R.A.: Introductory Combinatorics. Prentice Hall, New Jersey (2010). ISBN 0-13-602040-2

7. Calculator of bank fees (2015). http://www.bankovnipoplatky.com/kalkulator.html. Accessed 31 Dec 2015

8. Carmichel, F.: A Guide to Game Theory. Prentice Hall, Harlow (2005). ISBN 0-273-68496-5

9. Capgemini: World Retail Banking Report 2015 (2015). https://www.worldretailbankingre port.com/. Accessed 31 Dec 2015

10. CNB: Czech National Bank, Financial Sector (2015). https://www.cnb.cz/miranda2/export/ sites/www.cnb.cz/cs/financni_stabil-ita/zpravy_fs/fs_2014-2015/fs_2014-2015_financni_ sektor.pdf. Accessed 11 Dec 2015

11. CNB: Czech National Bank, Jak jsou na tom banky? (2015a). https://www.cnb.cz/cs/faq/ jak_jsou_na_tom_banky.html. Accessed 11 Dec 2015

12. Cohen, H.: Umění vyjednávat: jak dostat to, co chceš, 1. vydání Praha Pragma (1998). ISBN 80-7205-613-1

13. Draessler, J., Soukal, I., Hedvičáková, M.: Shluková analýza poptávkové strany trhu základních bankovních služeb. E+M Ekonomie a Manag. **14**(4), 102–114 (2011). ISSN 1212-3609

14. Fatima, S., Rahwan, I.: Negotiation and bargaining. In: Multiagent Systems, p. 143 (2013)

15. Fisher, R.: Jak dosáhnout souhlasu: zásady úspěšného vyjednávání, 2nd vyd, 173 s. Management Press, Praha (2004). Poradce pro praxi. ISBN 80-726-1100-3

16. Fisher, R., Ury, W., Patton, B.: Dohoda jistá: zásady úspěšného vyjednávání, 1st vyd, 174 s. Management Press, Praha (1994). Přeložil Aleš Lisa. ISBN 80-85603-48-9

17. Gintis, H.: Game Theory Evolving: A Problem-Centered Introduction to Modeling Strategic Interaction. Princeton University Press, New Jersey (2009). ISBN 978-0-691-14050-6

18. Government of the Czech Republic: Usnesení (2005). http://www.psfv.cz/assets/cs/media/ Usneseni_2005-1594_2005-12_O-zlepseni-podminek-v-bankovnim-sektoru.pdf. Accessed 9 Oct 2014

19. Hedvicakova, M.: Key study of bank accounts for young people with using multi-criteria optimization and fuzzy analysis. Appl. Econ. **49**(36), 3599–3610 (2017). https://doi.org/10. 1080/00036846.2016.1265073

20. Holá, L.: Mediace v teorii a praxi, 272 s. Grada Publishing, Praha (2011). ISBN 978-80-247-3134-6

21. Hovorka, J.: Jak velké jsou banky v Česku? Nový žebříček klientů i vkladů (2015). http:// zpravy.aktualne.cz/finance/jak-velke-jsou-banky-v-cesku-novy-zebricek-klientu-i-vkladu/ r~c6b9b70efe0211e499590025900fea04/. Accessed 30 Oct 2015

22. Chavan, J., Ahmad, F.: Factors affecting on customer satisfaction in retail banking: an empirical study. Int. J. Bus. Manag. Invention **2**(1), 55–62 (2013)

23. Keisidou, E., Lazaros, S., Maditions, D.I., Thalassinos, E.I.: Customer satisfaction, loyalty and financial performance: a holistic approach of the Greek banking sector. Int. J. Bank Mark. **31**(4), 259–288 (2013). https://doi.org/10.1108/IJBM-11-2012-0114

24. Munari, L., Lelasi, F., Bajetta, L.: Customer satisfaction management in Italian banks. Qual. Res. Financ. Markets **5**(2), 139–160 (2013). https://doi.org/10.1108/QRFM-11-2011-0028

25. Odell, J.: Negotiation and bargaining. In: Handbook of International Relations, vol. 2 (2011)

26. Plamínek, J.: Řešení konfliktů a umění rozhodovat. 1st Vyd, 198 s. Argo, Praha (1994). ISBN 8085794144

27. Plamínek, J.: Synergický management: vedení, spolupráce a konflikty lidí ve firmách a týmech, 328 s. Argo, Praha (2000). ISBN 80-7203-258-5

28. Soukal, I., Hedvičáková, M.: Klientsky index – metodika (2010). http://www. bankovnipoplatky.com/klientsky-index—metodika-12507.html. Accessed 19 Oct 2015

29. Tennant, D., Sutherland, R.: What types of banks profit most from fees charged? A cross-country examination of bank-specific and country-level determinants. J. Bank. Financ. **49**, 178–190 (2014). https://doi.org/10.1016/j.jbankfin.2014.08.023
30. Vega-Redondo, F.: Economics and the Theory of Games. Cambridge University Press, Cambridge (2003). 978-0-521-77590-8
31. Vodova, P.: Liquid assets in banking: what matters in the visegrad countries? E&M Ekonomie a Manag. **16**(3), 113–129 (2013)
32. Hedvicakova, M.: Unemployment and effects of the first work experience of university graduates on their idea of a job. Appl. Econ. **50**(31), 3357–3363 (2018). https://doi.org/10.1080/00036846.2017.1420895
33. Soukal, I., Draessler, J.: On the need for the next RCBS regulation. In: Soliman, K.S. (ed.) Proceedings of the 25th International Business Information Management Association Conference - Innovation Vision 2020: From Regional Development Sustainability to Global Economic Growth, IBIMA 2015, pp. 679–687 (2015)
34. Bank charges calculator. http://www.bankov-nipoplatky.com/kalkulator.html. Accessed 10 Feb 2018

# The Determinants of XBRL Adoption:
# An Empirical Study in an Emerging Economy

Tanja Lakovic[(✉)], Biljana Rondovic, Tamara Backovic-Vulic,
and Ivana Ivanovic

Faculty of Economics, University of Montenegro, Podgorica, Montenegro
{tanjavu,biljaro,tassabacc}@ucg.ac.me,
ivivanovic9@gmail.com

**Abstract.** The purpose of this paper is: (1) to analyze the current state of
financial reporting standardization; (2) to determine the impact of technical,
organizational and environmental factors on the level of adoption of XBRL;
(3) to investigate if there was a difference regarding the impact of the these
factors on financial companies, and regulatory bodies, in emerging countries, as
is Montenegro. Survey's data and the effect of the variables were tested using
the explorative factor analysis. In line with exceptions, results suggest that there
is a difference with regard to impact of analyzed factors on degree of acceptance
of standardized reporting forms. Environmental factors have the biggest influence, then the technical ones and at the end organizational factors. Obtained
findings can serve creators of national financial reporting strategies to understand impact of analyzed factors, properly identify challenges with regard
XBRL adoption and better manage with proactive or corrective initiatives.

**Keywords:** Financial reporting · XBRL · TOE · INT · Emerging economies

## 1 Introduction

eXtensible Business Reporting Language (XBRL) has been recognized, by many
regulators and professional organizations, as standardized format for electronic financial reporting [10, 14] with more benefits in the preparation, analysis, communication
and audit of business information [1, 7] than other reporting formats (e.g. Word, Excel,
PDF, XTML). Adopting of XBRL technology in the reporting process is a signal of
more disclosure and less information asymmetry [26] which will result in a reduction of
the cost of capital and in increase of company value [35] and improvement of business-
to-government reporting process [28]. These benefits are considered very important in
the context of well-known problems with transparency and accountability of financial
reporting, especially for emerging economies, as Montenegro, where sound financial
reporting system is imperative for their sound functioning and competitiveness.

According to Roztocki and Weistroffer [40], different factors affect the success of
the adoption and use of the new system in developed and developing economies.
Companies in emerging markets are usually faced with problems of lack of IT
capacities and managerial skills, limited access to funds, underdeveloped institutional
infrastructure and disclosure regimes etc., but also with lack of information on

© Springer Nature Switzerland AG 2019
M. Themistocleous and P. Rupino da Cunha (Eds.): EMCIS 2018, LNBIP 341, pp. 532–546, 2019.
https://doi.org/10.1007/978-3-030-11395-7_41

problems identification and solutions finding. For understanding the determinants of XBRL adoption, the authors linked two important theories of adoption and diffusion of innovations: Technology-organization-environment (TOE) framework and institutional (INT) theory. Separately, TOE framework [20] and institutional theory [16] have found a strong empirical foothold in this field of research. However, guided by the idea that multi-tiered approaches always lead to better results [32], the authors combined these two theories. The nine key factors (consisting of 22 attributes) were defined, based on which their individual impact on XBRL adoption was to be determined and measured. In order to identify the importance of these factors, the authors decided to apply factor analysis.

This research is focused on regulators, government bodies and financial companies. There are three main reasons for that: (1) The assumption that in the first phase of the XBRL implementation, more benefits will have users of financial statements, than the preparers of financial statements; (2) Most of the financial companies are part of the EU corporations, thus, the authors expect these companies will initiate introduction of this type of standardization; (3) Banks are primary source of capital for Montenegrin companies so they are, at the same time, users and analysts of company's data. In favor of this fact, the results of the study conducted by Yingchun and Baohua [47], also show that XBRL usage can be found in the financial industry prior to other industries.

This paper contributes to discussions on IT innovations in financial reporting because it provides findings on levels of technical and organizational readiness for adoption of technologies focused on standardization of financial reports, and also measuring the impact of institutional factors on speed of these technologies adoption in emerging countries as Montenegro. On the other side, with regard to practical implementation, this paper can help interested parties to more easily deal with the country-specific challenges in designing and implementation of strategies that will speed up the standardization of financial reports' electronic format.

The remainder of this article is organized as follow. Section 2 presents the results of the previous research on this topic and overview of the literature that has inspired this research. Section 3 describes research methodology and questions, the survey structure, the sample characteristics as well as applied factor analysis. Section 4 provides obtained results, which are then fully discussed in Sect. 4. Section 5 offers final conclusions, recommendations, limitations and guidelines for future research.

## 2 Literature Review

The efforts of the expert and scientists directed towards: (a) the analysis of the current situation of XBRL diffusion [16, 47], (b) proving the benefits of standardization of electronic financial reports [22] and (c) providing recommendations for XBLR implementation [15, 25], often shade the need for dedicated studies focused on factors influencing XBRL promotion and adoption. The authors believe that identifying and analyzing the influencing factors is of great importance, as the process of accepting XBRL as innovation does not take place everywhere and always in the same way.

In order to identify and analyze those factors, the authors have been focused on the literature based on theoretical frameworks from which those factors can be identified.

By studying the theoretical frameworks used in the studies conducted so far, it can clearly be noted that they differ depending on whether a study examines organizational adoption and use of IT innovation or it deals with its adoption and use by individuals, i.e., employees or consumers [37].

Since XBRL is technology, and since the problem of adopting new technology first appears on the enterprise level, and then on the level of individuals in the company [43], the authors analyzed theories consisting evidences for factors, from which XBRL acceptance by companies, depends on: TOE [7, 20, 38], Technology Acceptance Model-TAM [16, 34], Institutional Theory-INT [16, 20], Decomposed Theory of Planned Behavior-DTPB [36]. All these studies have in common to recognize three groups of factors on which adoption of XBRL depends on – technical, organizational and environmental factors, and also that there is a lack of consistent empirical evidences related to analyzed factors, influencing the degree of XBRL adoption.

By examining XBRL initiators and inhibitors in Australia, Troshani and Rao [44] noticed that enforced legal solutions and employees' skills as one of organizational factors supported XBRL usage, while scarce financial resources and technology inertia slowed down XBRL adoption in companies. Felden [16] developed a theoretical model based on the INT and TAM framework, and showed that the support of top management and social groups related activities are the most important drivers of XBRL's adoption in Germany. Also, research efforts are full of evidences that motives for XBRL adoption are duly connected to customer expectations related to: better transparency of financial information [26, 29]; better reliability, consistency, comparability, relevancy and availability of data [19]; higher degree of compliance with regulation, less production of misleading reports and need for better internal and external control [2]. Need for continuity and faster reporting [2] as well as for cost optimization by substitution of work and capital [33] are also recognized as important determinants for adoption of standardized reporting forms.

The authors agree that XBRL adoption assumes prior existence of software for conversion of financial reports into standardized format [16] and solved integration of existing and additional IS inside and outside of organization [3, 16]. These authors also agree that the integration and compatibility of the system are necessary for its easier and more successful use, and that they always impose the need for additional ICT expertise.

Comparing to the studies focused only on organizational and technical factors, step forward was made by adoption of Institutional theory. By examining factors influencing the adoption of XBRL in the context of the Securities Exchange Commission, Henderson et al. [20] showed that institutional factors are the most important for the adoption of this kind of innovations. On the other hand, by examining what influences the decision on XBRL adoption in Zeeland [7], it has been shown that no matter how strong the influence of government and regulatory bodies are, it would not be possible to accept these standards if the costs of system implementation exceed the benefits of its use. Previous studies have shown [7, 20] that regulatory bodies are those to push these standards' adoption by its regulations. However, there are evidences that in financial sector initiatives coming from banks' associations do not have to oblige, but can encourage acceptance and use of XBRL [46], while auditing companies can use their recommendations and advises to speed up the adoption process [23]. In the literature, it has also been recognized that company will adopt XBRL standard if it has been adopted by other companies in respective industry, to avoid gaining an epithet of non-innovative company [20], but also to imitate those who, thanks to the adopted innovation, have succeeded [42].

As in all above mentioned researches, factors from contexts of technological, organizational and external environments have been recognized, the authors thought that Framework of Technology-Organization-Environment–TOE [8] in combination with Institutional Theory (INT) can be further used for the purposes of this study.

Beside presented heterogeneity of given evidences, there is also evident need in the literature for creating complete picture on factors influencing XBRL adoption in emerging countries [13, 41]. This additionally motivated authors to conduct this research.

Doolin and Troshani [11] emphasize, that various adopters (producers and consumers of financial statements) are different in the way they benefit from XBRL. In that context, reviewing available literature, it can also be concluded that the opinions of representatives of regulatory bodies [7, 11], chartered accountants and managers [41] were most often considered. Taking into account the specific technical nature of XBRL, this survey additionally, also consider opinions of employees in IT sectors.

For the purpose of separating from the predecessors, and due to the heterogeneous results obtained in the abovementioned researches, the authors were motivated to do a research from which general conclusions could be derived for: (a) emerging countries, such as Montenegro; (b) finance companies that make a decision on XBRL adoption in order to convert their financial data into XBRL internally, and which would use XBRL for both internal and external purposes; (c) researches based on the integrated TOE and INT framework; (d) comparative analysis of the impact of technical, organizational and environmental factors between enterprises from an analyzed sector and regulatory agencies.

## 3  Methodology

### 3.1  Research Question and Selection of Criteria

According to the purpose of the research, the authors defined three research questions:

1. To what extent are the electronic format of financial statements currently standardized, and what is the level of demand for them?
2. To what extent technical, organizational and environmental factors influence the decision to accept standardized forms of financial statements, specifically XBRL?
3. To what extent the degree of influence of these factors in financial sector companies is different comparing to regulatory and government bodies?

In order to obtain the answer to the first research question, the authors analyzed:

- In which format was primary financial statements and the notes to the financial statements of the analyzed companies, submitted, and

- To what extent these formats contributed to the usefulness and transparency of financial statements for designated users (regulators and government bodies, and financial companies).

According to the Law on Accounting of Montenegro [27], a large and medium legal entity is obliged to submit financial reports and management report in written and electronic form to the Department of Public Revenues no later than March 31 of current year, for the previous year. Also, banks are obliged, to submit annual and quarterly financial reports in written and electronic form to the Central Bank of Montenegro, and the insurance companies also to the Insurance Supervision Agency. Since 2004, Montenegrin companies have submitted financial statements prepared in accordance with IFRS, so IASB Conceptual Framework [24] was used to assess accounting information usefulness. The level of relevant information disclosure is an important factor in the process of increasing trust on the relation of the "management-stakeholders groups", so the respondents were asked to identify the level of transparency and the usefulness of this information in the current financial statements.

In order to answer the second and the third research questions and based on the basic models (TOE and INT), 9 key factors (consisting of 22 attributes) impacting XBRL adoption were defined.

Technical factors describe characteristics of the ICT systems and the usage of underlying assumptions, on which the adoption of standardized forms of reporting depends. In accordance with previously studies [16, 17] in this research ICT infrastructure, IT integration and IT expertize are duly examined in technological context.

Organizational factors describe those attributes of a company that can influence decision-making on adoption of standardized reporting forms. Taking in consideration the literature review, authors have decided to analyze economic expectations [2, 29, 33]; inter-sectoral and inter-organizational cooperation [20].

Since the purpose of institutional theory is to focus on environmental factors that can have a decisive role in the adoption of innovation, the authors considered that mimetic, normative and coercive pressures could serve as variables for analyzing the problem of adopting the XBRL standard [7, 9, 20].

The observed attributes, obtained by integrating TOE framework and institutional theory, are shown in Fig. 1 which summarizes the design of the research model.

## 3.2   Data and Measurement

The authors conducted a survey taking into consideration the research questions and developed two forms of questionnaires, one form for financial companies and other form for regulatory and government bodies. Questionnaires for financial companies, were forwarded to accountants, IT employees and top management, while questionnaires for the regulatory bodies were forward to IT employees and top management (participant titles ranged from financial analyst to director for financial reporting). Questionnaires were chosen because they are mostly used in conducting quantitative research, where the researcher wants to count the frequency of occurrence of opinions and attitudes, experiences, processes, or predictions [39].

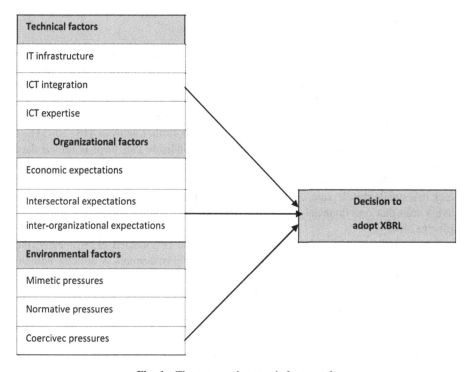

**Fig. 1.** The proposed research framework

The questionnaire survey consisted of two parts. Answers from the first part were used to obtain the answer to the first research question, and the answers from the second part of the questionnaire were used to obtain the answer to the second and third research questions. A 7-point Likert scale [21] was used to assess the current state of standardization of electronic financial statements and analyses of factors influencing future processes of their standardization with values varying from (1) "strongly disagree" to (7) "strongly agree". The survey lasted slightly more than 90 days and from 98 passed surveys, 52 fully completed surveys were returned (of which 45 for the first group and 7 for the second group of respondents). It makes the rate of return of 53.06%.

In order to obtain adequate answers to the first research question, authors used descriptive statistics, which was in line with a research's intention to explore the difference of reporting formats and opinions of the respondents on the comparability and transparency of financial reports. In order to obtain adequate answer to the second and the third research questions, nine independent variables were defined for the survey results analyses. Based on the question from the survey, 22 attributes are associated with these variables. The value of the variable is obtained as the average value of the corresponding attributes [5]. Control variables were two groups of respondents (financial companies and regulatory/governance bodies).

# 4   Results and Discussion

A reliability analysis, based on calculation of Cronbach's alpha, was carried out on the perceived task values scale comprising 9 items. It is necessary to note that the value of alpha is directly affected by the number of items that make up a scale and the sample size. Considering that in this study we have 9 items with the sample size of 52, Cronbach's alpha showed the questionnaire to reach acceptable reliability, $\alpha = 0.618$. According to the literature this is acceptable level for further analysis [18, 30, 31].

Answers received on the first research question indicate that there is no standard format for electronic reporting towards regulatory bodies in the system of financial reporting of Montenegro. In more cases, financial information are presented as a text block in a standard web page, spreadsheet, a printed document or a PDF document. We have a case that one financial company sends different reports in different formats to different users.

Results indicate that even if financial information is collected electronically, the integration of data elements from various data sources or formats is difficult without human intervention (retyping or extracting, mostly, from Excel files). Companies in the financial sector do not submit annual financial reports to XBRL format either to regulators or to parent companies, nor receive them from their clients (business entities). Companies in the financial sector, upon request of regulator, beside PDF files, submit primary financial statements and notes to financial statements in EXCEL or Word format, which clearly indicates need for interactive data existence. Financial companies are mostly submitted primary financial statements and notes to financial statements to their parent companies in Excel format (53% of the sample) than in PDF format (31%) and XML (16%). Compared to paper format, PDF format improves information accessibility, but it is document-centric format and it does not easily support system to system data transfer and analysis. In order to overcome the limitation of PDF format, the Central Bank and the Department of Public Revenues have developed their own system for their electronic filings of financial data for various analyzes since 2015. This is in line with ESMA's recommendations [14].

The obtained results indicate that there is room for further improvement in terms of transparency and usefulness of information, which is one of the benefits that XBRL should provide [26]. The survey found, that most respondents in the financial sector, on average, generally agreed that non unified reporting framework for individual users increased cost of reports preparation, decreased level of its understanding, and did not contribute to the standardization of the financial reporting process. The same opinion was shared by representatives of the regulatory agencies.

In order to get an answer to second question, the authors decided to apply explorative factor analysis to achieve two goals:

1. Tested the assumptions that all three factors are important and
2. Determined the individual significance of each of the previously mentioned factors.

To evaluate the justification of the application of factor analysis, the Kaiser-Meyer-Olkin test for all variables together, as well as Bartlett's spherical test, was applied. The results of the performed tests pointed out the fact that the application of the factor analysis for the given sample and the set of variables is justified, since the KMO measure is 0.764, therefore greater than the recommended lower limit, while the probability of making a mistake in rejecting the hypothesis of the existence of an identity matrix for the correlation matrix 0%.

**Table 1.** Justification of the use of factor analysis

| Kaiser-Meyer-Olkin measure of sampling adequacy | | .764 |
|---|---|---|
| Bartlett's test of sphericity | Approx. chi-square | 377.147 |
| | df | 36 |
| | Sig. | .000 |

On the basis of the correlation matrix, the authors concluded that it is justified to continue the implementation of factor analysis, since among the analyzed variables there is a sufficient number of coefficients of correlation whose values are greater than 0.3, as well as a sufficient number of statistically significant correlation coefficients.

In the further analysis, the common factors identified in the correlation coefficient table are recognized. This step is usually done by analyzing the main components. Factor rotation was done using the Varimax rotation with Keiser's normalization (Table 1).

**Table 2.** Extracting factors by the main component method

| Component | Initial eigenvalues | | | Extraction sums of squared loadings | | |
|---|---|---|---|---|---|---|
| | Total | % of variance | Cumulative % | Total | % of variance | Cumulative % |
| 1 | **4.171** | 46.349 | 46.349 | 4.171 | 46.349 | 46.349 |
| 2 | **2.448** | 27.198 | 73.547 | 2.448 | 27.198 | 73.547 |
| 3 | **1.053** | 11.705 | 85.252 | 1.053 | 11.705 | **85.252** |
| 4 | .466 | 5.180 | 90.432 | | | |
| 5 | .271 | 3.017 | 93.448 | | | |
| 6 | .249 | 2.768 | 96.216 | | | |
| 7 | .189 | 2.102 | 98.318 | | | |
| 8 | .098 | 1.084 | 99.402 | | | |
| 9 | .054 | .598 | 100.000 | | | |

The starting hypothesis defined three factors, which are important for the adoption of standardized forms of financial statements. This hypothesis is confirmed by research. Namely, by using the method of the main components, three factors with an eigenvalue of more than 1 have been extracted. These three factors explain 85.252% of the total variations.

Based on the results shown in Table 2, it is concluded that: the first factor has the highest load factor values for variables E1, E2 and E3, and is given the name

Environment Factor; the second factor has the highest factor load for the variables T1, T2 and T3, and is given the title Technical factor; the third factor has the highest factor load factor for the variables O1, O2 and O3, and is called Organizational Factor.

At the very end, it was necessary to see if all three factors, which were identified in both the theory and this analysis, were equally significant. The rotational sum of variance of factor loads has shown that these three factors explain 85.252% variations in the adoption of standardized forms of financial statements. Of these, the first factor, identified as the Environmental Factor, explains 30.239% variations, the other, the Technical Factor, explains 30.191% variations, while the third factor, the Organizational Factor is slightly less significant and explains 24.821% variations. In particular, the obtained results show that the transition to standardized reporting forms is currently largely dependent on external factors. Interestingly, the same ranking of an analyzed factors was recorded in another survey that was concerned with the research on this subject in Iranian companies [38].

**Table 3.** Factor loading after rotation

|  | Component | | |
|---|---|---|---|
|  | 1 | 2 | 3 |
| ICT infrastructure-T1 | −.125 | **.943** | −.025 |
| IT expertise-T2 | −.303 | **.907** | .069 |
| ICT integration-T3 | −.362 | **.822** | .090 |
| Economic expectations-O1 | .147 | .291 | **.765** |
| Intersectoral expectations-O2 | .008 | −.181 | **.925** |
| Inter-organizational expectations-O3 | .337 | .044 | **.825** |
| Mimetic pressures-E1 | **.817** | −.340 | .124 |
| Normative pressures-E2 | **.929** | −.240 | .137 |
| Coercive pressures-E3 | **.904** | −.188 | .254 |
| Factor loadings (rotation sums) | 2.722 | 2.717 | 2.234 |
| Rotation sums as % of variance | **30.239** | **30.191** | **24.821** |
| Rotation sums cumulative % | 30.239 | 60.430 | 85.252 |

This result is not uncommon when it comes to IT innovation and the introduction of standardized procedures [7, 38] and is in line with the author's expectations. Especially in developing countries, such as Montenegro, a direct or indirect impact of government, business partners and other regulatory institutions has to exist in order to create a favorable environment for accepting standards in reporting. Regulatory bodies with their obligatory acts, a professional associations, audit firms, parent corporations, etc., with their recommendations, suggestions and promotional efforts have to act towards facilitating easier adoption of XBRL or technologies similar to them. This support is important during phase of adoption of XBRL as well as at later stages of its integration with existing systems [20]. So, once again, it has been confirmed that ICT innovations have to be considered as part of the normative and as part of the corrective influences [4, 12] (Table 3).

This study also showed once again that Mimetic pressers do not always have to be very important for all types of IT diffusion [45], and in this way, this study provided only partial support institutional theory. It is obvious that in an analyzed companies, acceptance of this innovation will not come because of the need to imitate other companies (in order to avoid or minimize the risk of adopting technology, reducing the cost of its use, avoiding "childhood illnesses", etc.).

From the group of technical factors, which were in second place in significance, the acceptance of the XBRL standard has the greatest impact on the factor IT infrastructure (Factor load value is 0.943), and the smallest IT integration (Factor load value is 0.822). For the authors, this result was not surprising, regardless of the fact that the financial sector is considered to be the most information intensive [48], which is often treated as a leader in accepting IT innovations and where there is usually no problem of lack of IT infrastructure.

There are several possible reasons why this is the result of the analysis. First, the obtained results are in line with the results obtained in previous studies on IT innovation [48] and confirm the fact that the significance of this factor is precisely the highest in the phase of initiating the use of the system, and that it becomes smaller in each subsequent stage of the system's implementation, when, logically, the importance of IT integration should be greater. Second, even if the financial sector is well equipped with IT, it is possible that employees do not see the problem only in the existence of equipment, but in the scope and purpose of its use. It is also possible that employees are already aware that there is an adequate IT platform for current activities, but as such it is not sufficient to convert and convert financial reports into a standardized form, as has been shown in some previous research [16]. Being the factor of IT integration, the factor with the lowest significance, is normal in the phases of initiating the application of some IT innovation and it is logical that the significance of these factors will be greater with each subsequent phase, when logically, the focus from the possession of technology is increasingly shifted to shared use, i.e. IT integration [6].

Within the Organizational factors group, the most intimate relationship was measured with the O2 variant, which represents Inter-sectoral expectations, where the factor load value is 0.925. This finding is logical and consistent with previous research [2] and hence another confirmation that businesses, especially from this sector of the economy, have expressed the need to establish a common language of financial reporting, between sectors, between different internal business applications and between different accounting principles.

Since it was necessary to analyze the differences in the impact of individual factors for the two groups of subjects, enterprises and regulatory bodies, the use of the ANOVA test was not necessary, and a standard T-test was used. The size of the sample of regulatory and government bodies was significantly lower in relation to enterprises, it is logical that larger deviations of individual averages occurred in relation to the group average of the given variable, so the standard error of the average for this group of respondents was higher for each variable (Table 4).

**Table 4.** Descriptive statistics by variables

|  | Organization | N | Mean | Std. deviation | Std. error mean |
|---|---|---|---|---|---|
| ICT infrastructure-T1 | P | 44 | 5.20 | 1.250 | .188 |
|  | R | 8 | 5.13 | 1.727 | .611 |
| IT expertise-T2 | P | 44 | 5.32 | 1.235 | .186 |
|  | R | 8 | 6.00 | 1.069 | .378 |
| ICT integration-T3 | P | 44 | 4.95 | 1.200 | .181 |
|  | R | 8 | 5.75 | .886 | .313 |
| Economic expectations-O1 | P | 44 | 5.99 | .737 | .11 |
|  | R | 8 | 5.89 | 1.188 | .42 |
| Intersectoral expectations-O2 | P | 44 | 5.70 | 1.153 | .174 |
|  | R | 8 | 5.88 | .991 | .350 |
| Inter-organizational expectations-O3 | P | 44 | 6.36 | 1.123 | .169 |
|  | R | 8 | 6.00 | 1.195 | .423 |
| Mimetic pressures-E1 | P | 44 | 5.89 | 1.450 | .219 |
|  | R | 8 | 5.00 | 1.309 | .463 |
| Normative pressures-E2 | P | 44 | 6.432 | .8046 | .1213 |
|  | R | 8 | 4.750 | 1.1199 | .3960 |
| Coercive pressures-E3 | P | 44 | 6.363 | .794 | .119 |
|  | R | 8 | 4.479 | 1.059 | .374 |

**Table 5.** Test equivalence of variances and expected values by variables

|  | Levene's test for equality of variances | | t-test for equality of means | | |
|---|---|---|---|---|---|
| Variable | F | Sig. | T | df | Sig. (2-tailed) |
| ICT infrastructure-T1 | 1.592 | .213 | .156 | 50 | .877 |
| IT expertise-T2 | 1.172 | .284 | −1.463 | 50 | .150 |
| ICT integration-T3 | .390 | .535 | −1.782 | 50 | .081 |
| Economic expectations-O1 | 4.743 | .034 | .308 | 50 | .759 |
| Intersectoral expectations-O2 | .377 | .542 | −.392 | 50 | .697 |
| Inter-organizational expectations-O3 | .553 | .460 | .835 | 50 | .408 |
| Mimetic pressures-E1 | .438 | .511 | 1.611 | 50 | .113 |
| Normative pressures-E2 | 2.131 | .151 | 5.113 | 50 | **.000** |
| Coercive pressures-E3 | 1.505 | .226 | 5.862 | 50 | **.000** |

The results of the conducted tests showed that there are no differences in variations or the expected values for these two groups of subjects (Table 5). The exception was the Environment Factor and variables E2 and E3, which showed a deviation in the expected values of responses received from enterprises and regulatory bodies. Nevertheless, their variances remained the same. The final conclusion would be that, with the exception of the partial Environmental Factor (for the variable E1, the equivalence of expected values has been achieved), there is no difference in the relevance of these variables to the adoption of standardized forms of financial statements.

# 5  Conclusions, Implications and Limitation

Considering current reporting environment for financial entities in Montenegro, there is no standardized form of electronic reporting (single electronic format) in Montenegro and, up to date, there has been little encouragement from regulators or government departments to adopt XBRL. Only, the Insurance Supervisory Agency of Montenegro has planned to implement XBRL for financial reporting format for insurance companies until 2020.

Analyzing the measure of individual impacts of the identified factors from the group of environmental factors, it has been concluded that the normative pressures will have the greatest impact on the adoption of these standards. Yet, professional associations and auditors who have to invest additional efforts in promotion of these standards should not be ignored.

After the environmental factors, following in level of importance were technical factors, which means that the appropriate ICT platform and ICT expertise will also be crucial during the decision making on XBRL adoption, while each subsequent phase of the use of these standards will generally assume access to and routine use of the system, and therefore require a greater focus on IT integration.

The analysis showed that it was necessary to standardize financial reporting in the observed companies, but also that the same companies were not fully matured for the adoption of this standard. In other words, these companies need to continue with human resource resources and management capacities strengthening; changing the management attitude on standardization and codification of reporting which means insisting on their greater financial and moral supports. Also, following the obtained findings it is concluded that in the observed companies, the organizational issues with regard to IT competencies the allocation of financial resources for these purposes, the organization of IT supporting activities, etc. are probably not well resolved. In addition, it is obvious that in analyzed enterprises, work on campaigns raising awareness of economic and social benefits of XBRL or similar standards should continue.

This study offers both theoretical and practical implications. Theoretically, these results expand the base of empiric researches on the XBRL standards subject matter. This study may be an incentive for other researchers to address issues that will speed up the process of XBRL standards acceptance/adoption in countries, where this problem has not been resolved. In practical, this finding suggests that the observed companies should use external support as an instrument that can help in many ways, such as the ability to use a positive legal, political, institutional and investment climate to cooperate with other entities that have experience in the use of this standard; the ability to use government programs to promote standardization in financial reporting; through financial incentives in the processes of development and use of these standards; as a financial support in the field of consulting services in system development, hardware and software purchasing, etc., but also by providing ways to participate in international bodies so that employees in banks and other financial institutions can get acquainted with good international practice in the area of standardization of financial reporting. Also, the results obtained indicate that professional associations, audit firms, parent corporations, must increase awareness of the benefits of XBRL adoption, but also provide support at later stages use of systems.

This study has several limitations which brings further opportunities for future research. First, this study could be extended by analyzing the impact of technical, organizational and environmental factors at different stages of acceptance of standards (from initiation to routine practice) in different economic branches. Secondly, we do not know if the same results would be obtained by combining the TOE model with some other theoretical model for testing the determinants of accepting standardized forms of reporting. Third, the sample was relatively small because in Montenegro there is small number of financial companies. It would be interesting in future to work on a bigger sample which would include companies outside of financial sector. Lastly, the study does not address the reasons for the different effects of the proposed factors, so this limitation can also serve as an encouragement for researchers in the future.

# References

1. Alles, M., Piechocki, M.: Will XBRL improve corporate governance? A framework for enhancing governance decision making using interactive data. Int. J. Account. Inf. Syst. **13**, 91–108 (2012)
2. Baldwin, A.A., Trinkle, B.S.: The impact of XBRL: a delphi investigation. Int. J. Digit. Account. Res. **11**, 1–24 (2011)
3. Bizarro, P.A., Garcia, A.: XBRL-beyond the basics. CPA J. **80**(5), 62 (2010)
4. Bonsón, E., Cortijo, V., Escobar, T.: Towards the global adoption of XBRL using international financial reporting standards (IFRS). Int. J. Account. Inf. Syst. **10**, 46–60 (2009)
5. Bordonaba-Juste, V., Lucia-Palacios, L., Polo-Redondo, Y.: Antecedents and consequences of e-business adoption for European retailers. Internet Res. **22**(5), 532–550 (2012)
6. Chan, F.T., Chong, A.Y.L.: Determinants of mobile supply chain management system diffusion: a structural equation analysis of manufacturing firms. Int. J. Prod. Res. **51**(4), 1196–1213 (2013)
7. Cordery, C.J., Fowler, C.J., Mustafa, K.: A solution looking for a problem: factors associated with the non-adoption of XBRL. Pac. Account. Rev. **23**(1), 69–88 (2011)
8. Depietro, R., Wiarda, E., Fleischer, M.: The context for change: organization, technology and environment. Process. Technol. Innov. **199**, 151–175 (1990)
9. DiMaggio, P., Powell, W.W.: The iron cage revisited: collective rationality and institutional isomorphism in organizational fields. Am. Sociol. Rev. **48**(2), 147–160 (1983)
10. Directive 2013/50/EU of the European parliament and of the council, Official Journal of the European Union, L 294/13 (2013)
11. Doolin, B., Troshani, I.: Organizational adoption of XBRL. Electron. Mark. **17**(3), 199–209 (2007)
12. El-Haddadeh, R., Weerakkody, V., Al-Shafi, S.: The complexities of electronic services implementation and institutionalization in the public sector. Inf. Manag. **50**(4), 135–143 (2013)

13. Enachi, M.: XBRL–revolution in the digital financial reporting of the romanian organizations. Stud. Sci. Researches. Econ. Ed. **15**, 49–54 (2010)
14. European Securitas and Markets Authority (ESMA), Consultation Paper on the Regulatory Technical Standards on the European Single Electronic Format (ESEF) (2007). www.esma.europa.eu
15. Fang, J.: The progress of XBRL conversion. CPA J. **83**(2), 68 (2013)
16. Felden, C.: Characteristics of XBRL adoption in Germany. J. Manag. Control **22**(2), 161–186 (2011)
17. Garner, D., Henderson, D., Sheetz, S.D., Trinkle, B.S.: The different levels of XBRL adoption. Manag. Account. Q. **14**(2), 1 (2013)
18. Hair, J.F., Black, W.C., Babin, B.J., Anderson, R.E., Tatham, R.L.: Multivariate Data Analysis. Prentice Hall Pearson Education, Upper Saddle River (2006)
19. Hao, L., Zhang, J.H., Fang, J.: Does voluntary adoption of XBRL reduce cost of equity capital? Int. J. Account. Inf. Manag. **22**(2), 86–102 (2014)
20. Henderson, D., Sheetz, S.D., Trinkle, B.S.: The determinants of inter- organizational and internal in-house adoption of XBRL: a structural equation model. Int. J. Account. Inf. Syst. **13**(2), 109–140 (2012)
21. Ifinedo, P.: Internet/E-Business technologies acceptance in Canada's SMEs: focus on organizational and environmental factors. In: E-Business-Applications and Global Acceptance. In Tech (2012)
22. Ilias, A., Razak, M.Z.A., Rahman, R.A.: The expectation of perceived benefit of extensible business reporting language (XBRL): a case in Malaysia. J. Dev. Areas **49**(5), 263–271 (2015)
23. Ilias, A.: The practitioner's expectation of real-time reporting: case of the extensible business reporting language (XBRL). Glob. Bus. Manag. Res. **9**(3), 1–15 (2017)
24. International Accounting Standard Board (IASB), Conceptual Framework for Financial Reporting: The Objective of Financial Reporting and Qualitative Characteristics of Decision-useful Financial Reporting Information, London (2010)
25. Janvrin, D.J., No, W.G.: XBRL implementation: a field investigation to identify research opportunities. J. Inf. Syst. **26**(1), 169–197 (2012)
26. Kim, J.W., Lim, J.H., No, W.G.: The effect of first wave mandatory XBRL reporting across the financial information environment. J. Inf. Syst. **26**(1), 127–153 (2012)
27. Law on Accounting, Official Gazette of Montenegro, No. 052/16
28. Liu, C., Luo, X., Wang, L.F.: An empirical investigation on the impact of XBRL adoption on information asymmetry: evidence from Europe. Decis. Support Syst. **93**, 42–50 (2017)
29. Liu, C., Wang, T., Yao, L.J.: XBRL's impact on analyst forecast behavior: an empirical study. J. Account. Public Policy **33**(1), 69–82 (2014)
30. Moss, S., et al.: Reliability and validity of the PAS-ADD checklist for detecting psychiatric disorders in adults with intellectual disability. J. Intellect. Disabil. Res. **42**(2), 173–183 (1998)
31. Nagpal, J., Kumar, A., Kakar, S., Bhartia, A.: The development of quality of life instrument for Indian diabetes patients (QOLID): a validation and reliability study in middle and higher income groups. J. Assoc. Physicians India **58**, 295–304 (2010)
32. Nilashi, M., Ahmadi, H., Ahani, A., Ibrahim, O., Almaee, A.: Evaluating the factors affecting adoption of hospital information system using analytic hierarchy process. J. Soft Comput. Decis. Support. Syst. **3**(1), 8–35 (2016)
33. Pinsker, R.E., Li, S.: Costs and benefits of XBRL adoption: early evidence. Commun. ACM **51**(3), 47–50 (2008)

34. Pinsker, R.E: An Empirical Examination of Competing Theories to Explain Continuous Disclosure Technology Adoption Intentions Using XBRL as the Example Technology (2008)

35. Premuros, R.F., Bhattacharya, S.: Do early and voluntary filers of financial information in XBRL format signal superior corporate governance and operating performance? Int. J. Account. Inf. Syst. **9**, 1–20 (2008)

36. Rawashdeh, A., Selamat, M.H.: Critical success factors relating to the adoption of XBRL in Saudi Arabia. J. Int. Technol. Inf. Manag. **22**(2), 4 (2013)

37. Rondović, B., Djuričković, T., Kašćelan, L.: Drivers of e-business diffusion in tourism: a decision tree approach (2018)

38. Rostami, M., Nayeri, M.D.: Investigation on XBRL adoption based on TOE model. Br. J. Econ. Manag. Trade **7**(4), 269–278 (2015)

39. Rowley, J.: Designing and using research questionnaires. Manag. Res. Rev. **37**(3), 308–330 (2014)

40. Roztocki, N., Weistroffer, H.R.: Research trends in information and communications technology in developing, emerging and transition economies. Coll. Econ. Anal. **20**, 113–127 (2010)

41. Steenkamp, L.P., Nel, G.F.: The adoption of XBRL in South Africa: an empirical study. Electron. Libr. **30**(3), 409–425 (2012)

42. Teo, T.L., Chan, C., Parker, C.: Factors affecting e-commerce adoption by SMEs: a meta-analysis. In: ACIS 2004 Proceedings, p. 54 (2004)

43. Troshani, I., Doolin, B.: Drivers and inhibitors impacting technology adoption: a qualitative investigation into the Australian experience with XBRL. Paper Presented at 18th Bled e-Conference: e-Integration in Action, Bled, pp. 6–8 (2005)

44. Troshani, I., Rao, S.: Drivers and inhibitors to XBRL adoption: a qualitative approach to build a theory in under-researched areas. Int. J. E-Bus. Res. **3**(4), 98 (2007)

45. Tsai, M.C., Lai, K.H., Hsu, W.C.: A study of the institutional forces influencing the adoption intention of RFID by suppliers. Inf. Manag. **50**(1), 59–65 (2013)

46. Willis, M., Hannon, N.J.: Combating everyday data problems with XBRL. Strat. Financ. **87**(1), 57 (2005)

47. Yingchun, S., Baohua, T.: Research on the disclosure quality of financial reporting on the internet based on XBRL technology. In: International Conference on Computational and Information Sciences, pp. 605–608 (2010). https://doi.org/10.1109/iccis.2010.153

48. Zhu, K., Kraemer, K.L., Dedrick, J.: Information technology payoff in e-business environments: an international perspective on value creation of e-business in the financial services industry. J. Manag. Inf. Syst. **21**(1), 17–54 (2004)

# Mobile Technology Acceptance Model: An Empirical Study on Users' Acceptance and Usage of Mobile Technology for Knowledge Providing

Janusz Stal[✉] and Grażyna Paliwoda-Pękosz

Department of Computer Science, Cracow University of Economics,
Rakowicka 27, 31-510 Kraków, Poland
{janusz.stal,paliwodg}@uek.krakow.pl

**Abstract.** In this study we applied the technology acceptance model (TAM) to explain users' acceptance of mobile technology as a medium of knowledge providing. We adjusted the TAM by adding three new constructs: Access to Information, Information Quality, and Information Navigation. The model was tested on a population of 303 respondents using structural equation modeling (SEM). Our findings indicated that information quality and information navigation influence the perceived ease of use and, as a result, perceived usefulness of mobile technology usage that has an impact on the behavioral intention of use and the actual use of these devices. The developed model might comprise the basis for further research in the area of mobile technology usage for knowledge providing.

**Keywords:** Technology Acceptance Model (TAM)
Structural Equation Modeling (SEM) · Mobile technology
Knowledge providing

## 1 Introduction

Knowledge constitutes the driving force of changes affecting development in the modern economy. Knowledge-based development has taken place in the entire human history, but in the recent years there has been a noticeable increase in the phenomena of economic development related to wide application of knowledge. It starts to play a decisive role in stimulating social and economic development, determining the level and pace of changes. At present, the next stage in the development of the economy can be observed, in which the process of transition from industrial economy to a knowledge-based economy and new technologies takes place [15, 23, 31]. It is also suggested to develop lifelong learning in constant renewal, development and improvement of general and vocational qualifications as well as to improve the quality of education [7]. As it has been emphasized, one of the key elements contributing to the development of a knowledge-based economy is the development of technologies that process, store and transmit data in electronic form, which will allow the delivery of knowledge to the recipient.

© Springer Nature Switzerland AG 2019
M. Themistocleous and P. Rupino da Cunha (Eds.): EMCIS 2018, LNBIP 341, pp. 547–559, 2019.
https://doi.org/10.1007/978-3-030-11395-7_42

The development of various technologies affects the functioning of both individuals and organizations. Mobile technology's rapid growth can be observed in the last decade and offers several benefits including connectivity, flexibility, interactivity, and location awareness [27]. Literature contains numerous definitions of this concept and, at the same time, researchers also use interchangeable terms (e.g. mobile device, mobile computing) to describe mobile technology. Dearnley et al. [12] defines mobile technology as a coexistence of an easy-to-transport device that allows for instant access to information. Hussain and Adeeb [19] state that mobile technology refers to areas defined by mobile Internet connections and mobile devices. The latter can be defined as a portable, wireless computing device that is small enough to be used while held in the hand [8]. Today, billions of users have mobile devices that are opening up new possibilities in many areas providing access to information, processes, and communication anytime and anywhere [25, 40].

The changing technological environment calls for the development of new models in the area of knowledge provision both in the education and business domains. It should be noted, however, that the vast majority of existing studies focuses primarily on the use of mobile technology for providing knowledge in education [3, 11, 18]. Literature contains very few works dealing with the use of mobile technology for providing and acquiring knowledge in business. They are dealing with issues connected with agricultural knowledge delivery in rural areas [4, 21, 34], effects of mobile device usage on employees [32] or platforms for mobile knowledge delivery [28]. However, the research works concerning models of this technology acceptance are scarce [22]. In response to this gap, this article is an attempt to answer the question whether mobile devices can be an effective tool for providing knowledge in the professional area and what factors would affect this technology's acceptance. The paper is organized as follows. The next section provides the research background followed by an overview of the Technology Acceptance Model (TAM) and the development of a research model and hypotheses formulation. Next, research results and discussion are presented. The paper concludes with a summary and future research directions.

## 2   Research Background

The development of mobile technology has dramatically changed the way business is conducted, and we can observe the utilization of this technology in numerous domains [6, 20, 32, 33]. With a mobile connection, employees have the ability to access corporate resources anytime and anywhere, which leads to increasing their efficiencies owing to enhanced communication and connectivity [38]. Considering its properties (particularly access to information anytime and anywhere), mobile technology should operate well in the process of gathering, provision, and the use of knowledge [36, 37].

At the same time, along with the development and widespread availability of mobile technology, one can observe a constantly increasing willingness to use by enterprise employees of their own devices for access to corporate data of the organization. Bring your own device (BYOD) [16] is a strategy allowing employees to utilize a personally selected and purchased device to execute enterprise applications and access data. This trend has some benefits both for organizations and employees. In the

SWOT (Strengths, Weaknesses, Opportunities, Threats) analysis, Portela et al. [30] lists a number of factors that can influence BYOD on success in an organization, namely: (1) reduced IT cost for the company, (2) simplified IT infrastructure, (3) increased employee morale and satisfaction, (4) increased productivity, (5) flexible working culture, (6) bringing out a more efficient working tool, and (7) employees feeling comfortable while using their own devices.

# 3   Research Model and Hypotheses Formulation

As studies carried out in the area of information systems (IS) show, a variety of theories have been proposed to explain key factors affecting technology adoption. One of them, to provide an understanding of the determinants of technology usage, is a well-established theory of reasoned action (TRA) proposed by Fishbein and Ajzen [14]. Its aim is to explain the relationship between attitudes and behaviors within human action. TRA is used broadly to predict and explain how individuals will behave based on their pre-existing attitudes and behavioral intentions.

The Technology Acceptance Model (TAM), derived from TRA, is one of the most widely applied extensions of TRA that gained considerable support in understanding the process of new technology acceptance [9]. The original TAM consists of the following determinants for system use: PEOU (perceived ease of use), PU (perceived usefulness), ATU (attitude towards using), BI (behavioral intention to use), and AU (actual system use). In the subsequent research, Davis et al. [10] concludes that the explanatory power of TAM is equally good without using the ATU construct. As later studies show, it has become ubiquitous to exclude the attitude construct from TAM. In accordance with these arguments and research objectives, we excluded ATU from our considerations.

At the same time, many researchers pay attention to the need of using additional variables in TAM to complete the understanding of the phenomenon studied [41]. In previous studies, researchers have proposed more than 70 external variables for PU and PEOU to reveal how the individuals' perceptions are formed. In their study, Yousafzai et al. [42] have grouped all existing external variables into four categories: (1) organizational characteristics, (2) system characteristics, (3) user personal characteristics, and (4) other variables. We found a need of exploring more deeply the system characteristic as the most relevant to our research.

In spite of the undoubted advantages of mobile technology mentioned in the prior section, it has, however, a number of limitations that should be taken into account [39], namely: (1) the cost of mobile Internet access, (2) network speed and reliability, (3) access to mobile Internet, (4) content optimization for their correct display on mobile devices, (5) matching the content to the expectations of the mobile user, and (6) physical attributes of mobile devices (small mobile device display dimensions, lack of physical keyboard/mouse). These factors, in our opinion, can have a significant impact on the perceived ease of use and usefulness of mobile technology and have been included in the proposed research model (Fig. 1).

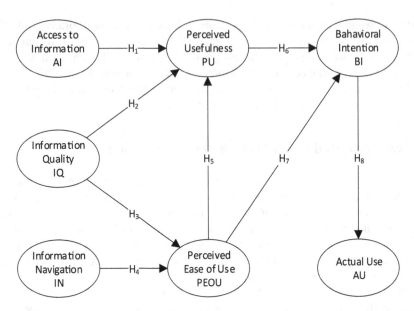

**Fig. 1.** The proposed research model of mobile technology acceptance in knowledge providing.

The external variable Access to Information (AI) refers to the possibility of access to mobile information resources (mobile network coverage, cost and speed) and has an impact on the perceived usefulness of mobile technology in knowledge providing. Information Quality (IQ) highlights the importance of content optimization intended for mobile devices (content tailored to the expectations of a mobile user) and affects PU and PEOU constructs. The last of external variables, Information Navigation (IN), refers to the possibility of navigation in the content presented on a mobile device and determines the ease of use of a mobile device (PEOU). Based on the proposed research model and taking into consideration previous studies, we defined a set of hypotheses describing the relationships between all constructs of the proposed model (Table 1).

# 4   Research Methodology

## 4.1   Instrument

For the needs of the research, a questionnaire consisting of 27 items was developed. The questionnaire was divided into two sections. The first one, comprising 21 questions, represented the measurement items of each of the seven constructs in the model (AI, IQ, IN, PU, PEOU, BI, AU). Every construct was represented by three questions, i.e. three items that were measured on a seven-point Likert-type scale ranging from 1 – "strongly disagree" to 7 – "strongly agree" (see Appendix). The second section, which included six questions, related to demographics information, which consisted of the following variables expressed on the nominal scale: gender, age, frequency of using a smartphone and a mobile Internet connection, professional experience, type of education, and work currently being performed by the respondent (related or non-related to IT).

**Table 1.** Research hypotheses.

| Hypothesis | Path | Statement |
|---|---|---|
| H1 | AI → PU | Access to mobile information has a significantly positive impact on the perceived usability of mobile devices for providing information |
| H2 | IQ → PU | The quality of mobile information has a significantly positive impact on the perceived usability of mobile devices for providing information |
| H3 | IQ → PEOU | The quality of mobile information has a significantly positive impact on the perceived ease of use of mobile devices in providing information |
| H4 | IN → PEOU | The characteristics of navigation of mobile information have a significantly positive impact on the perceived ease of use of mobile devices for providing information |
| H5 | PEOU → PU | The perceived ease of use of mobile devices has a significantly positive effect on their perceived usability for providing information |
| H6 | PU → BI | The perceived usefulness of mobile devices for providing information has a significantly positive impact on the intent of their use |
| H7 | PEOU → BI | The perceived ease of use of mobile devices for providing information has a significantly positive impact on the intent of their use |
| H8 | BI → AU | The behavioral intent to the use of mobile devices for providing information has a significantly positive impact on actual mobile device use |

The questionnaire was analyzed by four independent experts in the field of surveys, to improve its readability and comprehensibility. This allowed for the modification of the questionnaire, changing ambiguous or incomprehensible questions. The changes were introduced in the final version of the questionnaire. All measurement items in the survey questionnaire are available in the appendix. The survey was then developed and deployed in an electronic version (online survey) in the cloud using the Google Forms service in the Software as a Service model. The survey format has been adapted to the correct display on any device (desktop computer, laptop, tablet, smartphone).

## 4.2 Data Collection

Data for this study were collected from March to May 2018 by means of the developed survey. The questionnaire was made available electronically using the forum of courses run on the e-learning platform, social networking sites, and was distributed via e-mail. For the diversification of respondents, the survey was addressed to various groups of recipients. In particular, they were graduating and already mostly working students (the last year of undergraduate and graduate studies, both full-time and part-time students), scientific and research university staff, and public and private sector employees.

### 4.3   Data Analysis Methods

We followed the two-step approach for Structural Equation Modelling (SEM) proposed by Anderson and Gerbing [5] that has been applied successfully by other researches in the domain of ICT testing variations of the TAM model [2, 13, 24]. Firstly, a Confirmatory Factor Analysis (CFA) was performed that resulted in the development of the measurement model. Secondly, the proposed structural model that includes causal relationships between constructs (the model hypothesis) was tested using SEM. The analysis was performed using the Statistica software package (http://www.statsoft.com/Products/STATISTICA-Features).

## 5   Results

### 5.1   Data

A total of 303 respondents completed the questionnaire. No missing data were encountered since in the questionnaire it was obligatory to provide all the answers (the respective Google forms setting was in force). The demographic characteristics of respondents relevant to the current study (gender, age) together with an overview of their habits of using mobile devices for information access are presented in Table 2. Slightly greater share in the respondents' population are male than female. More than half of the respondents are between 21 and 30 years old, 80% of whom declared that they use smartphones numerous times per week for information access.

### 5.2   Reliability of the Measurement Model

The Cronbach's alpha for five latent variables ranges from 0.73 to 0.96 providing a good indication of internal consistency of measurement scales (Table 3). This

**Table 2.**  Respondents' characteristics.

| Variable | No. | % |
|---|---|---|
| *Gender* | | |
| Female | 126 | 42% |
| Male | 177 | 58% |
| *Age* | | |
| <20 | 10 | 3% |
| 21–30 | 185 | 61% |
| 31–40 | 30 | 10% |
| 41–50 | 37 | 12% |
| >50 | 41 | 14% |
| *Frequency of use* | | |
| 1–2 times a day | 22 | 7% |
| 1–2 times a week | 10 | 3% |
| Numerous times a day | 241 | 80% |
| Constantly | 27 | 9% |
| Never | 3 | 1% |

coefficient was around 0.6 for two remaining scales – considered to be poor but acceptable in the early stage of the measurement model development [35]. The correlation between latent variables ranged from 0.145 to 0.916 and but one (IN-AI) was significant at p = 0.01 (Table 4). The fit indices of the measurement model together with their recommended values are presented in Table 5.

**Table 3.** Reliability of the measurement scales.

| Variable | No. of items | Cronbach's alpha |
|---|---|---|
| Access to information (AI) | 3 | 0.73 |
| Information Quality (IQ) | 3 | 0.61 |
| Information Navigation (IN) | 3 | 0.57 |
| Perceived Usefulness (PU) | 3 | 0.77 |
| Perceived Ease of Use (PEOU) | 3 | 0.86 |
| Behavioral Intention (BI) | 3 | 0.80 |
| Actual Use (AU) | 3 | 0.96 |

**Table 4.** Correlations between the latent variables.

| | AI | IQ | IN | PU | PEOU | BI | AU |
|---|---|---|---|---|---|---|---|
| AI | 1 | | | | | | |
| IQ | 0.593 | 1 | | | | | |
| IN | 0.145** | 0.288 | 1 | | | | |
| PU | 0.199* | 0.383 | 0.317 | 1 | | | |
| PEOU | 0.484 | 0.661 | 0.453 | 0.477 | 1 | | |
| BI | 0.285 | 0.561 | 0.481 | 0.916 | 0.661 | 1 | |
| AU | 0.308 | 0.453 | 0.337 | 0.572 | 0.626 | 0.773 | 1 |

Note: * - significance at p = 0.003; ** - significance at p = 0.05; other values significant at p < 0.001.

**Table 5.** Fit indices of the measurement model.

| Fit indices | Recommended [13] | Results |
|---|---|---|
| Chi-square | Significant at p > 0.05 | p = 0.000 |
| Chi-square/degree of freedom | 2–5, <5 | 3.3 |
| RMSEA (Root Mean Square of Error of Approximation) | ≤0.06 | 0.090 |
| SRMR (Standardized Root Mean Residual) | ≤0.8 | 0.073 |
| CFI (Comparative Fit Index) | ≥0.9 | 0.893 |
| IFI (Incremental Fit Index) | ≥0.9 | 0.867 |
| NFI (Normed Fit Index) | ≥0.95, 0.9–0.95 - acceptable | 0.856 |

The Chi-square was significant at p = 0.0001 but for sample size greater than 250 this result is acceptable [17]. Other indices are close to the recommended level. Summing up, we decided that the measurement model might be used for further analysis.

## 5.3   Hypothesis Testing

The results of the structural model testing are presented in Fig. 2. The values on the arrows represent the regression coefficients. Out of eight hypothesis, two were rejected (H1 and H2).

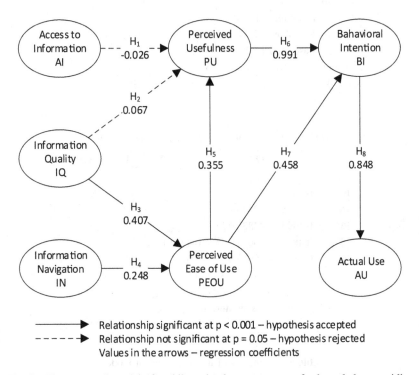

**Fig. 2.** The structural model of mobile technology acceptance for knowledge providing.

The study results did not confirm the hypothesis that Access to Information (AI) influences Perceived Usefulness (PU) and that Information Quality (IQ) influences Perceived Usefulness (PU).

## 6   Discussion

This study finds strong support of TAM in the context of mobile technology. Our results show that perceived usefulness and perceived ease of use indirectly influence the actual usage through behavioral intention to use which is in line with Davis [9]. Besides, the research results confirmed the positive influence of Information Quality (IQ) and the properties of mobile Information Navigation (IN) on Perceived Ease of Use (PEOU).

However, the study did not confirm a positive effect of Access to Information (AI) on Perceived Usefulness (PU). A possible explanation of this finding might be that the speed of mobile Internet and, above all, its availability, especially outside strongly urbanized areas, is still not satisfactory and there are still strong disparities between mobile and traditional access [1]. Another determinant of utilizing mobile devices for knowledge providing could be the cost of mobile Internet access. Despite the significant reduction in the cost of mobile Internet access in recent years [29], it is still perceived as too high, especially when compared to access via cable or fiber optic links. Surprisingly, the study did not support a possible effect of Information Quality (IQ) on Perceived Usefulness (PU). One of the possible explanations of this result might be that content displayed on smartphones is not tailored to the expectations of a mobile user. A typical approach is to develop content that can be displayed on any device, regardless of its type. However, mobile users expect content tailored to their mobility and, as Nicholas et al. suggest [26], typically light, shorter, and less interactive.

## 7 Limitations and Future Directions

The developed measurement model was useful for providing a preliminary analysis of the proposed structural model for mobile technology acceptance in knowledge providing. However, there seems to be still room for improvement judging by the comparatively low values of reliability scales measures (Cronbach alpha) for two constructs (Information Quality and Information Navigation) and some fit indices of the measurement model on the border of the acceptance level.

In future research we would like to enhance our measurement model and the questionnaire by adding more items that assess the structural model constructs. Besides, we would like to investigate whether there are any differences in mobile technology usage perception among different group of respondents: young vs older; IT professionals vs other professionals.

## 8 Conclusion

In our study, we developed and verified the acceptance of mobile technology for knowledge providing model. First, we extended the original TAM by adding three new constructs, in our opinion of high importance in the context of mobile technology: Access to Information, Information Quality, and Information Navigation. The adjusted TAM model comprises the proposed structural model. Next, we developed a measurement model that provided the background for survey development. The survey was distributed using electronic means. In total, 303 respondents completed the questionnaire and delivered their feedback concerning mobile technology usage for knowledge providing. The confirmatory factor analysis (CFA) was used to evaluate the reliability and validity of the measurement model, and then the structural equation modeling technique (SEM) was used to evaluate the proposed structural model. The study results indicate that mobile information navigation characteristics and information quality influence the perceived ease of use that in turn has an impact on the perceived usefulness and behavioral intention of mobile phones' usage. Summing up, the study indicates areas requiring special attention when using mobile technology in knowledge providing both in business and education.

**Funding**
This research has been financed by the funds granted to the Faculty of Management, Cracow University of Economics, Poland, within the subsidy for maintaining research potential.

# Appendix

Measurement items in the Survey Questionnaire

| Constructs (latent variables) | Measurement items | Questions |
|---|---|---|
| Access to Information (AI) | AI1 | In my opinion, the speed of mobile Internet is satisfactory |
| | AI2 | In my opinion, the availability of mobile Internet is satisfactory |
| | AI3 | In my opinion, the access cost to the mobile Internet is satisfactory |
| Information Quality (IQ) | IQ1 | I think that content intended for smartphones is optimized for their correct display |
| | IQ2 | I think that content displayed on smartphones is tailored to the expectations of a mobile user |
| | IQ3 | I think that it is possible to effectively present any type of content on a smartphone |
| Perceived Ease of Use (PEOU) | PEOU1 | I think that it's easy to use a smartphone |
| | PEOU2 | I think it would be easy for me to use a smartphone to get information |
| | PEOU3 | In general, I think that using a smartphone to get information would be easy |
| Information Navigation (IN) | IN1 | I think that small dimensions of a smartphone do not constitute an obstacle to effective navigation of the displayed information |
| | IN2 | I think that the lack of a traditional keyboard or mouse is not an obstacle to effective navigation of the presented information |
| | IN3 | In general, I think that the technical parameters of a smartphone should not be an obstacle to getting acquainted with the presented content |

*(continued)*

(*continued*)

| Constructs (latent variables) | Measurement items | Questions |
|---|---|---|
| Perceived Usefulness (PU) | PU1 | I believe that using a smartphone to obtain information can speed up the implementation of tasks |
| | PU2 | I believe that using a smartphone to obtain information can improve my work efficiency |
| | PU3 | In general, I think that using a smartphone to get information can be useful in my work |
| Behavioral Intention (BI) | BI1 | I intend to use a smartphone to retrieve information in the future |
| | BI2 | I intend to use a smartphone to get information as often as possible |
| | BI3 | I intend to use a smartphone to obtain information to support my work |
| Actual Use (AU) | AU1 | I used a smartphone to get information during the last week |
| | AU2 | I used a smartphone to get information during the last month |
| | AU3 | In general, I use a smartphone to get information |

# References

1. Alderete, M.V.: Mobile broadband: a key enabling technology for entrepreneurship? J. Small Bus. Manag. 55(2), 254–269 (2017)
2. Alharbi, S., Drew, S.: Using the technology acceptance model in understanding academics' behavioural intention to use learning management systems. Int. J. Adv. Comput. Sci. Appl. 5(1), 143–155 (2014)
3. Ally, M., Prieto-Blázquez, J.: What is the future of mobile learning in education? Int. J. Educ. Technol. High. Educ. 11(1), 142–151 (2014)
4. Anand, P.R., Kumaran, M.: Information seeking behaviour of shrimp farmers and their perception towards technology dissemination through mobile phones. J. Ext. Educ. 29(1), 5787–5796 (2017)
5. Anderson, J.C., Gerbing, D.W.: Structural equation modeling in practice: a review and recommended two-step approach. Psychol. Bull. 103(3), 411–423 (1988)
6. Barata, J., Da Cunha, P.R., Stal, J.: Mobile supply chain management in the Industry 4.0 era: an annotated bibliography and guide for future research. J. Enterp. Inf. Manag. 31(1), 173–192 (2018). https://doi.org/10.1108/JEIM-09-2016-0156
7. Brine, J.: Lifelong learning and the knowledge economy: those that know and those that do not – the discourse of the European Union. Br. Educ. Res. J. 32(5), 649–665 (2006)
8. Caudill, J.G.: The growth of m-learning and the growth of mobile computing: parallel developments. Int. Rev. Res. Open Distrib. Learn. 8(2), 1–13 (2007)
9. Davis, F.D.: Perceived usefulness, perceived ease of use, and user acceptance of information technology. MIS Q. 13(3), 319–340 (1989)

10. Davis, F.D., Bagozzi, R.P., Warshaw, P.R.: User acceptance of computer technology: a comparison of two theoretical models. Manag. Sci. **35**(8), 982–1003 (1989)
11. Davison, C.B., Lazaros, E.J.: Adopting mobile technology in the higher education classroom. J. Technol. Stud. **41**(1), 30–39 (2015)
12. Dearnley, C., et al.: Using mobile technologies for assessment and learning in practice settings: outcomes of five case studies. Int. J. E-Learn. **8**(2), 193–207 (2009)
13. Fathema, N., Shannon, D., Ross, M.: Expanding the Technology Acceptance Model (TAM) to examine faculty use of Learning Management Systems (LMSs) In higher education institutions. J. Online Learn. Teach. **11**(2), 210–232 (2015)
14. Fishbein, M., Ajzen, I.: Belief, Attitude, Intention and Behavior: An Introduction to Theory and Research. Addison-Wesley, Reading (1975)
15. Foray, D., Lundvall, B.: The knowledge-based economy: from the economics of knowledge to the learning economy. Econ. Impact Knowl. 115–121 (1998)
16. French, A.M., Guo, C., Shim, J.P.: Current status, issues, and future of Bring Your Own Device (BYOD). Commun. Assoc. Inf. Syst. (CAIS) **35**(10), 191–197 (2014)
17. Hair Jr., J.F., Black, W.C., Babin, B.J., Anderson, R.E., Tatham, R.L.: Multivariate Data Analysis, 6th edn. Prentice-Hall, Upper Saddle River (2006)
18. Heflin, H., Shewmaker, J., Nguyen, J.: Impact of mobile technology on student attitudes, engagement, and learning. Comput. Educ. **107**, 91–99 (2017)
19. Hussain, I., Adeeb, M.A.: Role of mobile technology in promoting campus-wide learning environment. TOJET: the Turk. Online J. Educ. Technol. **8**(3) (2009)
20. Junglas, I., Abraham, C., Ives, B.: Mobile technology at the frontlines of patient care: understanding fit and human drives in utilization decisions and performance. Decis. Support Syst. **46**(3), 634–647 (2009)
21. Kaske, D., Mvena, Z.S.K., Sife, A.S.: Mobile phone usage for accessing agricultural information in Southern Ethiopia. J. Agric. Food Inf. 1–15 (2017). https://doi.org/10.1080/10496505.2017.1371023
22. Kuciapski, M.: A model of mobile technologies acceptance for knowledge transfer by employees. J. Knowl. Manag. **21**(5), 1053–1076 (2017)
23. Lundvall, B.A., et al.: The New Knowledge Economy in Europe: A Strategy for International Competitiveness and Social Cohesion. Edward Elgar Publishing, Glos (2002)
24. Marangunić, N., Granić, A.: Technology acceptance model: a literature review from 1986 to 2013. Univ. Access Inf. Soc. **14**(1), 81–95 (2015)
25. Martin, F., Ertzberger, J.: Here and now mobile learning: an experimental study on the use of mobile technology. Comput. Educ. **68**, 76–85 (2013)
26. Nicholas, D., Clark, D., Rowlands, I., Jamali, H.R.: Information on the go: a case study of Europeana mobile users. J. Assoc. Inf. Sci. Technol. **64**(7), 1311–1322 (2013)
27. Nord, J.H., Koohang, A., Paliszkiewicz, J.: A report on the state of mobile technologies within organizations. Issues Inf. Syst. **17**(1), 70–79 (2016)
28. Núñez, D., Ferrada, X., Neyem, A., Serpell, A., Sepúlveda, M.: A user-centered mobile cloud computing platform for improving knowledge management in small-to-medium enterprises in the Chilean construction industry. Appl. Sci. **8**(4), 516 (2018)
29. Owczarek, M.: Analiza cen usług mobilnego dostępu do Internetu w Polsce. Urząd Komunikacji Elektronicznej, Warszawa (2018)
30. Portela, F., da Veiga, A.M., Santos, M.F.: Benefits of bring your own device in healthcare. In: Machado, J., Abelha, A., Santos, M.F., Portela, F. (eds.) Next-Generation Mobile and Pervasive Healthcare Solutions, pp. 32–45. IGI Global, Hershey (2018)
31. Prusak, L.: Knowledge in Organisations. Routledge, Abingdon (2009)

32. Román, S., Rodríguez, R., Jaramillo, J.F.: Are mobile devices a blessing or a curse? Effects of mobile technology use on salesperson role stress and job satisfaction. J. Bus. Ind. Mark. **33**(5), 651–664 (2018)
33. Rowles, D.: Mobile Marketing: How Mobile Technology is Revolutionizing Marketing, Communications and Advertising. Kogan Page Publishers, London (2017)
34. Roy, D.: Success factors of adoption of mobile applications in rural india: effect of service characteristics on conceptual model. In: Green Computing Strategies for Competitive Advantage and Business Sustainability, pp. 211–238. IGI Global, Hershey (2018)
35. Sekaran, U., Bougie, R.: Research Methods for Business: A Skill Building Approach. Wiley, Hoboken (2016)
36. Stal, J., Paliwoda-Pękosz, G.: Mobile technology in knowledge acquisition: a preliminary study. In: Ulman, P., Węgrzyn, R., Wójtowicz, P. (eds.) Knowledge, Economy, Society: Challenges and Tools of Modern Finance and Information Technology, pp. 123–132. Cracow, Poland (2017)
37. Stal, J., Paliwoda-Pękosz, G.: Towards Integration of mobile technology and knowledge management in organizations: a preliminary study. In: Kowal, J. et al. (eds.) Innovations for Human Development in Transition Economies. Proceedings of the International Conference on ICT Management for Global Competitiveness and Economic Growth in Emerging Economies, Wrocław, Poland, pp. 204–214 (2017)
38. Stal, J., Paliwoda-Pękosz, G.: Why M-learning might appeal to organisations? In: Themistocleous, M., Morabito, V., Ghoneim, A. (eds.) Proceedings of the 13th European, Mediterranean & Middle Eastern Conference on Information Systems, pp. 139–148. Cracow University of Economics, Kraków (2016)
39. Stal, J.: Data personalization in mobile environment: the content adaptation problem. In: Tvrdíková, M., Ministr, J., Rozehnal, P. (eds.). Proceedings of the 14th International Conference on Information Technology for Practice, pp. 181–188. Technical University of Ostrava (2011)
40. Stal, J.: Information and application management: implications for mobile business development. Int. J. Strateg. Manag. Decis. Support Syst. Strateg. Manag. **15**(4), 43–52 (2010)
41. Wu, J.H., Wang, S.C.: What drives mobile commerce?: an empirical evaluation of the revised technology acceptance model. Inf. Manag. **42**(5), 719–729 (2005)
42. Yousafzai, S.Y., Foxall, G.R., Pallister, J.G.: Technology acceptance: a meta-analysis of the TAM: Part 1. J. Model. Manag. **2**(3), 251–280 (2007)

# Author Index

Abdo, Jacques Bou  443
Aggelidis, Vasillis  302
Akinrolabu, Olusola  177
Alghamdi, Fahad  158
Amouri, Ali  369
Anaswah, Mohammed  457
Arreola González, Alejandro  464
Asimakis, Nikos  433
Astrova, Irina  59
Athanasis, Nikos  47

Backovic-Vulic, Tamara  532
Bahari, Mahadi  353
Barbar, Kablan  443
Bass, Julian  489
Belo, Orlando  80
Bernardino, Jorge  121
Berntzen, Lasse  91

Cai, Wenjie  272
Chaaya, Georges  443
Chaieb, Marwa  16
Chatzitheodorou, Christos  47
Chatzoglou, Prodromos  302
Chatzoudes, Dimitrios  302
Chiky, Raja  443
Clarisó, Robert  475

Demerjian, Jacques  443
Dennaoui, Hassan K.  283
Dhond, Varun  193
Dias, Luís S.  106

El-Gazzar, Rania  91
Elnagar, Samaa  405

Fakhfakh, Fairouz  144
Fernandes, João Miguel  106
Filep, Levente  131
Fosso Wamba, Samuel  38
Fourati, Hela  369

Gargouri, Faiez  369
Georgiou, Ifigenia  3
Grand-Brochier, Manuel  369
Gutierrez, Anabel  225

Hamdan, Allam  457
Hashim, Haslina  353
Hassan, Ahlam  457
Hedvicakova, Martina  518
Heine, Felix  59
Hussain, Hafez  353

Iosif, Elias  31
Ismail, Waidah  353
Ivanovic, Ivana  532

Jafni, Tiara Izrinda  353
Jaziri, Faouzi  369
Johannessen, Marius Rohde  91

Kacem, Ahmed Hadj  144
Kacem, Hatem Hadj  144
Kalabokidis, Kostas  47
Kaloyanova, Kalinka  114
Kamariotou, Maria  503
Kapassa, Evgenia  383
Karyda, Maria  258
Khamis, Reem  457
Kiourtis, Athanasios  383
Kiouvrekis, Yiannis  433
Kitsios, Fotis  503
Kokkinaki, Angelika I.  3, 283, 433
Koschel, Arne  59
Krcmar, Helmut  464
Kyriazis, Dimosthenis  383

Labidi, Taher  369
Lafourcade, Pascal  16
Lakovic, Tanja  532
Leonidas, Katelaris  185

Marco-Simó, Josep Maria    475
Marinos, Themistocleous    185
Martin, Andrew    177
Mavrogiorgou, Argyro    383
McKenna, Brad    193, 272
Megapanos, Christos    31
Meskauskiene, Vaida    331
Messaoudi, Rim    369
Métais, Elisabeth    443
Mtibaa, Achraf    369
Musleh Al-Sartawi, Abdalmuttaleb    457

New, Steve    177

Onwujekwe, Gerald    316
Öörni, Anssi    331

Paliwoda-Pękosz, Grażyna    547
Pedro, Luís    106
Pfaff, Matthias    464
Prazak, Pavel    518

Rahy, Scarlet    489
Rallis, Stellios    302
Richter, Shahper    193, 272
Robbana, Riadh    16
Roberto, Giovanni    185
Rodrigues, Mário    121
Rodríguez, José-Ramón    475
Rondovic, Biljana    532
Rossi, Elisa    72
Rubattino, Cinzia    72

Santos, Maribel Yasmina    106, 121
Sapuric, Svetlana    3
Sathye, Milind    158
Sell, Anna    331
Sharma, Dharmendra    158
Simão, José Pedro    80
Soja, Ewa    419
Soja, Piotr    419
Soukal, Ivan    211, 244
Stal, Janusz    547
Stefaneas, Petros    433
Stefanou, Kypros    31
Symeonidis, Symeon    302

Themistocleous, Marinos    31, 47, 383
Thomas, Manoj    405
Touloupou, Marios    383

Vacavant, Antoine    369
Vemou, Konstantina    258
Vieira, António A.C.    106
Viscusi, Gianluigi    72

Wang, Joanne Pei-Chung    225
Weistroffer, Heinz    316, 405

Yousfi, Souheib    16

Zeng, Xiaoxiao    272

Printed in the United States
By Bookmasters